MOSBY'S
REVIEW QUESTIONS
FOR NCLEX-RN

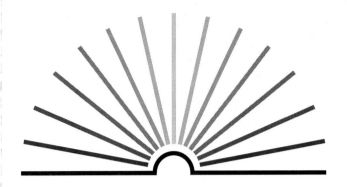

MOSBY'S
REVIEW QUESTIONS
FOR NCLEX-RN

SECOND EDITION

EDITOR
Dolores F. Saxton, R.N., B.S., M.A., M.P.S., Ed. D.

ASSOCIATE EDITORS
Phyllis K. Pelikan, R.N., A.A.S., B.S., M.A.
Patricia M. Nugent, R.N., A.A.S., B.S., M.S., Ed. M, Ed. D.
Selma K. Needleman, R.N., B.A., M.A.

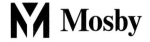

St. Louis Baltimore Boston Carlsbad Chicago Naples New York Philadelphia Portland
London Madrid Mexico City Singapore Sydney Tokyo Toronto Wiesbaden

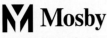

Senior Vice President, Editorial: Alison Harrison
Publisher: Nancy L. Coon
Editor: Susan Epstein
Senior Developmental Editor: Beverly J. Copland
Project manager: Linda Clarke
Production editor: Veda King
Designer: Nancy McDonald
Manufacturing Supervisor: Karen Lewis

SECOND EDITION

Printed in the United States of America
Composition by Mosby Electronic Production, Philadelphia
Printing/Binding by Von Hoffman Press

Mosby–Year Book, Inc.
11830 Westline Industrial Drive
St. Louis, MO 63146

Library of Congress Cataloging in Publication Data
Mosby's Review Questions for NCLEX-RN/editor, Dolores F. Saxton;
    associate editors, Phyllis K. Pelikan, Patricia M. Nugent, Selma R.
    Needleman—2nd ed.
Rev. ed. of: Mosby's Q & A for NCLEX-RN. ©1991.
Includes bibliographical references and index.
  ISBN 08151-7846-8
  1. Nursing—Examinations, questions, etc. I. Saxton, Dolores F.
  II. Mosby's Q&A for NCLEX-RN III. Title: Review Questions for
NCLEX-RN.
  {DNLM: 1. Nursing—examination questions. WY 18 M89448 1995}
  RT55.M65   1995
  610.73'076—dc20
  DNLM/DLC   94–26569
  for Library of Congress   CIP

95 96 97 98 99/ 9 8 7 6 5 4 3 2 1

CONTRIBUTORS

Janice M. Beitz, R.N., M.S.N., C.S., C.N.O.R.
Temple University
Philadelphia, Pennsylvania

Joann Blake, R.N., B.S., M.S., Ph.D.
Prairie View A&M University, College of Nursing
Houston, Texas

Carolyn Browne, R.N., M.A.
Olsten Kimberly QualityCare
East Meadow, New York

Darlene M. Cantu, R.N., B.S.N., M.S.N.
Baptist Memorial Hospital School of Nursing
San Antonio, Texas

**Karen D. Carpenter, R.N., B.S., M.S.N.,
M.Ed., Ph.D.**
University of South Carolina, School of Education and
Health Professions
Conway, South Carolina

Annie Sue Clift, R.N., B.S.N., M.R.E., M.N.
Brighton, Tennessee

Sherrilyn Coffman, R.N., D.N.S.
Florida Atlantic University, College of Nursing
Boca Raton, Florida

**Linda Carman Copel, R.N., M.S., M.S.N.,
Ph.D.**
Villanova University, College of Nursing
Villanova, Pennsylvania

Mary A. Crosley, R.N., B.S., M.S.
Suffolk County Community College
Brentwood, New York

**Teresa Marie Dobrzykowski, R.N., B.S.N.,
M.S.N.**
Indiana University at South Bend
South Bend, Indiana

Marsha Dowell, R.N., B.S.N., M.S.N.
University of Virginia, School of Nursing
Charlottesville, Virginia

Leann Eaton, R.N., B.S.N., M.S.N.
Jewish Hospital School of Nursing
St. Louis, Missouri

Carmel A. Esposito, R.N., B.S.N., M.S.N., Ed.D.
Ohio Valley Hospital School of Nursing
Steubenville, Ohio

JoAnn Festa, R.N., A.A.S., B.S., M.S., Ph.D.
Nassau Community College
Garden City, New York

Carol Flaugher, R.N., B.S., M.S.
State University of New York at Buffalo, School of Nursing
Buffalo, New York

Jane Flickinger, R.N., B.S., M.S.N.
Rochester Community College
Rochester, Minnesota

**Margaret Comerford Freda, R.N., B.S., B.S.N.,
M.A., Ed.D.**
Albert Einstein College of Medicine
Bronx, New York

Carol Coakley Genereux, R.N., B.S., M.S.
New England Baptist Hospital School of Nursing
Boston, Massachusetts

**Susan V. Gille, R.N., B.S.N., M.S.P.H.,
M.S.N., Ph.D.**
Missouri Western State College
St. Joseph, Missouri

Ruth Gouner, R.N., M.S.
Nichalls State University
Thibodaux, Louisiana

Rita M. Hammer, R.N., B.S., M.A.
Quinnipiac College
Hamden, Connecticut

**Barbara Fomenko Harrah, R.N., B.S.Ed.,
B.S.N., M.S.N.**
The Old Valley Hospital School of Nursing
Steubenville, Ohio

Janet T. Ihlenfield, R.N., B.S.N., M.S.N., Ph.D.
D'Youville College
Buffalo, New York

Sharon Isaac, R.N., B.S.N., M.S.N., Ed.D.
University of Indianapolis, School of Nursing
Indianapolis, Indiana

Bernadette Kahler, R.N., B.S.N., M.N.
Kansas Newman College
Wichita, Kansas

Christina Algiere Kasprisin, R.N., M.S.
University of Vermont
Burlington, Vermont

Laurie Gaspari Kaudewitz, R.N., B.S.N., M.S.N., R.N.C.
East Tennessee State Universtiy
Johnson City, Tennessee

Elaine M. Kelter, R.N., B.S.N., M.S.
New England Baptist Hospital School of Nursing
Boston, Massachusetts

Sheila M. Kyle, R.N., A.S., B.S.N., M.S., M.S.N.
St. Mary's Hospital School of Nursing
Huntington, West Virginia

Carole Labby, R.N., B.S.N., M.S.
College of the Mainland
Houston, Texas

Dorothy B. Lary, R.N., B.S.N., M.S.N.
Louisiana College
Pineville, Louisiana

Betty Jane Lee, R.N., M.S.N.
Albright College
Reading, Pennsylvania

Pamela M. Lemmon, R.N., B.S.N., M.S.N.
St. Elizabeth Hospital Medical Center
Youngstown, Ohio

Joan Cerniglia-Lowensen, R.N., B.S.N., M.S.N.
Union Memorial Hospital School of Nursing
Baltimore, Maryland

Judith A. McDonagh, R.N., B.S.N., M.S.
Simmons College
Boston, Massachusetts

Catherine Mechling, R.N., B.S.N., M.Ed.
Citizens General Hospital School of Nursing
New Kensington, Pennsylvania

Mary De Meneses, R.N., B.S.N., M.A., M.S., Ed.D.
Southern Illinois Universtiy at Edwardsville
School of Nursing
Edwardsville, Illinois

Sheila E. Miller, R.N., B.S.N., M.S.N.
Auburn Universtiy, School of Nursing
Auburn, Alabama

Jeanne M. Millett, R.N., B.S., M.S., F.N.P., Ed.D.
Albany Medical Center Hospital
Lifestar Regional Trauma System
Albany, New York

Marilyn M. Mohr, R.N., B.S.N., M.S.N.
Missouri Baptist Medical Center School of Nursing
St. Louis, Missouri

Rita Black Monsen, R.N., B.S.N., M.S.N., M.P.H., D.S.N.
Henderson State Universtiy
Arkadelphia, Arkansas

Anna P. Moore, R.N., B.S.N., M.S.
Southside Regional Medical Center School of Nursing
Petersburg, Virginia

Theresa A. Moran, R.N., A.A.S., B.S., Ed.M., Ed.D.
Nassau Community College
Garden City, New York

Cecilia Mukai, R.N., B.S., M.S.N.
University of Hawaii at Hilo
Hilo, Hawaii

Ann T. Muller, R.N., B.S., M.S., M.Ed., Ph.D.
Private Practice
Dallas, Texas

Ayda G. Nambayan, R.N., B.S.N., M.Ed., O.C.N.
University of Alabama at Birmingham, School of Nursing
Birmingham, Alabama

Doris E. Nicholas, R.N., M.S., Ph.D.
Howard Universtiy, College of Nursing
Washington, District of Columbia

Neil J. Nugent, A.A.S., B.S., M.B.A., M.S.W.
Nassau Community College
Garden City, New York

Elizabeth T. Payne, R.N., B.S.N., M.S.N.
Henderson Community College
Henderson, Kentucky

Margaret A. Phillips, R.N., B.S.N., M.A.Ed.
Jewish Hospital
St. Louis, Missouri

Mary Jane Reumann, R.N., B.S.N., M.S.N.
University of Alabama at Huntsville
Huntsville, Alabana

Lynn Rhyne, R.N., M.N.
Barnes Hospital School of Nursing
St. Louis, Missouri

Linda Owen Rimer, R.N., B.S.N., M.S.E.
University of Arkansas at Little Rock
Little Rock, Arkansas

Mary Ann S. Rogers, R.N., A.D.N., B.S.N., M.S.N., Ed.D.
University of South Carolina at Aiken
Aiken, South Carolina

Kathleen S. Rose, R.N., B.S.N.
Good Samaritan Hospital School of Nursing
Cincinnati, Ohio

Janice J. Rumfelt, R.N., M.S.N., Ed.D., R.N.C.
Southern Illinois University at Edwardsville
School of Nursing
Edwardsville, Illinois

Deborah Lekan Rutledge, R.N., M.S.N., Certified Gerontological Nursing
University of North Carolina
Chapel Hill, North Carolina

Mary Ann Hellmer Saul, R.N., A.A.S., B.S., M.S., Ph.D.
Nassau Community College
Garden City, New York

Carol G. Scott, R.N., A.S., B.S.N., M.S.N.
Lynchburg General Hospital School of Nursing
Lynchburg, Virginia

Cynthia C. Small, R.N., B.S.N., M.S.N.
Lake Michigan College
Benton Harbor, Michigan

Patricia Szczech, R.N., B.S., M.A.
Ohio Wesleyan University, School of Nursing
Delaware, Ohio

Anita Throwe, R.N., B.S.N., M.S.
Medical University of South Carolina, College of Nursing
Florence, South Carolina

Cecilia M. Tiller, R.N., B.S.N., M.N., D.S.N.
Medical College of Georgia, School of Nursing
Augusta, Georgia

Marita G. Titler, R.N., M.A.
Coe College
Cedar Rapids, Iowa

Vera Ellen Turner, R.N., A.D.N.
Baptist Memorial Hospital School of Nursing
Memphis, Tennessee

Judith A. Van Doren, R.N., B.S., M.Ed., M.S.N.
Good Samaritan Hospital School of Nursing
Cincinnati, Ohio

Carolyn H. Waltzer, R.N., B.S.N., B.A., M.A.
Parkersburg Community College
Parkersburg, West Virginia

Margaret T. Warren, R.N., B.A., B.S., M.A., M.S.
Rockland Community College
Suffern, New York

Mary H. West, R.N., M.S., Certified C.C.N.
Bob Jones Universtiy
Greenville, South Carolina

Judy E. White, R.N., B.S.N., M.A., M.S.N.
Rockland Community College
Suffern, New York

Deborah Williams, R.N., A.S., B.A., M.S.N.
Western Kentucky University
Bowling Green, Kentucky

Frances A. Wollner, R.N., B.S., B.S.N., M.N.
Grand Island, New York

Wanda Lee Wooten, R.N., B.S.N., M.A.Ed.
Eastern Kentucky University
College of Allied Health and Nursing
Richmond, Kentucky

Lynn M. Young, R.N., M.S.N.
Mohave Community College
Kingman, Arizona

Patricia E. Zander, R.N., B.S.N., M.S.N., R.N.C.
Viterbo College
LaCrosse, Wisconsin

PREFACE

This book was developed to meet the requests for "still more questions — with answers and rationales." We believe that, along with our other publications, *Mosby's Comprehensive Review of Nursing* and *Mosby's AssessTest*, this text completes the third leg of a strong tripod of study, self-evaluation, and review material on which students can base their study and review for both coursework and the NCLEX-RN. This second edition has been increased to over 2,600 single-item questions reflecting the NCLEX-RN format. The questions have been grouped by related content (categories of concern). A quiz follows each clinical chapter and two comprehensive examinations parallel the NCLEX-RN test plan. To enhance learning and preparation for the NCLEX-RN CAT, a computer disc with 100 additional questions is included.

To meet the needs of students with different study styles and learning needs, the questions in this book have been presented in four distinct formats:

- All of the clinical chapters group questions according to a Category of Concern. The category of concern reflects the specific content area within the broad clinical area from which the material in the question has been drawn. We have presented these questions in the traditional clinical groupings because we believe that, even when preparing for an integrated exam like the NCLEX-RN, most students will need to study all the distinct parts before attempting to put them together.

- At the end of each of the clinical chapters is a quiz that integrates the content from the various categories of concern within the chapter. These quizzes provide a bridge for moving from the clinical chapters to the comprehensive examinations.

- Two comprehensive examinations, consisting of 265 questions each, are provided to approximate the NCLEX-RN test plan. To parallel the NCLEX-RN, the first 75 questions reflect the minimal testing experience for students taking the NCLEX CAT. The total test of 265 questions reflects the maximum number of questions that a student will be asked on NCLEX-RN. Although NCLEX-RN is now computerized, the substance of the test remains constant. It is our belief that if students study the material and develop a strong knowledge base, the method of testing should not have a major influence on their performance.

- The enclosed computer disc contains 100 test items that can be used in both a study and test format. To reinforce learned information and build confidence, we suggest that students should practice answering questions on a computer to simulate the NCLEX-RN.

For each question in the book and on the disc, the reason why the correct answer is correct, as well as why each of the other options is incorrect, is included. In addition, each question has been analyzed as to the level of difficulty, the clinical area, the step in the nursing process, the area of client needs, and the category of concern (specific area of content). Questions incorporate material from the basic sciences, nutrition, and pharmacology, as well as current information relative to topics such as gerontology, rehabilitation, the DSM IV, and the delivery of health care.

All the questions in this book were developed by outstanding and experienced nursing educators and practitioners. The editorial panel reviewed all questions initially submitted, selecting and editing the most pertinent for inclusion in a mass field-testing project.

Students graduating from baccalaureate, associate degree, and diploma nursing programs in various locations in the United States and Canada provided a diverse testing group. The results were statistically analyzed; this analysis was used to select only the highest quality questions for inclusion in this book and to determine each question's level of difficulty.

We would like to take this opportunity to express our sincere appreciation to our many colleagues for their contributions; to Edith Augustson for her careful processing of the manuscript; to Susan Epstein, our editor, and Beverly Copland, our developmental editor, for their assistance and support; to Laurie Muench, Editorial Assistant, for her planning and supervision of field testing; and most of all to our families for their love, understanding, and encouragement.

Dolores F. Saxton
Phyllis K. Pelikan
Patricia M. Nugent
Selma R. Needleman

CONTENTS

5. Mental Health Nursing Review Questions

6. Comprehensive Examination 1

7. Comprehensive Examination 2

MOSBY'S
REVIEW QUESTIONS
FOR NCLEX-RN

CHAPTER 1

Preparing for the Licensure Examination

INTRODUCTION

Licensure examinations in the United States and Canada have been integrated and comprehensive for many years. Nursing candidates in both countries are required to answer questions that necessitate a recognition and understanding of the physiologic, biologic, and social sciences, as well as the specific nursing skills and abilities involved in a given client situation.

Both the United States and the Canadian tests contain objective multiple-choice questions based on the steps of the nursing process and recognition of client needs. To answer the questions appropriately, a candidate needs to understand and correlate certain aspects of anatomy and physiology, the behavioral sciences, basic nursing, the effects of medications administered, the client's attitude toward illness, and other pertinent factors (e.g., legal responsibilities). Most questions are based on nursing situations similar to those with which candidates have had experience, because both the United States and Canada emphasize the nursing care of clients with representative common national health problems. Some questions, however, require candidates to apply basic principles and techniques to clinical situations with which they have had little, if any, actual experience.

To prepare adequately for an integrated comprehensive examination, it is necessary to understand the discrete parts that compose the universe under consideration. This is one of the major principles of learning on which our review and study materials have been developed.

Using this concept, this text first presents for each major clinical area questions that test the student's knowledge of principles and theories underlying nursing care in a variety of situations (acute, critical, and long term), in a variety of settings (acute care hospitals, nursing homes, and the community), and with a variety of nursing approaches to promote health and prevent illness (including primary, secondary, and tertiary care). The book concludes with integrated comprehensive tests reflecting the licensure examinations. In other words, the questions require the student to cross clinical disciplines and respond to individual and specific needs associated with given health problems.

Answers to all of the questions, as well as rationales supporting the correct answers, are provided. Explanations are also presented to document why the other choices are inappropriate. Reviewing the rationales enables the student to verify information and reinforce knowledge.

HOW TO USE THIS BOOK IN STUDYING

A. Start in one clinical area. Answer all of the questions in the area. Record the answer by filling in the circle of the number you believe is correct. Do not worry if you select the same numbered answer repeatedly; there is usually no pattern to the answers.

B. As you answer each question, write a few words about why you think that answer was correct;

in other words, justify why you selected the answer.

C. If you guess at an answer in this book, you should make a special mark to identify it. This will permit you to recognize areas that need further review. It will also help you to see how correct your "guessing" can be.

D. Tear out the sheets with answers and rationales for the area you are reviewing and compare your answers with those provided. If you answered the item correctly, check your reason for selecting the answer with the rationale presented. If you answered the item incorrectly, read the rationale to determine why the one you selected was incorrect. In addition, you should review the correct answer and rationale for each item answered incorrectly. If you still do not understand your mistake, look up the theory pertaining to these questions. You should carefully review all questions and rationales for items you identified as guesses because you did not have mastery of the material being questioned.

E. Following the rationale for the correct answer you will find a number—1, 2, or 3—in parentheses. These numbers indicate the level of difficulty of the question and reflect the percentage of tested students answering the question correctly. These can serve as a guide in your studying. (See the sample questions on page 4.)

1. The number **1** signifies that 75% or more—but less than 89%—of the students in the testing group answered the question correctly. Sample question 3 is a level 1 question.

2. The number **2** signifies that 50% or more—but less than 75%—of the students in the testing group answered the question correctly. Sample questions 1 and 2 are level **2** questions.

3. The number **3** signifies that 25% or more—but less than 50%—of the students in the testing group answered the question correctly. Sample questions 4 and 5 are level **3** questions.

4. Questions that 89% or more or 24% or less of the students in the testing group answered correctly were not included in the book.

F. In addition to the level of difficulty of the question you will also find a grouping of letters that classify the question according to four categories: Clinical area; Nursing process; Client need; and Category of concern. This series of letters will always appear in the same order for each question in the book. The following descriptions and the five sample questions on p. 4 are presented to assist the reader in understanding and reviewing these classifications.

Clinical Area (*reflects the specialized area of nursing knowledge*)

1. **Medicine (ME).** These questions include the care of adult clients who have health problems that do not require surgical intervention or invasive techniques. Sample question 1 is a *medical nursing* question.

2. **Surgery (SU).** These questions include care of adult clients with health problems that require surgical intervention or invasive techniques. Sample question 5 is a *surgical nursing* question.

3. **Childbearing and Women's Health (CW).** These questions include the care of clients preparing for or experiencing childbirth and family planning. Sample question 2 is a *childbearing and women's health nursing* question.

4. **Pediatric (PE).** These questions include the care of clients from birth to young adulthood. Sample question 4 is a *pediatric nursing* question.

5. **Mental Health (MH).** These questions include the care of clients experiencing emotional stress with or without overt psychiatric behavior in all settings. Sample question 3 is a *mental health nursing* question.

Phases of the Nursing Process (*reflects types of behaviors of the nurse*)

1. **Assessment (AS).** The assessment phase requires the nurse to obtain objective and subjective data from primary and secondary sources, to identify and group significant data, and to communicate this information to other members of the health team. The information necessary for making nursing decisions is obtained through assessment. Sample question 1 is an *assessment* question.

2. **Analysis (AN).** This phase requires the nurse to interpret data gathered during the assessment phase. A nursing diagnosis must be made, client and family needs identified, and both short-term and long-term goals set to meet the identified needs. Sample question 2 is an *analysis* question.

3. **Planning (PL).** The planning phase requires the nurse to design a regimen with the client and family to achieve goals set during the analysis phase. It also requires setting priorities for nursing intervention. Sample question 3 is a *planning* question.

4. **Implementation (IM).** The implementation phase requires the nurse to provide care designed during the planning phase. The client may be given total care or may be assisted and encouraged to perform activities of daily living or follow the regimen prescribed by the physician. Implementation also includes activities such as counseling, teaching, and supervising. Sample question 4 is an *implementation* question.

5. **Evaluation (EV).** This phase requires the nurse to determine the effectiveness of nursing care. The goals of care are reviewed, the client's response to intervention identified, and a consideration made as to whether the client has achieved the predetermined goals. Evaluation also includes appraisal of the client's compliance with the health plan. Sample question 5 is an *evaluation* question.

Client Need (*reflects the health care need of the client that must be addressed by the nurse*)

1. **Support and promotion of physiological and anatomical equilibrium (PA).** Meeting this need includes reducing risks that interfere with physiologic or anatomic integrity, promoting comfort and mobility, and providing basic care to assist, modify, or limit physiologic and anatomic adaptations. Sample questions 1 and 5 reflect this client need.

2. **An environment that is safe and conducive to effective therapeutic care (TC).** The nurse must provide quality, goal-directed care that is coordinated, safe, and effective. Sample question 4 reflects this client need.

3. **Education and other forms of health promotion to prevent, minimize, or correct actual or potential health problems (ED).** Fulfilling this need involves supporting optimal growth and development to provide for the achievement of the highest levels of functioning. This includes encouraging use of support systems and self-care directed toward promoting the prevention, recognition, and treatment of disease throughout the life cycle. Sample question 3 reflects this client need.

4. **Support and promotion of psychosocial and emotional equilibrium (PS).** Addressing this need includes supporting individual emotional coping and adapting mechanisms to promote optimal emotional health while limiting or modifying those responses to crises that produce psychopathologic consequences. Sample question 2 reflects this client need.

Category of Concern (*reflects the specific content area within the broad clinical area from which the material in the question has been drawn.*)

1. **Medicine, Surgery, and Pediatrics**
   Blood and immunity (BI)
   Cardiovascular (CV)
   Drug-related responses (DR)
   Emotional needs related to health problems (EH)
   Endocrine (EN)
   Fluid and electrolyte (FE)
   Gastrointestinal (GI)
   Growth and development (GD)
   Integumentary (IT)
   Neuromuscular (NM)
   Respiratory (RE)
   Reproductive and genitourinary (RG)
   Skeletal (SK)

2. **Childbearing and Women's Health**
   Drug-related responses (DR)
   Emotional needs related to childbearing (EC)
   Healthy childbearing(HC)
   High-risk neonate (HN)
   High-risk maternal-fetal conditions affecting childbearing (HP)
   Normal neonate (NN)
   Reproductive choices (RC)
   Reproductive problems (RP)
   Women's health (WH)

3. **Mental Health**
   Anxiety, somatoform, and dissociative disorders (AX)
   Crisis situations (CS)
   Disorders first evident before adulthood (BA)
   Eating Disorders (EA)
   Disorders of mood (MO)
   Disorders of personality (PR)
   Drug-related responses (DR)
   Emotional problems related to physical health and childbearing (EP)
   Dementia, delirium, and other cognitive disorders (DD)
   Personality development (PD)
   Schizophrenic disorders (SD)

Substance abuse (SA)
Therapeutic relationships (TR)

SAMPLE QUESTIONS:

1. On a routine physical, a client is found to have a blood pressure of 150/96 and hypertension is suspected. In obtaining the health history an early sign of hypertension that the nurse should expect the client to complain of is:
   1. Swollen ankles
   2. Recent weight loss
   3. Palpitations of the heart
   4. Early morning headaches
   [Correct answer is 4. (2) (ME; AS; PA; CV)]

2. For a woman, identification with the parenting role begins:
   1. Early in life
   2. During adolescence
   3. After the baby has been born
   4. When pregnancy is confirmed
   [Correct answer is 1. (2) (CW; AN; PE; EC)]

3. A young male has a history of an antisocial personality disorder. His parents tell the nurse that their son is very manipulative and causes havoc in their home. The nurse should include in the teaching plan ways that they can cope with their son by using an approach that is:
   1. Rigid
   2. Flexible
   3. Accepting
   4. Consistent
   [Correct answer is 4. (1) (MH; PL; ED; PR)]

4. A 3-year-old girl is admitted for surgery. When her mother leaves, she begins to sob. The nurse should:
   1. Tell her to be a big girl, her mother will be right back
   2. Put up the side rails on the crib and let her calm down by herself
   3. Distract her with her teddy, expecting her to forget her mother has gone
   4. Hold her and explain that her mother had to go but will return in two hours
   [Correct answer is 3. (3) (PE; IM; TC; GD)]

5. Following a mastectomy, tamoxifen (Nolvadex) is prescribed for a client. The nurse knows that teaching about this drug was understood when the client states, "I will:

   1. Drink 4 glasses of milk every day while I am taking this drug."
   2. Expect pain at the site of the tumor when I am taking this drug."
   3. Take a stool softener every day while I am taking this medication."
   4. Rise from a sitting position slowly when I am taking this medication."
   [Correct answer is 2. (3) (SU; EV; PA; DR)]

G. A few days later, review the area again. If you miss the same question a second time, you need further study of the material.

H. After you have completed the clinical area questions, begin taking the comprehensive tests, because they will assist you in applying knowledge and principles from the specific clinical area to any nursing situation.
   1. Arrange a quiet, uninterrupted time span for each test in the comprehensive tests.
   2. Pace yourself during the testing period; allow about 1 minute per question.
   3. Do not rush.
   4. Answer every question.

I. Since most examinations have specified time limits, you will need to pace yourself during the practice testing period, working as quickly and accurately as possible. It is helpful to estimate the time that can be spent on each item and still complete the examination in the allotted time. You can obtain this figure by dividing the testing time by the number of items on the test. For example, with a 1-hour (60 minute) testing period and approximately 60 items, an average of 1 minute per item will be the appropriate pace.

J. To help analyze your mistakes on the comprehensive examinations and to provide a data base for making future study plans, two types of worksheets are included. One is designed to aid you in identifying and recording errors in the way you process information. The other is to help you identify and record gaps in knowledge. These worksheets follow the Answers and Rationales for each test in the Comprehensive Test Section and are on tear-out sheets. Instructions for their use appear on each worksheet.

K. After completing your worksheets, do the following:
   1. Use Worksheet 1 to identify the frequency

with which you made particular errors. As you review material in class notes or study material such as Mosby's Comprehensive Review of Nursing, pay special attention to correcting your most common problems.

2. Use Worksheet 2 to identify the topics you want to review. It might be helpful to set priorities; review the most difficult topics first so that you will have time to review them more than once.

L. Use this opportunity to learn from your mistakes.
   1. Because you receive immediate feedback on your performance, you have an excellent opportunity to learn from your mistakes. Answer every question. Do not leave any questions unanswered; use educated or pure guesses.
   2. The mistakes you make on the questions in this book will be as valuable to you as the confident feeling you get from answering correctly.

READINESS FOR THE LICENSURE EXAMINATION

A few individuals can improve their scores significantly by a highly concentrated period of study immediately before taking an examination. Most, however, profit by spreading their review over a much longer period of time. Cramming will not help. Identification of your own specific strengths and weaknesses should eliminate much of the anxiety of deciding what material to study by giving you a sense of direction and a means of setting priorities.

Reduce Stress
Stress is a part of life. While there is no way to prevent it, it is possible to reduce it by diffusing your emotional responses before stress gets the better of you. Controlling stress allows you to use it instead of being abused by it.

1. Talk it out but try to talk it out with someone who is not as stressed as you are. This relieves the burden of coping alone and helps put things in perspective. Try talking with people who have had the same experience and understand what you are going through.
2. Obtain as much information as you can. **STUDY!!!**
3. Keep fit. Good nutrition, regular exercise, and ample sleep help.

4. Try relaxation exercises. Relaxation is essential to reduce stress.
5. Sort out the important things. Take stock of your strengths. Set realistic deadlines. Drop the nonessentials.
6. Spend time on yourself and your needs outside of nursing.
7. Be greedy and put yourself first. Be flexible with yourself. Do not set rigid, unmanageable goals.
8. Discover your positive defenses and use them.
9. Become familiar with reading material on a computer screen. Familiarity reduces anxiety and limits errors.

Manage Test-Taking Time
The computerized NCLEX-RN is not a timed test per se although there is a minimum 1 $\frac{1}{2}$-hour to a maximum 5-hour time period. The computerized test has reportedly been designed to measure the individual's level of knowledge, skills, and abilities to determine that the competency level is achieved. The test length will vary depending on each candidate's performance but will be somewhere between 75 and 265 questions.

Although certain questions will be more difficult than others and will require more time, spending too much time on these difficult items may compromise your overall performance.

Do not be pressured into finishing early. Do not rush! Students who achieve higher scores on examinations are typically those who use all the time available.

Build Test-Taking Confidence
You should feel confident and competent if you have studied and reviewed the content to be tested and you are armed with methods for reading and answering questions. Your emotional state is vitally important when thinking about, preparing for, and taking any test. Think positively.

While you are taking the test, you may have problems with a question. On a written examination it is often best to move on to another question that you can answer. However, on the computerized NCLEX-RN you must answer the question before you can go on to the next question, so remain calm. Anxiety can block the recall of familiar information required to answer questions so control it early. Do not stop to think about gaps in your preparation nor waste time and emotional energy building anxiety. Focus on the positive. You have the ability to make sound "educated guesses." Now is the time to use it. Questions that seem complicated at first glance can often be answered by just such guesses. Remain calm and confident.

You will find that practice test-taking experiences will give you confidence for the actual examination. After you have completed studying in this book, you may wish to take a simulated examination such as *Mosby's AssessTest* before you take the licensure examination. The *AssessTest* is a computer-scored, multiple-choice examination designed to test nursing knowledge and evaluate your ability to apply that knowledge in clinical situations. The extensive computer analysis of your performance, which is the most outstanding feature of this test, will help you design effective and efficient plans for further study and review.

TAKING THE LICENSURE EXAMINATION

On the NCLEX-RN each of the 5 steps of the nursing process is represented by 15% to 25% of the questions. There are a variety of questions from each of the clinical areas. Recently there appears to have been a deemphasis of the areas of maternity (obstetric) nursing and severe mental illness. There seems to be a greater emphasis on medical-surgical principles and interpersonal skills, especially communication. In the category of client health care needs, approximately 42% to 48% of the questions reflect support and promotion of physiologic and anatomic equilibrium; 25% to 31% reflect the need for a therapeutic environment; 12% to 18% reflect the need for education and health promotion; and 9% to 15% reflect the need for support and promotion of psychosocial and emotional equilibrium. The score on the examination is reported as pass or fail.

The most crucial requisite for doing well on the licensure examination is a sound understanding of the subject and a high level of reading comprehension. Determination to do well and a degree of confidence will further enhance the well-prepared individual's chance of passing and achieving the recognition deserved.

At least three other requirements must be met if an individual's performance is to accurately reflect professional competence. First, the candidate must follow explicitly the directions given by the examiner and those appearing at the beginning of the test. Second, the candidate must read each question carefully before deciding how to answer it. Third, the candidate must record the answers in the manner specified.

The computerized NCLEX-RN is an individualized testing experience in which the computer chooses your next question based on the ability and competency you have demonstrated on previous questions. The minimum number of questions will be 75 and the maximum 265. You must answer each question before the computer will present the next question and you cannot go back to any previously answered questions. There is no deduction for incorrect answers so you are not penalized for guessing. You cannot leave an answer blank and since you have a 1 in 4 (25%) chance of guessing the correct answer, go for it. Remember, you do not have to get all the questions correct to pass.

You should also keep in mind that if you practice and learn the material the method of testing (oral, written, or computer) should not significantly influence your performance.

TEST-TAKING SKILLS

Test-taking skills and techniques are not a substitute for good study habits or an adequate grasp of the content and abilities measured in an examination. Memorization is of little help because few questions are simple recall and most require the use of higher, more complex thought processes. If you have a thorough understanding of the knowledge measured in an examination, however, good test-taking skills will enhance your overall performance.

The question in its entirety is called a test item. The portion of the test item that poses the question or problem is called the stem. Potential answers to the question or problem posed are called options. In well-constructed multiple-choice items there is only one correct answer among the options supplied; the incorrect options are called distractors. Remember, test questions are meant to measure your nursing knowledge. The items may be easy to read, but the answers to questions are not intended to be readily apparent. The questions draw on your ability to apply nursing knowledge from a variety of sources.

•Read Questions Carefully

Scores on tests are strongly affected by reading ability. In answering a test item, you should begin by carefully reading the stem and then asking yourself the following questions:

What is the question really asking?

Are there any key words?

What information relevant to answering this question is included in the stem?

How would I ask this question in my own words?

How would I answer this question in my own words?

After you have answered these questions, carefully read the options and then ask yourself the following questions:

Is there an option that is similar to the one I thought of?

Is this option the best, most complete answer to the question?

Deal with the question as it is stated, without reading anything into it or making assumptions about it. Answer the question asked, not the one you would like to answer. For simple recall items the self-questioning process will usually be completed quickly. For more complex items the self-questioning process may take longer, but it should assist you in clarifying the item and selecting the best response.

•Identify Key Words

Certain key words in the stem, the options, or both should alert you to the need for caution in choosing your answer. Because few things in life are absolute without exception, avoid selecting answers that include words such as always, never, all, every, only, must, no, except, and none, since answers containing these key word are rarely correct. They place special limitations and qualifications on potentially correct answers. For example:

All of the following are services of the National Kidney Foundation except:

1. Public education programs
2. Research about kidney disease
3. Fund-raising affairs for research activities
4. Identification of potential transplant recipients

This stem contains two key words: *all* and *except*. They limit the correct answer choice to the one option that does not represent a service of the National Kidney Foundation. When *except*, *not*, or a phrase such as *all but one of the following* appears in the stem, the inappropriate option is the correct answer—in this instance, option 4.

If the options in an item do not seem to make sense because more than one option is correct,

reread the question; you may have missed one of the key words in the stem. Also be on guard when you see one of the key words in an option; it may limit the context in which such an option would be correct.

•Pay Attention to Specific Details

The well-written multiple-choice question is precisely stated, providing you with only the information needed to make the question or problem clear and specific. Careful reading of details in the stem can provide important clues to the correct option. For example:

A male client is told that he will no longer be able to ingest alcohol if he wants to live. To effect a change in his behavior while he is in the hospital, the nurse should attempt to:

1. Help the client set short-term dietary goals
2. Discuss his hopes and dreams for the future
3. Discuss the pathophysiology of the liver with him
4. Withhold approval until the client agrees to stop drinking

The specific clause *to effect a change in his behavior while he is in the hospital* is critical. Option 2 is not really related to his alcoholism. Option 3 may be part of educating the alcoholic, but you would not expect a behavioral change observable in the hospital to emerge from this discussion. Option 4 rejects the client as well as his behavior instead of only his behavior. Option 1, the correct answer, could result in an observable behavioral change while the client is hospitalized; for example, he could define ways to achieve short-term goals relating to diet and alcohol while in the hospital.

•Eliminate Clearly Wrong Or Incorrect Answers

Eliminate clearly incorrect, inappropriate, and unlikely answers to the question asked in the stem. By systematically eliminating distractors that are unlikely in the context of a given question, you increase the probability of selecting the correct answer. Eliminating obvious distractors also allows you more time to focus on the options that appear to be potentially sound answers to the question. For example:

The four levels of cognitive ability are:

4. Medical nursing, surgical nursing, mental health nursing, child bearing and women's health nursing
3. Knowledge, comprehension, application, analysis

2. Knowledge, analysis, assessing, comprehension
1. Assessing, analyzing, applying, evaluating

Option 4 is clearly inappropriate, since the choices are all clinical areas. Option 1 contains both cognitive levels and nursing behaviors, thus eliminating it from consideration. Both options 2 and 3 contain levels of cognitive ability; however, option 2 includes assessing, which is a nursing behavior. Therefore, option 3 is correct. By reducing the plausible options, you reduce the material to consider and increase the probability of selecting the correct option.

•Identify Similar Options

When an item contains two or more options that are very similar in meaning, the successful test taker knows that all are correct, in which case it is a poor question, or that none is correct, which is more likely to be the case. The correct option will usually either include all the similar options or exclude them entirely. For example:

In teaching newly diagnosed diabetic clients about their condition, it is important to focus on:

1. Dietary modifications
2. Use of sugar substitutes
3. Their present understanding of diabetes
4. Use of diabetic nutritional exchange lists

Options 1, 2, and 4 deal only with the diabetic diet, involving no other aspect of diabetic teaching; it is impossible to select the most correct option because each represents equally plausible, though limited, answers to the question. Option 3 is the best choice, because it is most complete and allows the other three options to be excluded. As another example:

A child's intelligence is influenced by:

1. A variety of factors
2. Socioeconomic factors
3. Heredity and environment
4. Environment and experience

The most correct answer is option 1. It includes the material covered by the other options, eliminating the need for an impossible choice, since each of the other options is only partially correct.

•Identify Answer (Option) Components

When an answer contains two or more parts, you can reduce the number of potentially correct answers by identifying one part as incorrect. For example:

After a cholecystectomy the postoperative diet is usually:

1. Low fat, high protein
2. Low fat, high calorie
3. High fat, low protein
4. High fat, low calorie

If you know, for instance, that the diet after a cholecystectomy is usually low or moderate in fat, you can eliminate options 3 and 4 from consideration. If you know that the cholecystectomy client is most often overweight, you can eliminate option 2 from consideration. Therefore option 1 is correct.

•Identify Specific Determiners

When the options of a test item contain words that are identical or similar to words in the stem, the alert test taker recognizes the similarities as clues about the likely answer to the question. The stem word that clues you to a similar word in the option or that limits potential options is known as a specific determiner. For example:

The government agency responsible for administering the nursing practice act in each state is the:

1. Board of regents
2. Board of nursing
3. State nurses' association
4. State hospital association

Options 2 and 3 contain the closely related words *nurse* and *nursing*. The word *nursing*, used both in the stem and in option 2, is a clue to the correct answer.

•Identify Words In The Options That Are Closely Associated With Words In The Stem

Be alert to words in the options that may be closely associated with but not identical to a word or words in the stem. For example:

When a person develops symptoms of physical illness for which psychogenic factors act as causative agents, the resulting illness is classified as:

1. Dissociative
2. Compensatory
3. Psychophysiologic
4. Reaction formation

Option 3 ought to strike you as a likely answer, since it combines physical and psychologic factors, like those referred to in the stem.

•Watch For Grammatical Inconsistencies

If one or more of the options are not grammatically consistent with the stem, the alert test taker can frequently eliminate these distractors. The correct option must be consistent with the form of the question. If the question demands a response in the singular, plural options usually can be safely eliminated. When the stem is in the form of an incomplete sentence, each option should complete the sentence in a grammatically correct way. For example:

Communicating with a client who is deaf will be facilitated by:

1. Use gestures
2. Speaking loudly
3. Find out if he has a hearing aid
4. Facing the client while speaking

Options 1 and 3 do not complete the sentence in a grammatically correct way and can therefore be eliminated. Option 2 would be of no assistance with a deaf client, so option 4 is the correct answer.

•Be Alert To Relevant Information From Earlier Questions

Occasionally remembering information from one question may provide you with a clue for answering a later question. For example:

A client has a Cantor tube inserted for treatment of intestinal obstruction. Intestinal suction can result in excessive loss of:

1. Protein enzymes
2. Energy carbohydrates
3. Water and electrolytes
4. Vitamins and minerals

If you determined that the correct answer to this question was option 3, it may help you to answer a later question. For example:

Critical assessment of a client while a Cantor tube is draining should include observation for:

1. Edema
2. Nausea
3. Belching
4. Dehydration

The correct answer is option 4. If you knew that excessive loss of water and electrolytes may lead to dehydration, you could have used the clue provided in the earlier question to assist you in answering the later question.

•Make Educated Guesses

When you are unsure about the correct answer to a question, it is better to make an educated guess than not to answer the question. You can generally eliminate one or more of the distractors by using partial knowledge and the methods just

listed. The elimination process increases your chances of selecting the correct option from those remaining. Elimination of two distractors on a four-option multiple-choice item increases your probability of selecting the correct answer from 25% to 50%.

GENERAL STRATEGIES

1. Develop a plan for study and stick to it. A good plan is to allow one week per clinical area.
2. As you study, identify your problem areas that need attention.
3. Avoid planning things that will add stress to your life between now and the time you take the NCLEX-RN examination. Enough things will happen spontaneously; do not plan for them.
4. Do not change your pattern of study. It has obviously contributed to your being here, so it worked. If you have studied alone, continue to study alone. If you have studied in a group, form a study group.
5. Practice timed tests and stick to their suggested time frame. You usually will have about one minute per question on an examination.
6. Pace yourself during the testing period and work as accurately as possible. Do not rush. Excessive pressure on yourself early in the examination can result in early fade-out.
7. Although certain questions will be more difficult and will require more time, do not spend too much time on one question as it can compromise your overall performance.
8. If you find you tend to reread test answers and change the right ones to wrong ones, stop going back even if you are taking tests that permit you to go back. If you find that going back helps you to correct wrong answers, by all means go back and review your answers if the test permits you to go back. Remember; your first answer is usually correct and should not be changed without reason.
9. Do not read information into questions and avoid speculating. Reading into questions creates errors in judgment.
10. Make certain that the answer you select is reasonable and obtainable under ordinary circumstances and that the action can be carried out in the given situation.

11. Avoid selecting answers that state hospital rules or regulations as a reason or rationale for action.
12. Look for answers that focus on the client or are directed toward the client's feelings.
13. If the question asks for an immediate action or response, all the answers may be correct, so base your selection on identified priorities for action.
14. Do not select answers that contain exceptions to the general rule, controversial material, or degrading responses.
15. Do not be pressured into finishing early. Use all the time necessary without pressuring yourself.

CHAPTER 2

Medical–Surgical Nursing Review Questions

GROWTH AND DEVELOPMENT

1.   Developmentally, a 21-year-old male client who has sustained a spinal injury below the level of T6 will most likely have difficulty with:
     1. Mastering his environment
     2. Identifying with the male role
     3. Developing meaningful relationships
     4. Differentiating himself from the environment

2.   ✳ The anesthesiologist orders meperidine hydrochloride 100 mg IM preoperatively for a 76-year-old client. The priority nursing action would be to:
     1. Question the anesthesiologist about the order *Dose Toxic in elderly*
     2. Determine if the client is allergic to meperidine
     3. Administer the preoperative medication as ordered
     4. Raise the side rails after administering the medication

3.   When assessing a client with osteoporosis the nurse should recognize that most observable changes will occur in:
     1. Facial bones
     2. The long bones
     3. The vertebral column
     4. Joints of the hands and feet

Diet not adequate

✳ 4. The nurse recognizes that a client can best limit further progression of osteoporosis by:
     1. Taking supplemental calcium and vitamin D
     2. Taking supplemental magnesium and vitamin E
     3. Increasing the consumption of eggs and cheese
     4. Increasing the consumption of milk and milk products

✳ 5. A 70-year-old male client with ankylosing spondylitis asks the nurse if he should be taking multivitamin and mineral supplements. The nurse's best response would be:
     1. "Absolutely! They are a necessity as a person gets older."
     2. "Older people usually do need more vitamins, especially vitamin A."
     3. "There is no evidence that generally healthy older adults require added nutrient supplements."
     4. "If you took the supplement you could cut down on your food and help keep your weight down."

6. A day after an explanation of the effects of surgery to create an ileostomy, a 68-year-old male client remarks to the nurse, "It will be difficult for my wife to care for a helpless old man." These comments by the client regarding himself are an example of Erikson's conflict of:
1. Initiative vs guilt
2. Integrity vs despair
3. Industry vs inferiority
4. Generativity vs stagnation

7. The nurse should recognize that a genitourinary factor that may contribute to urinary incontinence in the elderly is:
1. A sensory deprivation
2. A urinary tract infection
3. The frequent use of diuretics
4. The inaccessibility of a bathroom

8. When correcting myths about aging, the nurse should teach that elderly people normally have:
1. Periods of confusion
2. An inflexible attitude
3. Some senile dementia
4. A slower reaction time

9. An elderly female is admitted to the hospital because of complications associated with severe dehydration. The client's daughter asks the nurse how her mother could have become dehydrated because she is alert and able to care for herself. The nurse's best response would be:
1. "The body's need for fluid decreases with age because of a change in the body composition."
2. "Access to fluid may be limited and insufficient to meet the daily needs of the older adult."
3. "Memory declines with age and the older adult may forget to ingest adequate amounts of fluid."
4. "The thirst reflex diminishes with age and therefore the recognition of the need for fluid is decreased."

10. An elderly female client tells the nurse that she read about a vitamin that may be related to aging because of its relationship to the structure of cell walls and wonders if she should be taking it. The nurse should recognize that the client is probably referring to:
1. Vitamin A
2. Vitamin C
3. Vitamin E
4. Vitamin B$_1$

11. A female client's osteoporosis has progressed dramatically in the last 5 years, and she is especially prone to falling. The statement that best reflects the client's understanding of why there is a greater risk for falls would be:
1. "I do not have the stamina that I used to have."
2. "At my age, I'm more prone to dizziness and falling."
3. "Because of the curvature of my spine, it is hard to keep my balance."
4. "Because I am bent over, I look down instead of up while I'm walking."

12. Nursing actions for the elderly should include health education and promotion of self-care. When dealing with the elderly the nurse should:
1. Encourage exercise and naps
2. Strengthen the concept of ageism
3. Reinforce clients' strengths and promote reminiscing
4. Teach about a high carbohydrate diet and focus on the present

13. The mental process most sensitive to deterioration with aging seems to be:
1. Judgment
2. Creativity
3. Intelligence
4. Short term memory

14. The nurse is preparing a health program for senior citizens in the community. The nurse teaches the group that physical findings that are normal in older people include:
1. A loss of skin elasticity and a decrease in libido
2. Impaired fat digestion and increased salivary secretions
3. An increase in body warmth and some swallowing difficulties
4. Increased blood pressure and decreased hormone production in women

15. An 89-year-old client with osteoporosis is admitted to the hospital with a compression fracture of the spine. The nurse understands that a factor of special concern when caring for an elderly client is the client's:
1. Inability to recall recent facts
2. Irritability in response to deprivation
3. Inability to maintain an optimal level of functioning
4. Gradual memory loss resulting from change in environment

EMOTIONAL NEEDS RELATED TO HEALTH PROBLEMS

16. A female client has just spent 5 minutes complaining to the nurse about numerous aspects of her hospital stay. The best initial nursing response would be to:
1. Attempt to explain the purpose of different hospital routines to the client
2. Explain to the client that becoming so upset dangerously blocks her need for rest
3. Refocus the conversation on the client's fears, frustrations, and anger about her condition
4. Permit the client to release feelings and then promptly leave to allow her to regain composure

17. A male client who has had a myocardial infarction asks the nurse, "What's the chance of my having another heart attack if I watch my diet and stress levels carefully?" The most appropriate initial response would be for the nurse to:
1. Suggest he discuss his feelings of vulnerability with his physician
2. Avoid giving him direct information and help him explore his feelings
3. Tell him that he certainly needs to be especially careful in these areas
4. Recognize that he is frightened and suggest he talk with the psychiatric nurse

18. A client who has recently had an abdomino-perineal resection and colostomy accuses the nurse of being uncomfortable during a dressing change, because the "wound looks terrible." The nurse recognizes that the client is using the defense mechanism known as:

1. Projection
2. Sublimation
3. Intellectualization
4. Reaction formation

19. A male client who has had an abdominoperineal resection and colostomy refuses to allow his wife to see the incision or stoma and ignores most of his dietary instructions. The nurse, when assessing this data, can assume that the client is experiencing:
1. Suicidal thoughts and should be seen by a psychiatrist
2. A reaction formation to his recent altered body image
3. Impotency due to the surgery and needs sexual counseling
4. A difficult time accepting reality and is in a state of denial

20. Three days after a below-the-knee amputation a client is refusing to eat, talk, or perform any rehabilitative activities. The best initial nursing approach would be to:
1. Frequently explain why there is a need to quickly increase activity
2. Emphasize repeatedly that with a prosthesis there will be a return to a normal life style
3. Appear cheerful and non-critical regardless of the client's response to attempts at intervention
4. Accept and acknowledge that the client's withdrawal is a normal and necessary part of initial grieving

21. The key factor in accurately assessing how a client will cope with body image changes is the:
1. Suddenness of the change
2. Obviousness of the change
3. Extent of body change present
4. Client's perception of the change

22. A client who was recently diagnosed as having myelocytic leukemia discusses the diagnosis by referring to statistics, facts, and figures. The nurse recognizes that the client is using the defense mechanism known as:
    1. Projection
    2. Sublimation
    3. Intellectualization
    4. Reaction formation

23. A female client who is dying jokes about the situation even though she is becoming sicker and weaker. The nurse's most therapeutic response would be:
    1. "Why are you always laughing?"
    2. "Your laughter is a cover for your fear."
    3. "Does it help to joke about your illness?"
    4. "She who laughs on the outside, cries on the inside."

24. When caring for a dying client who is in the denial stage of grief, the best nursing approach is to:
    1. Agree with and encourage the client's denial
    2. Reassure the client that everything will be okay
    3. Allow the denial but be available to discuss death
    4. Leave the client alone to confront feelings of impending loss

25. After a thymectomy for treatment of myasthenia gravis the nurse notes that a female client seems to be depressed. The nursing action that would be most appropriate at this point would be:
    1. Recognizing that depression often occurs after surgery
    2. Asking her physician to arrange for a psychological consultation
    3. Reassuring the client that she will feel better when her discharge date is set
    4. Talking with the client about her prognosis, emphasizing things that she can do

26. The home-care nurse supervisor makes an initial visit to a 60-year-old widowed client who has right ventricular failure. The client lives with her divorced, drug-addicted daughter and her seven grandchildren. The nurse finds the client feeding a 6-month-old granddaughter and preparing dinner for the rest of the family. A 14-year-old grandson, handicapped and in a wheelchair, states his mother is sleeping. The nurse should proceed by:
    1. Sitting down with the client and exchanging identifying data and information
    2. Accepting coffee when offered by the client and socializing for a few minutes
    3. Asking the client if it is alright to look around the apartment to evaluate environmental conditions
    4. Questioning the client to determine if there is a private place to take a health history and perform an examination

27. A client is taught how to change the dressing and how to care for a recently inserted nephrostomy tube. On the day of discharge the client states, "I hope I can handle all this at home; it's a lot to remember." The best response by the nurse would be:
    1. "I'm sure you can do it!"
    2. "Oh, a family member can do it for you."
    3. "You seem to be nervous about going home."
    4. "Perhaps you can stay in the hospital another day."

28. An 83-year-old client with non-insulin dependent diabetes mellitus is admitted to the hospital for elective cataract surgery. Before surgery the client asks the nurse, "How will my diabetes be managed during my hospitalization?" The best response by the nurse would be:
    1. "The anesthetist will take care of it."
    2. "What did your surgeon or the anesthetist tell you?"
    3. "Your surgeon will write orders for fluids and insulin."
    4. "I'm not quite certain I understand what you are asking."

29. A female client with nodular poorly differentiated lymphocytic lymphoma (NLPD), who has been treated with multiple chemotherapeutic agents, comes for her first radiation treatment. As the nurse prepares her for the therapy the client states, "I'm so discouraged" and starts to cry. The nurse should:

1. Leave her alone so that she can regain her composure
2. State, "It's difficult to deal with your diagnosis and treatment."
3. Complete the preparation and tell her, "We can talk about this later."
4. Explain the therapy and reiterate that it will cause only a little discomfort

30. A client's discouragement with the diagnosis of nodular poorly differentiated lymphocytic lymphoma (NLPD) continues during radiation therapy because of the long time required for treatment and its side effects. When assisting the client to plan for the future, the nurse should emphasize that:
1. Antidepressant medication can be prescribed
2. The client's feelings are normal and will lessen with time
3. A positive outlook can influence the outcome of cancer therapy
4. The prognosis for NLPD is more favorable than for other types

31. A client has just been given the diagnosis of multiple sclerosis. The client is obviously upset with the diagnosis and asks, "Am I going to die?" The nurse's best response would be:
1. "Most individuals with your disease live a normal life span."
2. "Is your family here? I would like to explain your disease to all of you."
3. "The prognosis is variable; most individuals experience remissions and exacerbations."
4. "Why don't you speak with your doctor who can give you more details about your disease."

32. A client refuses to go to the twice-a-day prescribed sessions in physical therapy. The nurse might best approach this problem by:
1. Having the client observe the progress of a more cooperative client with the same problem
2. Being the client's advocate and asking the physician if therapy can be decreased to once daily

3. Planning a conference with the client, the physical therapist, and the nurse to discuss the client's feelings
4. Assuring the client that analgesic medication will be administered before the scheduled physical therapy sessions

33. A 22-year-old male client with AIDS signs a Do Not Resuscitate (DNR) order when he is admitted to the hospital. When respiratory arrest occurs three weeks later the client is not resuscitated. A true statement about the legal aspects of a DNR order would be:
1. Age is an important factor in the decision not to resuscitate
2. The decision not to resuscitate resides with the client's physician
3. The status of the DNR order is contingent on the policies of the institution
4. Once the order has been signed, it remains in force for the entire hospitalization

34. The physician places a client with an infected surgical incision on strict isolation. After being taught about isolation, the client is seen sneaking out of the room to make telephone calls on the public phone. The most effective nursing intervention would be to:
1. Ensure regular visits by staff members
2. Explore what isolation means to the client
3. Report the situation to the infection control nurse
4. Reteach the entire isolation procedure to the client

35. The community health nurse makes a home visit to a 13-year-old boy who is handicapped and who has 3 siblings under 6 years of age. The nurse observes that the 6-month-old sister lies quietly in her crib, rarely smiles or vocalizes, and barely has her basic needs attended. The nurse should:
    1. Place an aide in the home to assist with chores and care for the infant
    2. Advise the mother that the child will be retarded if she is not stimulated
    3. Ask the 13-year-old handicapped brother to pay more attention to his sister
    4. Encourage purchasing appropriate toys manufactured for the baby's age level

36. The nurse should suspect that a male client, who has had a recent myocardial infarction, is experiencing denial when he:
    1. Attempts to minimize his illness
    2. Lacks an emotional response to his illness
    3. Refuses to discuss his condition with his wife
    4. Expresses displeasure with his activity program

37. A male client, who has had a subtotal gastrectomy for a peptic ulcer, and his wife attend the discharge conference with the nurse. This is helpful because, in addition to diet planning, they need to work together to plan:
    1. To maximize changes in his life-style
    2. Ways of dealing with stress in their environment
    3. To deal with long-term complications following surgery
    4. Methods of avoiding pernicious anemia following gastric surgery

38. A client is scheduled for a below-the-knee amputation of the right leg. Legally, the client may not sign the operative consent if:
    1. Ambivalent feelings regarding the operation are present
    2. Any sedative type of medication has recently been administered
    3. A discussion of alternatives with two physicians has not occurred
    4. A complete history and physical have not been performed and recorded

39. In the recovery room after a below-the-knee amputation a female client begins crying while feeling for her involved lower leg. The nurse should:
    1. Administer medication to induce sleep
    2. Allow the client to ventilate feelings of loss
    3. Ignore the behavior until the client is more alert
    4. Leave the client alone to provide additional time for privacy

40. The nurse raises a client's bedside rails at night. An alteration of the environment through the use of side rails may affect a client's psychologic status resulting in:
    1. A sense of security
    2. The prevention of falls
    3. Increased independence
    4. An alteration in proprioception

41. Teaching for clients who have sustained a sudden, traumatic, major loss is often most satisfactorily done during the acceptance or adaptation stage of coping. The nurse is aware that the rationale for this fact is that clients in this stage are:
    1. Ready for discharge and therefore in need of preparation
    2. At the peak of mental anguish and therefore open to change
    3. Less angry and therefore more compliant and easier to deal with
    4. Less anxious and more aware of reality and therefore ready to learn

42. On the fourth day after surgery for a fractured hip, a client appears angry and very restless and says, "I can't stand this another minute. There's a wrinkle in my sheet and my water is warm." The client changes position frequently and does not maintain eye contact with the nurse. The best initial interpretation of the client's behavior is that it indicates:
    1. Severe discomfort in the hip
    2. An increased level of anxiety
    3. Anger at the poor nursing care
    4. Frustration with the need for leg abduction

43. A post-surgical client complains about a variety of minor environmental factors, while frequently changing position and avoiding eye contact. The nurse responds to these observations by stating, "Let me get you some cold water and your pain pill and you'll be much better." The nurse's approach demonstrates the:
1. Empathetic recognition of anxiety
2. Introduction of the needs approach
3. Inappropriate use of the data presented
4. Use of problem identification and clarification

44. A client in thyroid storm tells the nurse, "I know I'm going to die. I'm very sick." The best response by the nurse would be:
1. "You must feel very sick and frightened."
2. "Tell me why you feel you are going to die."
3. "I can understand how you feel, but people do not die from this problem."
4. "If you would like, I will call your family and tell them to come to the hospital."

45. The nurse should be aware that sensory restriction in a client who is blind can:
1. Increase the use of daydreaming and fantasy
2. Heighten the client's decision-making ability
3. Decrease the client's restlessness and lethargy
4. Lead to the use of permanent neurotic behaviors

46. A young female client is diagnosed as having stage IIIA Hodgkin's disease with a grossly involved spleen and is scheduled for a splenectomy. After the nurse performs preoperative teaching the client appears very anxious. The best approach for the nurse to use at this time would be to:
1. Allow the client to regress at this time and let her rest quietly
2. State simply that she seems anxious and ask her if she would like to talk for awhile

3. Consider her reaction an unconscious response and inquire about her relations with her mother
4. Recognize that anxiety prevented the client from understanding and repeat the information in simpler terms

47. A female client with chronic renal failure has been on hemodialysis for 2 years. She relates to the nurse in dialysis in an angry, critical manner and is frequently noncompliant with medications and diet. The nurse can best intervene by first understanding that the client's behavior is most likely:
1. An attempt to punish the nursing staff
2. A constructive method of accepting reality
3. A defense against underlying depression and fear
4. An effort to maintain life to the fullest extent possible

48. The nurse observes another nurse changing a client's sterile dressing. The nurse changing the dressing uses the same pair of clean gloves to remove the soiled dressing and apply the new dressing. The observing nurse's initial action should be to:
1. Discuss the incident with the nurse
2. File an incident report about the action
3. Offer to demonstrate the proper technique
4. Report the individual to the nursing supervisor

49. Before major abdominal surgery for cancer the client says to the nurse, "I really don't think this is cancer at all. I'll bet they won't find anything." The nurse's most appropriate initial response would be:
1. "I can understand why you'd like to believe that."
2. "I hope you're right, but the tests do indicate cancer."
3. "It must be difficult to be facing such serious surgery."
4. "You think the doctor may have made a wrong diagnosis?"

50. A female client is diagnosed as having cancer of the breast and is admitted to the hospital for a lumpectomy to be followed by radiation. While being admitted to ambulatory surgery by the nurse, the client has tears in her eyes and her chin is quivering. In a shaky voice the client says, "I can't believe this is happening." The nurse's best response would be:
    1. "You can't believe this is happening?"
    2. "This must be a very scary time for you."
    3. "Do you have any questions at this time?"
    4. "Cancer of the breast has a high cure rate."

51. A client with a herniated nucleus pulposus at L4-5 is scheduled for a laminectomy. The night before surgery the client is extremely demanding, making frequent requests for about two hours. An empathetic nurse might best show understanding by saying:
    1. "You are being demanding tonight."
    2. "You are facing a rough day tomorrow."
    3. "Don't be so concerned, we'll take good care of you."
    4. "I know how scared you are, but this is routine surgery."

52. A nurse stops at the scene of an accident and finds a man with a deep laceration on his hand, a fractured arm and leg, and abdominal pain. The nurse wraps the man's hand in a soiled cloth and drives him to the nearest hospital. The nurse is:
    1. Negligent and can be sued for malpractice
    2. Practicing under guidelines of the Nurse Practice Act
    3. Protected for these actions, in most states, by the Good Samaritan Law
    4. Treating a health problem that can and should be handled by a physician

53. A male client hospitalized following a major automobile accident has no hospitalization insurance and is very worried about the medical bills. As the client is describing the accident to a friend, he becomes very restless, and his pulse and respirations increase sharply. It is most important for the nurse to recognize that these symptoms are probably related to:
    1. Bleeding from an undiscovered injury
    2. The client's method of seeking sympathy

    3. Delayed psychologic response to trauma
    4. A parasympathetic nervous system response to anxiety

54. A male client with pancreatic cancer is aware of the terminal nature of the illness. Behaviors that would indicate that he is accepting the fact of his impending death are:
    1. Alternately crying and talking openly about death
    2. Getting second, third, and fourth medical opinions
    3. Making out his will and planning a visit to a good friend
    4. Refusing to follow treatments and stating, "I'm going to die anyway."

55. A female client with terminal cancer decides to donate her eyes for organ transplantation after she dies. Statutes that address organ transplantation attempt to prevent abuse by:
    1. Permitting active euthanasia when necessary
    2. Preventing children from giving organs to others
    3. Allowing physicians to control both donor and recipient
    4. Requiring participating institutions to have review boards

56. A male client with thrombophlebitis is apprehensive about the possibility of a clot reaching his heart, causing sudden death. The nurse's initial intervention should be to:
    1. Clarify his misconception
    2. Explain preventive measures
    3. Teach recognition of early symptoms
    4. Encourage discussion of the client's concern

57. The physician discusses the need for an abdominoperineal resection and a colostomy with a male client. After the physician leaves, the client tells the nurse that he is pleased only minor surgery is necessary. The nurse recognizes that the client's reaction is an example of:
    1. Reflection
    2. Regression
    3. Repudiation
    4. Reconciliation

58. To be most effective when teaching colostomy care to a client, the nurse must first:
1. Wait until a family member is present
2. Assess barriers to learning ostomy care
3. Begin with simple written instructions concerning the care
4. Wait until the client has accepted the change in body image

59. During the evening after a paracentesis, the nurse notices that the client, although denying any discomfort, seems very anxious. The best nursing approach would be to:
1. Offer the client a back rub
2. Administer the prescribed narcotic
3. Reinforce the physician's explanation of the procedure
4. Explore the client's concerns and administer the ordered hypnotic

60. Individual nurses are responsible for their own professional actions. In addition, a hospital can be held legally responsible for the actions of a nurse employed by the hospital under the doctrine of:
1. In loco parentis
2. Respondeat superior
3. The state's department of health
4. The American Hospital Association's Review Board

61. After receiving diabetic education, a client with recently diagnosed diabetes mellitus states, "I feel bad. I don't seem to get along with my husband. He does not care about my diabetes." The nurse's most appropriate response would be:
1. "You don't get along with your husband?"
2. "I'm sorry, what can I do to make you feel better?"
3. "It's probably just temporary; he needs more time to adjust."
4. "You are unhappy. I wonder, have you tried to talk to your husband?"

62. A visitor from a room adjacent to a client asks the nurse what disease the client has. The nurse responds, "I will not discuss any client's illness with you. Are you concerned about it?" This response is based on the nurse's knowledge that to discuss a client's condition with someone not directly involved with that client is an example of:
1. Libel
2. Slander
3. Negligence
4. Invasion of privacy

63. When approaching homosexual clients with AIDS, it is most important for nurses to:
1. Have a strong sense of their own sexual identity
2. Admit their feelings of uncomfortableness to the client
3. Pay particular attention to establishing a meaningful rapport
4. Become aware of their own attitudes regarding homosexuality

64. A client with jaundiced skin and acute abdominal pain is refusing all visitors. The most therapeutic response would be to:
1. Listen to the client's fears
2. Encourage the client to socialize
3. Grant the client's request about visitors
4. Darken the client's room by pulling the drapes

65. A 26-year-old homosexual is diagnosed with AIDS. The primary nurse reports to the nursing team that the client wept when told of the diagnosis. One of the nursing assistants responds, "I don't feel sorry for him. He made his bed and now he can lie in it." This comment is most likely a result of the nursing assistant's:
1. Values and beliefs about sexual life-styles
2. Anger and mistrust of homosexual males in general
3. Discomfort with men who are unable to control their emotions
4. Hostility over having to care for someone with a sexually related disease

66. A client with AIDS comments to the nurse, "There are so many rotten people around. Why couldn't one of them get AIDS instead of me?" The nurse could best respond:
  1. "It seems unfair that you should be so ill."
  2. "I can understand why you're afraid of death."
  3. "Have you thought of speaking with a minister?"
  4. "I'm sure you really don't wish this on someone else."

67. A client is to be transferred from the coronary care unit to a progressive care unit. The client asks the nurse, "Are you sure I'm ready for this move?" From this statement the nurse ascertains that the client is most likely experiencing:
  1. Fear
  2. Depression
  3. Dependency
  4. Ambivalence

68. A client who is suspected of having a brain tumor is scheduled for a CT scan. Before the test the nurse should:
  1. Withhold routine medications
  2. Describe the equipment involved
  3. Administer the prescribed sedative
  4. Explain that no radiation will be involved

69. During the assessment interview a client suspected of having an aldosteronoma states, "I don't know why the doctor doesn't just give me a prescription for high blood pressure pills. I'm missing work by being here for these tests." The nurse's best response would be:
  1. "It might not be high blood pressure. We have to be sure."
  2. "I know it's frustrating, but you need to be here for these tests."
  3. "It's frustrating to miss work and not know for sure what's wrong."
  4. "Did you ask your doctor if the tests could be done on an outpatient basis?"

70. During a home visit the nurse discovers that a child in the household has a handicap and has been experiencing convulsions. In addition the child's mother not only was unresponsive to the child's needs but also failed to obtain needed medication or follow-up of medical attention. The mother also seems to provoke convulsive episodes by harsh verbal exchanges with the child. The nurse believes that intervention by an appropriate community resource is indicated. A referral should be made to:
  1. The outpatient clinic
  2. The hospital pediatric unit
  3. The Bureau of Child Welfare
  4. The Bureau of the Handicapped

FLUIDS AND ELECTROLYTES

71. During an 8 hour shift a client drinks two 6 ounce cups of tea and vomits 125 ml of fluid. During this 8 hour period the client's fluid balance would be:
  1. +55 ml
  2. +137 ml
  3. +235 ml
  4. +485 ml

72. A client weighed 210 pounds on admission to the hospital. After 2 days of diuretic therapy the client weighs 205.5 pounds. The nurse could estimate that the amount of fluid the client has lost is:
  1. 0.5 L
  2. 1.0 L
  3. 2.0 L
  4. 3.5 L

73. A male client with a history of congestive heart failure and atrial fibrillation comes to the clinic for his regular 2 week visit. The client is 9 pounds heavier than his usual weight. The nurse interprets that the most likely cause of this sudden weight gain is:
  1. Fluid retention
  2. Urinary retention
  3. Renal insufficiency
  4. Abdominal distension

74. After a surgical procedure for cancer of the pancreas a client is to receive the following intravenous fluids over 24 hours: 1000 ml D5W; 0.5 liter normal saline; 1500 ml D5NS. In addition, an antibiotic piggyback in 50 ml D5W is ordered every 8 hours. The nurse cal-

culates that the client's IV fluid intake for 24 hours will be:
1. 3150 ml
2. 3200 ml
3. 3650 ml
4. 3750 ml

75. The dietary practice that will help a client reduce the dietary intake of sodium is:
1. Increasing the use of dairy products
2. Using an artificial sweetener in coffee
3. Avoiding the use of carbonated beverages
4. Using catsup for cooking and flavoring foods

76. An ECG is performed before a client is to have a cardiac catheterization, and hypokalemia is suspected. To confirm the presence of hypokalemia the nurse would expect the physician to order:
1. Blood cultures times 3
2. A complete blood count
3. A serum electrolyte level
4. An X-ray film of long bones

77. A client is to receive an intravenous solution containing potassium chloride. When starting this IV infusion the nurse should select:
1. The antecubital vein in the client's arm
2. The largest possible vein in the client's arm
3. A vein in the back of the client's dominant hand
4. A vein in the back of the client's non-dominant hand

78. When evaluating a client's response to fluid replacement therapy, the observation that indicates adequate tissue perfusion to vital organs is:
1. Urinary output of 30 ml in an hour
2. Central venous pressure reading of 2 cm H$_2$O
3. Pulse rates of 120 and 110 in a 15-minute period
4. Blood pressure readings of 50/30 and 70/40 within 30 minutes

79. When administering albumin intravenously, the nurse is aware that body water will shift from the:

1. Interstitial compartment to the extracellular compartment
2. Intravascular compartment to the interstitial compartment
3. Intracellular compartment to the extracellular compartment
4. Extracellular compartment to the intracellular compartment

80. A client with chronic renal failure cannot use salt substitutes in the diet because:
1. A person's body tends to retain fluid when a salt substitute is included in the diet
2. Limiting salt substitutes in the diet prevents a build up of waste products in the blood
3. Salt substitutes contain potassium which must be limited to prevent abnormal heart beats
4. A substance in the salt substitute interferes with the transfer of fluid across capillary membranes resulting in anasarca

81. The nurse is aware that total parenteral nutrition is a more desirable therapy than just intravenous fluids for clients with gastrointestinal problems. The nurse understands that clients receiving only IV fluids lose weight because of:
1. Lack of bulk in the diet
2. Deficient carbohydrate intake
3. Insufficient intake of water-soluble vitamins
4. Increased concentrations of electrolytes in cells

82. A client's clinical symptoms indicate a possible gastric ulcer. Considering the symptoms of epigastric pain, vomiting, dehydration, weakness, lethargy, and shallow respirations, and the laboratory results which demonstrate metabolic alkalosis, the primary nursing diagnosis for this client would be:
1. Impaired gas exchange related to pain
2. High risk for injury related to weakness
3. Fluid volume deficit related to vomiting
4. Pain related to hypersecretion of gastric acids

83. A client with hypertension is being taught to restrict the intake of sodium. The nurse would evaluate that the teaching about foods low in sodium was understood when the client states, "I can eat:
   1. Broiled scallops."
   2. A bologna sandwich."
   3. Shredded wheat cereal."
   4. Carrot and celery sticks."

84. An elderly client is diagnosed as having acute renal failure secondary to dehydration, and the physician orders an IV infusion of 50% glucose and regular insulin. The nurse understands that this is ordered for a client in renal failure to:
   1. Prevent cardiac arrest
   2. Increase urinary output
   3. Prevent respiratory acidosis
   4. Decrease serum calcium levels

85. When monitoring for hyponatremia, the nurse should assess the client for:
   1. Dry skin
   2. Confusion
   3. Tachycardia
   4. Pale coloring

86. A client with an acute episode of ulcerative colitis is admitted to the hospital. Blood studies reveal that the chloride level is low. This electrolyte deficiency can best be corrected by:
   1. A low-residue diet
   2. Hyperalimentation
   3. Intravenous therapy
   4. An oral electrolyte solution

87. Clients with insulin dependent diabetes mellitus may experience a fluid imbalance. The primary fluid shift that occurs in diabetes mellitus is:
   1. Intravascular to interstitial because of glycosuria
   2. Extracellular to interstitial because of hypoproteinemia
   3. Intracellular to intravascular as a result of hyperosmolarity
   4. Intercellular to intravascular as a result of increased hydrostatic pressure

88. Serum albumin is to be administered intravenously to a client with ascites. The expected outcome of this treatment will be a decrease in:
   1. Urinary output
   2. Abdominal girth
   3. Serum ammonia level
   4. Hepatic encephalopathy

89. A client with a history of cardiac dysrhythmias is admitted to the hospital with the diagnosis of dehydration. The nurse should anticipate that the physician will order:
   1. A glass of water every hour until hydrated
   2. Small frequent intake of juices, broth, or milk
   3. Short-term NG replacement of fluids and nutrients
   4. A rapid IV infusion of an electrolyte and glucose solution

90. A client with chronic renal failure who is receiving dialysis is prescribed a protein-, sodium-, and potassium-restricted diet. The nurse would know that the dietary teaching was effective when the client says:
   1. "I cannot add seasonings to my food."
   2. "I should avoid using salt substitutes."
   3. "I can eat canned, no-salt vegetables."
   4. "I should get the protein I eat from meat."

91. Before administering a prescribed intravenous solution that contains potassium chloride, the assessment by the nurse that should be brought to the physician's attention would be:
   1. Poor skin turgor with "tenting"
   2. Behaviors indicating irritability and confusion
   3. A urinary output of 200 ml during the previous shift
   4. An oral intake of 300 ml of fluid during the previous shift

92. A client with hyperpyrexia, who has just been started on IV antibiotics, has a diminished urine output. The nurse should recognize that this is probably the result of:
   1. A declining blood pressure
   2. Bacterial invasion of the kidneys
   3. Nephrotoxicity from antimicrobial agents
   4. A normal compensatory response to fever

93. The nurse, when assessing the adequacy of a client's fluid replacement during the first 2 to 3 days following full-thickness burns to the trunk and right thigh, would be aware that the most significant data would be obtained from recording:
    1. Weights every day
    2. Urinary output every hour
    3. Blood pressure every 15 minutes
    4. Extent of peripheral edema every 4 hours

94. A client with diabetes mellitus develops ketoacidosis. The arterial blood gas report that is representative of diabetic ketoacidosis is:
    1. P_{CO_2} 49, HCO_3 32, pH 7.50
    2. P_{CO_2} 26, HCO_3 20, pH 7.52
    3. P_{CO_2} 54, HCO_3 28, pH 7.30
    4. P_{CO_2} 28, HCO_3 18, pH 7.28

95. The most effective way for the nurse to assess a client's response to ongoing serum albumin therapy for cirrhosis of the liver is to:
    1. Monitor the client's vital signs frequently
    2. Measure the client's urine output every half hour
    3. Obtain the client's weight at least once each day
    4. Determine the client's urine albumin level each shift

96. A client is placed on a low sodium diet. The family asks if they can bring some snacks from home. The nurse suggests that they bring foods low in sodium such as:
    1. Ice cream
    2. Celery sticks
    3. Fresh oranges
    4. Peanut butter cookies

97. A client with ascites has a paracentesis and 1500 ml of fluid is removed. Immediately following the procedure it is most important for the nurse to observe for:
    1. A rapid, thready pulse   Shock
    2. Decreasing peristalsis
    3. Respiratory congestion
    4. An increase in temperature

98. A 79-year-old client is admitted for dehydration, and an IV infusion of normal saline at 125 ml/hr is started. One hour later the client begins screaming, "I can't breathe." The nurse should:
    1. Call the physician to order a sedative
    2. Discontinue the IV and call the physician
    3. Elevate the head of the bed and obtain vital signs
    4. Assess the client for allergies and change the IV to a heparin lock

99. A client has been receiving 2500 ml of IV fluid and 300 to 400 ml of oral intake daily for two days. The client's urine output has been decreasing and now has been less than 40 ml per hour for the past three hours. The nurse should initially:
    1. Catheterize the client to empty the bladder
    2. Assess breath sounds and obtain the client's vital signs
    3. Check for dependent edema and continue to monitor I and O
    4. Decrease the IV flow rate and increase oral fluids to compensate

100. The nurse is aware that the shift of body fluids associated with the intravenous administration of albumin occurs by the process of:
    1. Osmosis
    2. Diffusion
    3. Filtration
    4. Active transport

101. A client on a 2 g sodium 1600 calorie ADA diet complains about the bland food and refuses to eat dinner. The nurse should first:
    1. Ask the client what foods are usually eaten at home
    2. Explain to the client that the diet will eventually have to be accepted
    3. Provide the client with several packets of lemon juice and one packet of salt
    4. Urge the client to eat to become accustomed to the diet that must be eaten at home

102. Following a gastrojejunostomy (Billroth II) for cancer of the stomach, a client progresses to a regular diet. After eating lunch the client becomes diaphoretic and has palpitations. The symptoms are probably the result of:
   1. An intolerance to fatty foods
   2. The dehiscence of the surgical incision
   3. An extracellular fluid shift into the bowel
   4. Diminished peristalsis in the small intestine

103. After abdominal surgery a client should be encouraged to turn from side to side and to carry out deep-breathing exercises. These activities are essential to prevent:
   1. Metabolic acidosis
   2. Metabolic alkalosis
   3. Respiratory acidosis
   4. Respiratory alkalosis

104. A client's arterial blood gases (ABGs) show a PO_2 of 89 mmHg; a PCO_2 of 35 mmHg; and a pH of 7.37. These findings indicate that the client is in:
   1. Fluid balance
   2. Oxygen depletion
   3. Metabolic acidosis
   4. Acid-base balance

105. A client is diagnosed as having metabolic acidosis. The nurse understands that in metabolic acidosis the:
   1. Blood pH is increased
   2. Plasma bicarbonates are increased
   3. Respiratory center in the medulla is depressed
   4. Excess number of hydrogen ions are excreted in the urine

106. A client appears very anxious with respirations that are shallow and very rapid (40 per minute). The client complains of feeling dizzy and light-headed and of having tingling sensations of the fingertips and around the lips. The nurse should recognize that the client's complaints are probably related to:
   1. Eupnea
   2. Hyperventilation
   3. Kussmaul respirations
   4. Carbon dioxide intoxication

107. Nursing intervention for a client who is hyperventilating should focus on providing reassurance and:
   1. Administering oxygen
   2. Using an incentive spirometer
   3. Having the client breathe into a paper bag
   4. Administering an IV containing bicarbonate ions

108. A client is hospitalized with epigastric pain, nausea, and vomiting of 4 days duration. The following laboratory data are noted: a plasma pH of 7.51; a PCO_2 of 50 mmHg; an HCO_3 of 58 mEq/L; a Cl of 55 mEq/L; a K^+ of 3.8 mEq/L. The nurse recognizes that the collected data indicate:
   1. Hyperkalemia
   2. Hyperchloremia
   3. Metabolic alkalosis
   4. Respiratory acidosis

109. Following a gastrectomy a client has a nasogastric tube to low continuous suction. The client begins to hyperventilate. The nurse should be aware that this pattern will alter the client's arterial blood gases by:
   1. Increasing PO_2
   2. Decreasing pH
   3. Increasing HCO_3
   4. Decreasing PCO_2

110. When a client is in profound (late) hypovolemic shock the nurse should assess the client's laboratory values, especially the arterial blood gases, because people in late shock will develop:
   1. Hypokalemia
   2. Decreased PCO_2
   3. Metabolic acidosis
   4. Respiratory alkalosis

111. When a client develops respiratory alkalosis, the nurse should expect the laboratory values to reflect:
   1. An elevated pH, elevated PCO_2
   2. A decreased pH, elevated PCO_2
   3. An elevated pH, decreased PCO_2
   4. A decreased pH, decreased PCO_2

112. When assessing a client's arterial blood gases the nurse would know that the client was in

compensated respiratory acidosis when the pH is 7.34 and the:

1. PO_2 is 80 mmHg
2. HCO_3 is 50 mEq/L
3. PCO_2 is 60 mmHg
4. Serum potassium is 4 mEq/L

113. Surgery is performed on a client with a parotid tumor. The postoperative arterial blood gas values are pH 7.32; PCO_2 53 mmHg; HCO_3 25 mEq/L. The nurse should:

1. Obtain a medical order for the administration of a diuretic
2. Encourage the client to breathe into a rebreather bag at a slow rate
3. Encourage the client to cough productively and take deep breaths
4. Obtain a medical order for the administration of sodium bicarbonate

114. After surgery a client is to receive an antibiotic by IV piggyback in 50 ml of D5W. The piggyback is to infuse in 20 minutes. The drop factor of the IV set is 10 gtt/ml. The nurse should set the piggyback to flow at:

1. 25 gtt/min
2. 30 gtt/min
3. 35 gtt/min
4. 45 gtt/min

115. Forty-eight hours after a client sustained a burn injury the physician orders 2 liters of IV fluid to be administered q12h. The drop factor of the tubing is 10 gtt/ml. The nurse should set the flow to provide:

1. 18 gtt/min
2. 28 gtt/min
3. 32 gtt/min
4. 36 gtt/min

116. A client's IV fluid orders for 24 hours are 1500 ml D5W followed by 1250 ml of NS. The IV tubing has a drop factor of 15 gtt/ml. To administer the required fluids, the nurse should set the drip rate at:

1. 13 gtt/min
2. 16 gtt/min
3. 29 gtt/min
4. 32 gtt/min

117. The physician orders a client's IV fluids to be delivered at 80 ml/hour. To adjust the drip

rate when administering the IV via gravity, the nurse must know the:

1. Total volume of fluid in the IV bag
2. Size of the needle or catheter in the vein
3. Drops per milliliter delivered by the infusion set
4. Diameter of the tubing being used to instill the fluid

118. A client is to receive D5RL 850 ml every 8 hours. The drop factor of the tubing is 10 gtt/ml. The nurse should set the flow to provide:

1. 12 gtt/min
2. 18 gtt/min
3. 24 gtt/min
4. 36 gtt/min

119. The physician orders 1250 ml of IV fluid every 8 hours. The drop factor of the tubing is 15 gtt/ml. The nurse should set the flow to provide:

1. 36 gtt/min
2. 39 gtt/min
3. 40 gtt/min
4. 42 gtt/min

120. The physician orders IV fluids and gentamicin sulfate (Garamycin) 100 mg IVPB q8h for a client. The nurse, using gravity to instill the IV, hangs the piggyback gentamicin higher than the primary IV bag. When the piggyback bag is empty, the client observes air in the tubing of the IVPB and becomes frightened. The nurse should explain that:

1. Air in the tubing, even if it got into the vein, would not be fatal unless it was a large amount
2. The gentamicin and now the air are flowing into the large IV bag not into the venous system directly
3. The solution from the large IV bag will begin to flow when the solution from the smaller bag ceases to flow
4. The clamps on the tubing leading from both bags can be closed for a few minutes to prevent air from entering the vein

121. A client is admitted to the surgical unit, and intravenous fluids are ordered. The client is to receive 100 ml D5W at 90 ml per hour. If the drop factor is 15 gtt/ml, the nurse should set the drip rate at:
1. 15 gtt/min
2. 23 gtt/min
3. 25 gtt/min
4. 30 gtt/min

BLOOD AND IMMUNITY

122. Twelve hours after a female client is admitted to the critical care unit following motorcycle injuries she begins to complain of increased abdominal pain in the left upper quadrant. A ruptured spleen is diagnosed, and she is scheduled for an emergency splenectomy. When preparing the client for surgery the nurse should emphasize the:
1. Complete safety of the procedure
2. Expectation of postoperative bleeding
3. Risk of the procedure with the other injuries
4. Presence of abdominal drainage for several days after the surgery

123. After abdominal surgery a client develops internal hemorrhaging. During further assessments, the nurse should expect the client to exhibit:
1. Polyuria
2. Bradypnea
3. Tachycardia
4. Hypertension

124. Immediately following abdominal surgery a client begins to hemorrhage. The nurse should observe the client for signs of progressive hypovolemia, which include:
1. Oliguria
2. Bradypnea
3. Pulse deficit
4. Hyperkalemia

125. A client is brought to the emergency room after an automobile accident. The client's blood pressure is 100/60 mmHg and the physical assessment suggests a ruptured spleen. Based on this information, the nurse should assess the client for an early sign of decreased arterial pressure, such as:
1. Warm, flushed skin
2. Confusion and lethargy
3. Increased pulse pressure
4. Reduced peripheral pulses

126. When a client is experiencing hypovolemic shock with decreased tissue perfusion, the body initially attempts to compensate by:
1. Producing less ADH
2. Producing more red blood cells
3. Maintaining peripheral vasoconstriction
4. Decreasing mineral corticoid production

127. After sustaining multiple internal injuries from being hit by a car, the client's blood pressure suddenly drops to 80/60 mmHg. The nurse should realize that this is probably caused by:
1. A reduction in the circulating blood volume
2. Diminished vasomotor stimulation to the arterial wall
3. Vasodilation resulting from diminished vasoconstrictor tone
4. Cardiac decompensation resulting from electrolyte imbalance

128. The nurse is aware that shock associated with a ruptured abdominal aneurysm is called:
1. Vasogenic shock
2. Neurogenic shock
3. Cardiogenic shock
4. Hypovolemic shock

129. A client has emergency surgery for a ruptured appendix. After assessing that the client is manifesting symptoms of shock the nurse should:
1. Prepare for a blood transfusion
2. Notify the physician immediately
3. Elevate the head of the bed 30 degrees
4. Administer the oxygen prescribed postoperatively

130. In the progressive stage of shock, anaerobic metabolism occurs. The nurse must be aware that this initially causes:
1. Metabolic acidosis
2. Metabolic alkalosis
3. Respiratory acidosis
4. Respiratory alkalosis

131. A client who is in hypovolemic shock has a hematocrit of 20%. The nurse should anticipate that the physician will order:
1. Serum albumin
2. Ringer's lactate
3. Blood replacement
4. High molecular dextran

132. The physician orders 2 units of blood to be infused for a client who is bleeding. Before blood administration the nurse's highest priority should be:
1. Obtaining the client's vital signs
2. Allowing the blood to reach room temperature
3. Monitoring the hemoglobin and hematocrit levels
4. Determining proper typing and cross-matching of blood

133. When administering blood, it is important for the nurse to:
1. Administer each unit within a 6 hour period
2. Use a volume control infusion pump to administer blood
3. Run the blood at a slower rate during the first 5 to 10 minutes
4. Draw blood samples from the client immediately after each unit is transfused

134. While receiving a blood transfusion a client develops flank pain, chills, fever, and hematuria. The nurse recognizes that the client is probably experiencing:
1. An allergic transfusion reaction
2. A hemolytic transfusion reaction
3. A pyrogenic transfusion reaction
4. An anaphylactic transfusion reaction

135. Halfway through the administration of a unit of blood, a client complains of lumbar pain. The nurse should:
1. Obtain vital signs
2. Stop the transfusion
3. Assess the pain further
4. Increase the flow of normal saline

136. A client comes to the clinic complaining of weight loss, fatigue, and a low grade fever. Physical examination reveals a slight enlarge-

ment of the cervical lymph nodes. To assess possible causes for the fever, it would be most appropriate for the nurse to initially ask:
1. "Have you been sexually active lately?"
2. "Do you have a sore throat at the present time?"
3. "Have you been exposed recently to anyone with an infection?"
4. "When did you first notice that your temperature had gone up?"

137. The nursing staff has a team conference on AIDS and discusses the routes of transmission of the human immunodeficiency virus (HIV). The discussion reveals that an individual has no risk of exposure to HIV when that individual:
1. Has intercourse with just the spouse
2. Makes a donation of a pint of whole blood
3. Limits sexual contact to those without HIV antibodies
4. Uses a condom each time there is sexual intercourse

138. The nurse knows that a positive diagnosis for HIV infection is made based on:
1. A history of high risk sexual behaviors
2. A positive ELISA and Western blot test
3. Evidence of extreme weight loss and high fever
4. Identification of an associated opportunistic infection

139. Blood screening tests of the immune system of a client with AIDS would indicate:
1. A decrease in CD_4 and T cells
2. An increase in thymic hormones
3. An increase in immunoglobulin E
4. A decrease in the serum level of glucose-6 phosphate dehydrogenase

140. When taking the blood pressure of a client who has AIDS the nurse must:
1. Wear clean gloves
2. Use barrier techniques
3. Wear a mask and gown
4. Wash the hands thoroughly

141. A client with acquired immunodeficiency syndrome (AIDS) and cryptococcal pneumonia is incontinent of feces and urine and is producing copious sputum. When providing care for this client the nurse's priority should be to:
    1. Wear goggles when suctioning the client
    2. Use gown, mask, and gloves when bathing the client
    3. Use gloves to administer oral medications to the client
    4. Wear a gown when assisting the client with the bedpan

142. In addition to *Pneumocystis carinii*, a client with AIDS also has an ulcer 4 cm in diameter on a leg. Considering the client's total health status, the most critical nursing diagnosis would be:
    1. Social isolation
    2. Impaired skin integrity
    3. Impaired gas exchange
    4. Altered nutrition: less than body requirements

143. A client with AIDS is to receive palliative treatment. A palliative approach would involve planning measures to:
    1. Restore the client's health
    2. Promote the client's recovery
    3. Relieve the client's discomfort
    4. Support the client's significant others

144. A Schilling test is ordered for a client who is suspected of having pernicious anemia. The nurse recognizes that the primary purpose of the Schilling test is to determine the client's ability to:
    1. Store vitamin B_{12}
    2. Digest vitamin B_{12}
    3. Absorb vitamin B_{12}
    4. Produce vitamin B_{12}

145. When explaining the therapeutic regimen of vitamin B_{12} for pernicious anemia to a client the nurse should explain that:
    1. Weekly Z-track injections provide needed control
    2. Daily intramuscular injections are required for control

    3. Intramuscular injections once a month will maintain control
    4. Oral tablets of vitamin B_{12} taken daily will keep the symptoms under control

146. The nurse knows that the teaching regarding the use of vitamin B_{12} injections to treat pernicious anemia is understood when a client states, "I must take the drug:
    1. When feeling fatigued."
    2. Until my symptoms subside."
    3. Monthly for the rest of my life."
    4. During exacerbations of anemia."

147. A client with Hodgkin's disease enters a remission and remains symptom free for 6 months when a relapse occurs. The Hodgkin's disease is diagnosed at stage IV. The therapy option the nurse should expect to be implemented at this time is:
    1. Radiation therapy
    2. Combination chemotherapy
    3. Radiation with chemotherapy
    4. Surgical removal of the affected nodes

148. The physician has decided to use total nodal irradiation in conjunction with chemotherapy for a young female client with stage IIIA Hodgkin's disease. The client tells the nurse she wants to have children and is quite concerned that the radiation therapy include the pelvic nodal areas. When questioned about this, the nurse should refer the client to the physician, because the nurse should be aware that:
    1. The ovaries can be surgically moved and placed in a shielded area
    2. Intense radiation to the area always causes permanent sterilization
    3. The radiation used is not radical enough to destroy ovarian function
    4. Ovarian function will be temporarily destroyed but will return in about 6 months

149. The nurse should plan to teach a client with pancytopenia caused by chemotherapy to:
    1. Begin a program of aggressive, strict mouth care
    2. Avoid traumatic injuries and exposure to any infection

3. Increase oral fluid intake to a minimum of 3000 ml daily
4. Report any unusual muscle cramps or tingling sensations in the extremities

150. An elderly client develops severe bone marrow depression from chemotherapy for cancer of the prostate. The nurse should:
1. Monitor him for signs of alopecia
2. Increase his daily intake of fluids
3. Monitor his intake and output of fluids
4. Use a soft toothbrush for his oral hygiene

151. The laboratory results for a client following chemotherapy for cancer indicate bone marrow depression. The nurse should encourage the client to:
1. Use an electric razor when shaving
2. Drink citrus juices frequently for nourishment
3. Sleep with the head of the bed slightly elevated
4. Increase the activity level and ambulate frequently

152. A client who is suspected of having leukemia has a bone marrow aspiration. Immediately following the procedure, the nurse should:
1. Apply brief pressure to the site
2. Ask the client to lie on the affected side
3. Swab the site with an antiseptic solution
4. Monitor the vital signs every hour for 4 hours

153. When obtaining a health history from a young client with probable acute lymphocytic leukemia (ALL), the clinical manifestations the nurse should expect to be present are
1. Petechiae, alopecia
2. Anorexia, insomnia
3. Anorexia, petechiae
4. Alopecia, bleeding gums

154. A 26-year-old client with a history of chronic myelogenous leukemia and splenomegaly is admitted to the hospital. The nurse should expect this client to have:
1. An increased urinary output
2. A tender mass in the left upper abdomen

3. Polydipsia, increased appetite, and frequency
4. Increased erythrocytes, platelets, and granulocytes

155. The diagnostic finding most specific for multiple myeloma is:
1. Low serum calcium levels
2. Bence-Jones protein in the urine
3. Occult and frank blood in the stool
4. Positive bacterial culture of sputum

156. A client with multiple myeloma is scheduled to have a chest x-ray examination and a bone scan. For this client, the primary responsibility of the nursing and radiology staff is to:
1. Explain the procedure and its purpose
2. Observe the client for shortness of breath
3. Provide for rest periods during the procedure
4. Handle the client with supportive movements   *Due to Fragile Bones*

157. A client who is newly diagnosed with multiple myeloma asks the physician what treatment will be necessary. The nurse should expect the physician to reply:
1. "Human leukocyte interferon therapy."
2. "Radiotherapy on an outpatient basis."
3. "Surgery to remove the lesion and lymph nodes."
4. "Chemotherapy employing a combination of drugs."

158. A young adult plans to enter a private college. To meet the admission requirements for the school and to ensure immunity, the student must have proof of having had:
1. One dose of diphtheria toxoid; one dose of oral poliomyelitis, live measles, live rubella, and mumps vaccines
2. Two doses of diphtheria toxoid and oral poliomyelitis vaccine; one dose of live measles, live rubella, and mumps vaccines
3. Three doses of diphtheria toxoid; two doses of oral poliomyelitis vaccine; one dose of live measles, live rubella, and mumps vaccines
4. Three doses of diphtheria toxoid; three doses of oral poliomyelitis vaccine; one dose of live measles, live rubella, and mumps vaccines

159. A client steps on a rusty nail and the puncture becomes swollen and painful. Tetanus antitoxin is prescribed. The nurse explains that this is used because it:
    1. Provides antibodies
    2. Stimulates plasma cells
    3. Produces active immunity
    4. Facilitates long-lasting immunity

160. A tuberculin skin test with purified protein derivative of tuberculin (PPD) is performed as part of a routine physical examination. The nurse should instruct the client to make an appointment so the test can be read in:
    1. 3 days
    2. 5 days
    3. 7 days
    4. 10 days

161. A client is admitted with cellulitus of the left leg and a temperature of 103°F. The physician orders IV antibiotics. Before instituting this therapy, the nurse should:
    1. Determine if the client has any allergies
    2. Apply a warm, moist dressing over the area
    3. Measure the amount of swelling in the client's leg
    4. Obtain the results of the culture and sensitivity tests

162. Following multiple bee stings a client has an anaphylactic reaction. The nurse is aware that the symptoms the client is experiencing are caused by:
    1. Respiratory depression and cardiac stand-still
    2. Bronchial constriction and decreased peripheral resistance
    3. Decreased cardiac output and the dilation of major blood vessels
    4. Constriction of capillaries and a decrease in peripheral circulation

INTEGUMENTARY

163. A client has been in a coma for 2 months and is maintained on bedrest. The nurse understands that to prevent the effects of shearing force the head of the bed should be at an angle of:
    1. 30 degrees
    2. 45 degrees
    3. 60 degrees
    4. 90 degrees

164. The physician orders bedrest for a client after surgery. The nurse is aware that the most beneficial method of preventing skin breakdown while the client is confined to bed is to:
    1. Massage the skin with cream
    2. Use a sheepskin pad on the bed
    3. Promote passive range of motion
    4. Encourage independent movement

165. The physician orders bedrest for a client with cellulitis of the leg. The nurse under-stands that the primary purpose of bedrest for this client is to:
    1. Decrease catabolism to promote healing at the site of injury
    2. Lower the metabolic rate in an attempt to help reduce the fever
    3. Reduce the energy demands on the body in the presence of infection
    4. Limit muscle contractions that would force causative organisms into the blood stream

166. The nurse is preparing to change a client's dressing. The statement that best explains the basis of surgical asepsis that the nurse will follow in this procedure is:
    1. Keep the area free of microorganisms
    2. Protect self from microorganisms in the wound
    3. Confine the microorganisms to the surgical site
    4. Keep the number of opportunistic microorganisms to a minimum

167. The equipment that will be used by the nurse during central venous catheter site care for a client receiving total parenteral nutrition is:
    1. Double sterile gloves
    2. Mask and sterile gloves
    3. Gown and sterile gloves
    4. Mask, gown, and sterile gloves

168. An extremely obese client must self-administer insulin at home. The nurse should teach the client to:

1. Bunch the tissue and inject at a 45-degree angle
2. Bunch the tissue and inject at a 60-degree angle
3. Spread the tissue and inject at a 45-degree angle
4. Spread the tissue and inject at a 90-degree angle

169. A client develops an infection at a catheter insertion site. The nurse uses the term iatrogenic when describing this infection because it resulted from:
1. Poor physical hygiene
2. A therapeutic procedure
3. Inadequate dietary patterns
4. The client's developmental level

170. A client develops an infection of an abdominal incision and overhears the nurses say that it is a nosocomial infection. The client asks the nurse what this means. The nurse should reply:
1. "The infection you had prior to hospitalization has flared up."
2. "You acquired the infection after being admitted to the hospital."
3. "This is a highly contagious infection requiring protective procedures."
4. "As a result of medical treatment, you have developed a secondary infection."

171. A male client is admitted to the hospital for intravenous antibiotic therapy and an incision and drainage of an abscess that developed at the site of a puncture wound. The nurse should begin teaching wound care to the client:
1. In the preoperative period
2. A few days before discharge
3. On the first postoperative day
4. During the first dressing change

172. The nurse is aware that research has shown that malnutrition occurs in as many as 50% of hospitalized clients. In view of a postoperative client's poor appetite, the nurse should observe for:
1. Dependent edema
2. "Spoon" shaped nails
3. Loose, decayed teeth
4. Delayed wound healing

173. The primary nurse tells a client with an infected wound that the nurse epidemiologist will visit daily. The client asks what the nurse epidemiologist does. The nurse could correctly explain the role by saying: "The nurse epidemiologist:
1. Decides what antibiotics should be prescribed for infections."
2. Works in the laboratory to identify bacteria causing infection."
3. Helps physicians and hospital personnel to control infections."
4. Is responsible for doing cultures of all infections and drainages."

174. Following a choledocholithotomy a client complains that the skin around the T-tube is raw and excoriated. After assessing the skin the nurse should plan to:
1. Reinforce the dressings when they are wet
2. Cleanse the area with an antiseptic solution
3. Use a skin barrier around the T-tube exit site
4. Change the type of adhesive tape used on the dressing

175. When teaching older adults how to limit the itching that results from dry skin, the nurse should instruct them to:
1. Take hot tub baths
2. Wear warm clothes
3. Utilize a moisturizer
4. Expose skin to the air

176. A client with jaundice complains of severe pruritus. To relieve the discomfort, the nurse would expect the physician to order:
1. Sponge baths with alcohol
2. Applications of talcum powder
3. Baths with sodium bicarbonate solution
4. Applications of baby oil to the involved areas

177. A client with a long history of bilateral varicose veins questions the nurse about the brownish discoloration of the skin of the lower extremities. The nurse should explain that this is probably the result of:
    1. An inadequate arterial blood supply
    2. Delayed healing of tissues after an injury
    3. Leakage of RBCs through the vascular wall
    4. Increased production of melanin in the area

178. A client arrives at the emergency room after being bitten by a stray dog. The bite involved tearing of skin and deep soft tissue injury. The client says the dog was foaming at the mouth and afterward ran away. The first nursing action is to:
    1. Ask the client about horse serum allergy
    2. Notify the police department to capture the dog
    3. Assess the client's injury, vital signs, and past history
    4. Inoculate the client with human rabies immune globulin

179. A client comes to the clinic after being bitten by a raccoon in the woods in an area where rabies is endemic. The nurse recalls that rabies is:
    1. An acute bacterial infection characterized by encephalopathy and opisthotonos
    2. An acute bacterial septicemia that results in convulsions and a morbid fear of water
    3. A nonspecific immunoresponse to organisms deposited under the skin by an animal bite
    4. An acute viral infection, characterized by convulsions and difficult swallowing, that affects the nervous system

180. A client who is to receive radiation therapy for cancer says to the nurse, "My family said I will get a radiation burn." The best response by the nurse would be:
    1. "It will be no worse than a sunburn."
    2. "A localized skin reaction usually occurs."
    3. "Have they had experience with this type of radiation?"
    4. "Daily application of an emollient will prevent the burn."

181. A client is to begin radiation therapy for cancer. When teaching about skin care to the irradiated area, the nurse should instruct the client to:
    1. Apply warm compresses to the site
    2. Apply no lotions or powders to the area
    3. Cover the area with a sterile gauze bandage
    4. Lie on the back and unaffected side when sleeping

182. Irradiation to the chest wall on an outpatient basis is prescribed for a client following removal of a tumor in the right lung. When teaching skin care to the client the nurse should emphasize:
    1. Frequent washing to remove desquamated cells
    2. Massaging 4 times a day to increase circulation
    3. Keeping the skin dry and protected from abrasions
    4. Using skin lotion twice daily to keep the skin supple

183. A client with scleroderma complains of having difficulty chewing and swallowing. When providing dietary counseling, the nurse should advise the client to:
    1. Liquefy food in a blender
    2. Puree all foods before eating
    3. Take frequent sips of water with meals
    4. Use a local anesthetic mouthwash before eating

184. A female client with scleroderma tells the nurse that she frequently has numbness and tingling in her hands followed by blanching of her fingers. The nurse recognizes that the client has Raynaud's phenomenon, a condition frequently associated with scleroderma. The nurse should advise the client to:
    1. Bathe her hands frequently in hot water
    2. Keep her hands warm by wearing gloves
    3. Briskly rub her hands to increase circulation
    4. Take the anticoagulants that will be prescribed to prevent attacks

185. As part of the teaching plan for a client with scleroderma the nurse should include the

need for special skin care. The nurse should plan to advise the client to:
1. Use calamine lotion for pruritus
2. Keep the skin well lubricated with oil
3. Apply warm soaks to the inflamed areas
4. Take frequent baths to remove scaly lesions

186. The physician orders a regimen of daily exercises for a client with scleroderma. The nurse understands that with this client exercises are performed to:
1. Preserve muscle strength
2. Promote tissue regeneration
3. Prevent spread of the disease
4. Promote a sense of well-being

187. When lighting a barbecue with lighter fluid, the individual's shirt bursts into flames. To extinguish the flames most effectively, with as little further damage as possible, it is best to:
1. Remove the burning clothes
2. Slap the flames with the hands
3. Log-roll the person in the grass
4. Pour cold liquid over the flames

188. A person's bathrobe ignites while cooking in the kitchen on a gas stove. Once the flames are extinguished, it is most important to:
1. Give the person sips of water
2. Assess the person's breathing
3. Cover the person with a warm blanket
4. Calculate the extent of the person's burns

189. A person sustains burns of the arms from a barbecue accident in the park. A bystander emerges from the crowd and suggests to a nurse that has come to the person's assistance that butter be applied to the burns. An appropriate response by the nurse would be, "Thanks, but:
1. We'll just wait for the ambulance."
2. It is better to use some first aid cream."
3. I'll just use a tablecloth as a blanket for now."
4. We should apply ice. Could you go get me some?"

190. A worker is involved in an explosion of a steam pipe and receives a scalding burn to the chest and arms. The burned areas are painful, mottled red, weeping, and edematous. These burns would be classified as:
1. Eschar
2. Full-thickness burns
3. Deep partial-thickness burns
4. Superficial partial-thickness burns

191. A client is burned on the anterior part of both legs, from the knees to the feet. Using the rule of nines, the nurse estimates the burn surface to be:
1. 4.5%
2. 9%
3. 18%
4. 27%

192. A client is admitted for treatment of partial- and full-thickness burns of the entire right lower extremity and the anterior portion of the right upper extremity. Performing an immediate appraisal, using the rule of nines, the nurse estimates that the percent of body surface burned is:
1. 4.5%
2. 9%
3. 18%
4. 22.5%

193. When a female client who has partial-thickness burns on her chest, abdomen, and right leg from a fire at her workplace arrives in the emergency room the nurse's first responsibility should be to:
1. Carefully remove all of the client's clothing
2. Evaluate whether heat inhalation had occurred
3. Apply sterile saline dressings on all burned surfaces
4. Determine the extent of the burns, using the rule of nines

194. In the evaluation of the condition of a client with burns of the upper body, an assessment that would indicate potential respiratory obstruction is:
1. Deep breathing
2. Pink tinged, frothy sputum
3. Hoarse quality to the voice
4. Rapid abdominal breathing

195. During the first 48 hours following a thermal injury, the nurse should assess the client for:
     1. Hypokalemia and hyponatremia
     2. Hyperkalemia and hyponatremia
     3. Hypokalemia and hypernatremia
     4. Hyperkalemia and hypernatremia

196. A severely burned client has been hospitalized for 2 days. Until now recovery has been uneventful, but the client begins to exhibit extreme restlessness. The nurse recognizes that this most likely indicates that the client is developing:
     1. Renal failure
     2. Hypervolemia
     3. Cerebral hypoxia
     4. Metabolic acidosis

197. A client's partial-thickness (second degree) burns differ from full-thickness (third degree) burns in that with partial thickness burns the burned area will:
     1. Require grafting before it can heal
     2. Be painful, reddened, and have blisters
     3. Have total destruction of the epidermis and dermis
     4. Take months of extensive treatment before healing occurs

198. A client with burns develops a wound infection. The nurse knows that local wound infections are primarily treated with:
     1. Oral antibiotics
     2. Topical antibiotics
     3. Intravenous antibiotics
     4. Intramuscular antibiotics

199. The method of treatment chosen for a client's burns is the exposure method with application of mafenide (Sulfamylon) bid. When applying this medication the nurse should plan to:
     1. Use medical asepsis
     2. Apply a dry sterile dressing
     3. Monitor liver function studies
     4. Give ordered pain medication

200. A client tells the nurse that the doctor mentioned doing skin grafts after a burn and asks when they will be done. The most appropriate response by the nurse would be:

1. "Within 7 days."
2. "What did your doctor tell you?"
3. "As soon as scar formation occurs."
4. "As soon as signs of infection disappear."

201. A client with a partial-thickness burn complains of chilling. To limit this adaptation, the nurse should:
     1. Limit the occurrence of drafts
     2. Keep room temperature over 90°F
     3. Maintain room humidity below 40%
     4. Place a sterile top sheet over the client

202. A temporary heterograft (pig skin) is used to treat burns because this graft will:
     1. Debride necrotic epithelium
     2. Be sutured in place for better adherence
     3. Relieve pain and promote rapid epithelialization
     4. Frequently be used concurrently with topical antimicrobials

203. When planning care to prevent deformities and contractures in a client with burns, the nurse should expect to begin routine range-of-motion exercises when the client's:
     1. Pain has lessened
     2. Vital signs are stable
     3. Skin grafts are healed
     4. Emotional status stabilizes

204. After a subtotal gastrectomy for cancer of the stomach, the pathology report describes the tumor as "well-differentiated, grade I." After the physician discusses this finding with the client and family, the nurse should:
     1. Provide statistics about the 5-year survival rates for this type cancer
     2. Support a positive outlook, as the tumor cells showed little dysplasia
     3. Teach the client and family how to observe for the development of a primary lesion at another site
     4. Be supportive and assist the client and family to prepare for a rapidly advancing terminal outcome

205. A client returns from surgery with an incisional dressing and a catheter that is attached to a portable wound drainage system exiting from the operative site. The nurse recognizes

that the principle underlying the function of a portable drainage system is:
1. Gravity
2. Osmosis
3. Active transport
4. Negative pressure

206. After surgery for cancer, a client is to receive adjuvant chemotherapy. When teaching the client about the side effects of chemotherapy, the nurse should emphasize that the occurrence of alopecia is:
1. Usually rare
2. Never permanent
3. Frequently prolonged
4. Sometimes preventable

SKELETAL

207. A male college basketball player comes to the infirmary complaining of a "click" in his knee when walking. He states that it occasionally gives way when he is running and sometimes locks. He does not recall any specific injury. The nurse suspects that he may have:
1. Cracked the patella
2. A ruptured Achilles tendon
3. Injured the cartilage in the knee
4. A stress fracture of the tibial plateau

208. A client is scheduled for an arthroscopy of the knee in the morning and asks the nurse about the procedure. The statement by the nurse that best describes the procedure would be:
1. "You will be anesthetized and not remember anything about the procedure."
2. "It is a direct visualization of the joint to diagnose the extent of the knee injury."
3. "It is a radiologic procedure that will help diagnose the extent of the knee injury."
4. "The procedure will determine the type of treatments the physician will prescribe."

209. A client is scheduled for a bone scan to determine the presence of metastases. The nurse is aware that teaching prior to a scheduled bone scan was effective when the client states that:

1. "X-rays will be taken to identify where I may have lost calcium from my bones."
2. "A portion of my bone marrow will be removed and examined for cell composition."
3. "A radioactive chemical will be injected into my vein which will destroy cancer cells present in my bones."
4. "A substance of low radioactivity will be injected into my vein, and my body will be inspected by an instrument to detect where it is deposited."

210. Clients who have casts applied to lower extremities must be monitored for complications. Therefore, the nurse should assess the extremities of these clients for:
1. Warmth
2. Numbness
3. Skin desquamation
4. Generalized discomfort

211. A client's right tibia is fractured in an automobile accident, and a cast is applied. To assess for damage to major blood vessels from the fractured tibia, the nurse should monitor the client for:
1. Swelling of the right thigh
2. An increased blood pressure
3. A decreased dorsalis pedis pulse
4. Increased skin temperature of the foot

212. Three days after a cast is applied to a client's fractured tibia, the client states that there is a burning pain over the ankle. The cast over the ankle feels warm to the touch and the pain is not relieved when the client changes position. The nurse's priority action should be to:
1. Obtain an order for an antibiotic
2. Explain that it is a typical response to a cast
3. Report the client's complaint to the physician
4. Administer the prescribed medication for pain relief

213. After a long leg cast is removed, the client should be instructed to:
    1. Report any discomfort or stiffness of the ankle
    2. Cleanse the leg by scrubbing with a brisk motion
    3. Elevate the leg when sitting for longer periods of time
    4. Put the entire leg through a full range of motion once daily

214. The nurse performs full range of motion on a client's extremities. When putting an ankle through range of motion the nurse must perform:
    1. Flexion, extension, left and right rotation
    2. Abduction, flexion, adduction, and extension
    3. Pronation, supination, rotation, and extension
    4. Dorsiflexion, plantar flexion, eversion, and inversion

215. The physician orders nonweight bearing with crutches for a client with a leg injury. The nurse understands that, before ambulation is begun, the most important activity to facilitate walking with crutches is:
    1. Sitting up in a chair to help strengthen back muscles
    2. Keeping the unaffected leg in extension and abduction
    3. Exercising the triceps, finger flexors, and elbow extensors
    4. Using the trapeze frequently to strengthen the biceps muscles

216. The nurse would recognize that the demonstration of crutch walking with a tripod gait was understood when the client places weight on the:
    1. Axillary regions
    2. Palms of the hands
    3. Feet which are set wide apart
    4. Palms of the hands and axillary regions

217. An x-ray film of a client's arm reveals a comminuted fracture of the left radial bone. The nurse understands that with a comminuted fracture:

    1. There is a break in the skin and the bone is protruding
    2. Splintering has occurred on one side and bending on the other
    3. The bone has broken into several fragments, but the skin is intact
    4. The bone is broken into two parts, and the skin may or may not be broken

218. A client with osteomyelitis of the leg is to have a debridement of the infected bone. When planning for postoperative care the nurse knows that:
    1. Frequent range-of-motion exercises will be needed
    2. Septicemia is a common postoperative complication
    3. The client's leg will be immobilized in a cast or a splint
    4. The client will be allowed out of bed after the first postoperative day

219. A client has painful swelling of multiple joints and a tentative diagnosis of rheumatoid arthritis is made. During a subsequent visit the client tells the nurse, "I'm so confused. The doctor said I probably have arthritis, but my lab tests were negative. I don't see how that can be when I'm always so uncomfortable." The nurse's best response would be:
    1. "It might help if you try not to think about your discomfort."
    2. "Don't let that upset you; eventually the tests will turn positive."
    3. "Laboratory tests are often negative in the early stages of arthritis."
    4. "Did the doctor say that the laboratory tests were going to be repeated?"

220. A client with rheumatoid arthritis asks the nurse about ways to decrease morning stiffness. The nurse should suggest:
    1. Wearing loose but warm clothing
    2. Avoiding excessive physical stress and fatigue
    3. Taking a hot tub bath or shower in the morning
    4. Planning a rest break periodically for about 15 minutes

221. A client is admitted to the hospital for an acute episode of rheumatoid arthritis. During the initial assessment the nurse observes that the client's finger joints are swollen. The nurse understands that this swelling is most likely related to:
1. Urate crystals in the synovial tissue
2. Inflammation in the joint's synovial lining
3. Formation of bony spurs on the joint surfaces
4. Escaped fluid from the capillaries, increasing interstitial fluids

222. As an acute episode of rheumatoid arthritis subsides, active and passive range-of-motion exercises are ordered for the client. The nurse should avoid applying direct pressure to the client's joints because this may precipitate:
1. Pain
2. Swelling
3. Nodule formation
4. Tophaceous deposits

223. The physician orders bedrest for a client with acute arthritis who has bilateral, painful, swollen knee and wrist joints. To prevent flexion deformities during the acute phase, the client's positioning schedule should include placement in the:
1. Sims' position
2. Prone position
3. Contour position
4. Trendelenburg position

224. A client with acute rheumatoid arthritis improves and the physician changes the order for bedrest to out of bed as tolerated. This client should be assisted out of bed to a:
1. Low soft lounge chair
2. Straight-back arm chair
3. Wheelchair with foot rests
4. Recliner chair with both legs elevated

225. After a painful exacerbation of rheumatoid arthritis, a client is to begin a walking and exercise program. An appropriate outcome would be that the client:

1. Avoids exercising when there is some discomfort
2. Is pain free while engaging in the activity program
3. Walks and exercises even when the pain is severe
4. Exercises unless the discomfort becomes too great

226. A client with lower back pain is tentatively diagnosed as having a herniated intervertebral disc. When assessing this client's back pain, the nurse should ask:
1. "Is there any tenderness in the calf of your leg?"
2. "Have you had any burning sensation on urination?"
3. "Do you have any increase in pain during bowel movements?"
4. "Does the pain begin in your flank and move around to the groin?"

227. A client, who is diagnosed as having a herniated intervertebral disc, complains of pain. The nurse recognizes that the pain is caused by the:
1. Inflammation of the lamina of the involved vertebrae
2. Shifting of two adjacent vertebral bodies out of proper alignment
3. Compression of the spinal cord by the extruded nucleus pulposus
4. Increased pressure of cerebrospinal fluid within the vertebral column

228. A client is awaiting surgery for a ruptured lumbar nucleus pulposus. The nurse's teaching should include that the pain will most likely increase if the client:
1. Lies on the side
2. Flexes the knees
3. Coughs excessively
4. Sits for long periods

229. A male client who develops degenerative joint disease of the vertebral column is taught to turn himself from his back to his side keeping his spine straight. The least effort will be exerted if he does this by crossing his arm over his chest and:
    1. Pulling himself to one side by using his night table
    2. Bending his top knee to the side to which he is turning
    3. Crossing his ankles and turning with both his legs straight
    4. Flexing his bottom knee to the side to which he wishes to turn

230. A client is scheduled for a laminectomy. Preoperatively the nurse should demonstrate the:
    1. Use of a trapeze
    2. Contour position
    3. Traction apparatus
    4. Log-rolling technique

231. Following a laminectomy, the nurse should monitor the client's vital signs and:
    1. Logroll the client to the prone position
    2. Check circulation and sensation of the feet
    3. Observe bowel movements and voiding patterns
    4. Encourage the client to drink a moderate amount of fluid

232. When two nurses are getting a client out of bed for the first time following a laminectomy, the client complains of feeling faint and light-headed. The nurses should have this client:
    1. Slide slowly to the floor, to prevent a fall and injury
    2. Sit on the edge of the bed and hold the client upright
    3. Bend forward, because it will increase the blood flow to the brain
    4. Lie down immediately, so they can take the client's blood pressure

233. When preparing a client for discharge after a laminectomy, the nurse would know that further health teaching is necessary when the client says, "I should:

    1. Sleep on a firm mattress to support my back."
    2. Spend most of the day sitting in a straight-back chair."
    3. Avoid lifting heavy objects until the doctor tells me that I can."
    4. Put a pillow under my knees when sleeping in bed on my back."

234. A back brace is prescribed for a client who has had a laminectomy. The nurse should include in the teaching plan instructions to:
    1. Use the brace when the back feels tired
    2. Apply the brace before getting out of bed
    3. Put the brace on while in the sitting position
    4. Wear the brace when performing twisting exercises

235. After an amputation of a limb a client begins to experience extreme discomfort in the area where the limb once was. An appropriate nursing diagnosis at this time would be:
    1. Ineffective coping
    2. Pain related to amputation
    3. Sensory-perceptual alteration
    4. Hopelessness related to altered life-style

236. After an amputation the client's stump is snugly bandaged throughout the postoperative period. The main purpose for this is to:
    1. Promote stump shrinkage
    2. Prevent injury to the stump
    3. Prevent suture line infection
    4. Promote drainage of secretions

237. A client with an above-the-knee amputation asks why the stump needs to be wrapped with an elastic bandage. The nurse explains that it:
    1. Decreases phantom-limb pain
    2. Limits the formation of blood clots
    3. Prevents hemorrhage and covers the incision
    4. Supports the soft tissue and minimizes edema

238. A client has an above-the-knee amputation because of a gangrenous leg ulcer. After the second postoperative day, to prevent deformities the nurse should:

1. Keep the client's stump elevated on a pillow
2. Place an abduction pillow between the client's legs
3. Encourage the client to lie in the supine or prone position
4. Teach the client to press the stump against a hard surface frequently

239. The nurse should teach a client with an above-the-knee amputation a variety of postoperative activities. The activity designed to aid in the use of crutches is:
1. Stump care
2. Weight lifting
3. Changing bed position
4. Phantom-limb exercise

240. A client requires a below-the-knee amputation. A major advantage of an immediate postoperative prosthesis is that it:
1. Decreases phantom limb sensations
2. Encourages a normal walking pattern
3. Reduces the incidence of wound infection
4. Allows for the fitting of the prosthesis before discharge

241. When assessing a client using a prosthesis following an above-the-knee amputation, the finding that indicates that the prosthesis fits correctly is:
1. Shrinking of the stump
2. Absence of phantom pain
3. Darkened skin areas on the stump
4. Uneven wearing down of the heels

242. At the scene of an accident, the nurse can minimize the immediate life-threatening systemic complication of injury to the long bones of the injured person by:
1. Elevating the affected limb
2. Handling and transporting gently
3. Maintaining functional alignment
4. Encouraging deep breathing and coughing

243. An elderly client is hospitalized after falling and fracturing a hip. The physician applies Buck's traction until surgery can be performed to replace the head of the femur with a prosthesis. When checking the client's Buck's traction, the nurse should be aware that:

1. The spreader bar should fit snugly around the foot
2. Weights greater than eight pounds will cause skin damage
3. The moleskin is placed on the anterior and posterior aspects of the leg
4. Tape must cover the malleoli to adequately secure the weights to the leg

244. After a client with multiple fractures of the left femur is admitted to the hospital for surgery, the client demonstrates cyanosis, tachycardia, dyspnea, and restlessness. Initially the nurse should:
1. Administer oxygen by mask (has fat embulle)
2. Immediately call the physician
3. Place the client in the supine position
4. Place the client in the high Fowler's position

245. After surgery for a fractured hip a client complains of pain. The nurse should:
1. Notify the physician
2. Use distraction techniques
3. Medicate the client as ordered
4. Perform a complete pain assessment

246. A client has an open reduction and internal fixation of a fractured hip. To prevent the most common complication following this type of surgery, the nurse should expect the physician's order to state:
1. Turn from side to side q2h
2. Apply sequential compression stockings
3. Encourage isometric exercises to the extremities
4. Perform passive range of motion to the affected extremity

247. A client is admitted to the hospital for a total hip replacement. The nurse's preoperative teaching plan for the early postoperative period should include instructions related to:
1. Abduction of the operative hip
2. Adduction of the operative hip
3. Turning 45 degrees onto the operative side
4. Hip flexion of 90 degrees on the operative side

248. When assisting a client who has had a total hip replacement onto the bedpan on the first postoperative day, the nurse should instruct the client to:
1. Turn toward the operative side
2. Flex both knees and slowly lift the pelvis
3. Extend both legs and pull on the trapeze to lift the pelvis
4. Flex the unoperative knee and pull on the trapeze to lift the pelvis

249. A client with a distal femoral shaft fracture is at risk for developing a fat embolism. A distinguishing sign that is unique to a fat embolism is:
1. Oliguria
2. Dyspnea
3. Petechiae
4. Confusion

250. Twelve days after a left total hip replacement a client is permitted to sit for short periods. After assisting the client out of bed the nurse should place the client in a:
1. Soft armchair with left leg straight out in front
2. Firm armchair with left leg elevated on a stool
3. Firm chair with left foot flat on the floor's surface
4. Soft chair with enough pillows to keep the hip at a right angle

251. Four weeks following a total hip replacement, a client asks when daily walks can be resumed. The nurse bases the answer on the knowledge that after surgery:
1. Full-weight bearing is usually permitted after 6 weeks
2. Full-weight bearing is usually restored after 4 months
3. Partial weight-bearing restrictions will be enforced for at least 12 weeks
4. Partial weight-bearing and positional restrictions will be in effect for 2 months

NEUROMUSCULAR

252. When assessing trigeminal nerve function the nurse should evaluate:

1. Corneal sensation
2. Smiling and frowning
3. Ocular muscle movement
4. Shrugging of the shoulders

253. When assessing a client's vagal nerve (cranial nerve X) function, the nurse will need:
1. A tuning fork
2. Tongue depressors
3. An ophthalmoscope
4. Cotton and a safety pin

254. The nurse is caring for a client who is about to have a lumbar puncture. Planned care following the procedure should include:
1. Having the client lie in the supine position for 6 to 12 hours
2. Encouraging the client to ambulate every hour for 6 to 8 hours
3. Maintaining the client in the Trendelenburg position for 4 hours
4. Placing the client in high Fowler's position immediately after the procedure

255. A client with pain and paresis of the left leg is scheduled for an electromyography. Before the test, the nurse should explain that:
1. The involved area will be shaved immediately before testing
2. The client's heart rate and rhythm will be frequently monitored
3. Needles will be inserted into the affected muscles during the test
4. The client will be kept in a recumbent position after the procedure

256. The nurse recognizes that the most specific diagnostic test that the physician can perform for a client who is suspected of having myasthenia gravis is:
1. An electromyography (EMG)
2. The pyridostigmine (Mestinon) test
3. The edrophonium chloride (Tensilon) test
4. A thorough history and physical assessment

257. When assessing a client with myasthenia gravis, the nurse would expect the client to demonstrate:

1. Partial improvement of muscle strength with mild exercise
2. Fluctuating weakness of muscles innervated by the cranial nerves
3. Little or no change in muscle strength regardless of therapy initiated
4. Dramatic worsening in muscle strength with anticholinesterase drugs

258. A young female client comes to the physician because she has been experiencing fatigue and double vision. The physician suspects myasthenia gravis. When obtaining information from the client, the nurse would expect her to report that:
1. Her level of fatigue has been constant
2. The longer she rests the weaker she feels
3. Her strength increases with progressive activity
4. The symptoms seem more severe in the evening

259. When talking with a client who has been diagnosed as having myasthenia gravis, the nurse observes that the client has:
1. Problems with cognition
2. Difficulty swallowing saliva
3. Intention tremors of the hands
4. Non-intention tremors of the extremities

260. The priority nursing diagnosis for a client who is in myasthenic crisis would be:
1. Activity intolerance
2. Impaired physical mobility
3. Ineffective breathing pattern
4. Sensory-perceptual alteration: visual

261. The basis of the nursing care plan for a client with myasthenia gravis is the fact that:
1. Muscle weakness decreases with hot baths
2. Muscle weakness decreases with muscle use
3. Muscle strength improves immediately after meals
4. Muscle strength decreases with repeated muscle use

262. When assisting a client who has myasthenia gravis with a bath, the nurse notices that the client's arms become weaker with sustained movement. The nurse should:

1. Continue the bath while supporting the client's arms
2. Encourage the client to rest for short periods of time
3. Gradually increase the client's activity level each day
4. Administer an additional dose of Mestinon to the client

263. A client with myasthenia gravis improves and is discharged from the hospital. The discharge medications include Mestinon 10 mg every 6 hours. The nurse would know that the drug regimen was understood when the client says, "I should:
1. Take milk with each dose of Mestinon."
2. Take the Mestinon on an empty stomach."
3. Set my alarm clock to take my medication."
4. Take my pulse and respirations before taking the drug."

264. A client with myasthenia gravis comes to the neurology clinic for a routine visit. During an assessment the nurse should expect the client will have:
1. Tremors of the hands when attempting to lift objects
2. Partial improvement of muscle strength with mild exercise
3. Fluctuating weakness of muscles innervated by the cranial nerves
4. Involvement of the distal muscles rather than the proximal muscles

265. During a routine clinic visit of a female client who has myasthenia gravis the nurse reinforces previous teaching about the disease and self-care. The nurse would evaluate that the teaching was effective when the client recognizes that she should:
1. Plan activities for later in the day
2. Avoid people with respiratory infections
3. Eat meals in a semi-recumbent position
4. Take muscle relaxants when she is under stress

266. A client is scheduled to have a series of diagnostic studies for myasthenia gravis, including a Tensilon test. The nurse should explain to the client that the diagnosis of myasthenia gravis will be confirmed if the administration of Tensilon produces a:
1. Brief exaggeration of symptoms
2. Prolonged symptomatic improvement
3. Rapid but brief symptomatic improvement
4. Symptomatic improvement of just the ptosis

267. The physician has ordered a diagnostic work-up for a client who may have myasthenia gravis. The initial nursing goal for the client during the diagnostic phase would be that, "The client will:
1. Adhere to a teaching plan."
2. Achieve psychologic adjustment."
3. Maintain present muscle strength."
4. Prepare for the appearance of myasthenic crisis."

268. The most significant initial nursing assessment associated with myasthenia gravis includes the client's:
1. Ability to chew and speak distinctly
2. Degree of anxiety about the diagnosis
3. Ability to smile and to close the eyelids
4. Respiratory exchange and ability to swallow

269. A client with myasthenia gravis begins to experience increased difficulty in swallowing. To prevent aspiration of food, the most effective nursing action would be to:
1. Change the client's diet order from soft to clear liquid
2. Place an emergency tracheostomy set in the client's room
3. Assess the client's respiratory status before and after meals
4. Coordinate the client's meal schedule with the peak effect of Mestinon

270. A female client with myasthenia gravis is concerned about her fluctuating physical condition and generalized weakness. When planning for this client's care it would be most important to:

1. Have a family member stay with her
2. Space her activities throughout the day
3. Restrict her activities and encourage bed rest
4. Teach her the limitations imposed by her disease

271. A client with myasthenia gravis is scheduled for a thymectomy. When preparing the client for surgery, the nurse should emphasize:
1. A detailed explanation of the procedure
2. The experimental nature of this procedure in myasthenia gravis
3. The difficulty of predicting the degree of improvement after the operation
4. An explanation of the usual postoperative complications of a thymectomy

272. The nurse notes that a client exhibits the characteristic gait associated with Parkinson's disease. When recording on the client's chart, the nurse should describe this gait as:
1. Ataxic
2. Spastic
3. Shuffling
4. Scissoring

273. While performing the history and physical examination of a client with Parkinson's disease, the nurse should assess the client for:
1. Frequent bouts of diarrhea
2. Hyperextension of the neck
3. A low-pitched, monotonous voice
4. A recent increase in appetite and weight gain

274. When assessing a client with Parkinson's disease, a common adaptation the nurse would expect to find is:
1. Leaning toward the affected side
2. Blank facies or lack of expression
3. Tremors of the hand on movement
4. Hyperextension of the affected extremity

275. The nurse might expect a client with multiple sclerosis to complain about the most common initial symptom which is:
1. Diarrhea
2. Headaches
3. Skin infections
4. Visual disturbances

276. A client with multiple sclerosis is informed that it is a chronic progressive neurologic condition. The client asks the nurse, "Will I experience pain?" The nurse's best response would be:
1. "Tell me about your fears regarding pain."
2. "Analgesics will be ordered to control the pain."
3. "Let's make a list of the things you need to ask your doctor."
4. "Pain is not a characteristic symptom of this disease process."

277. A client asks for an explanation about glaucoma. The nurse explains that with glaucoma there is:
1. An increase in the pressure within the eyeball
2. An opacity of the crystalline lens or its capsule
3. A curvature of the cornea that becomes unequal
4. A separation of the neural retina from the pigment retina

278. When obtaining the nursing history from a client who has open-angle (chronic) glaucoma, a complaint that the nurse should expect is:
1. Flashes of light
2. Intolerance to light
3. Seeing floating specks
4. Loss of peripheral vision

279. A client who has open-angle (chronic) glaucoma is scheduled for eye surgery to promote aqueous humor outflow. The nurse would evaluate that the client understands the preoperative teaching about the first 24 hours after surgery when the client states, "I should:
1. Cough and deep breathe."
2. Lie on my unaffected side."
3. Move around freely in bed."
4. Elevate the head of my bed."

280. Preoperative teaching for a client who is to have an extracapsular cataract extraction with an intraocular lens implant should include the importance of:
1. Remaining in bed for 48 hours
2. Breathing and coughing deeply
3. Avoiding bending from the waist
4. Lying in supine position for 12 hours

281. A client has an extracapsular cataract extraction with an intraocular lens implant. Postoperatively the nurse should provide for the client's safety by:
1. Putting the side rails up when the client is in bed
2. Darkening the room by closing the window shades
3. Applying a vest restraint until the dressing is removed
4. Immobilizing the head by placing a sandbag on each side

282. After cataract surgery a client complains of feeling nauseated. The nurse should:
1. Give the client some dry crackers to eat
2. Administer the antiemetic drug as ordered
3. Explain that this is expected following surgery
4. Instruct the client to deep breathe until the nausea subsides

283. A client is being prepared for discharge from an ambulatory surgical unit following a cataract removal with an intraocular lens implant. The statement by the client that suggests to the nurse that discharge teaching was effective is:
1. "I'm driving home since I feel so good."
2. "I can't wait until I get home to wash my hair."
3. "I can expect to see bright flashes of light for awhile."
4. "I'll call the surgeon if the analgesic doesn't relieve the pain."

284. After cataract surgery, a client is taught how to self-administer eyedrops before discharge. The nurse approves the technique when the client:
1. Holds the dropper tip above the eye
2. Places the drops on the cornea of the eye
3. Raises the upper eyelid with gentle traction
4. Squeezes the eye shut after instilling the eye drops

285. After an automobile accident, a client complains of seeing frequent flashes of light. The nurse should suspect:
1. Scleroderma
2. Acute glaucoma
3. A detached retina
4. A cerebral concussion

286. A client with a detached retina is scheduled for surgery to reattach the retina. The nurse explains that the procedure employed involves the use of:
1. Radiation
2. Burr holes
3. Dermabrasion
4. Lasar technique

287. A construction worker fell off the roof of a 2 story building and is brought to the hospital unconscious. The nurse would be most concerned if assessment reveals:
1. Reactive pupils
2. A depressed fontanel
3. Bleeding from the ears
4. An elevated temperature

288. Following an anterior fossa craniotomy a client is placed on controlled mechanical ventilation. To ensure adequate cerebral blood flow the nurse should:
1. Clear the ear of draining fluid
2. Monitor the serum carbon dioxide
3. Discontinue anticonvulsant therapy
4. Elevate the head of the bed 30 degrees

289. A client has a supratentorial craniotomy for a tumor in the right frontal lobe of the cerebral cortex. Postoperatively the position that would be most appropriate for this client would be:
1. High Fowler's with knee gatch raised
2. Flat with a small pillow under the nape of the neck
3. Head of the bed elevated 20 degrees with the head turned to the operative side
4. Head of the bed elevated 45 degrees with a large pillow under the head and shoulders

290. A client undergoes a supratentorial craniotomy with burr holes after sustaining a head injury in an automobile accident. Because of

the presence of burr holes, the client is at risk for developing an infection. An early clinical manifestation of meningeal irritation is:
1. Sunset eyes
2. Kernig's sign
3. Homan's sign
4. The plantar reflex

291. After a three month rehabilitation period following a craniotomy a female client is still having some motor speech difficulty. To promote the client's use of speech the nurse should:
1. Correct her mistakes immediately
2. Respond to her crude efforts of speaking
3. Reexplain why she is having difficulty speaking
4. Speak to her in simple words and short sentences

292. A client with a history of hypertension is admitted with aphasia. A bruit is heard over the left carotid artery and the pulse is irregular. The nurse is aware that complete occlusion of the branches of the middle cerebral artery resulting in aphasia may occur because of:
1. A history of hypertensive disease
2. Emboli associated with atrial fibrillation
3. Developmental defects of the arterial wall
4. Inappropriate paroxysmal neural discharge

293. A client has a history of progressive carotid and cerebral atherosclerosis and transient ischemic attacks (TIAs). The nurse understands that TIAs are:
1. Temporary episodes of neurologic dysfunction
2. Periods of alternating exacerbations and remissions
3. Transient attacks caused by multiple small emboli
4. Ischemic attacks that result in progressive neurologic deterioration

294. A client has carotid atherosclerotic plaques and a right carotid endarterectomy is performed. Two hours after surgery, the client demonstrates progressive hypotension. The nurse should:

1. Increase the IV flow rate
2. Raise the head of the bed
3. Notify the physician immediately
4. Position the client in slight Trendelenburg

295. After a carotid endarterectomy, the client should be monitored for the complication of cranial nerve dysfunction. To monitor for this complication, the nurse should assess the client for:
1. Labored breathing
2. Edema of the neck
3. Difficulty in swallowing
4. Alteration in blood pressure

296. A client is admitted to the hospital with weakness in the right extremities and a slight speech problem. Vital signs are normal. During the first 24 hours the nurse should give priority to:
1. Checking the client's temperature
2. Evaluating the client's motor status
3. Monitoring the client's blood pressure
4. Obtaining a urine specimen from the client

297. On the evening before discharge from the hospital, a client has a hypertensive crisis and has a cerebral vascular accident. Initially, the nurse should place the client in a:
1. Supine position
2. Contour position
3. Side-lying position
4. Slight Trendelenburg position

298. Initially, after a cerebral vascular accident, a clients' pupils are equal and reactive to light. Later the nurse assesses that the right pupil is reacting more slowly than the left and the systolic blood pressure is beginning to rise. The nurse recognizes that these adaptations are suggestive of:
1. Spinal shock
2. Hypovolemic shock
3. Transtentorial herniation
4. Increasing intracranial pressure

299. A client who has had a cerebrovascular accident is admitted to the hospital with right-sided hemiplegia. It is important for the nurse to consider any restrictions of mobility or neuromuscular abnormalities that are observed because:
1. Disuse hypertrophy of the muscles will eventually result
2. Shortening and eventual fibrosis of the muscles will occur
3. Rigid extension can occur making therapy painful and difficult
4. Decreased movement on the affected side predisposes to infection

300. A female client manifests a right hemianopsia as a result of a cerebrovascular accident. The nurse should:
1. Correct the client's misuse of equipment
2. Instruct the client to scan her surroundings
3. Provide tactile stimulation to the client's affected extremities
4. Teach the client to look at the position of her right extremities

301. The wife of a client who has had a cerebrovascular accident tells the home-health nurse that her husband cries easily and without provocation. She asks why he is so emotionally labile. The nurse should explain that:
1. Her husband can remember only depressing events from the past
2. This is a way of getting attention and the behavior should be ignored
3. Her husband feels guilty about the demands he is making on his family
4. This behavior is a common response over which he has very little control

302. The husband of a client with aphasia as a result of a cerebrovascular accident asks if his wife's speech will ever return. The nurse should respond:
1. "You will have to ask your doctor."
2. "It should return to normal in 2 or 3 months."
3. "It is hard to say how much improvement will occur."
4. "This will probably be the extent of her speech from now on."

303. When assisting the family to help an aphasic member to regain as much speech as possible, the nurse should instruct them primarily to:
    1. Speak louder than usual to the client during visits
    2. Tell the client to use the correct words when speaking
    3. Give positive reinforcement for correct communication
    4. Encourage the client to speak while being patient with all attempts

304. A client, employed as a carpenter, has trouble holding tools because of carpal tunnel syndrome. Because the client continues to work, the nursing diagnosis of most concern would be:
    1. Pain
    2. Anxiety
    3. High risk for injury
    4. Self esteem disturbance

305. A client has a seizure. The first intervention by the nurse during the tonic-clonic phase of the seizure should be to:
    1. Call the client's physician
    2. Protect the client's head from injury
    3. Note the condition of the client's pupils
    4. Check the client's pulse and respirations

306. A client sustains a vertebral fracture at the T1 level as a result of diving into shallow water. On admission to the emergency room a detailed neurological assessment is performed. The nurse should expect to find:
    1. Inability to move the lower arm
    2. Normal biceps reflexes in the arm
    3. Loss of pain sensation in the hands
    4. Difficulty breathing and a flaccid diaphragm

307. The nurse is aware that autonomic dysreflexia is a complication associated with some spinal cord injuries. The nurse plans to observe for signs of this problem in a client who sustained a spinal cord injury at the T2 level because:
    1. The injury has resulted in loss of all reflexes
    2. The injury is above the sixth thoracic vertebra

    3. There has been a partial transection of the cord
    4. There is a flaccid paralysis of the lower extremities

308. The nurse is aware that a client with a spinal cord injury is developing autonomic dysreflexia when the client has:
    1. Flaccid paralysis and numbness
    2. Absence of sweating and pyrexia
    3. Escalating tachycardia and shock
    4. Paroxysmal hypertension and bradycardia

309. During the first week after a spinal cord injury at the T3 level, a male client and the nurse identify a short-term goal. An appropriate short-term goal for this client would be, The client will:
    1. Understand his limitations
    2. Consider alternate life-styles
    3. Perform independent ambulation
    4. Carry out personal hygiene activities

310. A client, who is recuperating from a spinal cord injury at the T4 level, wants to use a wheelchair. In preparation for this activity the client should be taught:
    1. Leg lifts to prevent hip contractures
    2. Push ups to strengthen arm muscles
    3. Balancing exercises to promote equilibrium
    4. Quadriceps-setting exercises to maintain muscle tone

ENDOCRINE

311. When obtaining a health history from a client recently diagnosed with non-insulin dependent diabetes mellitus (NIDDM) the nurse should expect the client to mention symptoms associated with the classic signs of diabetes mellitus such as:
    1. Polydipsia, polyuria, irritability
    2. Polyphagia, confusion, polyuria
    3. Polydipsia, polyphagia, polyuria
    4. Polydipsia, nocturia, weight loss

312. When assessing the laboratory values of a client with non-insulin dependent diabetes mellitus (NIDDM), the nurse should expect the results to reveal:

1. Ketones in the blood but not the urine
2. Glucose in the urine but not in the blood
3. Urine negative for ketones and 4⁺ for glucose
4. Urine and blood positive for both glucose and ketones

313. The nurse should explain to a client with diabetes mellitus that self blood glucose monitoring is preferred to urine glucose testing because it is:
1. More accurate
2. Easier to perform
3. Done by the client
4. Not influenced by drugs

314. A client is diagnosed as having non-insulin dependent diabetes mellitus (NIDDM). The priority teaching goal would be, The client will be able to:
1. Perform foot care
2. Administer insulin
3. Test urine for sugar and acetone
4. Identify hypoglycemia and hyperglycemia

315. The nurse teaches a client with non-insulin dependent diabetes mellitus (NIDDM) how to provide self care to prevent infections of the feet. The nurse recognizes that the teaching was effective when the client says, "I should:
1. Massage my feet and legs with oil or lotion."
2. Apply heat intermittently to my feet and legs."
3. Eat foods high in kilocalories of protein and carbohydrates."
4. Control my diabetes through diet, exercise, and medication."

316. A client with non-insulin dependent diabetes mellitus (NIDDM) is taking one glyburide (Micronase) tablet daily. The client asks if an extra pill should be taken before exercise. The nurse should reply:
1. "You will need to decrease your exercise."
2. "An extra pill will help your body use glucose correctly."
3. "Your diet and medicine will not be affected by exercise."
4. "No, but observe for signs of hypoglycemia while exercising."

317. A client who is taking an oral hypoglycemic daily for non-insulin dependent diabetes mellitus (NIDDM) develops the flu and is concerned about the need for special care. The nurse should advise the client to:
1. Skip the oral hypoglycemic pill, drink plenty of fluids, and stay in bed
2. Avoid food, drink clear liquids, take a daily temperature, and stay in bed
3. Eat as much as possible, increase fluid intake, and call the office again the next day
4. Take the oral hypoglycemic pill, drink warm fluids, and perform a fingerstick for glucose ac and hs

318. A client with non-insulin dependent diabetes mellitus (NIDDM) asks about the use of alcohol or special "dietetic" food in the diet. The client should be taught that:
1. Alcohol can be used with its calories accounted for in the diet
2. Unlimited amounts of sugar substitutes can be used as desired
3. Alcohol should not be used in cooking because it adds too many calories
4. Special "dietetic" foods are needed because many regular foods cannot be used

319. A client with non-insulin dependent diabetes mellitus (NIDDM) travels frequently and asks how to plan meals during trips. The nurse's most appropriate response would be:
1. "You can order diabetic foods on most airlines and in restaurants."
2. "You should plan your food ahead and carry it with you from home."
3. "Make regular food choices, wherever you are, following your food plan."
4. "You can monitor your blood sugar level frequently and can eat accordingly."

320. A client with newly diagnosed diabetes mellitus indicates a hatred for asparagus, broccoli, and mushrooms. When reviewing the exchange list with the client, the nurse would know that the teaching about the exchange list was understood when the client states, "Instead of these foods I can eat:
1. String beans, beets, or carrots."
2. Corn, lima beans, or dried peas."
3. Corn muffin, corn chips, or pretzels."
4. Baked beans, potatoes, or parsnips."

321. While hospitalized a client with diabetes mellitus is observed picking at callouses on the feet. The nurse should immediately:
1. Warn the client of the danger of infection
2. Suggest that the client wear white cotton socks
3. Check the client's shoes for proper fit in the area of the callouses
4. Demonstrate and teach the importance of proper foot care to the client

322. Four hours after surgery, the blood glucose level of a client, who has insulin dependent diabetes mellitus (Type I), is elevated. The nurse should expect to:
1. Administer an oral hypoglycemic
2. Institute urine glucose monitoring
3. Give supplemental doses of regular insulin
4. Decrease the rate of the intravenous infusion

323. A client who has insulin dependent diabetes mellitus is admitted for major surgery. Prior to surgery the client's insulin requirements are elevated but well controlled. Postoperatively the nurse would anticipate that the client's insulin requirements will:
1. Fluctuate widely
2. Increase sharply
3. Remain elevated
4. Decrease immediately

324. A client is admitted to the hospital with diabetic ketoacidosis. The nurse understands that the elevated ketone level present with this disorder is caused by the incomplete oxidation of:
1. Fats
2. Protein

3. Potassium
4. Carbohydrates

325. The serum potassium level of a client who has diabetic ketoacidosis is 5.4 mEq/L. When monitoring the ECG tracing, the nurse would expect to observe:
1. Abnormal P waves and depressed T waves
2. Peaked T waves and widened QRS complexes
3. Abnormal Q waves and prolonged ST segments
4. Peaked P waves and increased number of T waves

326. A client with insulin dependent diabetes is placed on an insulin pump. The most appropriate short-term goal in teaching this client to control the diabetes is "The client will:
1. Adhere to the medical regimen."
2. Remain normoglycemic for 3 weeks."
3. Demonstrate the correct use of the insulin pump."
4. List 3 self-care activities necessary to control the diabetes."

327. When the nurse plans to teach a client with insulin dependent diabetes mellitus (IDDM) about the use of an insulin pump, it is of major importance that the client understand:
1. That the needle needs to be changed every 24 hours
2. That glucose monitoring will only be necessary once daily
3. That the pump is an attempt to mimic the way a healthy pancreas works
4. That the pump will be implanted in a subcutaneous pocket near the abdomen

328. For proper foot care, the nurse should provide a client with non-insulin dependent diabetes mellitus with instructions to:
1. Remove all corns and stop smoking
2. Always wear shoes and use natural fiber socks
3. Wear nylon socks and wash feet in warm water
4. Wear shoes that are slightly larger and avoid using corn removers

329. Besides the individual who has insulin dependent diabetes mellitus, the nurse is aware that acute hypoglycemia can also develop in the client who is diagnosed with:
1. Liver disease
2. Hypertension
3. Type II diabetes
4. Hyperthyroidism

330. A client with insulin dependent diabetes mellitus of long duration takes Humulin N and Humulin R insulin every morning. At noon, before eating lunch, the client is admitted to the emergency room with an acute myocardial infarction. Two hours later, the client's serum glucose drops to 30 mg/dl and insulin shock is diagnosed. The nurse understands the reason for the development of acute hypoglycemia in this client is that:
1. The stress brought on by the chest pain increases the use of glucose available to the client
2. Glycogenolysis was accelerated when the client failed to eat lunch after taking Humulin N insulin
3. Glucose levels that are controlled by insulin drop more quickly than those controlled by oral antidiabetics
4. The client's body became sensitive to the prescribed dose of insulin after long use, and the blood glucose dropped erratically

331. A client with insulin dependent diabetes mellitus of several years duration takes 40 U of NPH and 20 U of regular insulin each AM. The client's serum glucose level averages about 130 mg/dl. When the client complains of symptoms of hypoglycemia, the nurse should suspect that the client's serum glucose is:
1. About 100 mg/dl
2. Between 50 and 70 mg/dl
3. Between 100 and 120 mg/dl
4. At least 20 mg/dl below the norm

332. When assessing a client who is experiencing hypoglycemia, the nurse should expect to find:
1. Lethargy
2. Tachycardia

3. Warm, dry skin
4. Increased respirations

333. A client with diabetic ketoacidosis who is receiving intravenous fluids and insulin complains of tingling and numbness of the fingers and toes and shortness of breath. The cardiac monitor shows the appearance of a U wave. The nurse should recognize that these symptoms indicate:
1. Hypokalemia
2. Hyponatremia
3. Hypoglycemia
4. Hypercalcemia

334. The nurse recognizes that a client with diabetes mellitus understands the teaching about the treatment of hypoglycemia when the client says, "If I become hypoglycemic I should initially eat:
1. Hard candy and fruit juice."
2. A slice of bread and sugar."
3. Chocolate candy and a banana."
4. Peanut butter crackers and a glass of milk."

335. A client with hypertension is scheduled for a medical workup including a scan for an aldosteronoma. The nurse recognizes that this scan is ordered to rule out disease of the:
1. Thyroid
2. Kidneys
3. Pituitary
4. Adrenals

336. A client who is scheduled to have surgery to remove an aldosterone-secreting adenoma wonders what will happen if the surgery is refused. The nurse would base a response on the fact that:
1. The tumor must be removed to prevent heart and kidney damage
2. Surgery will prevent the tumor from metastasizing to other organs
3. Radiation therapy can be just as effective as surgery if the tumor is small
4. Chemotherapy is as reliable as surgery to treat adenomas of this type in some cases

337. Late in the postoperative period following the removal of an aldosteronoma, the nurse would expect the client's blood pressure to:
1. Gradually return to near normal levels
2. Rise quickly above the preoperative levels
3. Fluctuate greatly during this entire period
4. Drop very low, then rise rapidly to normal levels

338. Following removal of an aldosteronoma, a client's wife tells the nurse, "I hope this is the end of this problem, and my husband will be back to work soon." Based on an understanding of the health problem, the nurse should:
1. Caution the wife against setting her expectations too high, since the outcome for this problem is variable
2. Explain that her husband's surgery is curative, since the other adrenal gland is meeting the body's needs
3. Advise the wife to investigate other occupational alternatives for her husband if he plans to return to work
4. Tell her that although her husband will require hormone supplements for the rest of his life, he should be able to work

339. When scheduling thyroid function tests, the nurse should ask if in the last month the client has had a:
1. Mammogram
2. Chest x-ray film
3. Cholecystogram
4. Glucose tolerance test

340. A female college freshman visits the health center because she feels nervous, irritable, and extremely tired. She complains that, although she eats large amounts of food, she has frequent bouts of diarrhea and is losing weight. The nurse observes a fine hand tremor, an exaggerated reaction to external stimuli, and a wide-eyed expression. The laboratory tests that might be ordered to determine what may be causing this client's symptoms are the:
1. T_3 and T_4
2. PTT and PT
3. VDRL and CBC
4. Serum barbiturate levels

341. When assessing a client with Graves' disease the nurse should expect to find:
1. Constipation, dry skin, and weight gain
2. Lethargy, weight gain, and forgetfulness
3. Weight loss, exophthalmos, and restlessness
4. Weight loss, protruding eyeballs, and lethargy

342. When assessing a client with Graves' disease the nurse would expect to find a history of:
1. Diaphoresis
2. Menorrhagia
3. Dry, brittle hair
4. Sensitivity to cold

343. The nurse teaches a client with exophthalmos how to reduce discomfort and prevent corneal ulceration. The nurse recognizes that the teaching is understood when the client states, "I should:
1. Eliminate excessive blinking."
2. Not move my extraocular muscles."
3. Elevate the head of my bed at night."
4. Avoid using a sleeping mask at night."

344. A client is scheduled to have a thyroidectomy for cancer of the thyroid. When providing preoperative teaching for the postoperative period, the nurse should teach the client to:
1. Cough and deep breathe every 2 hours
2. Perform range-of-motion exercises of the head and neck
3. Support the head with the hands when changing position
4. Apply gentle pressure against the incision when swallowing

345. When planning for a client's return from the operating room after a subtotal thyroidectomy the nurse should consider that in this surgery:
1. The entire thyroid gland is removed
2. A small part of the gland is left intact
3. One parathyroid gland is also removed
4. A portion of the thyroid and four parathyroids are removed

346. The nurse plans to set up emergency equipment at the bedside of a client in the imme-

diate postoperative period following a thyroidectomy. The nurse should include:
1. A crash cart with bed board
2. A tracheostomy set and oxygen
3. An airway and rebreathing mask
4. Two ampules of sodium bicarbonate

347. Immediately after a subtotal thyroidectomy the nurse plans to assess a female client for unilateral injury of the pharyngeal nerve every 30 to 60 minutes by:
1. Checking her throat for swelling
2. Observing her for signs of tetany
3. Asking her to state her name out loud
4. Palpating the side of her neck for blood seepage

348. When planning care for a client who has had a thyroidectomy, the nursing action that should be given highest priority during the first 24 hours postoperatively is:
1. Humidifying the room air continuously
2. Performing range-of-motion neck exercises every 4 hours
3. Assessing for hoarseness and voice weakness every 2 hours
4. Checking vital signs every 2 hours after they have stabilized

349. When planning care for a client in the first 24 hours after a thyroidectomy, the nurse should include:
1. Checking the back and sides of the operative dressing
2. Supporting the head during mild range of motion exercises
3. Encouraging the client to ventilate feelings about the surgery
4. Advising the client that normal activities can be resumed immediately

350. After a client has a thyroidectomy the nurse should observe for possible complications. The nurse should be aware that if tingling and numbness of the fingers and toes, muscle twitching, or muscle spasms occur the client may be:
1. Hypokalemic
2. Hypocalcemic

3. In thyroid crisis
4. In hypovolemic shock

351. Following a thyroidectomy the client exhibits carpopedal spasm and some tremors. The client complains of tingling in the fingers and around the mouth. The nurse should notify the physician and expect to administer:
1. Potassium iodide
2. Calcium gluconate
3. Magnesium sulfate
4. Potassium chloride

352. After a thyroidectomy a client should be observed for the possible complication of thyroid crisis which would be evidenced by:
1. An increased pulse deficit
2. A decreased blood pressure
3. A decreased pulse rate and respirations
4. An increased temperature and pulse rate

353. Following a thyroidectomy a client is treated with 131^1 to eradicate residual thyroid tissue. Because of this treatment the nurse should:
1. Maintain universal precautions and limit visitors
2. Consider all discharges including urine and feces to be radioactive
3. Use strict isolation procedures to prevent contamination of the client
4. Provide frequent contact to prevent feelings of abandonment, but maintain an appropriate distance

354. When preparing a client for discharge after a thyroidectomy, the nurse should teach the signs of hypothyroidism. The nurse would be aware that the client understands the teaching when the client says, "I should call my physician if I develop:
1. Dry skin and intolerance to cold."
2. Muscle cramping and sluggishness."
3. Fatigue and an increased pulse rate."
4. Tachycardia and an increase in weight."

355. A client who has had a subtotal thyroidectomy does not understand how hypothyroidism could develop when the problem was hyperthyroidism. The nurse should base a response on the knowledge that:
1. Hypothyroidism is a gradual slowing of the body's function
2. There will be a decrease in pituitary thyroid-stimulating hormone
3. There is less thyroid tissue to supply thyroid hormone after surgery
4. Atrophy of tissue remaining after surgery reduces secretion of thyroid hormones

356. Prior to a client's discharge following a thyroidectomy, the nurse teaches the client to observe for signs of surgically induced hypothyroidism. The nurse would know that the teaching was understood when the client states that the physician should be notified if:
1. Dry skin and fatigue occur
2. Intolerance to heat is present
3. Insomnia and excitability develop
4. Progressive weight loss is evident

RESPIRATORY

357. The description that should be used for the soft swishing sounds of normal breathing heard when the nurse auscultates a client's chest would be:
1. Fine crackles
2. Adventitious sounds
3. Vesicular breath sounds
4. Diminished breath sounds

358. The nurse auscultates a client's lungs and notes a fine crackling sound in the left lower lung during respiration. If crackles and rhonchi in left lower lung were charted on the nurse's notes, the notation would be:
1. A nursing diagnosis
2. A correct nursing notation
3. An inaccurate interpretation
4. Correct if palpation ruled out crepitus

359. The nurse's physical assessment of a client with congestive heart failure reveals tachypnea and bilateral crackles (rales). The nurse should:
1. Initiate oxygen therapy
2. Assess for a pleural friction rub

3. Obtain a chest x-ray film immediately
4. Position the client in the Fowler's position

360. A client arrives in the emergency room with multiple crushing wounds of the chest, abdomen, and legs. The assessments that assume the greatest priority are:
1. Level of consciousness and pupil size
2. Abdominal contusions and other wounds
3. Pain, respiratory rate, and blood pressure
4. Quality of respirations and presence of pulses

361. A client is admitted to the intensive care unit with a diagnosis of adult respiratory distress syndrome. When assessing this client, the nurse should expect to find:
1. Hypertension
2. Tenacious sputum
3. An altered mental status
4. A slowed rate of breathing

362. A client's respiratory status necessitates endotracheal intubation and positive pressure ventilation. The most immediate nursing intervention for this client at this time would be to:
1. Prepare the client for emergency surgery
2. Facilitate the client's verbal communication
3. Assess the client's response to the equipment
4. Maintain sterility of the ventilation system the client is using

363. A client is placed on a ventilator. Because hyperventilation can occur when mechanical ventilation is used, the nurse should monitor the client for signs of:
1. Hypoxia
2. Hypercapnia
3. Metabolic acidosis
4. Respiratory alkalosis

364. A client is on a ventilator. One of the nurses asks what should be done when condensation due to humidity collects in the ventilator tubing. The best response to this question would be to:
1. "Notify the respiratory therapist."
2. "Empty the fluid from the tubing."

3. "Decrease the amount of humidity."
4. "Measure the fluid and record it on the I&O."

365. A tracheostomy is performed for a client with respiratory distress. After the procedure, the client should be placed in the:
1. Supine position
2. Orthopneic position
3. High Fowler's position
4. Semi-Fowler's position

366. The nurse knows that when a client has a tracheostomy tube with a high volume, low pressure cuff, it is used primarily to prevent:
1. Lung infection
2. Leakage of air
3. Mucosal necrosis
4. Tracheal secretion

367. A client with emphysema is short of breath and using accessory muscles of respiration. The nurse recognizes that the client's difficulty in breathing is caused by:
1. Spasm of the bronchi that traps the air
2. An increase in the vital capacity of the lungs
3. A too rapid expulsion of the air from the alveoli
4. Difficulty in expelling the air trapped in the alveoli

368. The nurse should observe a client with chronic obstructive pulmonary disease for early indications of respiratory acidosis, which include:
1. Bradypnea
2. Bradycardia
3. Restlessness
4. Lightheadedness

369. The physician orders oxygen given in low concentration and intermittently, rather than in high concentration and continuously, for a client with COPD to prevent:
1. A decrease in red cell formation
2. Rupture of emphysematous bullae
3. Depression of the respiratory center
4. An excessive drying of the respiratory mucosa

370. The position that would provide for the greatest respiratory capacity for a client with dyspnea would be the:
1. Sims' position
2. Supine position
3. Orthopneic position
4. Semi-Fowler's position

371. The breathing exercises that the nurse teaches to a client with emphysema (COPD) should include:
1. An inhalation that is longer than an exhalation
2. Abdominal exercises to limit the use of accessory muscles
3. Sit-ups to strengthen the abdominal and intercostal muscles
4. Diaphragmatic exercises to improve contraction of the diaphragm

372. The nurse is aware that a client understands the instructions about an appropriate breathing technique for COPD when the client:
1. Inhales through the mouth
2. Increases the respiratory rate
3. Holds each breath for a second at the end of inspiration
4. Progressively increases the length of the inspiratory phase

373. A client who has had emphysema (COPD) for many years develops an enlarged liver. The nurse understands that this results from:
1. Liver hypoxia
2. Hepatic acidosis
3. Esophageal varices
4. Portal hypertension

374. A client with chronic obstructive pulmonary disease (COPD) complains of a weight gain of 5 pounds in 1 week. The complication of COPD that may have precipitated this weight gain is:
1. Polycythemia
2. Cor pulmonale
3. Compensated acidosis
4. Left ventricular heart failure

375. A client with a history of chronic obstructive pulmonary disease (COPD) develops cor pulmonale. When teaching about nutrition, the nurse should encourage this client to:
1. Eat small meals six times a day to limit oxygen needs
2. Lie down after eating to permit energy to be used for digestion
3. Drink large amounts of fluids to help liquefy respiratory secretions
4. Increase protein intake to decrease intravascular hydrostatic pressure

376. When inspecting a dressing following a partial pneumonectomy for cancer of the lung, the nurse observes some puffiness of the tissue around the area. When the area is palpated, the tissue feels spongy and crackles. When charting, the nurse should describe this assessment as:
1. Stridor
2. Crepitus
3. Pitting edema
4. Chest distention

377. On the first day following a right pneumonectomy a male client suddenly sits straight up in bed. His respirations are labored, and he is making a crowing sound. His skin is pale, cool, and moist. Immediately the nurse should:
1. Notify the physician
2. Auscultate the left lung
3. Inspect the incision for bleeding
4. Check the chest tube for patency

378. When turning a client following a right pneumonectomy the nurse should plan to place the client in either the:
1. Right or left side-lying position
2. High Fowler's or supine position
3. Supine or right side-lying position
4. Left side-lying or low Fowler's position

379. The nurse should be vigilant for the unique complications associated with a pneumonectomy by observing the client for:
1. Signs of cardiac overload
2. Increased pulse and respirations
3. Cardiac irregularities with premature beats
4. Increased BP, decreased temperature, and cold, moist skin

380. After a client undergoes a lobectomy, the nurse should observe for symptoms of the most life-threatening complication, which is:
1. Hemothorax due to decreased thoracic drainage
2. Dyspnea due to increased intrathoracic pressure
3. Decreased cardiac output due to mediastinal shift
4. Pneumothorax due to increased abdominal pressure

381. A female client develops increased respiratory secretions because of radiation therapy to the lung. When teaching postural drainage, the nurse should explain that the client will know that it is effective when she:
1. Is free of crackles
2. Can breathe deeply
3. Has a productive cough
4. Is able to expectorate saliva

382. A client with oat cell lung cancer is scheduled for a mediastinoscopy with biopsy. The nurse should:
1. Tell the client that chest tubes will be present after the procedure
2. Explain that the procedure will visualize the lungs and the chest cavity
3. Advise the client of the npo status after midnight the night before the test
4. Inform the client that some pleural fluid will be removed during the procedure

383. A client is to have a thoracentesis for a pleural effusion. The nurse knows that:
1. A thoracentesis is generally followed by instillation of a sclerosing agent
2. A thoracentesis is usually contraindicated in clients with a history of COPD
3. The rapid removal of large amounts of pleural fluid may precipitate cardiovascular collapse
4. The client usually has a temporary increase in dyspnea immediately following the procedure

384. When assessing a client with pleural effusion the nurse should expect to find:

1. Moist crackles at the back of the lungs
2. Deviation of the trachea toward the involved side
3. Reduced or absent breath sounds at the base of the lung
4. Increased resonance with percussion of the involved area

385. A client with chronic obstructive pulmonary disease is admitted to the hospital with a tentative diagnosis of pleuritis. When caring for this client the nurse should plan to:
1. Assess for signs of pneumonia
2. Administer pain medication frequently
3. Administer medication to suppress coughing
4. Limit fluid intake to prevent pulmonary edema

386. After a thoracentesis for pleural effusion a client returns to the physician's office for a follow-up visit. The nurse would suspect a recurrence of pleural effusion when the client says:
1. "Lately I can only breathe well if I sit up."
2. "During the night I sometimes have a fever and chills."
3. "I get a sharp, stabbing pain when I take a deep breath."
4. "I'm coughing up larger amounts of thicker mucus for the last two days."

387. Immediately after a thoracentesis a client's right lung collapses. A chest tube is inserted and attached to a three chamber closed drainage system. The nurse knows that the chest tube is functioning properly when fluid:
1. Is bubbling gently in the chest drainage chamber *Air leak*
2. Remains constant in the chest drainage chamber *obstruction*
3. Is bubbling vigorously in the suction control chamber *suction too high*
4. Rises in the tube of the waterseal chamber on inspiration

388. Before a scheduled bilateral herniorrhaphy, the nurse should teach the client that postoperatively the client will:
1. Have a nasogastric tube in the nose
2. Have a portable wound drainage system
3. Turn and change positions every 2 hours
4. Perform coughing and deep breathing exercises

389. The nurse performs preoperative teaching related to a subtotal thyroidectomy. The nurse would know that the client understands the teaching about the local effects of general anesthesia when the client states, "Immediately after surgery I will experience:
1. Feelings of chilliness."
2. Transient headaches."
3. Difficulty swallowing."
4. Paroxysmal hiccoughs."

390. Following a gastroscopy the nurse should assess the client for the return of the gag reflex by:
1. Touching the pharynx with a tongue depressor
2. Giving a small amount of water using a syringe
3. Observing for when the client spits out the airway
4. Instructing the client to breathe deeply and cough gently

391. When caring for clients in the operating room the nurse knows that the last physiologic function the client loses during the induction of anesthesia is:
1. Gag reflex
2. Corneal reflex
3. Consciousness
4. Respiratory movement

392. A client has an aneurysm resected and replaced with a graft. On arrival in the recovery room, the client is in shock. The nursing priority should be:
1. Assessing the client's respiratory status
2. Monitoring the client's hourly urine output
3. Putting several warm blankets on the client
4. Placing the client in the Trendelenburg position

393. When a client returns from a bronchoscopy, the nurse should withhold food and fluid for several hours to prevent:
1. Aspiration of food
2. Projectile vomiting
3. Abdominal distention
4. Dysphasia and dyspepsia

394. A client has a bronchoscopy. The nurse should assess for return of the gag reflex by:
1. Having the client say a few words
2. Giving the client a small swallow of water
3. Touching the pharynx with a tongue depressor
4. Instructing the client to breathe deeply and cough gently

395. Following surgery, the physician orders an incentive spirometer for a client. The nurse would evaluate that the client was using the spirometer correctly when observing that the client:
1. Coughs twice before inhaling deeply through the mouthpiece
2. Uses the incentive spirometer for 10 consecutive breaths per hour
3. Inhales deeply, seals the lips around the mouthpiece, and exhales
4. Inhales deeply through the mouthpiece, relaxes, and then exhales

396. A client is scheduled for coronary artery bypass surgery. The nurse explains to the client that underwater seal chest tubes will be inserted during surgery to:
1. Drain fluid from the pericardial sac
2. Prevent atelectasis postoperatively
3. Reestablish negative intrapleural pressure
4. Monitor the amount of blood loss after surgery

397. When giving a client care on the first day postoperatively following coronary artery bypass surgery, the nurse notes that the fluid in the water seal chamber of the drainage device (Pleurevac) stops fluctuating. The nurse should:
1. Increase the amount of suction
2. Look for obstructions of the tube
3. Add sterile water to the chamber
4. Consider this a normal occurrence

398. The nurse is instructed to measure and document the amount of drainage from a client's chest tube. The nurse should:
1. Aspirate fluid from the collection chamber of the disposable water-seal drainage system (Pleurevac) with a needle and syringe and measure the drainage
2. Clamp the chest tube, empty the collection chamber of the disposable water-seal drainage system (Pleurevac) into a measuring cup and reconnect the drainage system
3. Connect a new Pleurevac, measure the drainage in the collection chamber of the old disposable water seal drainage system (Pleurevac) and dispose of the old drainage system
4. Place a piece of tape on the outside of the collection chamber of the disposable waterseal drainage system (Pleurevac) and mark the fluid level and the time of measurement

399. After thoracic surgery a client has a chest tube connected to a three-bottle water-seal drainage system. When excessive bubbling is noted in the water-seal bottle, the nurse should:
1. Check the system for air leaks
2. Decrease the amount of suction pressure
3. Recognize the system is functioning correctly
4. "Milk" the chest tube toward the collection chamber

400. A client is performing postthoracotomy exercises. The least productive exercise for this client would be:
1. Extending the arm up and back and out to the side and back
2. Climbing a wall with the fingers until the arm is fully extended
3. Tying a rope to a doorknob and swinging the arm in wide circles
4. Extending the arm out and bringing it up to touch the nose with the finger

401. A chest tube is inserted following a crushing chest injury. The observation that indicates a desired response to treatment of the client's chest injury would be:

1. Increased breath sounds
2. Increased respiratory rate
3. Crepitus detected on palpation of chest
4. Constant bubbling in drainage chamber

402. The nurse knows that a closed water-seal drainage system connected to a client's pleural chest tube is functioning properly when the fluid in the water-seal chamber of the drainage system:
1. Contains many small air bubbles
2. Bubbles vigorously on inspiration
3. Rises with inspiration and falls with expiration
4. Remains at a constant level during the respiratory cycle

403. A client sustains a stab wound to the chest and a chest tube with water-seal drainage is inserted. Later, the client's chest tube seems to be obstructed. The most appropriate nursing action would be to:
1. Gently squeeze the tube
2. Clamp the tube immediately
3. Prepare for chest tube removal
4. Arrange for a stat chest x-ray film

404. On the way to x-ray a client with a chest tube becomes confused and pulls the chest tube out. The nurse's immediate action should be to:
1. Place the client in the Trendelenburg position
2. Hold the insertion site open with a Kelly clamp
3. Obtain sterile Vaseline gauze to cover the opening
4. Cover the opening with the cleanest material available

405. A client has a chest tube for a pneumothorax. The nurse finds the client in respiratory difficulty with the chest tube separated from the drainage system. The nurse should:
1. Obtain a new sterile drainage system
2. Clamp the drainage tubing with two clamps
3. Reconnect the client's tube to the drainage system
4. Place the client in the high Fowler's position immediately

406. To best promote continued improvement in a client's respiratory status after chest drainage is discontinued, the nurse should:
1. Continue observing for dyspnea and crepitus
2. Encourage frequent coughing and deep breathing
3. Turn the client from side to side at least every 2 hours
4. Encourage bedrest with active and passive range-of-motion exercises

407. A chronically ill, elderly female client tells the home-care nurse that the daughter with whom she lives seems run-down and disinterested in her own health as well as the health of her children, ages 2, 5, 7, and 12. The client tells the nurse that her daughter coughs a good deal and does a lot of sleeping. In this situation the nurse should pursue the daughter's condition for potential case finding because:
1. Children younger than 12 are very susceptible to tuberculosis
2. Deaths from tuberculosis have been generally on the decrease
3. Tuberculosis has been dramatically rising in the general population
4. Aging clients with chronic illness are most adversely affected by tuberculosis

408. During a routine physical examination, a client's chest x-ray film reveals a lesion in the right upper lobe. When the nurse obtains a history from the client the information that supports the physician's tentative diagnosis of pulmonary tuberculosis is:
1. Frothy sputum and fever
2. Dry cough and pulmonary congestion
3. Night sweats and blood-tinged sputum
4. Productive cough and engorged neck veins

409. The nurse notes 12 mm of induration at the site of a Mantoux test when a client returns to the health office to have it read. The nurse should explain to the client that this:
1. Test result is negative, and no follow-up is needed
2. Test was used for screening and a Tine test will now be given
3. Skin test is inconclusive and will have to be repeated in 6 weeks
4. Result indicates a need for further tests, including a chest x-ray film examination

410. To make a definitive diagnosis of tuberculosis, the nurse understands that the physician must order a:
1. Chest x-ray film
2. Tuberculin skin test
3. Pulmonary function test
4. Sputum for acid-fast testing

411. A client with pulmonary tuberculosis is being treated on an outpatient basis. The nurse should expect that the physican will order a diet that:
1. Includes liquid protein supplements
2. Has frequent small high-calorie meals
3. Is low in calories but high in carbohydrates
4. Contains foods high in calories and low in protein

412. A client with pulmonary tuberculosis is being treated in the home. To help control the spread of the disease, the client should be instructed to:
1. Have visitors sit at least eight feet away
2. Keep personal articles away from the rest of the family
3. Open the windows slightly to allow a good airflow throughout the house
4. Avoid putting used dishes in the dishwasher with the rest of the family's dishes

413. A client's Tine test and chest x-ray film indicate pulmonary tuberculosis. The physician orders sputum specimens for acid fast bacilli. The nurse should teach the client that the sputum specimens should be:
1. Coughed up from deep in the lungs
2. Collected in the early morning hours

3. Copius in amount for adequate testing
4. Refrigerated until brought to the laboratory

414. A client's sputum smears for acid-fast bacillus (AFB) are positive and the client is placed on isolation. The nurse should instruct visitors to:
1. Limit contact with nonexposed family members
2. Avoid contact with any objects present in the client's room
3. Wear an Ultra-Filter mask when they are in the client's room
4. Put on a gown and gloves before going into the client's room

415. When teaching a client with tuberculosis about recovery after discharge from the hospital, the nurse should reinforce that the treatment measure with the highest priority is:
1. Having sufficient rest
2. Getting plenty of fresh air
3. Changing the current life-style
4. Consistently taking prescribed medication

CARDIOVASCULAR

416. To determine the status of a client's carotid pulse, the nurse should palpate:
1. In the lateral neck region
2. Immediately below the mandible
3. At the anterior neck lateral to the trachea
4. At the base of the neck along the clavicle

417. During auscultation of the heart, the nurse would expect the first heart sound (S_1) to be the loudest at the:
1. Apex of the heart
2. Base of the heart
3. Left lateral border
4. Right lateral border

418. When auscultating a client's heart the nurse understands that the first heart sound is produced by the closure of the:
1. Mitral and tricuspid valves
2. Aortic and tricuspid valves
3. Mitral and pulmonic valves
4. Aortic and pulmonic valves

419. Thrombus formation is a danger for all postoperative clients. The nurse should act independently to prevent this complication by:
1. Applying elastic stockings
2. Massaging gently with lotion
3. Encouraging in-bed exercises
4. Providing adequate fluids intake

420. Oxygen by nasal cannula is prescribed for a client. The nurse plans to use safety precautions in the room because oxygen:
1. Is flammable
2. Supports combustion
3. Has unstable properties
4. Converts to an alternate form of matter

421. An electrocardiogram is ordered for a client complaining of chest pain. An early finding in the lead over an infarcted area would be:
1. Flattened T waves (hypokalemia)
2. Absence of P waves
3. Elevated ST segments
4. Disappearance of Q waves

422. The nurse can assist the physician with the safe insertion of a central venous catheter by instructing the client to:
1. Void 15 minutes before the procedure is started
2. Take nothing by mouth for two hours before the procedure
3. Breathe out slowly and use the "purse-lip" breathing technique
4. Breathe deeply, hold the breath, and bear down with the mouth closed

423. A client has a Swan-Ganz catheter inserted for monitoring cardiovascular status. With the Swan-Ganz catheter the most accurate measurement of the client's left ventricular pressure would be the:
1. Right atrial pressure
2. Cardiac output by thermodilution
3. Pulmonary artery diastolic pressure
4. Pulmonary capillary wedge pressure

424. A thallium scan is performed on a client with a history of chest pain to:
1. Monitor action of the heart valves
2. Determine myocardial muscle viability
3. Visualize ventricular systole and diastole
4. Determine adequacy of electrical conductivity

425. A client's diet is modified to eliminate foods that act as cardiac stimulants. The nurse should teach the client to avoid:
1. Yogurt
2. Club soda
3. Chocolate
4. Red meats

426. A client is placed on the "Prudent Diet" proposed by the American Heart Association. The nurse should be aware that the caloric distribution of this diet includes:
1. 50% fat (20% saturated), 20% carbohydrate, 30% protein
2. 10% fat (5% saturated), 80% carbohydrate (50% complex), 10% protein
3. 45% fat (15% saturated), 40% carbohydrate (20% complex), 15% protein
4. 30% fat (<10% saturated), 50% carbohydrate (35% complex), 20% protein

427. A female client tells the nurse that the doctor just told her that her triglycerides and cholesterol are excessively elevated. The client appears discouraged and says, "Well, I guess I'd better cut out all the fat and cholesterol in my diet." The nurse's most appropriate response would be:
1. "Well yes, that would certainly lower the amount of your blood fats."
2. "That's good, but be sure to compensate by adding more proteins and carbohydrates."
3. "You need some fat to supply a necessary fatty acid, so it's mainly just a need for cutting down the amount."
4. "You need some cholesterol in your diet because your body cannot manufacture it, so just avoid excessive amounts."

428. To help reduce a client's risk factors for heart disease, the nurse, in discussing dietary guidelines, should teach the client to:
1. Avoid eating between meals
2. Decrease the amount of unsaturated fat
3. Decrease the amount of fat-binding fiber
4. Increase the ratio of complex carbohydrates

429. When preparing a client for a cardiac catheterization, the nurse should advise the client that:
1. The procedure will take fifteen minutes
2. The client will be npo six to eight hours before the procedure
3. Ambulation will be permitted within 1 hour after the procedure
4. Complete sedation will be maintained throughout the procedure

430. Before a cardiac catheterization the nurse should assess and mark the location of pedal pulses with a ballpoint pen on the client's feet to:
1. Establish baseline data
2. Identify the site for arterial cannulation
3. Assess the extent of any residual edema
4. Check the effectiveness of venous return

431. A client returns from a cardiac catheterization with a pressure dressing over the left groin. The client is to be flat in bed for 6 hours with the leg straight. These measures are important to prevent:
1. Orthostatic hypotension
2. Headache and disorientation
3. Bleeding at the arterial puncture site
4. Infiltration of radiopaque dye into tissue

432. For the first several hours following a cardiac catheterization, it would be most essential for the nurse to:
1. Keep the head of the client's bed elevated 45 degrees
2. Monitor the client's apical pulse and blood pressure frequently
3. Encourage the client to cough and deep breathe every 2 hours
4. Check the client's temperature every hour until it returns to normal

433. The finding that would most significantly indicate that a client is hypertensive is:
1. An extended Korotkoff sound
2. A regular pulse of 92 beats per minute
3. A systolic pressure ranging from 140 to 150 mmHg
4. A diastolic pressure that remains greater than 90 mmHg

434. The nurse would expect a client, diagnosed as having hypertension, to report experiencing the most common symptom associated with this disorder, which is:
1. Fatigue
2. Headache
3. Nosebleeds
4. Flushed face

435. A businessman makes many long airplane trips. He confides to the nurse at his place of business that he is concerned because his legs swell on these long flights. The nurse should advise him to:
1. Relax in a reclining position
2. Sit upright with legs extended
3. Walk about the cabin at least once every hour
4. Sit in any position that relieves pressure on the legs

436. A client with a history of hypertension develops pedal edema and demonstrates dyspnea on exertion. The nurse recognizes that the client's dyspnea on exertion is probably:
1. Caused by cor pulmonale
2. A result of left ventricular failure
3. A result of right ventricular failure
4. Associated with wheezing and coughing

437. A client who has been admitted to the cardiac care unit with a myocardial infarction complains of chest pain. The nursing intervention that would be most effective in relieving the client's pain would be to administer the ordered:
1. Morphine sulfate 2 mg IV
2. Oxygen per nasal cannula
3. Nitroglycerin sublingually
4. Lidocaine hydrochloride 50 mg IV bolus

438. The nurse admitting a client with a myocardial infarction to the ICU understands that the pain the client is experiencing is a result of:
1. Compression of the heart muscle
2. Release of myocardial isoenzymes
3. Inadequate perfusion of the myocardium
4. Rapid vasodilation of the coronary arteries

439. A male client who is hospitalized following a myocardial infarction asks the nurse why he is receiving morphine. The nurse replies that morphine:
1. Dilates coronary blood vessels
2. Relieves pain and prevents shock
3. Decreases anxiety and restlessness
4. Helps prevent fibrillation of the heart

440. Isoenzyme laboratory studies are ordered for a client following a myocardial infarction. The isoenzyme test that is the most reliable early indicator of myocardial insult is:
1. AST
2. LDH
3. SGOT
4. CPK-MB

441. Several days following surgery a client develops pyrexia. The nurse should monitor the client for other adaptations related to the pyrexia including:
1. Dyspnea
2. Chest pain
3. Increased pulse rate
4. Elevated blood pressure

442. When a client has a myocardial infarction, one of the major manifestations is a decrease in the conductive energy provided to the heart. When assessing this client the nurse understands that the existing action potential is in direct relationship to the:
1. Heart rate
2. Refractory period
3. Pulmonary pressure
4. Strength of contraction

443. Because a client with a myocardial infarction can develop left ventricular failure, the nurse should assess this client for:

1. Distended neck veins
2. Anorexia and weight loss
3. Paroxysmal nocturnal dyspnea
4. Right upper quadrant tenderness

444. A client who has had a myocardial infarction experiences a noticeably decreased pulse pressure. The nurse should immediately recognize this as a possible indication of:
1. Increased blood volume
2. Hyperactivity of the heart
3. Increased cardiac sufficiency
4. Decreased force of contraction

445. The nurse notes premature ventricular beats (PVBs) on a client's cardiac monitor and recognizes that these complexes are a sign of:
1. Atrial fibrillation
2. Cardiac irritability
3. Impending heart block
4. Ventricular tachycardia

446. The wife of a client who has had emergency coronary artery bypass surgery asks why her husband has a dressing on his left leg. The nurse explains that:
1. This is the access site for the heart lung machine
2. A filter is inserted in the leg to prevent embolization
3. The saphenous vein is used to bypass the coronary artery
4. The arteries in distal extremities are examined during surgery

447. It is determined that a client will require implantation of a permanent pacemaker to assist heart function. In response to the client's inquiries as to why this is necessary, the nurse's best response would be:
1. "It shocks the AV node to contract."
2. "It will cause a normal heartbeat to occur."
3. "It will work the valves of your heart better."
4. "It will slow down the heart to a more normal rate."

448. The nurse recognizes that a pacemaker is indicated when a client is experiencing:
1. Angina
2. Chest pain
3. Heart block
4. Tachycardia

449. A client's wife arrives at the cardiac care unit and is informed that her husband needs a pacemaker. The wife expresses the concern that her husband could accidentally become electrocuted. The nurse's best response would be:
1. "No one has been electrocuted yet by a pacemaker."
2. "The new technology prevents electrocution from occurring."
3. "Pacemakers are pretested for safety before being inserted."
4. "The voltage emitted is not strong enough to electrocute him."

450. A client with a history of hypertension and left ventricular failure arrives for a scheduled clinic appointment and tells the nurse, "My feet are killing me. These shoes got so tight." The nurse's best initial action would be to:
1. Weigh the client
2. Notify the physician
3. Take the client's pulse rate
4. Listen to the client's breath sounds

451. When assessing a client with a diagnosis of left ventricular heart failure (congestive heart failure), the nurse should expect to find:
1. Crushing chest pain
2. Dyspnea on exertion
3. Jugular vein distention
4. Extensive peripheral edema

452. The teaching plan for a client receiving digoxin for left ventricular failure should include having the client:
1. Sleep flat in bed
2. Rest during the day
3. Follow a low-potassium diet
4. Take the pulse three times a day

453. After the acute phase of left ventricular failure (congestive heart failure), the nurse

should expect the dietary management of the client to include the restriction of:
1. Sodium
2. Calcium
3. Potassium
4. Magnesium

454. A client is admitted to the intensive care unit with pulmonary edema. When performing the admission assessment, the nurse should expect:
1. A decreased blood pressure
2. Radiating anterior chest pain
3. A pulse that is weak and rapid
4. Crackles at the base of each lung

455. The physician orders "Bathroom privileges only" for a client with pulmonary edema. The client becomes irritable and asks the nurse if it is really necessary to stay in bed so much. The nurse's best reply would be:
1. "Why do you want to be out of bed?"
2. "Yes. Bedrest plays a role in most therapy."
3. "Rest will help your body direct energy to healing."
4. "Not always. Ask your physician to change the order."

456. When assessing a client for signs of right ventricular failure, the nurse should expect to note:
1. A slowed pulse rate
2. A pleural friction rub
3. Neck vein distention
4. Increasing hypotension

457. The nurse suggests that a client with right ventricular failure should:
1. Take a hot bath before bedtime
2. Avoid sleeping in an air-conditioned room
3. Avoid emotionally stressful situations when possible
4. Exercise daily until the pulse rate exceeds 100/minute

458. The home care nurse is assessing a client with cardiac insufficiency. The nurse notes that the client's pulse rate increases from 70 to 92 beats/minute while climbing the stairs. The nurse should immediately instruct the client to:

1. Continue climbing
2. Stand still and rest
3. Walk down the stairs
4. Climb at a slower rate

459. During a routine physical examination, an abdominal aortic aneurysm is diagnosed. The client is immediately admitted to the hospital, and surgery is scheduled for the next morning. When performing the admission assessment, the nurse should expect:
1. Severe radiating abdominal pain
2. Cyanosis and symptoms of shock
3. A pattern of visible peristaltic waves
4. A palpable pulsating abdominal mass

460. A client is admitted for resection of an abdominal aortic aneurysm. During the evening before surgery, the client suddenly develops symptoms of shock. The nurse should:
1. Prepare for blood transfusions
2. Notify the physician immediately
3. Give the client nothing by mouth
4. Administer the prescribed sedative

461. To prevent thrombus formation after most surgery, the nurse should plan to:
1. Keep the bed gatched to elevate the client's knees
2. Have the client dangle the legs off the side of the bed
3. Have the client use an incentive spirometer every hour
4. Encourage the client to ambulate with assistance as needed

462. When performing a physical assessment the nurse identifies bilateral varicose veins. The symptom the nurse should expect the client to report is:
1. Increased sensitivity to cold
2. Pallor of the lower extremities
3. Calf pain when foot is dorsiflexed
4. Increasing ankle edema over the day

463. During an office visit to a physician a client, who is considering sclerotherapy, asks the nurse to explain what causes varicose veins. The nurse's best response would be, "They are caused by:
1. Incompetent valves of superficial veins."
2. Decreased pressure within the deep veins."

3. Atherosclerotic plaque formation in the veins."
4. Abnormal configurations of the vascular system."

464. The physician orders knee length elastic support stockings for a client with varicose veins. When teaching the client about these stockings, the nurse should explain that:
1. It is best to apply them before getting out of bed
2. The stockings should come up to the middle of the knee
3. The stockings should be applied at the first sign of discomfort
4. Elastic bandages are more economical and may be substituted

465. When collecting data from a client with varicose veins who is to have sclerotherapy, the nurse should expect the client to report:
1. A feeling of heaviness in both legs
2. Calf pain on dorsiflexion of the foot
3. Intermittent claudication of the legs
4. Hematomas of the lower extremities

466. When assessing the lower extremities of a client with multiple varicosities who is to have sclerotherapy, the nurse should expect to find:
1. Pallor
2. Ankle edema
3. Yellowed toe nails
4. Diminished pedal pulses

467. Before having sclerotherapy for varicose veins, a female client, who states she is fearful of a chemical injection, asks the nurse to explain what would be involved if she insisted on a ligation and stripping to correct the problem. The nurse should explain that this surgery involves:
1. Removing the dilated saphenous veins
2. Cleaning out plaque from within the vessels
3. Anastomosing superficial veins to deep veins
4. Placing an umbrella filter in the large affected veins

468. A client with a history of thrombophlebitis and varicosities is to have a herniorrhaphy for an incarcerated hernia. The client's past medical history and present diagnosis indicate to the nurse that a primary responsibility following surgery is to:
1. Raise the foot of the bed
2. Get the client out of bed twice daily
3. Maintain body alignment with firm support of the extremities
4. Encourage the client to turn often and to exercise the legs regularly

469. Before discharging a client who has had an inguinal herniorrhaphy, the nurse teaches the client about exercising to prevent venous stasis. For best results, the nurse should:
1. Demonstrate specific exercises
2. Suggest frequent moving of the legs
3. Advise against sitting for prolonged periods
4. Suggest that the client change position frequently

470. A client who has been hospitalized for thrombophlebitis asks how future attacks can best be prevented. The nurse should teach the client to:
1. Follow the program of exercises
2. Take prophylactic anticoagulants
3. Apply warm soaks to the legs daily
4. Apply elastic stockings before arising

471. A client is suspected of having thrombophlebitis of the left lower extremity. During the initial assessment the nurse should specifically observe the client for:
1. Edema of the left leg
2. Mobility of the left leg
3. A positive left-sided Babinski reflex
4. Presence of peripheral arterial pulses

472. A client with an ischemic foot needs to understand that the pain in the foot is a result of inadequate blood supply, which may be further diminished by:
1. Drinking alcohol
2. Lowering the limb
3. Smoking cigarettes
4. Consuming excessive fluid

473. A male client with intermittent claudication asks the nurse why he is not allowed to smoke. The nurse's best response would be:

1. "The policy states that the hospital is a smoke-free environment."
2. "Nicotine causes arteries to go into spasm, which decreases circulation."
3. "Cigarette smoking is not allowed for clients who have venous problems."
4. "The doctor may allow you to begin smoking again after you are feeling better."

474. An essential nursing function in the care of a client with arterial insufficiency in the left foot caused by generalized arteriosclerosis should be to:
1. Maintain elevation of the legs
2. Massage the legs when painful
3. Check arterial pulses frequently
4. Apply a hot water bottle to the feet

475. A client develops a nonhealing ulcer of the right lower extremity and complains of leg cramps after walking short distances. The client asks the nurse what causes these leg pains. The nurse's best response would be:
1. "Muscle weakness occurs in the legs because of a lack of exercise."
2. "Edema and cyanosis occur in the legs because they are dependent."
3. "Pain occurs in the legs while walking because there is a lack of oxygen to the muscles."
4. "Pressure occurs in the legs because of vasodilation and pooling of blood in the extremity."

476. The physician prescribes a progressive exercise program, that includes walking, for a client with a history of diminished arterial perfusion to the lower extremities. The nurse should explain to the client that, if leg cramps occur while walking, the client should:
1. Take one aspirin twice a day
2. Stop and rest until the pain resolves
3. Walk more slowly while pain is present
4. Take one nitroglycerin tablet sublingually

477. A client comes to the outpatient clinic with a painful leg ulcer. The symptom that supports the diagnosis of arterial ulcer is:
1. Pain at the ulcer site
2. Bleeding around the ulcer area

3. Dependent edema of the extremities
4. Stasis dermatitis on affected extremity

478. A client is admitted with a large leg ulcer and a femoral angiogram is performed. After this procedure the nurse should:
1. Provide passive ROM to all extremities
2. Elevate the foot of the bed for 36 hours
3. Assist the client to stand if unable to void
4. Apply pressure to the catheter insertion site

479. A client with impaired peripheral pulses and signs of chronic hypoxia in a lower extremity has a femoral angiogram. After the angiogram the nurse should:
1. Elevate the foot of the bed
2. Have the client void within two hours
3. Keep the client in the high Fowler's position
4. Perform a neurovascular assessment of the affected extremity

480. Six hours after a femoral-popliteal bypass graft, the client's blood pressure becomes severely elevated. The nurse should notify the physician primarily because the client's:
1. Blood pressure could cause the graft to occlude
2. Hypervolemia needs to be corrected immediately
3. Intraabdominal pressure could compromise the viability of the graft
4. Cardiovascular status could precipitate a cerebral vascular accident

481. A client has a femoral-popliteal bypass graft. When the vital signs are assessed, the client's blood pressure is 200/110. The nurse should notify the physician immediately because the:
1. Graft could rupture
2. Client is anaphylactic
3. Client is hypervolemic
4. Graft may be occluded

482. A client with a history of severe intermittent claudication has a femoral-popliteal bypass graft. An appropriate postoperative intervention on the day after surgery would be to:
1. Keep the client on bedrest

2. Have the client sit in a chair
3. Assist the client with ambulation
4. Encourage the client to keep the legs elevated

483. The nurse provides discharge teaching for a client with a history of hypertension who has had a femoral-popliteal bypass graft. The nurse is aware that the teaching is effective when the client says, "I should:
1. Massage my calves gently every day."
2. Keep my foot elevated when I am in bed."
3. Sit in a hot bath for 25 minutes twice a day."
4. Assess the color and pulses of my legs every day."

REPRODUCTIVE AND GENITOURINARY

484. A female client is tentatively diagnosed as having cystitis pending laboratory results. The nurse recognizes that *Escherichia coli* is a common causative agent in cystitis because it is:
1. A particularly virulent bacteria
2. Commonly found in the kidneys
3. Usually found in the intestinal tract
4. A competitor with *Candida* for host sites

485. A client is scheduled for an intravenous pyelogram (IVP). The nurse explains that on the day before the IVP the client must:
1. Eat a fat free dinner
2. Drink a large amount of fluids
3. Omit dinner and limit beverages
4. Take a laxative before going to bed

486. During an exacerbation of multiple sclerosis a client complains of urinary urgency and frequency. The initial nursing measure should be to:
1. Palpate the suprapubic area
2. Begin teaching self-catheterization
3. Develop a plan to ensure high fluid intake
4. Initiate a regimen to monitor urinary output

487. To facilitate micturition in a male client with renal calculi the nurse should instruct him to:
1. Use a urinal for voiding
2. Drink cranberry juice daily
3. Wash his hands after voiding
4. Assume the normal position for voiding

488. A client with multiple trauma is admitted to the intensive care area, IV fluids are instituted, and a Foley catheter is inserted. With an indwelling catheter, urinary infection is a potential danger. The nurse can best plan to avoid this problem by:
1. Assessing urine specific gravity
2. Maintaining the ordered hydration
3. Collecting a weekly urine specimen
4. Emptying the drainage bag frequently

489. As the nurse assesses a client's kidney function after surgery, the components of urine will be monitored. Essential to this process is the knowledge that the normal kidney filters a number of blood components and urine should not contain:
1. Urea nitrogen
2. Large proteins
3. Sodium chloride
4. Potassium chloride

490. When a client has surgery for cancer of the uterus, the nurse must be concerned with the prevention of postoperative thrombosis because the majority of pulmonary emboli begin as deep vein thromboses of the:
1. Calf of the leg
2. Thoracic cavity
3. Pelvis and thighs
4. Extremities and abdomen

491. Postoperatively, the nursing care plan for a client who has had pelvic surgery should include:
1. Encouraging the client to ambulate in the hallway
2. Elevating the client's lower extremities by gatching the bed
3. Assisting the client to dangle the legs over the side of the bed
4. Maintaining the client on bedrest until the bandages are removed

492. A client complains of urinary problems. Cholinergic medications are prescribed. The nurse is aware that this type of medication is prescribed to prevent:
1. Kidney stones
2. A flaccid bladder
3. A spastic bladder
4. Urinary tract infections

493. Twenty-four hours after a penile implant the client's scrotum is edematous and painful. The nurse should:
1. Assist the client with a sitz bath
2. Apply warm soaks to the scrotum
3. Elevate the scrotum using a soft support
4. Prepare for a possible incision and drainage

494. A male client comes to the emergency room because he has a discharge from his penis. The physician suspects gonorrhea and orders a culture and sensitivity test to assist with the diagnosis. To obtain the culture the nurse should:
1. Instruct client to provide a semen specimen
2. Swab the discharge as it appears on the prepuce
3. Obtain a mucosal scraping from the anterior urethra
4. Teach the client how to obtain a clean catch specimen of urine

495. A client comes to the infectious disease clinic because a sexual partner was recently diagnosed as having gonorrhea. The health history reveals that the client has engaged in receptive anal intercourse. The nurse should assess the client for:
1. Melena
2. Anal itching
3. Constipation
4. Ribbon shaped stools

496. A young male client comes to the clinic complaining of a sore throat and a rash. Because of the client's active sexual history, serologic testing is performed to confirm the diagnosis of syphilis. The symptoms indicate that the client's syphilis can be classified as:

1. Late
2. Latent
3. Primary
4. Infectious

497. To limit the spread of syphilis and to treat those with the disease, the sexual contacts of a client with infectious syphilis must be investigated to locate those who may have infected the client or been infected during sexual relations with the client. The nurse should ask the client with infectious syphilis about sexual contacts during the past:
1. 21 days
2. 30 days
3. 3 months
4. 6 months

498. The physician diagnoses that a client has late stage syphilis. When obtaining a health history, the nurse recognizes that the statement by the client that would most support this diagnosis would be:
1. "I noticed a wart on my penis."
2. "I have sores all over my mouth."
3. "I've been losing a lot of hair lately."
4. "I'm having trouble keeping my balance."

499. A 45-year-old client develops acute glomerulonephritis following a streptococcal infection. When performing the health assessment the nurse would expect the client to report a history of:
1. Nocturia
2. Mild headache
3. A recent weight loss
4. An increased appetite

500. A client with acute glomerulonephritis complains of thirst. The nurse should offer:
1. Ginger ale
2. Hard candy
3. A milk shake
4. A cup of broth

501. To prevent future attacks of glomerulonephritis, the nurse should instruct a female client to:
1. Take showers instead of bubble baths
2. Avoid situations that involve physical activity

3. Continue the restrictions concerning fluid intake
4. Seek early treatment for respiratory tract infections

502. The nurse is aware that the most serious complication for a client with acute renal failure is:
1. Anemia
2. Infection
3. Weight loss
4. Platelet dysfunction

503. The factor in a client's history that may have contributed to a present problem of renal calculi is:
1. A high cholesterol diet
2. Excess ingestion of antacids
3. An excessive exercise program
4. Frequent consumption of alcohol

504. A client is admitted to the hospital with severe flank pain, nausea, and hematuria caused by a ureteral calculus. A lithotripsy is scheduled. The initial nursing action should be to:
1. Strain all urine output
2. Increase the oral fluid intake
3. Obtain a urine specimen for culture
4. Administer the prescribed analgesic

505. When taking the admitting history of a client with a left ureteral calculus who is scheduled for a transurethral ureterolithotomy, the nurse would expect the client to report:
1. A boring pain in the left flank
2. Pain that intensifies on urination
3. Pain that is dull and constant in the costovertebral angle
4. Spasmodic pain on the left side radiating to the suprapubis

506. The laboratory values of a client with renal calculi reveal a serum calcium within normal limits and an elevated serum purine. The nurse should recognize that these stones are probably composed of:
1. Cystine
2. Struvite
3. Oxalate
4. Uric acid

507. A female client, who is scheduled for a lithotripsy later in the week, is admitted to the hospital with severe renal colic caused by a ureteral calculus. Later that evening, the client's urinary output is much less than her intake. When it is noted that her bladder is not distended, the nurse should suspect the development of:
1. Oliguria
2. Hydroureter
3. Renal shutdown
4. Urethral obstruction

508. A client with a calculus in the right renal pelvis is admitted for its removal. The nurse prepares the client for the procedure by explaining that:
1. The right ureter will be removed
2. A suprapubic catheter will be in place
3. Surgery will be performed transurethrally
4. A small incision will be present in the flank area

509. Before discharge after a ureterolithotomy, the nurse discusses the need to avoid urinary tract infections with a male client who has had recurring renal calculi. The nurse knows that the signs of infection are understood when the client says he will report:
1. Urgency or frequency on urination
2. The inability to maintain an erection
3. Pain radiating to the external genitalia
4. An increase in alkalinity or acidity of urine

510. The person at highest risk of developing prostate cancer is a:
1. 55-year-old Black male
2. 55-year-old Asian male
3. 45-year-old Hispanic male
4. 45-year-old Caucasian male

511. Prior to a transurethral resection of the prostate, a client asks the nurse about the postoperative recovery period. The most appropriate response by the nurse would be:
1. "You will have an abdominal incision and a dressing."
2. "You can expect your urine to be pink and free of clots."

3. "You will have an incision between your scrotum and rectum."
4. "You can expect an indwelling catheter and possibly a continuous bladder irrigation."

512. A client is scheduled for a transurethral resection of the prostate. As part of the preoperative teaching, the nurse should explain that after surgery:
1. Urinary control may be permanently lost to some degree
2. The client's ability to perform sexually will be permanently impaired
3. Urinary drainage will be dependent on a urethral catheter for 24 to 48 hours
4. Frequency and burning on urination will last while the cystostomy tube is in place

513. After a transurethral resection of the prostate, a client's nursing care should include:
1. Changing the abdominal dressing
2. Maintaining patency of the cystostomy tube
3. Maintaining patency of a 3-way Foley catheter
4. Observing for hemorrhage and wound infection

514. After a transurethral resection of the prostate the client's retention catheter is secured to his leg, causing slight traction of the inflatable balloon against the prostatic fossa. This is done to:
1. Limit discomfort
2. Provide hemostasis
3. Reduce bladder spasms
4. Promote urinary drainage

515. When planning care for a client with a continuous bladder irrigation the nurse should:
1. Measure the output hourly
2. Monitor the specific gravity of the urine
3. Irrigate the catheter with saline three times daily
4. Exclude the amount of irrigant instilled from the output

516. In the early postoperative period following a transurethral resection of the prostate, the most common complication the nurse should observe for is:

1. Sepsis
2. Hemorrhage
3. Leakage around the catheter
4. Urinary retention with overflow

517. Twenty-four hours after having had a transurethral resection of the prostate, a client tells the nurse he has lower abdominal discomfort. The nurse notes that catheter drainage from the continuous bladder irrigation has stopped. The nurse's initial action should be to:
1. Notify the physician
2. Remove the catheter
3. Milk the catheter tubing
4. Irrigate the catheter with saline

518. Following a prostatectomy the client's Foley catheter is pulled taut and taped to the thigh. The client complains that the catheter is pulled too tight. The nurse's best initial action would be to:
1. Adjust the tension on the catheter to relieve pressure
2. Untape the Foley and retape it closer to the urinary meatus
3. Assess the degree of tension on the catheter and call the physician
4. Explain to the client that the traction is required to help control bleeding

519. Three days following prostate surgery a client's Foley catheter and continuous bladder irrigation (CBI) is to be removed, and the nurse discusses what to expect with the client. The nurse recognizes that the teaching has been understood when the client states, "After the catheter is removed I may:
1. Have dilute urine."
2. Exhibit dark red urine."
3. Be unable to pass my urine."
4. Experience some burning on urination."

520. The nurse would know that a client who has had a transurethral resection of the prostate understood his discharge teaching when he says, "I should:
1. Attempt to void every 3 hours when I'm awake."
2. Get out of bed into a chair for several hours daily."

3. Call the physician if my urinary stream decreases."
4. Avoid vigorous exercise for 6 months after surgery."

521. In answer to a client's question, the nurse explains that a suprapubic prostatectomy differs from other surgical procedures of the prostate in that:
1. The postoperative convalescent period is shorter
2. An indwelling catheter is not required after surgery
3. An incision is made directly into the urinary bladder
4. A major complication, that of sexual impotence, may occur

522. Following a suprapubic prostatectomy, the nurse understands that a client's plan of care must include the prevention of postoperative deep vein thrombosis. This can best be achieved by increasing the:
1. Coagulability of the blood
2. Velocity of the venous return
3. Effectiveness of internal respiration
4. Oxygen-carrying capacity of the blood

523. An acute, life-threatening complication that the nurse should assess a client for in the early postoperative period following a partial nephrectomy would be:
1. Sepsis
2. Hemorrhage
3. Renal failure
4. Paralytic ileus

524. The nurse's postoperative plan of care for a client who has had a partial nephrectomy should include:
1. Giving the client a regular diet on the first postoperative day
2. Clamping the nephrostomy tube when the client is out of bed
3. Turning the client from the back to the operated side every 2 to 3 hours
4. Leaving the client's original dressing in place for at least the first 48 hours

525. Following a partial nephrectomy the observation about the client's urinary output that the nurse should recognize as normal is that urine:
1. Output will be less than 30 ml per hour
2. Specific gravity will remain below 1.010
3. Will remain dark red with clots for 3 to 4 days
4. Will drain from the wound for at least several days

526. Following a partial nephrectomy a client is being discharged with the nephrostomy tube in place. The nurse should instruct the client to:
1. Limit the intake of fluids
2. Remain on bedrest at home
3. Irrigate the nephrostomy tube
4. Change the dressings frequently

527. A client with chronic renal failure is on a restricted protein diet and is taught about high biological value protein foods. An understanding of the rationale for this diet is demonstrated when the client states that high biologic value protein foods are:
1. Needed to increase weight gain
2. Necessary to prevent muscle wasting
3. Used to increase urea blood products
4. Responsible for controlling hypertension

528. The nurse would be aware that a client with chronic renal failure recognizes an adequate source of high biological value protein when the food the client selected from the menu was:
1. Apple juice
2. Raw carrots
3. Cottage cheese
4. Whole wheat bread

529. A client with a history of chronic renal failure is hospitalized. The nurse assesses the client for symptoms of related renal insufficiency, which include:
1. Facial flushing
2. Edema and pruritus
3. Dribbling after voiding
4. Diminished force and caliber of stream

530. A client with uremic syndrome has the potential to develop many complications. The complication that the nurse should anticipate in such a client is:
1. Hypotension
2. Hypokalemia
3. Flapping hand tremors
4. An elevated hematocrit

531. The physician decides to treat a client with a history of chronic renal failure with continuous ambulatory peritoneal dialysis (CAPD). When assessing the client before the institution of CAPD, the nurse should be alert for the presence of:
1. Motivation
2. Dysrhythmias
3. Emotional lability
4. Pulmonary problems

532. A client who is to begin continuous ambulatory peritoneal dialysis (CAPD) asks the nurse what this treatment entails. The explanation should include information that:
1. Peritoneal dialysis is done in an ambulatory care clinic
2. There is continuous hemodialysis and peritoneal dialysis
3. There is continuous contact of dialysate with peritoneal membrane
4. About a quarter of a liter of dialysate is maintained intraperitoneally

533. Diet instruction for a client who is being treated with continuous ambulatory peritoneal dialysis (CAPD) for chronic glomerulonephritis should include the need for:
1. Low calorie foods
2. High quality protein
3. Increased fluid intake
4. Foods rich in potassium

534. A client with chronic glomerulonephritis will begin to perform continuous ambulatory peritoneal dialysis (CAPD) at home. To decrease the discomfort of the peritoneal dialysis, the nurse should teach the client to:
1. Eat a diet that is very low in fiber
2. Instill 2 liters of dialysate solution quickly
3. Keep the outflow bag level with the abdomen
4. Apply a heating pad to the abdomen during inflow

535. A client with renal insufficiency is to have peritoneal dialysis. Preparation for insertion of the peritoneal dialysis catheter includes:
1. IV pyelogram, vital signs, emptying the bladder
2. Catheterization, general anesthetic, IV pyelogram
3. Cleansing enema, consent form, general anesthetic
4. Cleansing enema, emptying the bladder, consent form

536. Nursing measures related to the inflow of dialysate fluid include:
1. Infusing the dialysate solution over 2 hours
2. Slightly warming solution before instilling
3. Positioning the client in the side-lying position
4. Withholding medication until all solution is administered

537. If a client on peritoneal dialysis develops symptoms of severe respiratory difficulty during the infusion of the dialysate solution, the nurse should:
1. Slow the rate of infusion
2. Auscultate the lungs for breath sounds
3. Drain the fluid from the peritoneal cavity
4. Place the client in a low Fowler's position

538. The nurse should monitor the client on peritoneal dialysis for complications such as:
1. Fever, oliguria, and hemorrhage
2. Pruritus, hemorrhage, and cloudy outflow
3. Abdominal pain, tachycardia, and pruritus
4. Tachycardia, cloudy outflow, and abdominal pain

539. A client is scheduled for the creation of an internal arteriovenous fistula and the placement of an external arteriovenous shunt to be used until the fistula heals. The nurse should keep in mind that:
1. Blood pressure readings will be higher in the arm with the fistula than in the arm with the shunt
2. The shunt is more subject to the complications of hemorrhage, clotting, and infection than the fistula

3. IV fluids should not be infused in the arm with the shunt, but they are permitted in the arm with the fistula
4. A light surgical dressing can be applied over the fistula incision, but the shunt should be thoroughly covered with a heavier dressing

540. A client has end stage renal disease and is on hemodialysis. During dialysis, the client complains of nausea and a headache. In addition, the nurse notes the client seems confused. The dialysis nurse, operating on standing protocols, should:
1. Administer an antiemetic
2. Attempt to reorient the client
3. Decrease the rate of dialysis (Disequilibrium)
4. Monitor for changes in vital signs

541. A client with chronic renal failure is accepted for a kidney transplant and attends a group educational program for potential transplant candidates. The client asks the nurse which kidney will be removed. The nurse's best response would be:
1. "Neither of your kidneys will be removed unless they are infected."
2. "It is up to the surgeon as to which kidney is replaced with the new one."
3. "The kidney that is the most diseased is removed and replaced with the new one."
4. "Your right kidney will be removed because it has a longer renal vein making transplant easier."

542. A client who is to have a kidney transplant should be taught to expect:
1. A colonoscopy
2. An appendectomy
3. A partial gastric resection
4. An intravenous cystogram

543. When a client returns from the recovery room after a kidney transplant, the nurse should plan to measure the client's urinary output every:
1. 15 minutes
2. 30 minutes
3. 60 minutes
4. Two hours

544. The most important test used to determine if a client's newly transplanted kidney is working is a:
1. Renal scan
2. Serum creatinine
3. 24 hour urine output
4. White blood cell count

545. A client with a transplanted kidney is taught the signs of rejection. The nurse would know that the teaching was effective when the client says that a sign of rejection would be:
1. Weight loss
2. A subnormal temperature
3. An elevated blood pressure
4. An increased urinary output

546. A client who has had a kidney transplant develops leukopenia 3 weeks after surgery. The nurse should be aware that the leukopenia is probably caused by:
1. A bacterial infection
2. High creatinine levels
3. Rejection of the kidney
4. The antirejection medications

GASTROINTESTINAL

547. A client has decided to become a total vegetarian (vegan) and wishes to plan a diet to ensure adequate protein quality. To provide guidance, the nurse should instruct this client to:
1. Add milk to grains to provide complete proteins
2. Use eggs with plant foods to provide essential amino acids
3. Plan a careful mixture of plant proteins to provide a balance of amino acids
4. Add cheese to grains and beans to increase the quality of the protein consumed

548. An obese client asks the nurse how to lose weight. Before answering, the nurse should remember that long-term weight loss occurs best when:
1. Fats are limited in the diet
2. Eating patterns are altered
3. Carbohydrates are regulated
4. Exercise is part of the program

549. To motivate an obese client to eventually include aerobic exercises in a weight reduction program, the nurse should discuss exercise and its relationship to weight loss. The nurse would know that this teaching was effective when the client states, "I know that exercise will:
1. Raise my heart rate."
2. Decrease my appetite."
3. Lower my metabolic rate."
4. Increase my lean body mass."

550. A client is admitted with complaints of frequent, loose, watery stools; anorexia; malaise; and a considerable weight loss over the past month. Laboratory findings indicate leukocytosis and an elevated sedimentation rate. The nurse recognizes that the presenting symptoms in conjunction with the laboratory findings could be indicative of:
1. The consistent, long-term use of an irritant-type laxative
2. An emotional response that has resulted in physical symptoms
3. Systemic responses of the body to a localized inflammatory process
4. Poor dietary practices that have resulted in an alteration of bowel function

551. When assessing a client's abdomen, the nurse palpates the area directly above the umbilicus. This area is known as the:
1. Iliac area
2. Epigastric area
3. Hypogastric area
4. Suprasternal area

552. An adaptation after a gastroscopy that indicates a major complication is:
1. Difficulty swallowing
2. Increased GI motility
3. Abdominal distention
4. Nausea and vomiting

553. A client is scheduled for a barium swallow; the nurse should:
1. Ask the client about allergies to iodine
2. Ensure a laxative is ordered after the test
3. Give only clear fluids on the day of the test
4. Administer cleansing enemas before the test

554. Routine postoperative intravenous fluids are designed to supply hydration and electrolytes and only limited energy. Since 1 L of a 5% dextrose solution contains 50 g of sugar, 3L/day would supply approximately:
1. 400 kilocalories
2. 600 kilocalories
3. 800 kilocalories
4. 1000 kilocalories

555. After abdominal surgery a client is placed on a progressive post-surgical diet. This diet is characterized by progressive alterations in the:
1. Caloric content of food
2. Nutritional value of food
3. Texture and digestibility of food
4. Variety of food and fluids included

556. The diet ordered for a client permits 190 g of carbohydrates, 90 g of fat, and 100 g of protein. The nurse understands that this diet contains approximately:
1. 2200 calories
2. 2000 calories
3. 1800 calories
4. 1600 calories

557. A client's serum albumin is 2.8 g/dl. The nurse should evaluate client teaching as successful when the client says, "For lunch I am going to have:
1. Fruit salad."
2. Sliced turkey."
3. Spinach salad."
4. Clear beef broth."

558. A client who is a heavy smoker is placed on a high-calorie, high-protein diet. In light of the history of smoking the client should also be encouraged to eat foods high in:
1. Niacin
2. Thiamin
3. Vitamin C
4. Vitamin B$_{12}$

559. A client is cautioned to avoid vitamin D toxicity while increasing protein intake. The nurse would know that the teaching was understood when the client states, "I must increase my intake of:
1. Tofu products."
2. Fruit and eggnog."
3. Powdered whole milk."
4. Cottage cheese custard."

560. When helping a client plan a therapeutic diet, the nurse is aware that an excellent food source of vitamin C is:
1. Apples
2. Lettuce
3. Broccoli
4. Apricots

561. The physician tells a client that an increase in vitamin E and beta carotene is important for healthier skin. The nurse teaches the client that excellent food sources of both of these substances are:
1. Spinach and mangoes
2. Fish and peanut butter
3. Oranges and grapefruits
4. Carrots and sweet potatoes

562. While the nurse is teaching a client with diabetes mellitus about the ordered 1800 calorie ADA diet, the client states, "I do not like broccoli." The nurse suggests that the client could substitute:
1. $^1/_3$ cup of corn
2. $^1/_2$ cup of lima beans
3. $^1/_2$ cup of green peas
4. $^1/_2$ cup of green beans

563. Because of multiple physical injuries and emotional concerns, a hospitalized client is at high risk to develop a stress (Curling's) ulcer. The nurse should know that stress ulcers are usually evidenced by:
1. Unexplained shock
2. Melena for several days
3. A gradual drop in hematocrit
4. A sudden massive hemorrhage

564. To prevent bleeding after pelvic surgery, a client should be instructed to avoid straining on defecation. The nurse evaluates that the related teaching has been understood when the client states, "I must increase my intake of:
1. Milk products."
2. Ripe bananas."
3. Green vegetables."
4. Creamed potatoes."

565. A client with Parkinson's disease complains about a problem with elimination. The nurse should encourage the client to:
1. Eat a banana daily
2. Decrease fluid intake
3. Take cathartics regularly
4. Increase residue in the diet

566. The physician orders three stool specimens for occult blood from a client who complains of blood-streaked stools and a ten pound weight loss in 1 month. To ensure valid test results the nurse should instruct the client to:
1. Avoid eating red meat before testing
2. Test the specimen while it is still warm
3. Discard the first stool of the day and use the next three stools
4. Take three specimens from different sections of the fecal sample

567. When a client develops steatorrhea, the nurse should describe this stool as:
1. Dry and rock-hard
2. Clay colored and pasty
3. Bulky and foul smelling
4. Black and blood-streaked

568. A client is admitted to the hospital with a diagnosis of acute pancreatitis. The physician's orders include nothing by mouth and total parenteral nutrition. When the client asks for an explanation for this therapy, the nurse's most accurate response would be:
1. "It is the easiest method for staff to administer needed nutrition."
2. "It is the safest method for meeting your daily nutritional requirements."
3. "It will satisfy your desire for food without the discomfort associated with eating."
4. "It will meet your nutritional needs without causing the discomfort associated with eating."

569. The physician orders total parenteral nutrition (TPN) 1L q 12 hours. The primary nursing responsibility should be to monitor the client's:
1. Electrolytes
2. Urinary output
3. Administration rate
4. Serum glucose levels

570. Six hours after the initiation of total parenteral nutrition the client's serum glucose is 240 mg/dl. When considering this client's elevated serum glucose, the nurse should recognize that it is probably related to the fact that the:
1. Infusion is flowing too rapidly
2. Prescribed solution is too concentrated
3. Rise is an expected response that will eventually subside
4. Infusion is too slow to meet the client's total nutritional needs

571. In preparing a client to go home with total parenteral nutrition (TPN) the nurse should help the client plan:
1. Which days will be used for administration
2. For daily insertion of the circulatory access
3. For professional help to administer the daily TPN
4. A schedule of administration around normal activity

572. A client presents with symptoms associated with salmonellosis. Relevant data to gather from this client is a history of:
1. Rectal cancer in the family
2. All foods eaten in the past 24 hours
3. Any recent extreme emotional stress
4. An upper respiratory infection in the past 10 days

573. Enteric precautions for a client with salmonellosis include:
1. Isolation in a private room
2. Wearing a gown if soiling is likely
3. Limiting visiting hours during the acute phase
4. Wearing a mask when emptying the client's bedpan

574. A client who is suspected of having salmonellosis asks how the diagnosis is confirmed. The nurse should respond that the diagnosis is established by a:
1. CBC
2. Urinalysis
3. Stool culture
4. Febrile agglutinin test

575. A client is admitted to the hospital with the diagnosis of acute salmonellosis. The nurse would expect that the client will be receiving:
1. Antacids
2. Electrolytes *(prevent dehydration)*
3. Antidiarrheics
4. Antispasmodics

576. During a health symposium, a nurse teaches the group how to prevent food poisoning. The nurse evaluates that the teaching has been understood when one of the participants states:
1. "All meats and cream-based foods need to be refrigerated."
2. "Once most food is cooked it does not need to be refrigerated."
3. "Poultry should be stuffed and then refrigerated before cooking."
4. "Cooked food should be cooled before being put into the refrigerator."

577. The laboratory values of a client with cancer of the esophagus show a hemoglobin of 7 g/dL, hematocrit of 29%, and RBC count of 2.5 million/mm^3. Considering these data, the most appropriate nursing diagnosis for the client at this time is:
1. Altered nutrition: less than body requirements related to dysphagia
2. Ineffective airway clearance related to tumor growth and metastasis
3. Pain related to pressure of tumor on surrounding tissues and nerves
4. High risk for injury related to possible metastasis and subsequent airway obstruction

578. Immediately after esophageal surgery the priority nursing assessment concerns the client's:
1. Incision
2. Respirations
3. Level of pain
4. Nasogastric tube

579. A client with achalasia is to have bougienage to dilate the lower esophagus and cardiac sphincter. Following the procedure the nurse should assess the client for esophageal perforation, which is indicated by:
1. Faintness and feelings of fullness
2. Diaphoresis and cardiac palpitations
3. Increased heart rate and thoracic pain
4. Increased blood pressure and frequent burping

580. A client with a hiatal hernia asks the nurse how to best prevent esophageal reflux. The nurse's best response would be:
1. "Increase your intake of fat with each meal."
2. "Lie down after you have eaten to help your digestion."
3. "Reduce your caloric intake to foster weight reduction."
4. "Drink several glasses of fluid during and immediately after each of your meals."

581. When performing the initial history and physical of a client with a tentative diagnosis of peptic ulcer, the nurse would expect the client to describe the pain as:
1. Gnawing epigastric pain or boring pain in the back
2. Sudden, sharp abdominal pain, increasing in intensity
3. Heartburn and substernal discomfort when lying down
4. Located in the right shoulder and preceded by nausea

582. A client develops gastric bleeding and is hospitalized. An important etiologic clue for the nurse to explore while taking this client's history would be:
1. Any recent foreign travel
2. The client's usual dietary pattern
3. Any change in status of family relationships
4. The medications that the client has been taking

583. Once a client's gastric bleeding is controlled, the physician orders individual dietary management. The meal pattern that would probably be most appropriate for this client would be:
1. A flexible plan according to the client's appetite
2. Limited food and fluid intake when pain is present
3. Regular meals and snacks to limit gastric discomfort
4. Three meals large enough to supply adequate energy

584. Following an acute episode of upper GI bleeding, a client vomits undigested antacids and complains of severe epigastric pain. The nursing assessment reveals an absence of bowel sounds, pulse rate of 134, and shallow respirations of 32 per minute. In addition to calling the physician, the nurse should:
1. Start O_2 per nasal cannula at 3 to 4 L per minute
2. Keep the client npo in preparation for possible surgery
3. Ask the client if any red or black stools have been noted
4. Place the client in the supine position with the legs elevated

585. Following a subtotal gastrectomy (Billroth I) a client begins to eat more food in varied forms. After meals the client experiences a cramping discomfort and a rapid pulse with waves of weakness, which are frequently followed by nausea and vomiting. The nurse recognizes that this response is known as the "dumping syndrome" and is caused by:
1. A slowed passage of food dumping into the small intestine
2. A rapid passage of dilute food mixture into the small intestine
3. Rapid passage of hyperosmolar food solution into the small intestine
4. Food that is less concentrated than surrounding extracellular fluid entering the small intestine

586. A client with gastric cancer asks if this cancer will spread. The nurse recognizes that the client is looking for reassurance, but knows that gastric cancers are most likely to metastasize to the:
1. Liver and lung
2. Bone and brain
3. Pancreas and brain
4. Lymph nodes and blood

587. Twelve hours after a subtotal gastrectomy, the nurse notes large amounts of bloody drainage from the client's nasogastric tube. The nurse should:
1. Instill 30 ml of iced normal saline into the tube
2. Clamp the tube and call the physician immediately
3. Report the type and quantity of drainage to the physician
4. Continue to monitor the drainage and record the observations

588. After a client has a total gastrectomy, the nurse should plan to include in the discharge teaching the need for:
1. Weekly injections of vitamin B_{12}
2. Regular daily use of a stool softener
3. Monthly injections of iron dextran (Imferon)
4. Daily replacement therapy of pancreatic enzymes

589. The nurse discusses dietary needs with a client who has had a gastroduodenostomy (Billroth I). The nurse knows that the teaching was understood when the client states, "I will plan:
1. Five or six small meals every day, limiting bulk."
2. A diet of blenderized foods for an indefinite period."
3. To gradually resume my normal eating routine and diet."
4. A diet high in carbohydrates, proteins, and fats to replace lost nutrients."

590. After 2 months of self-management for symptoms of gastritis is unsuccessful, a client goes to the physician and extensive carcinoma of the stomach is diagnosed. The client asks the nurse how the disease got so advanced. The nurse's explanation should be based on the knowledge that carcinoma of the stomach is:

1. Difficult to accurately diagnose until late in the disease process
2. Painful in early stages and often misdiagnosed as myocardial infarction
3. Usually diagnosed following the discovery of enlarged lymph nodes in the epigastric area
4. Rarely diagnosed early because the symptoms are usually nonspecific until late in the disease

591. A client with extensive gastric carcinoma is to be admitted to the hospital for an esophagojejunostomy. When preparing this client for surgery, the nurse should include information about the possibility that:
1. A chest tube will be in place in addition to a nasogastric tube
2. Liquids by mouth may be permitted the evening after surgery
3. Complete bedrest may be necessary for 48 hours after surgery
4. The Trendelenburg position will be used on the first day after surgery

592. When teaching a client how to avoid the dumping syndrome following a gastrectomy, the nurse should emphasize:
1. Increasing activity after eating
2. Avoiding excess fluids with meals
3. Eating heavy meals to delay emptying
4. Providing carbohydrates with each meal

593. Immediately after a subtotal gastrectomy a client returns to the surgical unit. The nurse irrigates the nasogastric tube and notes small blood clots in the return. The nurse should:
1. Clamp the nasogastric tube
2. Consider this a normal event
3. Irrigate the tube with iced saline
4. Notify the physician of this finding

594. On the third postoperative day after a subtotal gastrectomy, a client complains of severe abdominal pain. The nurse palpates the client's abdomen and notes rigidity. The nurse should first:

1. Assist the client to ambulate
2. Assess the client's vital signs
3. Administer the prescribed analgesic
4. Encourage the use of the spirometer

595. To determine when a client who has had a subtotal gastrectomy can begin oral feedings after surgery, the nurse must assess for the:
1. Presence of flatulence (Bowel sounds)
2. Extent of incisional pain
3. Stabilization of hematocrit
4. Occurrence of dumping syndrome

596. A client who has had a gastric ulcer asks what to do if the epigastric pain occurs. The nurse would know that the teaching was effective when the client states, "I will:
1. Increase my food intake."
2. Take the aspirin with milk."
3. Eliminate fluids with meals."
4. Take an antacid preparation."

597. A client is diagnosed as having a peptic ulcer. When teaching about peptic ulcers, the nurse should instruct the client to report any stools that appear:
1. Frothy
2. Ribbon shaped
3. Pale or clay colored
4. Dark brown or black

598. Following abdominal surgery a client returns to the unit with a nasogastric tube in place. The physician has ordered Phenergan 50 mg IM q6h prn for nausea. When the client complains of nausea the first action by the nurse should be to:
1. Notify the physician of the problem
2. Administer the ordered Phenergan IM
3. Check for placement of the nasogastric tube
4. Irrigate the nasogastric tube with normal saline

599. A male client has a subtotal gastrectomy because of a perforated gastric ulcer. Postoperatively he has a nasogastric tube to low suction and IV fluids. Three hours after surgery the client complains of nausea and abdominal pain, his abdomen appears distended, and there are no bowel sounds. Considering the type of surgery and the orders for pain medication and irrigation of the NG tube, the nurse should first:
1. Irrigate the nasogastric tube
2. Give the prn pain medication
3. Check stools and gastric drainage for blood
4. Notify the physician of absent bowel sounds

600. The nurse notes some bright red blood in a client's nasogastric drainage four hours after a subtotal gastrectomy. The nurse should:
1. Gently irrigate the tube with 30 ml normal saline
2. Clamp the nasogastric tube and call the physician
3. Continue to monitor the drainage from the tube and record the observations
4. Reduce the pressure on the suction and record observations of the drainage

601. The day before a client who has had a subtotal gastrectomy is to be discharged, the client complains of perspiring and having epigastric discomfort about a half hour after eating lunch. The symptoms disappear within a few minutes. The nurse recognizes that the teaching about prevention is understood when the client states, "I can limit these symptoms by:
1. Increasing fluids with each meal."
2. Avoiding spicy, gas-forming meals."
3. Resting before and after each meal."
4. Eating small, low carbohydrate meals."

602. Following a subtotal gastrectomy a client develops the dumping syndrome. In addition, about 2 hours after the initial postmeal attack, the client experiences a second period of discomfort, feeling somewhat "shaky." The nurse recognizes that this later follow-up effect, which is precipitated by the dumping syndrome, is caused by:

1. The increased use of simple carbohydrates in meals creating a more prolonged glucose rise
2. The increased fat content and larger amount of seasoned food creating digestive discomfort
3. Hyperglycemia from a rapidly absorbed glucose load which overwhelms the insulin-adjusting mechanism
4. Mild hypoglycemia from an overproduction of insulin that occurs in response to the postprandial blood glucose rise

603. The characteristics that would alert the nurse that a client is at increased risk of developing gallbladder disease would be:
1. Female, over the age of 40, obese
2. Male, under the age of 40, past history of hepatitis
3. Male, over the age of 40, low serum cholesterol level
4. Female, under the age of 40, family history of gallstones

604. A client with a tentative diagnosis of cholecystitis is discharged from the emergency room with instructions to make an appointment for a more definitive diagnostic workup. The recommendation that would produce the most valuable diagnostic information would be:
1. "Keep a journal related to your pain."
2. "Save all stool and urine for inspection."
3. "Follow the doctor's orders exactly without question."
4. "Keep a record of the amount of fluid you drink daily."

605. The nurse asks a client to make a list of the foods that cause dyspepsia. If the client has cholecystitis, the foods that are most likely to be included on this list would be:
1. Nuts and popcorn
2. Meatloaf and baked potato
3. Chocolate and boiled shrimp
4. Fried chicken and buttered corn

606. The physician orders a modified diet for a client with cholecystitis. The nurse understands that with cholecystitis:

1. Soft-textured foods are used to reduce the digestive burden
2. Low-cholesterol foods are used to avoid further formation of gallstones
3. Fat is decreased to avoid stimulation of the cholecystokinin mechanism for bile release
4. Increased protein and kilocalories are necessary to promote tissue healing and provide energy

607. A client develops a gallstone that becomes lodged in the common bile duct. The physician schedules an endoscopic sphincterotomy. Preoperative teaching should include information that for the procedure the client will:
1. Have spinal anesthesia
2. Have general anesthesia
3. Receive an epidural block
4. Receive an intravenous sedative

608. A client has cholelithiasis with possible obstruction of the common bile duct. Before the scheduled cholecystectomy, nutritional deficiencies and excesses should be corrected. A nutritional assessment should be conducted to determine if the client:
1. Is deficient in vitamins A, D, and K
2. Eats adequate amounts of dietary fiber
3. Consumes excessive amounts of protein
4. Has excessive levels of potassium and folic acid

609. A client undergoes an abdominal cholecystectomy with common duct exploration. In the immediate postoperative period, the nursing action that should assume the highest priority for this client is:
1. Irrigating the T-tube frequently
2. Changing the dressing at least bid
3. Encouraging coughing and deep breathing
4. Promoting an adequate fluid intake by mouth

610. The nurse is aware that a client's T-tube has been inserted during a resection of the pancreas to:
1. Divert the bile flow to the cystic duct
2. Drain blood and pus from the operative site
3. Prevent postoperative infection at the site of the incision
4. Facilitate bile drainage while the common duct is edematous

611. A client returns from surgery after a resection of the pancreas for cancer with a T-tube in place. The nurse recognizes that immediately after this surgery the position that would provide the most comfort for the client is the:
1. Sims' position
2. Supine position
3. Side-lying position
4. Low Fowler's position

612. Because of prolonged bile drainage, a client may develop symptoms related to a lack of fat-soluble vitamins such as:
1. Easy bruising
2. Muscle twitching
3. Excessive jaundice
4. Tingling of the fingers

613. A client with cholelithiasis is scheduled for a lithotripsy. Preoperative teaching should include the information that:
1. Narcotics will be available for postoperative pain
2. A fever is a common response after this intervention
3. Heart palpitations frequently occur after the procedure
4. Analgesics and anesthetics are not necessary during the procedure

614. Following a laparoscopic laser cholecystectomy a client is to be discharged. The nurse would recognize that the discharge instructions were understood when the client states:
1. "I can change the bandages every day."
2. "I should remain on a full liquid diet for 3 days."
3. "I should not bathe the surgical sites for a week."
4. "I may have mild shoulder pain for about a week."

615. After a cholecystectomy, a client asks if there are any dietary restrictions that must be followed. The nurse would recognize that the dietary teaching was understood when the client tells a family member:
1. "I will need to avoid fatty foods for the rest of my life."
2. "I should not eat those foods that upset me before I had surgery."
3. "Most people can tolerate a regular diet after this type of surgery."
4. "Most people need to eat a high protein diet for several months after surgery."

616. A client with cancer of the pancreas has surgery and the Whipple procedure is performed. After surgery, the nurse should expect the client to have a:
1. Chest tube
2. Intestinal tube
3. Nasogastric tube
4. Gastrostomy tube

617. A client has an extensive surgical revision of the head of the pancreas because of cancer. After surgery, to decrease the chance of hemorrhage at the operative site the nurse should:
1. Keep the client in the supine position
2. Maintain patency of the nasogastric tube
3. Replace fat-soluble vitamins as necessary
4. Administer the ordered tube feeding slowly

618. When teaching a client about the diet following a Whipple procedure performed for cancer of the pancreas, the statement the nurse should include would be:
1. "There are no dietary restrictions; you may eat what you desire."
2. "Your diet should be low in calories to prevent taxing your diseased pancreas."
3. "Meals should be restricted in protein because of your compromised liver function."
4. "Low-fat meals should be eaten because of interference with your fat digestion mechanism."

619. A long-term complication that a client must be made aware of following a Whipple procedure for cancer of the pancreas is hypoinsulinism. The nurse would know that the teaching about hypoinsulinism is understood when the client states, "I should seek medical supervision if I experience:
1. Oliguria."
2. Anorexia."
3. Weight gain."
4. Increased thirst."

620. After revision of the pancreas because of cancer, total parenteral nutrition is instituted via a central venous infusion route. During the fourth hour of the first infusion the client complains of nausea, fatigue, and a headache. The hourly urine output is twice the amount of the previous hour. The nurse should call the physician and:
1. Stop the infusion and cover the insertion site
2. Slow the infusion and check the serum glucose level
3. Prepare the client for immediate surgery for possible bowel obstruction
4. Increase fluids via a peripheral IV route and give analgesics for the headache

621. A client is to be discharged with a percutaneous catheter for home administration of total parenteral nutrition (TPN). The nurse should help the client to:
1. Learn how to change the percutaneous catheter
2. Determine which days to self-administer the TPN
3. Schedule the TPN administration around meal times
4. Arrange professional help to monitor the administration of the TPN

622. After surgery for cancer of the pancreas, the client's nutritional and fluid regimen will be influenced by the remaining amount of functioning pancreatic tissue. Considering both the exocrine and endocrine functions of the pancreas, the client's postoperative regimen would primarily include managing the intake of:
1. Alcohol and caffeine
2. Vitamins and minerals
3. Fluids and electrolytes
4. Fats and carbohydrates

623. A client with a 20 year history of excessive alcohol use is admitted to the hospital with jaundice and ascites. A priority nursing action during the first 48 hours after the client's admission will be to:
1. Monitor the client's vital signs (withdrawal)
2. Increase the client's fluid intake
3. Improve the client's nutritional status
4. Identify the client's reasons for drinking

624. The nurse, aware of a client's 25 year history of excessive alcohol use, would expect the physical assessment to reveal a:
1. Hepatitis A
2. Low blood ammonia
3. Small liver with a rough surface
4. High fever with a generalized rash

625. A male client with liver dysfunction reports that his gums bleed spontaneously. In addition, the nurse notes small hemorrhagic lesions on his face. The nurse recognizes that the client needs additional:
1. Bile salts
2. Folic acid
3. Vitamin A
4. Vitamin K

626. A client with ascites is scheduled for a paracentesis. To prepare the client for the abdominal paracentesis the nurse should:
1. Medicate the client for pain
2. Encourage the client to drink fluids
3. Shave and prep the client's abdomen
4. Instruct the client to empty the bladder

627. A client is admitted with the diagnosis of hepatitis A. The information from the client's history that is most likely linked to hepatitis A is:
1. Working for a local plumber
2. Washing dishes at a local restaurant
3. Working in a hemodialysis unit of a hospital
4. Being exposed to arsenic compounds at work

628. A client with jaundice associated with hepatitis expresses concern over the change in skin color. The nurse should recognize that this color change is due to:

1. Stimulation of the liver to produce an excess quantity of bile pigments
2. The inability of the liver to remove normal amounts of bilirubin from blood
3. Increased destruction of the red blood cells during the acute phase of the disease
4. Decreased prothrombin levels, leading to multiple sites of spontaneous intradermal bleeding

629. After an acute episode of hepatitis a client is to be discharged to continue recovery at home. The nurse should expect that the diet the physician will order will be:
1. Low-calorie, high-protein, low-carbohydrate, low fat
2. High-calorie, low-protein, high-carbohydrate, high-fat
3. Low-calorie, low-protein, low-carbohydrate, moderate-fat
4. High-calorie, high-protein, high-carbohydrate, moderate-fat

630. A mother whose son has hepatitis A states that there is only one bathroom in their home and she is worried that other members of the family could get hepatitis. The nurse's best reply would be:
1. "I suggest that you buy a commode exclusively for your son's use."
2. "There is no problem with your son sharing the same bathroom with everyone."
3. "Your son may use the bathroom, but you need to use disposable toilet seat covers."
4. "It is important that your son and all family members wash their hands after using the bathroom."

631. The physician orders enteric precautions for a client with hepatitis A. In addition to universal precautions the isolation procedures that must be followed are:
1. A private room is required, and the door must be kept closed
2. Persons entering the room must wear a gown, a mask, and gloves
3. Gowns and gloves must be worn only when handling the client's soiled linen, dishes, or utensils
4. A gown and gloves must be worn when handling articles possibly contaminated by urine and/or feces

632. A client has a temporary diagnosis of primary biliary cirrhosis. Symptoms include jaundice, ascites, and peripheral edema. When performing the physical assessment, the skin change the nurse would expect to observe is:
1. Vitiligo
2. Hirsutism
3. Melanuria
4. Telangiectasis

633. Immediately following a liver biopsy, a client is placed on the right side. The nurse explains that this position should be maintained for 60 to 90 minutes because it will:
1. Help stop bleeding if any occurs
2. Restore circulating blood volume
3. Be the position of greatest comfort
4. Help reduce fluid trapped in the biliary ducts

634. Following a liver biopsy the nurse checks the client's dressing and notices a moderately large amount of bile-colored drainage. The client also complains of right upper quadrant pain. The nurse should recognize that:
1. Fluid is leaking into the intestine
2. The pancreas has been lacerated
3. A biliary vessel has been penetrated
4. This is the normal, expected response

635. The serum ammonia level of a client with cirrhosis is elevated. As a priority the nurse should:
1. Weigh the client daily
2. Observe for increasing confusion
3. Measure the urine specific gravity
4. Restrict the client's oral fluid intake

636. A client with esophageal varices has severe hematemesis, and the physician is going to insert a Sengstaken-Blakemore tube. The nurse is aware that this tube is a:
1. Single-lumen tube for gastric lavage
2. Double-lumen tube for intestinal decompression
3. Triple-lumen tube used to compress the esophagus
4. Multi-lumen tube for gastric and intestinal decompression

637. A client develops peritonitis and sepsis following the surgical repair of a ruptured diverticulum. The nurse should expect an assessment of the client to reveal:
1. Bradycardia
2. Hypertension
3. Abdominal rigidity
4. Increased bowel sounds

638. One month after abdominal surgery a client is readmitted with recurrent abdominal pain and fever. The diagnosis is fistula formation with peritonitis. The nurse should place the client in the:
1. Supine position
2. Right Sims' position
3. Semi-Fowler's position
4. Position that is most comfortable

639. A client with colitis inquires as to whether surgery will ever be necessary. When teaching about the disease and its treatment, the nurse should emphasize that:
1. Medical treatment for colitis is curative, and surgery is not needed
2. Surgery for colitis is considered only as a last resort for most clients
3. Surgery for colitis is done early in the course of the disease for most clients
4. Medical treatment is all that will be needed if the client can acquire some emotional stability

640. After surgery for creation of an ileostomy the client is to be discharged. Before discharge the primary nursing intervention should be to:
1. Coax the client into caring for the ileostomy
2. Evaluate the client's ability to care for the ileostomy
3. Ensure that the client understands the dietary limitations that must be followed
4. Have the client change the dry sterile dressing on the incision without assistance

641. When teaching a client about the signs of colorectal cancer, the nurse stresses that the most common complaint of persons with colorectal cancer is:

1. Abdominal pain
2. Rectal bleeding
3. Change in bowel habits
4. Change in caliber of stools

642. A client with a diagnosis of cancer of the sigmoid colon is to have an abdominoperineal resection with a permanent colostomy. Before surgery a low-residue diet is ordered. The nurse explains that this is necessary to:
1. Lower the bacterial count in the GI tract
2. Limit production of flatus in the intestine
3. Prevent irritation of the intestinal mucosa
4. Reduce the amount of stool in the large bowel

643. An abdominoperineal resection with a colostomy is scheduled for a client with cancer of the rectum. The nurse recognizes that the physician will need the client to sign a consent for a:
1. Permanent sigmoid colostomy
2. Permanent ascending colostomy
3. Temporary double-barrel colostomy
4. Temporary transverse loop colostomy

644. A client has a permanent sigmoid colostomy because of cancer. The physician orders daily colostomy irrigations. The nurse should explain to the client that the primary purpose of these irrigations is to:
1. Prevent straining at passage of stool
2. Establish a regular elimination schedule
3. Decrease the amount of flatus in the bowel
4. Limit the amount of fluid lost from the intestine

645. To promote perineal wound healing after an abdominoperineal resection, the nurse should encourage the client to assume the:
1. Knee-chest position
2. Left or right Sims' position
3. Dorsal recumbent position
4. Left or right side-lying position

646. The nurse plans to teach a client to irrigate a new colostomy when the:
1. Abdominal incision is closed and contamination is no longer a danger
2. Stool starts to become formed, around the seventh postoperative day

3. Client can lie on the side comfortably, about the third postoperative day
4. Perineal wound heals and the client can sit comfortably on the commode

647. The discharge teaching for a client with a colostomy should include instructing the client that the problem during colostomy irrigation at home that should be reported to the physician is:
1. Abdominal cramps during fluid inflow
2. A difficulty in inserting the irrigating tube
3. Passage of flatus during expulsion of feces
4. An inability to complete the procedure in an hour

648. A client returns from surgery with a permanent colostomy. During the first 24 hours the colostomy does not drain. The nurse should realize this is a result of:
1. Intestinal edema following surgery
2. A presurgical decrease in fluid intake
3. The absence of gastrointestinal motility
4. Proper functioning of nasogastric suction

649. When preparing to teach a male client how to irrigate his colostomy, the nurse should plan to perform the procedure:
1. At least 2 hours before visitors
2. Prior to breakfast and morning care
3. After the client accepts his altered body image
4. When the client would have normally had a bowel movement

650. When observing a return demonstration of a colostomy irrigation, the nurse knows that more teaching is required if the client:
1. Clamps off the flow of fluid when feeling uncomfortable
2. Lubricates the tip of the catheter prior to inserting it into the stoma
3. Discontinues the insertion of fluid after only 500 ml of fluid have been instilled
4. Hangs the irrigation bag on the bathroom door clothes hook during fluid insertion

651. The nurse is aware that teaching about colostomy care is understood when the client states, "I will contact my physician and report:
1. If I notice a loss of sensation to touch in the stoma tissue."
2. When mucus is passed from the stoma between irrigations."
3. The expulsion of flatus while the irrigating fluid is running out."
4. If I have any difficulty in inserting the irrigating tube in the stoma."

652. The nurse would know that dietary teaching for a client with a colostomy had been effective when the client states, "It is important that I eat:
1. Food low in fiber so that there is less stool."
2. Bland foods so that my intestines do not become irritated."
3. Everything I ate before the operation while avoiding foods that cause gas."
4. Soft foods that are more easily digested and absorbed by my large intestine."

653. A client is admitted for repair of bilateral inguinal hernias under general anesthesia. Before surgery the nurse would assess the client for signs that strangulation may have occurred. An early sign of strangulation would be:
1. Increased flatus
2. Projectile vomiting
3. Sharp abdominal pain
4. Decreased bowel sounds

654. After a bilateral herniorrhaphy a male client should be observed for the development of:
1. A hydrocele
2. Paralytic ileus
3. Urinary retention
4. Thrombophlebitis

DRUG RELATED RESPONSES

655. The physician orders 8 mg of morphine sulfate to be given by injection. The vial on hand is labeled 1 ml = 10 mg. The nurse should administer:
1. 8 minims
2. 10 minims
3. 12 minims
4. 15 minims

656. The nurse should be aware that hydroxyzine hydrochloride (Vistaril) is administered as a preoperative sedative to:
1. Inhibit peristalsis
2. Promote unconsciousness
3. Limit the development of dysrhythmias
4. Reduce the amount of necessary narcotics

657. The physician orders 0.2 mg of cyanocobalamin (vitamin B_{12}) IM for a client with pernicious anemia. A vial of the drug labeled 1 ml = 100 mcg is available. The nurse should administer:
1. 0.5 ml
2. 1.0 ml
3. 1.5 ml
4. 2.0 ml

658. The physician orders lidocaine HCl 1.5 mg per minute for a client whose ECG tracing reveals multiple PVBs. The nurse adds 500 mg of lidocaine HCl to 100 ml of D5W. The drop factor of the IV set is 60 gtt/ml. To administer the correct amount of medication the nurse should set the IV at:
1. 10 gtt/minute
2. 12 gtt/minute
3. 14 gtt/minute
4. 18 gtt/minute

659. The physician orders cefazolin sodium (Kefzol) 375 mg IVPB every 8 hours. The vial of powder contains 500 mg of the drug. This must be reconstituted with 2 ml of 0.9% sodium chloride. In the resulting solution 1 ml equals 225 mg of Kefzol. The nurse should administer:
1. 1.2 ml
2. 2.2 ml
3. 20 minims
4. 25 minims

660. The physician orders aminocaproic acid (Amicar Elixir) 4 grams po for a client with an intracerebral hemorrhage. The bottle is labeled 250 mg/ml. The nurse should administer:
1. 16 ml
2. 1.6 ml

3. 0.16 ml
4. 0.016 ml

661. The physician orders 250 mg of an antibiotic IVPB. A vial containing 1 g of the powdered form of the drug must be reconstituted with 2.8 ml of diluent to form a withdrawable volume of 3 ml. Using this solution, the nurse should administer:
1. 8 minims
2. 10 minims
3. 12 minims
4. 17 minims

662. The physician orders Humulin N insulin 30 U every AM. The nurse has Humulin N insulin 100 U/ml but no insulin syringe. The nurse should administer:
1. 3 minims
2. 5 minims
3. 7 minims
4. 9 minims

663. The physician orders penicillin G benzathine suspension (Bicillin L-A) 2.45 million units for a client with a sexually transmitted disease. The drug is available in a multidose vial of 10 ml in which 1 ml= 300,000 units. The nurse should administer:
1. 8.8 ml
2. 8.2 ml
3. 0.8 ml
4. 0.008 ml

664. The physician orders 1000 mcg of procainamide (Pronestyl) IV per minute. The directions state 500 mg of the drug should be added to 500 ml of D5W. The IV set has a drop factor of 60 gtt/ml. To administer the medication correctly the nurse should set the flow rate at:
1. 30 gtt/min
2. 60 gtt/min
3. 90 gtt/min
4. 120 gtt/min

665. The physician orders 1200 mg of an antibiotic to be added to 50 ml D5W qid IVPB via a Heplock. The vial contains 5 g of powdered antibiotic to which 12 ml of diluent is to be

added. The resulting solution contains 1 gram of drug per 3 ml. The nurse should use:
1. 0.7 ml
2. 1.2 ml
3. 2.9 ml
4. 3.6 ml

666. Tuberculosis is confirmed and isoniazid (INH) and rifampin (Rifadin) therapy is prescribed for a client. The client says, "I've never had to take so much antibiotic for an infection before." The nurse should explain:
1. "Rifampin prevents side effects from INH."
2. "This type of organism is difficult to destroy."
3. "You'll need only one medication when you get better."
4. "Your infection is well advanced and needs aggressive therapy."

667. A client with tuberculosis is started on a chemotherapy protocol that includes rifampin (Rifadin). The nurse knows the teaching about rifampin was effective when the client states:
1. "I will have my hearing tested while I take this medicine."
2. "I will drink large amounts of fluid while I take this medicine."
3. "A skin rash is normal with rifampin and nothing to worry about."
4. "It's normal for my urine to be orange colored from this medication."

668. The physician prescribes vitamin B_6 and isoniazid (INH) as part of the chemotherapy protocol for a client with tuberculosis. The nurse understands that vitamin B_6 is used because it:
1. Improves the nutritional status of the client
2. Enhances the tuberculostatic effect of isoniazid (INH)
3. Accelerates the destruction of dormant tubercular bacilli
4. Counteracts the peripheral neuritis that isoniazid may cause

669. A client with a diagnosis of tuberculosis has been receiving isoniazid (INH) as part of a chemotherapy protocol. During a subsequent clinic visit the nurse should recognize that prompt intervention is required when the client develops:
1. Yellow sclera
2. Orange stools
3. A temperature of 96.8°F
4. A weight gain of 5 pounds

670. A client is diagnosed as having pulmonary tuberculosis and one of the drugs the physician orders is pyrazinamide (PZA). The nurse evaluates that the teaching concerning the drug was effective when the client says, "I will:
1. Drink at least 2 quarts of fluid a day."
2. Take the medication 2 hours after each meal."
3. Report any changes in vision to the physician."
4. Expect a discoloration of my urine, sweat, and tears."

671. A client is diagnosed with tuberculosis associated with HIV infection. The test results that are crucial for the nurse to review before starting antitubercular pharmacotherapy are:
1. Liver function studies
2. Pulmonary function studies
3. Electrocardiogram and echocardiogram
4. White blood cell counts and sedimentation rate

672. A client with AIDS is receiving Azidothymidine (AZT). It is most important for the nurse to monitor the client's:
1. Cardiac enzymes
2. Serum electrolytes
3. HIV antibody levels
4. Complete blood count

673. A client with HIV associated *Pneumocystis carinii* pneumonia is to receive pentamidine isethionate (Pentam) IV once daily. To ensure client safety the nurse should:
1. Mix the drug with sterile saline without a preservative
2. Monitor the blood pressure for hypertension during therapy
3. Administer the drug over a period of twenty to thirty minutes
4. Assess blood glucose levels daily during therapy and several times after therapy

674. A client who is receiving mechanical ventilation begins to "fight" the respirator and the physician orders atracurium (Tracrium). The most important nursing action for a client receiving Tracrium is to:
1. Decrease anxiety
2. Monitor skin integrity
3. Promote urinary output
4. Maintain mechanical ventilation

675. The physician orders 50 U of insulin to be added to an IV of glucose and water for a preoperative client with diabetes mellitus. The nurse understands that the only insulin that can be used is:
1. NPH insulin
2. Lente insulin
3. Regular insulin
4. Ultralente insulin

676. A client, newly diagnosed as a non-insulin dependent diabetic, is receiving glyburide (Micronase) and asks the nurse how this drug works. The nurse answers the question about Micronase by telling the client it acts by:
1. Stimulating the beta cells to produce insulin
2. Accelerating the liver's release of stored glycogen
3. Increasing glucose transport across the cell membrane
4. Lowering blood sugar in the absence of beta cell function

677. A client is diagnosed as having non-insulin dependent diabetes mellitus and the physician prescribes chlorpropamide (Diabinese). While taking this medication, the client should be taught to observe for:
1. Ketonuria
2. Weight loss
3. Ketoacidosis
4. Hypoglycemia

678. A client with insulin dependent diabetes mellitus receives NPH insulin (Humulin N)

every morning at 8 AM. The nurse recognizes that the client understands the action of this insulin when the client says, "I should be alert for signs of hypoglycemia between:
1. 10 AM and Noon."
2. 2 PM and 4 PM."
3. 4 PM and 6 PM."
4. 8 PM and 10 PM."

679. A client with newly diagnosed insulin dependent diabetes mellitus is in a self-care teaching group. The nurse has confidence that the client is able to recognize hypoglycemia when the client states, "I will drink orange juice and eat a slice of bread when I feel:
1. Nervous and weak."
2. Flushed and short of breath."
3. Thirsty and have a headache."
4. Nauseated and have abdominal cramps."

680. A client with hyperthyroidism is treated first with propylthiouracil (PTU). When teaching the client about this medication, the nurse should include the information that:
1. This medication will have to be taken for the remainder of life
2. Symptoms may not subside for several days or weeks after the start of therapy
3. Milk should be taken with the medication so that gastric irritation does not occur
4. The medication should be taken between meals so that it is more readily absorbed

681. A client receiving allopurinol (Zyloprim) for gout is also diagnosed as having non-insulin dependent diabetes mellitus (NIDDM) and the physician orders chlorpropamide (Diabinese). At a follow-up visit the following week the client states, "I've been fainting and sweating a lot in the past week." The nurse should realize that the:
1. Diabinese should be changed to insulin
2. Diabinese dosage may have to be reduced
3. Zyloprim and Diabinese should be alternated daily
4. Zyloprim should be eliminated from the medication regimen

682. On a clinic visit an elderly client with rheumatoid arthritis tells the nurse that the prescribed aspirin to reduce pain has helped. The client asks if the arthritis could have moved to the ears because both ears now are buzzing. The nurse recognizes that ringing in the ears is:
1. A symptom of otitis media
2. A normal part of the aging process
3. Evidence of eighth cranial nerve damage
4. Caused by an accumulation of cerumen in the ear

683. The physician orders ibuprofen (Motrin) 800 mg po tid for a client with rheumatoid arthritis. The nurse would know that the teaching about the side effects of Motrin was effective when the client:
1. Makes an appointment for blood work in 1 month
2. Recognizes that exercise must be balanced with rest
3. Realizes that any position changes should be made slowly
4. Understands that the medication must be taken between meals

684. A client who takes 4 tablets of buffered aspirin 4 times a day for arthritis complains of dizziness and ringing in the ears. The nurse should recognize that the client is probably experiencing:
1. Salicylate toxicity
2. An allergic reaction
3. Withdrawal symptoms
4. Acetaminophen overdose

685. A client who has had a long leg cast applied is to be discharged. When discussing pain management, the nurse should advise the client to take the prescribed prn Tylenol with codeine:
1. Just as a last resort
2. Before going to sleep
3. When the discomfort begins
4. As the pain becomes intense

686. A client had a laminectomy and is receiving a skeletal muscle relaxant that will be continued after discharge. After teaching the client about the skeletal muscle relaxant, the nurse recognizes that no further health teaching is necessary when the client says:
1. "If the medication makes me sleepy, I'll stop taking it."
2. "I'm going to take the medication 3 hours after I've eaten."
3. "If the medication upsets my stomach, I'll take it with milk."
4. "I'll take an extra dose of the medication before I do anything active."

687. The physician orders a low dosage of narcotic to relieve the pain of a client with deep partial-thickness burns. The nurse recognizes that the preferred mode of administration is:
1. Oral
2. Rectal
3. Intravenous
4. Intramuscular

688. A female client is receiving Ethylestrenol (Maxibolin), an anabolic steroid, for the treatment of the catabolic processes associated with a burn injury. The nurse should observe the client for signs of:
1. Lethargy
2. Virilization
3. Hyponatremia
4. Hyperglycemia

689. The nurse applies mafenide acetate cream (Sulfamylon) to a client's burns as ordered by the physician. This medication will:
1. Inhibit bacterial growth
2. Relieve pain from the burn
3. Prevent scar tissue formation
4. Provide chemical debridement

690. The physician prescribes isosorbide dinitrate (Sorbitrate) 10 mg prn tid and a nitroglycerin transdermal disc once a day for a client with chronic angina pectoris. The client asks the nurse why the Sorbitrate is prescribed. The nurse's best response would be:
1. "It prevents the blood from clotting."
2. "It suppresses irritability in the ventricles."
3. "It allows more oxygen to get to the heart tissue."
4. "It increases the force of contraction of the heart."

691. When teaching a client about isosorbide dinitrate (Sorbitrate), the nurse should plan to include instructions about how to prevent:
1. Bradycardia
2. Constipation
3. Respiratory distress
4. Postural hypotension

692. The nurse teaches a client about the side effects of furosemide (Lasix) which has just been prescribed. The nurse assesses that the teaching was understood when the client states, "I should:
1. Wear dark glasses."
2. Avoid lying flat in bed."
3. Avoid eating citrus fruits."
4. Change my position slowly."

693. At each clinic visit, the nurse should assess a client taking furosemide (Lasix) for:
1. Tinnitus
2. Xanthopsia
3. Hyporeflexia
4. Bronchospasm

694. A client with a history of hypertension comes to the emergency room with double vision and a blood pressure of 260/120. In addition to other drugs, the physician orders a nitroprusside (Nipride) infusion. The nurse recognizes that Nipride decreases blood pressure by:
1. Increasing cardiac output
2. Decreasing the heart rate
3. Increasing peripheral resistance
4. Relaxing venous and arterial muscles

695. A client is receiving clonidine (Catapres) for hypertension. The nurse would recognize that the discharge instructions were understood when the client states, "I will call the doctor if I develop:
1. Pruritus."
2. Diarrhea."
3. Euphoria."
4. Photosensitivity."

696. A client with hypertensive heart disease, who had an acute episode of congestive heart failure, is to be discharged on propranolol HCl (Inderal) and digoxin (Lanoxin). The nurse should be aware that Inderal, when administered with Lanoxin, may:
1. Produce a headache
2. Precipitate bradycardia
3. Increase the blood pressure
4. Stimulate nodal conduction

697. The physician adjusts a client's dosages of digoxin and Warfarin sodium (Coumadin). The antidote for Coumadin that the nurse should keep in the client's medicine drawer is:
1. Vitamin K
2. Fibrinogen
3. Prothrombin
4. Protamine sulfate

698. A client who recently has had a myocardial infarction is to continue to take digoxin (Lanoxin) following discharge from the hospital. The nurse would know the teaching concerning digoxin is understood when the client states, "I should:
1. Increase my intake of vitamin K."
2. Not eat foods high in potassium."
3. Check my pulse rate and rhythm daily."
4. Adjust my dosage according to my activities."

699. The physician orders furosemide (Lasix) for a client with hypervolemia. The nurse understands that Lasix exerts its effects in the:
1. Distal tubule
2. Collecting duct
3. Glomerulus of the nephron
4. Ascending limb of Henle's loop

700. A client has been receiving a cardiac glycoside, a diuretic, and a vasodilator and is on bedrest. The client's apical pulse rate is 44. The nurse concludes that this pulse rate is most likely a result of the:
1. Diuretic
2. Vasodilator
3. Bedrest regimen
4. Cardiac glycoside

701. A physician orders a tissue plasminogen activator to be administered intravenously over 1 hour for a client experiencing a myocardial infarction. The nursing priority that is specific to the use of this drug is the assessment of the client's:
1. Respiratory rate
2. Peripheral pulses
3. Level of consciousness
4. Intravenous insertion site

702. A client who has had a myocardial infarction is digitalized, and a nitroglycerin patch is ordered. The nurse recognizes that the purpose of the nitroglycerin is to decrease:
1. Peripheral resistance by dilating coronary arteries
2. Cardiac output, thereby reducing cardiac workload
3. Pulse rate, thereby strengthening cardiac contractility
4. Preload of the heart, thereby reducing cardiac workload

703. When administering the ordered digoxin (Lanoxin) 0.25 mg po qd to a client with a history of insulin dependent diabetes mellitus who is now in congestive heart failure, the nurse should:
1. Give it with orange juice
2. Monitor for dysrhythmias
3. Withhold it if the apical pulse is 90
4. Administer it 1 hour after the AM insulin

704. A client develops premature ventricular beats (PVBs). The nurse should anticipate that the client will receive:
1. Epinephrine
2. Atropine sulfate
3. Sodium bicarbonate
4. Lidocaine hydrochloride

705. When administering an intravenous titrated drip of lidocaine HCl to a client, a serious side effect that must be reported to the physician immediately is:
1. Tremors
2. Anorexia
3. Tachycardia
4. Hypertension

706. The physician prescribes furosemide (Lasix) 40 mg qd in conjunction with digoxin (Lanoxin) for a client. The nurse recognizes that potassium supplements are essential with this combination of drugs because:
1. Digoxin causes significant potassium depletion
2. Potassium is destroyed by the liver as digoxin is detoxified
3. Lasix requires adequate serum potassium to promote diuresis
4. Digoxin toxicity occurs rapidly in the presence of hypokalemia

707. The nurse would know that a client understands the side effects of hydrochlorothiazide (HydroDIURIL) when the client states, "I should call the physician if I develop:
1. Insomnia."
2. A stuffy nose."
3. Increased thirst."
4. Generalized weakness."

708. The physician orders potassium supplements for a client on diuretic therapy. The nurse recognizes that the client understands the teaching about the potassium when the client states, "I should:
1. Use salt substitutes with food."
2. Report any abdominal distress."
3. Take the drug on an empty stomach."
4. Increase the dosage if I have muscle cramps."

709. A client with Hodgkin's disease is started on MOPP therapy. Mechlorethamine HCl (Mustargen) is given IV. With this drug the client is most likely to develop:
1. Hair loss
2. Transient nausea
3. Urinary incontinence
4. Neurological dyskinesia

710. A client is to receive doxorubicin (Adriamycin) as part of a chemotherapy protocol. The major life-threatening side effect of Adriamycin that the nurse should assess the client for is:
1. Pancytopenia
2. Cardiotoxicity
3. Pulmonary fibrosis
4. Ulcerative stomatitis

711. Specific nursing intervention for a client who is receiving doxorubicin (Adriamycin) for acute myelogenous leukemia should include:
1. Giving frequent oral hygiene and increasing oral fluids
2. Serving hot liquids, such as broths or tea, with each meal
3. Administering medications IM and increasing activity level
4. Emphasizing that the disease will be cured when this treatment is completed

712. A client with cancer develops pancytopenia during the course of chemotherapy. The client asks the nurse why this has occurred. The nurse should explain that:
1. Normal cells are also susceptible to the effects of chemotherapeutic drugs
2. Steroid hormones have a depressant effect on the spleen and the bone marrow
3. Dehydration caused by nausea, vomiting, and diarrhea results in hemoconcentration
4. Lymph node activity is depressed by the radiation therapy used prior to chemotherapy

713. A client is receiving busulfan (Myleran) for chronic myelogenous leukemia. When assessing for complications of alkylating agents, the nurse should be alert for:
1. Stomatitis and nausea
2. Feminization or masculinization
3. Fluid retention and hyperglycemia
4. Leukopenia and thrombocytopenia

714. When a client who is receiving methotrexate (Folex) for acute lymphocytic leukemia (ALL) develops a temperature of 101°F, the physician is notified. Aspirin 650 mg q4h prn is ordered. The nurse should:
1. Ask the physician for an antacid order
2. Question the type of antipyretic ordered
3. Question the dosage ordered by the physician
4. Withhold the aspirin until the temperature reaches 102°F

715. A client with cancer is receiving a multiple chemotherapy protocol. Included in the proto-

col is leucovorin calcium (Wellcovorin). The nurse recognizes that this drug is administered to:
1. Potentiate the effect of alkylating agents
2. Diminish the toxicity of folic acid antagonists
3. Limit the occurrence of nausea and vomiting associated with chemotherapy
4. Interfere with cell division at a different stage of cell division than the other drugs

716. A client with metastatic melanoma is being treated with Interferon. The nurse is aware that the teaching about this drug is understood when the client states:
1. "I will increase my fluid intake to 2 to 3 liters daily."
2. "I need to discard any reconstituted solution at the end of the week."
3. "I can continue driving my car as before, as long as I have the stamina."
4. "I should be able to continue my usual activity while taking this medication."

717. The physician prescribes cimetidine (Tagamet) and Maalox for a client with a peptic ulcer. The nurse should teach the client to take these drugs:
1. At the same time
2. At least 1 hour apart
3. One immediately before the other
4. Together with milk or orange juice

718. A client is admitted for abdominal surgery for cancer of the pancreas. Before surgery, meperidine (Demerol) is ordered for pain. The nurse recognizes that morphine sulfate would be contraindicated for this client because it:
1. Causes respiratory excitement
2. Stimulates pancreatic duct secretion
3. Causes spasm of the pancreatic ducts
4. Stimulates the sympathetic nervous system

719. The physician prescribes oral pancreatic enzymes for a client. The nurse would know that the teaching about the enzymes is understood when the client states, "I will take them:
1. At bedtime."
2. With meals."

3. One hour before meals."
4. On arising each morning."

720. The medication order that should be questioned by the nurse if it is prescribed for a client with acute pancreatitis is:
1. Tagamet
2. Phenergen
3. Morphine sulfate
4. Meperidine hydrochloride

721. Following an acute episode of GI bleeding a peptic ulcer is confirmed by a gastroscopy and upper GI series. The physician orders ranitidine (Zantac) 150 mg bid with meals. The nurse should check this order with the physician because:
1. This is less than the recommended dose
2. Zantac is contraindicated for peptic ulcer
3. Zantac may be given by a variety of routes
4. This drug is usually given on an empty stomach

722. Prednisone, an adrenal steroid, is ordered for a client with an exacerbation of colitis. When administering the first dose, the nurse should stress that this drug:
1. Will protect the client from getting an infection
2. May decrease the client's appetite causing weight loss
3. Is not curative but does cause a suppression of the inflammatory process
4. Is relatively slow in effecting a response, but is effective in reducing symptoms

723. Immediately following a bilateral adrenalectomy, a client is placed on corticosteroids which are to be continued after discharge. The nurse should recognize a need for further teaching when the client states:
1. "I need to have periodic tests of my blood for sugar."
2. "I must take the pills between meals on an empty stomach."
3. "Hopefully, the dosage will be regulated so I can take them once or twice a day."
4. "I should tell the doctor if I am overly restless, depressed, or have trouble sleeping."

724. Neomycin is prescribed for a client with cirrhosis. The nurse recognizes that this drug is given to:
  1. Reduce intestinal edema
  2. Reduce abdominal distention
  3. Provide a prophylactic antibiotic
  4. Reduce the blood ammonia level

725. The physician orders meperidine hydrochloride (Demerol) 50 mg q6h for a client after a laparotomy. The client asks the nurse why this medicine is necessary. The nurse replies that Demerol is given to:
  1. Relieve abdominal pain
  2. Facilitate oxygen utilization
  3. Dilate the coronary blood vessels
  4. Decrease anxiety and restlessness

726. The physician orders docusate sodium (Colace) every day for a client. The nurse recognizes that this drug is ordered specifically to:
  1. Lubricate the feces and GI tract
  2. Create an osmotic effect in the GI tract
  3. Lower the surface tension in the GI tract
  4. Stimulate the motor activity of the GI tract

727. The physician orders Maalox by mouth and cimetidine (Tagamet) by IVPB for a client with crushing injuries caused by a train accident. The client asks why these medications are being administered. The nurse's best response would be:
  1. "They decrease irritability of the bowel."
  2. "They limit acidity in the stomach and intestine."
  3. "They're ordered for all clients with multiple trauma."
  4. "They're what your doctor ordered to calm your stomach."

728. The physician orders bedrest, Maalox, and cimetidine (Tagamet) for a client who has just had major surgery. After several days of this regimen, the client complains of diarrhea. The nurse recognizes that the diarrhea is most likely caused by:
  1. Bedrest
  2. The Maalox
  3. The cimetidine
  4. Diet alteration

729. Atropine is to be given preoperatively to an elderly client. The nurse should specifically assess for the presence of glaucoma before administering this medication because it causes:
  1. Deviation of the eye
  2. Increased heart rate
  3. Pupillary constriction
  4. Increased intraocular pressure

730. When caring for a client who has open-angle (chronic) glaucoma the eye drops the nurse should expect to administer would be:
  1. Tetracaine (Pontocaine)
  2. Cyclopentolate (Cyclogyl)
  3. Atropine sulfate (Atropisol)
  4. Pilocarpine hydrochloride (Pilocarpine)

731. Levodopa is prescribed for a client with Parkinson's disease. The sign or symptom that would be unrelated to the administration of levodopa would be:
  1. Nausea
  2. Anorexia
  3. Bradycardia
  4. Mental changes

732. A client taking levodopa should be taught about the signs of levodopa toxicity. The client and family should be instructed to contact the physician if they note the development of:
  1. Nausea
  2. Twitching
  3. Dizziness
  4. Constipation

733. L-Deprenyl (Eldepryl) is prescribed for a client with Parkinson's disease who had had a poor response to levodopa therapy. When teaching the client and family about this drug, the nurse should explain that:
  1. If a severe headache occurs it should be reported to the physician immediately
  2. The side effects of levodopa will decrease when these drugs are taken concurrently

3. The dosage of the drug can be adjusted daily depending on the client's response that day
4. Blood studies should be performed monthly to measure therapeutic blood levels of the drug

734. Dexamethasone (Decadron) is ordered for the early management of a client's cerebral edema. This treatment is effective because it:
1. Acts as a hyperosmotic diuretic
2. Increases tissue resistance to infection
3. Reduces the inflammatory response of tissues
4. Decreases the formation of cerebral spinal fluid

735. When a client is receiving dexamethasone (Decadron), the nurse should observe for the development of a negative side effect by:
1. Auscultating for bowel sounds
2. Culturing respiratory secretions
3. Measuring blood glucose levels
4. Monitoring deep tendon reflexes

736. The wife of a client with an intracranial bleed asks why her husband is not receiving anticoagulant therapy. The nurse explains that in her husband's situation anticoagulant therapy:
1. Will be started if necessary to enhance circulation
2. May be necessary to prevent pulmonary thrombosis
3. Is contraindicated because bleeding would be increased
4. Is inadvisable because it would mask signs and symptoms

737. To prevent excessive bruising when administering heparin subcutaneously the nurse should:
1. Avoid rubbing the injection site after the injection
2. Dilute the heparin with 2 ml of sterile normal saline
3. Inject the medication into the subcutaneous tissue quickly
4. Utilize the Z-track technique for administering the injection

738. In the event of excessive bleeding in a client who is receiving heparin sodium, the nurse should be prepared to administer:
1. Vitamin K
2. Panheparin
3. Warfarin sodium
4. Protamine sulfate

739. The nurse knows discharge teaching in relation to warfarin sodium (Coumadin) therapy has been understood when the client states, "I will:
1. Take Tylenol for my occasional headaches."
2. Spend most of the day working at my desk."
3. Make an appointment to have a CBC drawn."
4. Ask the doctor for antibiotics before going to the dentist."

740. After a short hospitalization for an episode of a transient ischemic attack (TIA) related to hypertension a client is discharged on a regimen that includes chlorothiazide (Diuril). The nurse should instruct the client to:
1. Take protein supplements
2. Increase the intake of potassium
3. Avoid eating fruits and vegetables
4. Return to normal eating habits once home

741. One month after an endarterectomy the physician instructs the client to take 5 grains of aspirin a day. The nurse evaluates that the reason for taking this drug is understood when the client says, "It will:
1. Limit the inflammation around my incision."
2. Help to prevent further clogging of my arteries."
3. Lower the slight fever I have had since surgery."
4. Reduce the discomfort I feel at the surgical site."

742. A client is diagnosed as having myasthenia gravis and pyridostigmine bromide (Mestinon) therapy is started. During the first week of therapy, while the dosage is being adjusted, the nurse's priority intervention is to:
    1. Administer the medication exactly on time
    2. Administer the medication with food or with milk
    3. Evaluate the client's psychological responses between doses
    4. Evaluate the client's muscle strength hourly after administration

743. A client with myasthenia gravis is admitted to the emergency room in crisis. To distinguish between myasthenic crisis and cholinergic crisis the nurse should prepare to administer:
    1. Atropine sulfate
    2. Protamine sulfate
    3. Naloxone (Narcan)
    4. Edrophonium chloride (Tensilon)

744. A client with myasthenia gravis has been receiving pyridostigmine bromide (Mestinon). Because of inadequate symptomatic control the physician begins long-term steroid therapy. When this type of therapy is being initiated, it is especially important to:
    1. Increase the client's sodium intake
    2. Place the client on protective isolation
    3. Decrease the client's fluid intake to 1000 ml daily
    4. Observe the client for an exacerbation of symptoms

745. The physician orders neostigmine (Prostigmin) for a client with myasthenia gravis. The nurse would know that the client understands the teaching about this drug when the client says:
    1. "I should keep the drug refrigerated in a tight container."
    2. "I should take the drug at the exact time specified by my doctor."
    3. "The peak action of the drug occurs 3 to 4 hours after ingestion."
    4. "The drug should be taken between meals to promote it's absorption."

746. Oxacillin sodium (Bactocill) 500 mg every 6 hours is ordered by the physician for a client who is to be discharged. The nurse would know that the teaching about the Bactocill is understood when the client says:
    1. "I will take the medication with meals."
    2. "I should drink a glass of milk with each pill."
    3. "I should drink at least 6 glasses of water every day."
    4. "I will take the medication 1 hour before or 2 hours after meals."

747. Two days after surgery a client's temperature is normal and an IVPB of gentamicin q8h started earlier is discontinued. The physician orders a clear liquid diet and OOB ad lib. After lunch the client complains of dizziness when walking to go to the bathroom. The nurse should recognize that the dizziness is probably related to:
    1. Bedrest
    2. The liquid diet
    3. The gentamicin
    4. Postanesthesia hypotension

748. The physician orders peak and trough levels of gentamicin for a client who is receiving the medication IVPB. For peak levels the nurse should have the laboratory obtain a blood sample from the client:
1. Between 30 to 60 minutes after the IVPB
2. Halfway between 2 IVPB administrations
3. Immediately before administering the IVPB
4. Anytime it is convenient for the client and laboratory

749. When planning discharge teaching for a client who has had a kidney transplant, the nurse should explain the drug regimen that will be needed to prevent rejection of the kidney. The drugs of choice usually include:

1. Ancef, methotrexate, and citric acid
2. Lasix, neomycin, and cyclosporine (Sand-immune)
3. Methylprednisolone (Solu-Medrol), Dilantin, and insulin
4. Prednisone, cyclophosphamide (Cytoxan), and azathioprine (Imuran)

750. In relation to a client's treatment with the drug erythropoietin (Epogen), the data that would be considered significant is an:
1. Elevated liver panel
2. Elevated hematocrit
3. Increase in the WBC counts
4. Increase in Kaposi sarcoma lesions

Answers and Rationales for Medical–Surgical Nursing Questions

GROWTH AND DEVELOPMENT

1. 3 This is the young-adult task associated with intimacy vs isolation. (2) (SU; AN; ED; GD)

    1 This is a toddler's task associated with autonomy vs shame and doubt.

    2 This is a school-ager's task associated with initiative vs guilt.

    4 Same as answer 1.

2. 1 This dose could be excessive in the elderly because detoxification and excretion of the drug take longer. (2) (SU; AN; TC; GD)

    2 Although this would be appropriate if the medication is administered, the nurse should first question the order because the dosage is excessive for an elderly client.

    3 This dosage could excessively depress the elderly client; the nurse has a responsibility to question the order.

    4 Same as answer 2.

3. 3 Compression fractures of the vertebrae are the most frequent fractures in clients with osteoporosis; a gradual collapse of vertebrae may be asymptomatic and only observed as kyphosis. (1) (ME; AS; PA; GD)

    1 This is untrue; it is not supported by statistics.

    2 Same as answer 1.

    4 Same as answer 1.

4. 1 Research demonstrates that women past menopause need 1500 mg of calcium a day, which is almost impossible to obtain through dietary sources because the average daily consumption of calcium is 300 to 500 mg; vitamin D promotes the deposition of calcium into the bone. (2) (ME; AN; PA; GD)

    2 If large amounts of magnesium are present, calcium absorption is impeded because magnesium and calcium absorption are competitive; vitamin E is unrelated to osteoporosis.

    3 These do not contain adequate calcium to meet requirements to prevent osteoporosis; these do not contain vitamin D unless fortified.

    4 This does not contain adequate calcium and vitamin D to meet requirements to prevent osteoporosis.

5. 3 Data support supplementation in the elderly only in illness or debilitated states to help restore tissue integrity and function; the progression of spondylitis usually decreases after 50 years of age. (2) (ME; IM; ED; GD)

    1 This is untrue; a well-balanced diet that contains a variety of foods as recommended by the food pyramid is adequate.

    2 The elderly do not need supplemental vitamins and minerals as long as their diet is adequate.

    4 This is untrue; the best source of all nutrients is from natural foods rather than supplements; loss of weight results from reduction of calories, not by the addition of vitamins and minerals.

6. 2 According to Erikson, poor self-concept and feelings of despair are conflicts manifested in the 65-and-older age group. (3) (SU; EV; ED; GD)

    1 These are conflicts manifested in early childhood between 3 and 6 years.

    3 These are conflicts manifested during the ages from 6 to 11 years.

    4 These are conflicts manifested during middle adulthood, 45 to 65 years.

7. 2 Urinary tract infections affect the genito-urinary tract and interfere with the voluntary control of micturition. (3) (ME; AS; ED; GD)
1 This is a neurologic, not a genitourinary, factor.
3 These are iatrogenic factors.
4 This is an environmental factor.

8. 4 A decrease in neuromuscular function slows reaction time. (1) (ME; IM; ED; GD)
1 Confusion is not a normal process of aging, but occurs for various reasons such as multiple stresses, perceptual changes, or medication side effects.
2 The ability to be flexible has nothing to do with age, but with character.
3 The majority of older adults do not have organic mental disease.

9. 4 For reasons that are still unclear, the thirst reflex diminishes with age and this leads to a concomitant decline in fluid intake. (1) (ME; IM; ED; GD)
1 There are no data to support this statement.
2 This would not be true for an alert person who is able to meet the activities of daily living.
3 Research does not support progressive memory loss in normal aging as a contributor to decreased fluid intake.

10. 3 Vitamin E hinders oxidative breakdown of structural lipid membranes in body tissues caused by free radicals in the cells. (2) (ME; AN; PA; GD)
1 This assists in the formation of visual purple needed for night vision.
2 This is used for formation of collagen, which is important for maintaining capillary strength, promoting wound healing, and resisting infection.
4 This is necessary for protein and fat metabolism and normal function of the nervous system.

11. 3 Kyphosis alters the center of gravity which contributes to alterations in balance and gait. (3) (ME; EV; ED; GD)
1 Decreased endurance and fatigue should not change the center of gravity or alter the gait; a lack of stamina by itself should not cause falls.
2 Age is incidental; one should not accept falls as an inescapable aspect of aging.
4 Although kyphosis alters the line of vision downward, this by itself would not cause increased falls.

12. 3 Reinforcing strengths promotes self esteem; reminiscing is a therapeutic tool which provides a life review that assists adaptation and helps achieve the task of intregrity associated with the elderly. (ME; IM; ED; GD)
1 Exercise should be encouraged, but naps tend to interfere with adequate sleep at night.
2 Reinforcing ageism would enhance devaluation of the older adult.
4 A well balanced diet that also includes protein and fiber should be encouraged; the elderly need to put the past in perspective and a positive self-assessment should be supported.

13. 4 In the aged, there is a progressive atrophy of the convolutions with a decrease in the blood flow to the brain, which may produce a tendency to become forgetful, a reduction in short-term memory, and susceptibility to personality changes. (1) (ME; AS; ED; GD)
1 People with a normal aging process show little or no change in their judgment.
2 Creativity is not affected by aging; many people remain creative until very late in life.
3 There is little or no intellectual deterioration; intelligence scores show no decline up to the age of 75-80.

14. 4 With aging, there is a significant increase in the systolic blood pressure and a slight increase in the diastolic blood pressure; hormone production is decreased with menopause. (3) (ME; IM; ED; GD)
1 There are no changes in libido with aging; there is a loss of skin elasticity.

2   Salivary secretions decrease, not increase, causing more difficulty with swallowing; there is some impairment of fat digestion.

3   There is a decrease in subcutaneous fat, decreasing body warmth; some swallowing difficulties occur because of decreased secretions.

15. 3   The onset of disabling illness will divert an aged person's energies, making it difficult to maintain an optimum level of functioning. (3) (ME; AN; ED; GD)

1   This can result from the aging process and the change in environment; it is not as important as the loss of function.

2   This would be an expected response.

4   A gradual memory loss and some confusion can be expected; a sudden memory loss would be cause for alarm.

EMOTIONAL NEEDS RELATED TO HEALTH PROBLEMS

16. 3   This provides the opportunity for the client to verbalize the feelings underlying behavior. (2) (ME; IM; PS; EH)

1   This has no effect on decreasing the client's anxiety or allowing ventilation.

2   Explanation will not decrease anxiety so that the client can rest.

4   Although allowing release of feelings is therapeutic, leaving immediately denies the client the opportunity for verbalization and discussion.

17. 2   The nurse must analyze the feelings that are implied in the client's question and reflect these to help the client verbalize and explore them; the focus is on collecting more data. (1) (ME; IM; PS; EH)

1   This is avoiding the responsibility of helping the client explore feelings; it cuts off communication.

3   Although this may be true, it does not respond to the feelings implicit in the client's comment.

4   No data presented at this time suggest that such a referral is warranted; this also cuts off communication when the client has expressed a need; the nurse is avoiding responsibility for assisting the client.

18. 1   Projection is the attribution of unacceptable feelings and emotions to others. (2) (SU; AN; PS; EH)

2   Sublimation is the substitution of socially acceptable feelings or instincts that, if expressed, would be threatening to the ego.

3   Intellectualization is the use of mental reasoning processes to deny facing emotions and feelings involved in a situation.

4   A reaction formation is the unconscious reversal of feelings or behavior unacceptable to the self image and the assumption of opposite feelings or behavior.

19. 4   As long as no one else confirms the presence of the stoma and the client does not need to adhere to a prescribed regimen, the client's denial is supported. (2) (SU; AS; PS; EH)

1   There is no evidence presented that suicidal thoughts are present or will be acted out.

2   There is no evidence to document that reaction formation is being used.

3   There are no data to support this conclusion; the client should be able to function sexually as before.

20. 4   The withdrawal provides time for the client to assimilate what has occurred and integrate the change in the body image. (2) (SU; IM; PS; EH)

1   The client is not ready to hear these explanations until assimilation of the accident and surgery has occurred.

2   This does not acknowledge that the client must grieve; it also does not allow the client to express any feelings that may be present that life will never be normal again.

3   The client would feel that the nurse had no comprehension of the situation or understanding of feelings.

21. 4 It is not reality, but the client's feeling about the change, that is the most important determinant in the ability to cope. (3) (SU; AN; PS; EH)
 1 This is not relevant to the client's ability to deal with a change in body image.
 2 Same as answer 1.
 3 The extent of change is not relevant; it is whether the client perceives the change as enormous or minuscule.

22. 3 Intellectualization is the use of reasoning and thought processes to avoid the emotional aspects of a situation; this is a defense against anxiety. (1) (ME; AN; PS; EH)
 1 Projection is denying unacceptable traits and regarding them as belonging to another person.
 2 Sublimation is a defense wherein the person redirects the energy of unacceptable impulses into socially acceptable behaviors or activities.
 4 Reaction formation is behavior exactly opposite to what the person is feeling.

23. 3 This nonjudgmentally points out the client's behavior. (2) (ME; IM; PS; EH)
 1 This is too confrontational; client may not be able to answer the question.
 2 This is too confrontational and an assumption by the nurse.
 4 This is too judgmental, an assumption, and a stereotypical response.

24. 3 This does not take away the client's only way of coping, and it permits future movement through the grieving process when the client is ready. (2) (ME; PL; PS; EH)
 1 The client's denial should be neither supported nor taken away; encouraging denial is a form of false reassurance.
 2 This is false reassurance.
 4 The client must not be abandoned; the nurse's presence is a form of emotional support.

25. 4 Honest discussion with emphasis on functional and psychologic abilities helps promote adjustment. (2) (SU; IM; PS; EH)

 1 Postoperative depression is not a characteristic feature of thymectomy.
 2 This is too soon; it may eventually be necessary if the client has trouble adjusting to the chronicity of this condition.
 3 This provides false reassurance; there is no guarantee the client will feel better on discharge.

26. 4 The medical history could be obtained during assessment, and a relationship could be established if they were uninterrupted. (3) (ME; IM; PS; EH)
 1 Agency information and data could be obtained after the assessment data had been obtained and rapport established.
 2 Accepting coffee may be an imposition and is not the best way to develop trust.
 3 Assessment of the environment could be less obviously done while obtaining the history and physical data.

27. 3 Reflection conveys acceptance and encourages further communication. (2) (SU; IM; PS; EH)
 1 This is false reassurance that does not help to reduce anxiety.
 2 This provides false reassurance that also removes the focus from the client's needs.
 4 This is unrealistic and it is a little late to think of this.

28. 4 The nurse needs to know specifically what the client is asking; this response permits clarification. (2) (SU; IM; PS; EH)
 1 This assumes that the client is referring to the diabetes in relation to surgery and sidesteps the question.
 2 This collects more information, but it will not clarify what the client wants to know.
 3 The nurse is making an assumption about medical management.

29. 2 This response focuses on the client's feelings of despair and provides the opportunity to talk about them. (1) (ME; IM; PS; EH)
 1 This abandons the client and leaves the client with no support.
 3 This response avoids a pressing problem

and misses an opportunity for discussion of feelings.

4   This focuses on the nurse's interpretation of the problem, not the client's.

30. 4   This is true; it could be the foundation for developing a positive mental outlook. (2) (ME; IM; PS; EH)

1   There is no indication that the client needs drugs to combat depression.

2   This is a patronizing response that does not recognize the despair.

3   This is probably true, but this response belittles the client's actual concern and physical discomfort.

31. 3   This is a truthful answer that provides some realistic hope. (1) (ME; IM; PS; EH)

1   This provides false reassurance; there are frequent remissions and exacerbations that may reduce the life span.

2   This response avoids the client's question; the family did not ask.

4   This avoids the client's question and transfers responsibility to the physician.

32. 3   This includes the client in the problem solving process. (2) (SU; PL; PS; EH)

1   This does not include the client in the problem solving process; more data should be obtained from the client before deciding on an intervention, which may or may not be appropriate.

2   Same as answer 1.

4   Same as answer 1.

33. 3   Policies relative to DNR orders vary among hospitals and the nurse must adhere to the policies within the institution. (2) (ME; AN; PS; EH)

1   This is untrue; the wish of the client is the deciding factor.

2   The decision resides with the client.

4   This may not be true for all hospitals or states; the information does not indicate this is so in this situation; these orders are reviewed periodically.

34. 2   Communication facilitates joint solution of the problem; the nurse must first determine the client's understanding and per-

ceptions before solutions to the problem can be attempted. (2) (SU; AS; PS; EH)

1   This will not collect data about why the client is leaving the room.

3   This abdicates the responsibility of the primary nurse.

4   This may be done, but not until further assessment is done to determine the reason why the client is leaving the room.

35. 1   Placing an aide in the home will allow the mother to rest and provide the child with attention. (3) (ME; IM; TC; EH)

2   Making the mother feel guilty will only increase anxiety and will not be constructive.

3   The handicapped sibling requires attention, and this responsibility may increase jealousy, rivalry, and resentment.

4   Elaborate toys need not be employed for sensory stimulation; household objects can serve as well.

36. 1   This is a classic sign of denial; by reducing the importance or extent of the problem the individual is able to cope; not acknowledging that it is really a problem is a form of denial. (2) (ME; AS; PS; EH)

2   This indicates repression of affect rather than denial.

3   Failure to communicate is insufficient evidence to diagnose denial; the husband/wife relationship may be strained, or the husband may be worried about upsetting the wife.

4   This usually indicates displacement of anger, not denial.

37. 2   It is helpful to minimize stress to limit further ulcer development; this is most effective if the family is involved. (2) (SU; PL; PS; EH)

1   Maximizing changes in life-style can increase stress and is contraindicated for clients with ulcers.

3   Most clients recover from gastric surgery without complications.

4   Although pernicious anemia can occur as the result of gastric surgery, there is little that can be done to prevent it.

38. 2 Any client who has been sedated, or who is not fully conscious, may not sign the consent for a surgical procedure. (2) (SU; AN; PS; EH)
  1 Many clients face contradictory feelings regarding their impending surgery, but their consent is legal unless they withdraw the consent.
  3 A second opinion is not required for a consent to be legal.
  4 A complete history and physical are needed before surgery, but they do not affect the legality of consent.

39. 2 Allowing the client to grieve for the lost limb often aids acceptance of the loss. (1) (SU; IM; PS; EH)
  1 Sedation will prevent the client from facing the problem.
  3 Behavior should never be ignored.
  4 This behavior may be interpreted by the client as rejection.

40. 1 Because the hospital beds are narrower and higher than the beds clients sleep in at home, side rails frequently create a sense of security. (1) (ME; EV; PS; EH)
  2 This relates to the physical status, not the psychologic status, of the client.
  3 On the contrary, this will cause the client to feel more dependent.
  4 Bed rails are unrelated to proprioception, which is knowing the location of a body part when it is out of the field of vision.

41. 4 This is a true statement; anxiety and/or anger associated with other stages interferes with learning. (3) (ME; AN; ED; EH)
  1 Too late to start preparation for discharge and teaching; many factors influence readiness for learning; planning for teaching must begin on the day of admission.
  2 The anxiety associated with mental anguish would interfere with the ability to process new information; mental anguish is associated with an earlier stage.
  3 Although clients in the acceptance or adaptation phase are less angry, the reason teaching is most effective is not because of their compliance but because new information can be processed more easily.

42. 2 When a client is anxious and has a decreased ability to cope, minor environmental irritants are magnified; eye contact is avoided to decrease additional stimuli. (3) (SU; EV; PS; EH)
  1 This would be indicated by complaints of pain, splinting, refusal to move, and alterations in vital signs.
  3 If the client were angry, eye contact would be maintained; prolonged eye contact may be used as a form of intimidation or aggression.
  4 If this were so, the client would be verbalizing about the need to continue the abduction, not about a variety of other annoyances.

43. 3 The nurse never clarified if the client was in pain; also, this offers false reassurance. (2) (SU; EV; PS; EH)
  1 The nurse's response denies the client's anxiety; it identifies pain as the problem.
  2 The nurse's response denies the client's needs; the client needs to discuss concerns and feelings.
  4 The nurse inappropriately identifies the problem and never clarifies the need.

44. 1 This reflects the client's feelings and encourages a further exploration of concerns. (3) (SU; IM; PS; EH)
  2 This response does not reflect the feeling tone of the client's statement; also, the client may not be able to answer this question.
  3 This is false reassurance; thyroid storm is capable of causing death.
  4 This could reinforce the client's anxiety and avoids discussing the client's concerns; it cuts off communication.

45. 1 Internal self-stimulation increases as external stimuli decrease. (3) (ME; AN; PS; EH)
  2 Blindness is an added stress that could increase anxiety, which impairs decision making; lack of visual stimuli limits data for decision making.
  3 Lack of visual stimuli would increase restlessness, lethargy, and apathy.
  4 Blindness would not precipitate neurotic

behavior unless other emotional factors were present.

46. 2 This provides an opportunity for the client to explore concerns with the nurse. (2) (SU; IM; PS; EH)

1 The data do not indicate regression; the client is anxious, not regressed.

3 The nurse is basing the response on an incorrect interpretation of the data.

4 The data do not indicate that the client does not understand; the nurse should attempt to provide for consensual validation before coming to this conclusion.

47. 3 Hostility and noncompliance are both forms of anger that are associated with grieving. (2) (ME; AN; PS; EH)

1 This is not a conscious attempt to hurt others, but a way to relieve and reduce anxiety within the self.

2 This is a self-destructive method of coping, which could result in death.

4 This is an effort to maintain control over a situation that is really controlling the client; it is an unconscious method of coping and may be a form of denial.

48. 1 This is the first action; the nurse should be aware that the technique is not safe, and it provides an opportunity to correct the technique being used; the dressing should be immediately and correctly changed; the priority is to protect the client. (3) (ME; IM; TC; EH)

2 This depends on the policy of the institution and might be done later.

3 This may or may not be done by the observing nurse; it could be done by an in-service educator.

4 Same as answer 2.

49. 1 This response indicates recognition of the client's need to use denial and opens the way for discussion of feelings. (3) (SU; IM; PS; EH)

2 This forces reality on the client and blocks discussion of feelings.

3 This reply focuses on the surgery, which is not the concern expressed by the client.

4 This changes the subject and moves away from the client's feelings.

50. 2 This identifies the client's feelings and provides an opportunity for further discussion. (2) (SU; IM; PS; EH)

1 Although this echoes the client's statement, it does not identify a feeling.

3 This denies the client's feelings and focuses on information; the client may be too emotionally distraught to be able to construct or verbalize questions.

4 This provides false reassurance and cuts off communication; introduction of the word "cancer" could increase anxiety.

51. 2 This identifies the underlying client concern in a non-judgmental way by not actually addressing the behavior; it provides the opportunity for an exploration of concerns and feelings. (2) (SU; IM; PS; EH)

1 Although it points out behavior, this is aggressive and may produce a defensive response instead of an exploration of concerns and feelings.

3 This response minimizes the client's feelings and provides false reassurance.

4 Same as answer 3.

52. 1 The nurse at the scene of an accident should function in a responsible and prudent manner; the use of a soiled cloth on an open wound is not prudent, nor is the independent transfer of an accident victim from the scene. (2) (ME; EV; PS; EH)

2 Although the Nurse Practice Act defines nursing, it does not provide detailed standards for practice; the nurse's action was not prudent.

3 The nurse's action was not what a reasonably prudent nurse would do and the nurse is therefore not protected.

4 The nurse's intervention was not prudent and placed the client in jeopardy; the nurse was not practicing medicine, but attempting to provide first aid.

53. 3   Reliving the experience brings back the feelings, such as anxiety and fear, associated with it; the symptoms described reflect sympathetic nervous system activity. (2) (ME; AN; PA; EH)

1   The increased pulse and restlessness could indicate bleeding; however, the other data presented support anxiety; additional assessment would be necessary to identify bleeding.

2   Not enough data are present to recognize the client's usual method of seeking sympathy.

4   These symptoms are indicative of a sympathetic, not a parasympathetic, response.

54. 3   These are realistic, productive, and constructive ways of using this time. (1) (ME; AN; PS; EH)

1   These are signs of depression.

2   Going from physician to physician demonstrates disbelief, denial, or desperation.

4   This indicates anger and hopelessness, not acceptance.

55. 4   This is a legal requirement of participating institutions to protect the individuals involved. (1) (SU; AN; PS; EH)

1   Active euthanasia is a direct act to shorten a person's life and is illegal.

2   This is untrue; no age restrictions exist.

3   Legal statutes make certain the opposite is true.

56. 4   This helps the client express concerns and examine feelings. (1) (ME; IM; PS; EH)

1   The client's apprehension is legitimate and should be explored; the misconception that the clot will hurt the heart can be explored later.

2   This was not the client's question and would not meet the need to explore feelings; this could be done later.

3   This is inappropriate; it disregards the client's expressed fears and would increase anxiety.

57. 3   A refusal to recognize anticipated loss in an attempt to protect oneself against the overpowering stress of illness is called

repudiation. (2) (SU; AN; PS; EH)

1   The data do not suggest that the client has contemplated consequences related to the illness.

2   There are no data to support that the client is demonstrating behavior characteristic of an earlier stage of development.

4   The data do not suggest that the client has made a realistic adjustment to the illness.

58. 2   Before a teaching plan can be developed, the factors that interfere with learning must be identified. (2) (SU; AS; ED; EH)

1   Although family members can be helpful, client involvement in care is important for promoting independence and self-esteem.

3   This is premature; assessment comes before intervention; written instructions may not be the most appropriate teaching modality.

4   This may be an unrealistic expectation; the client may never accept the change but must learn to manage care.

59. 4   Sharing concerns and talking about them often releases anxieties; giving the ordered hypnotic would produce relaxation. (1) (SU; IM; PS; EH)

1   This might relax the client but may not reduce the client's level of anxiety.

2   The client is not in pain at this time but needs to share concerns.

3   The procedure is over; this might be appropriate before the paracentesis; also, there are no data to support that this is the client's concern.

60. 2   Respondeat superior is a doctrine that states employers may be held liable for torts committed by their employees. (3) (ME; AN; PS; EH)

1   In loco parentis refers to another person or agency assuming responsibility for a minor in the absence of the minor's parents.

3   The department of health sets standards and evaluates if these are met; the hospital's responsibility for safe care under respondeat superior is a legal one.

4   This is unrelated to respondeat superior or to a hospital's legal responsibility to its clients.

61.   4   This response identifies the client's feelings and accepts them but also points out the responsibility of the client to take action. (1) (ME; IM; PS; EH)
1   Although this response identifies one of the client's concerns, the identification of the underlying feeling would be more therapeutic.
2   This response makes the nurse responsible for changing the situation, which is not appropriate or therapeutic.
3   This response denies the client's feelings and provides false reassurance.

62.   4   The release of information to an unauthorized person, gossiping about a client's activities, and the nurse's unwanted intrusion into private family matters constitute invasion of privacy. (1) (ME; AN; PS; EH)
1   Libel occurs when a person writes false statements about another that may injure the individual's reputation.
2   Slander occurs when a person verbally defames, detracts from, or maligns another's reputation.
3   Negligence is a careless act of omission or commission that results in injury to another.

63.   4   Before nurses can help others they must understand themselves first, particularly on issues that may impact on clients; this is the first step toward providing nonjudgmental care. (1) (ME; AS; PS; EH)
1   Although it is beneficial for nurses to understand themselves, this does not necessarily mean that the care will be nonjudgmental.
2   Although truthfulness is important in a therapeutic relationship, the nurse should attempt to be nonjudgmental; a nurse who feels uncomfortable should not be caring for the client in the first place.
3   Although this is important for all therapeutic relationships, it follows a thorough self-assessment of attitudes, values, and beliefs.

64.   1   Voicing fears often reduces the associated anxiety. (1) (ME; IM; PS; EH)
2   Socialization when feelings need exploration is not therapeutic.
3   Although this should be done, simply accepting the client's wishes is not by itself therapeutic.
4   This avoids the problem and is not therapeutic.

65.   1   This statement reflects values and beliefs regarding homosexuality as being bad and deserving of punishment. (2) (ME; EV; PS; EH)
2   There is not enough evidence presented to justify drawing this conclusion.
3   Same as answer 2.
4   Although this may be true, no information is given to suggest that the nursing assistant has been assigned to care for this client.

66.   1   The client is in the anger or "why me" stage; encouraging the expression of feelings will help resolve them while moving toward acceptance. (2) (ME; IM; PS; EH)
2   This does not reflect on what the client said; introducing the topic of death may not be therapeutic.
3   This abdicates the responsibility of talking with the client; suggesting speaking with a minister ignores the client's present concerns.
4   This is judgmental, which may precipitate feelings of guilt and block the nurse-client relationship.

67.   1   Fear of recurrent myocardial infarct or sudden death is common when the client's environment is to be changed to one that appears less vigilant. (3) (ME; AN; PS; EH)
2   Depression is exhibited by withdrawal, crying, anorexia, and apathy and usually becomes more evident after discharge from the hospital.
3   Dependency would be exhibited by an unwillingness to increase exercise or perform tasks.
4   Ambivalence is exhibited by contrasting emotions; the client's statement does not demonstrate this.

68. 2 Knowing what to expect decreases anxiety. (2) (ME; IM; ED; EH)
1 Routine medications are not withheld unless ordered by the physician.
3 A sedative is not necessary for this test.
4 A small amount of radiation is emitted during the scan; the client should be assured the procedure is safe.

69. 3 This indicates the nurse has heard the client's verbal message and has empathy; it encourages further verbalization. (2) (ME; IM; PS; EH)
1 This may increase anxiety.
2 This minimizes the client's concerns.
4 This depersonalizes the client's concerns; it focuses on the test and the setting rather than the client's concerns.

70. 3 The Bureau of Child Welfare handles cases of child abuse and neglect, of which the child seems to be a victim. (2) (ME; IM; TC; EH)
1 The clinic would observe the client medically but the Bureau of Child Welfare would handle the child abuse and other social problems.
2 The hospital would probably not admit the child unless an immediate medical incident required it.
4 The Bureau of the Handicapped would be concerned with equipment and supplies required for the individual with a handicap.

FLUIDS AND ELECTROLYTES

71. 3 The client's intake was 360 (12 oz × 30 ml) and loss was 125 ml of fluid; loss is subtracted from intake. (1) (ME; EV; TC; FE)
1 This is an inaccurate calculation; the client has a more positive fluid balance.
2 Same as answer 1.
4 This is an inaccurate calculation; this answer added the output to the intake.

72. 3 One liter of fluid weighs approximately 2.2 pounds; therefore, a 4.5 pound weight loss equals approximately 2 liters. (2) (ME; EV; PA; FE)
1 This is approximately a 1 pound weight loss.
2 This is approximately a 2.2 pound weight loss.
4 This is approximately a 7.5 pound weight loss.

73. 1 With the client's history and the large weight gain, this is the most likely cause of the increase in weight. (1) (ME; AN; PA; FE)
2 This occurs in the bladder, not the tissues, and would not account for the large weight gain.
3 This can occur with CHF but it is not the primary etiology of the fluid retention.
4 Abdominal distention is usually caused by gas and should not contribute to this large a weight gain; if the abdomen is enlarged assessment by ballotement should be done to determine if enlargement is caused by fluid.

74. 1 The client receives 1000 ml + 500 ml + 1500 ml from the main IV and 150 ml in piggybacks (3 × 50 ml). (1) (SU; AN; TC; FE)
2 This is an incorrect computation; this is more than the amount of fluid ordered.
3 Same as answer 2.
4 Same as answer 2.

75. 3 Carbonated beverages are generally high in sodium and should be avoided. (1) (ME; PL; ED; FE)
1 Many of these products contain sodium.
2 Same as answer 1.
4 Same as answer 1.

76. 3 Hypokalemia is suspected when the T wave on an ECG tracing is depressed or flattened; serum potassium below 3.5 mEq/L indicates hypokalemia. (1) (ME; AS; PA; FE)
1 This would have no significance in diagnosing a potassium deficit.
2 Same as answer 1.
4 Same as answer 1.

77. 2 Potassium is irritating to veins; larger veins can accommodate irritating substances for longer periods of time than small veins can. (2) (ME; IM; PA; FE)

1 Using the antecubital space would restrict client movement unnecessarily because the arm would have to be kept extended to prevent piercing the vein which would result in an infiltration.

3 The back of the hand does not have veins large enough to accommodate a potassium infusion; using the dominant hand would restrict movement unnecessarily.

4 The back of the hand does not have veins large enough to accommodate a potassium infusion.

78. 1 A rate of 30 ml/hr is considered adequate for perfusion of the kidneys, heart, and brain. (1) (SU; EV; PA; FE)

2 A central venous pressure reading of 2 cm H_2O indicates hypovolemia.

3 This indicates improvement but not necessarily adequate tissue perfusion.

4 Same as answer 3.

79. 3 Albumin intravenously increases colloid osmotic pressure resulting in a pull of fluid from the interstitial and intracellular compartments to the intravascular compartment. (3) (SU; AN; PA; FE)

1 The interstitial compartment is part of the extracellular compartment.

2 This is opposite to the actual shift of fluids.

4 Same as answer 2.

80. 3 Salt substitutes usually contain potassium which would lead to symptoms of hyperkalemia, such as an abnormal heart beat. (3) (ME; AN; PA; FE)

1 Sodium in the diet causes retention of fluid.

2 Salt substitutes do not contain substances that influence BUN and creatinine levels; these are the result of protein metabolism.

4 There is no such substance in salt substitutes.

81. 2 Intravenous fluids supply minimal calories; a client on only IV therapy will lose weight and become malnourished. (1) (ME; EV; PA; FE)

1 This is not related to weight; lack of bulk in the diet results in constipation.

3 Vitamins are not related to weight loss.

4 Intracellular electrolytes are not related to weight loss.

82. 3 The stomach produces about 3 L of secretions per day; fluid lost through vomiting can produce a fluid volume deficit. (2) (SU; AN; TC; FE)

1 The shallow respirations are not related to a primary respiratory problem or pain; they are a compensatory mechanism to conserve CO_2 to combine with H^+ to form carbonic acid (H_2CO_3) and lower the plasma pH.

2 Although this diagnosis is related it is not the priority.

4 This would be true for duodenal ulcer; the gastric acid secretory rate is normal in persons with gastric ulcers; in gastric ulcers there is a decreased resistance of the gastric mucosa to acid-pepsin injury and a reflux of bile-containing duodenal contents back into the stomach; the priority is fluid volume deficit, which can lead to dysrhythmias and death.

83. 3 This has a low sodium content. (3) (ME; EV; ED; FE)

1 Shellfish is high in sodium.

2 Processed meats are high in sodium.

4 These vegetables are high in sodium.

84. 1 This treats the hyperkalemia associated with renal failure; it moves potassium from the intravascular compartment into the intracellular compartment. (3) (ME; AN; TC; FE)

2 This would not increase urinary output.

3 This is not a treatment for respiratory acidosis.

4 Insulin and glucose do not decrease serum calcium levels.

85. 2 Cellular swelling and cerebral edema are associated with hyponatremia; as the extracellular sodium level decreases, the cellular fluid becomes relatively more concentrated and pulls water into cerebral cells. (2) (ME; AS; PA; FE)
1 This is not a symptom of hyponatremia; it may indicate dehydration.
3 This is associated with hypovolemia, not hyponatremia.
4 This is not a symptom of hyponatremia; it may indicate anemia.

86. 3 This ensures a rapid, well-controlled technique for electrolyte (chloride) replacement. (3) (ME; AN; PA; FE)
1 There is no assurance that adequate chloride will be ingested and absorbed.
2 Hyperalimentation is not necessary at this point, although it may eventually be used.
4 This is not a rapid or well-controlled method to correct electrolyte deficiencies.

87. 3 The osmotic effect of hyperglycemia pulls fluid from cells, resulting in cellular dehydration. (3) (ME; AN; PA; FE)
1 The opposite is true; hyperglycemia pulls fluid from the interstitial compartment to the intravascular compartment.
2 Interstitial fluid is part of the extracellular compartment; the osmotic pull of glucose exceeds other osmotic forces.
4 An increase in hydrostatic pressure results in an intravascular to interstitial shift.

88. 2 An increased serum albumin level increases the osmotic effect and pulls fluid back into the intravascular compartment, thereby increasing renal flow and diuresis. (3) (ME; EV; PA; FE)
1 This therapy will increase blood volume and blood flow to the kidney, thereby increasing urinary output.
3 Albumin therapy has no effect on blood ammonia levels.
4 Albumin will not lower the blood ammonia level; an elevated blood ammonia level causes hepatic encephalopathy.

89. 2 This would provide gradual replacement of both fluid and electrolytes without overloading the intravascular compartment. (2) (ME; PL; PA; FE)
1 Water does not supply the necessary electrolytes and hyponatremia could result.
3 No data are presented to indicate that the client cannot take fluids orally; an NG tube is not necessary when the client can take fluids by mouth.
4 This is unsafe; rapid correction of a fluid and electrolyte imbalance is dangerous; therapy should promote a gradual correction.

90. 2 Commercially prepared salt substitutes are usually high in potassium. (2) (SU; EV; ED; FE)
1 Nonsalt seasonings, such as lemon juice and pepper, can be used to make food more palatable.
3 These contain high concentrations of potassium.
4 Some complete protein foods must be included in the diet but, on a restricted protein diet, proteins will also come from other sources.

91. 3 A decreased urinary output will result in the retention of potassium causing hyperkalemia. (3) (ME; AS; TC; FE)
1 Reporting this is unnecessary; this is a sign of dehydration which can be corrected with appropriate hydration.
2 Reporting this is unnecessary; these indicate dehydration, which is probably the rationale for the fluid ordered.
4 Reporting this is unnecessary; this can precipitate dehydration or compound an existing dehydration and can be prevented by appropriate hydration.

92. 4 Pyrexia increases fluid loss through the skin; to maintain balance, the body compensates by reducing urinary output. (1) (ME; AN; PA; FE)
1 Blood pressure is not directly affected by antimicrobials, and there are no data to suggest blood pressure is decreasing.
2 This is unlikely; the client would have to become septic before this could occur.
3 This represents a possible, but not probable, side effect of antimicrobial agents;

also, nephrotoxicity would not be evident so soon.

93. 2 Urinary output reflects circulating blood volume; it is the most reliable, immediately available information to assess fluid needs. (1) (SU; EV; PA; FE)
   1 Daily weights reflect fluid retention or loss; however, other factors beside fluid affect weight; this is not as immediately accurate as hourly urines.
   3 This may indicate hypervolemia or hypovolemia, but is not as accurate an indicator of insufficient fluid replacement as hourly urine output.
   4 Peripheral edema may have many causes; it is not an effective indicator of fluid balance.

94. 4 A low pH and bicarbonate reflect metabolic acidosis; a low $P{CO_2}$ indicates compensatory hyperventilation. (3) (ME; AS; PA; FE)
   1 An elevated pH and bicarbonate reflect metabolic alkalosis; an elevated $P{CO_2}$ indicates compensatory hypoventilation.
   2 An elevated pH and a low $P{CO_2}$ reflect hyperventilation and respiratory alkalosis.
   3 A low pH and elevated $P{CO_2}$ reflect hypoventilation and respiratory acidosis.

95. 3 The increased osmotic effect following the administration of albumin increases intravascular volume and urinary output; weight loss reflects fluid loss. (2) (ME; EV; TC; FE)
   1 Vital signs do not change drastically; "frequently" is a nonspecific time frame.
   2 Urinary output is measured hourly, q8h, and q24h; half-hour outputs are insignificant in this instance.
   4 Serum albumin levels would be significant; albumin in the urine indicates kidney dysfunction, not liver dysfunction.

96. 3 An orange only contains trace amounts of sodium. (3) (ME; IM; PA; FE)
   1 One cup of ice cream contains approximately 115 milligrams of sodium.
   2 One cup of celery contains approximately 106 milligrams of sodium .

4 Four peanut butter cookies contain 142 milligrams of sodium.

97. 1 Fluid shifts from the intravascular compartment into the abdominal cavity, causing hypovolemia; a rapid, thready pulse is a compensatory response to this shift. (2) (SU; EV; PA; FE)
   2 Assessing for shock is the priority.
   3 After a paracentesis, intravascular fluid shifts into the abdominal cavity, not the lungs.
   4 Same as answer 2.

98. 3 Verbalization indicates the client is breathing; elevating the head of the bed facilitates breathing by decreasing pressure against the diaphragm; checking the vital signs after this is the first step in assessing the cause of the distress. (2) (ME; PL; TC; FE)
   1 There is not enough information to support this option; further assessment is required.
   2 Discontinuing the IV access line may cause unnecessary discomfort and expense if it must be restarted; there are too little data to call the physician at this time.
   4 There is no information to support this option; assessment for allergies should be done on admission.

99. 2 The imbalance in intake and output, with a decreasing urinary output, may indicate renal failure with an increase of body fluid and the incipient development of congestive heart failure; assessing breath sounds and vital signs are the first steps when monitoring for these complications. (3) (ME; EV; TC; FE)
   1 There are no data to support a problem with excretion of urine; the problem is with insufficient production.
   3 These are appropriate assessments after respirations and vital signs are evaluated.
   4 It is immaterial whether the fluid is given orally or intravenously; if there is hypervolemia, fluid intake would be decreased.

100. 1 Osmosis is the movement of water from an area of lesser solute concentration to an area of greater solute concentration. (3) (SU; AN; PA; FE)

2 Diffusion is the movement of particles across a semipermeable membrane from an area of greater concentration of particles to an area of lesser concentration of particles.

3 Filtration is the passage of fluid through a material that prevents the passage of certain constituents; hydrostatic pressure, the pressure exerted within a closed system, is known as filtration force; this force moves fluid by pressure and concentration gradients.

4 In active transport, molecules move against a concentration gradient; this differs from diffusion and osmosis because metabolic energy is expended.

101. 1 This attempts to collect adequate data to plan the most appropriate intervention. (2) (ME; AS; TC; FE)

2 This alone will not guarantee compliance once the client goes home; the client has the right to accept or reject therapy.

3 Table salt is contraindicated on a 2 g sodium diet.

4 Same as answer 2.

102. 3 Hypertonic food increases osmotic pressure and pulls fluid from the intravascular compartment into the intestine (dumping syndrome). (2) (SU; AN; TC; FE)

1 Increased carbohydrates, not fats, are responsible for the increased osmotic pressure often associated with dumping syndrome.

2 This is separation of the wound edges, usually accompanied by a gush of pink-tinged fluid.

4 While peristalsis may be decreased because of surgery, it would not account for the symptoms.

103. 3 Shallow respirations, bronchial tree obstruction, and atelectasis compromise gas exchange in the lungs; an elevated carbon dioxide level leads to acidosis. (1) (SU; AN; PA; FE)

1 Metabolic acidosis is seen in diarrhea with loss of base from the lower gastrointestinal tract.

2 Metabolic alkalosis is caused by excessive loss of hydrogen ions from gastric decompression or excessive vomiting.

4 Respiratory alkalosis is caused by increased expiration of carbon dioxide, a component of carbonic acid.

104. 4 All data are within normal limits; Po_2 is 80 to 100 mmHg, Pco_2 is 35 to 45 mmHg, and the pH is 7.35 to 7.45. (1) (SU; AN; PA; FE)

1 None of the data are indicators of fluid balance.

2 Oxygen is within normal limits of 80 to 100 mmHg.

3 The pH would have to be below 7.35

105. 4 The body fights acidosis by H^+ exchange, which results in excretion of excess H^+ in the urine, a compensatory mechanism to raise serum pH. (3) (ME; AN; PA; FE)

1 In acidosis the pH of the blood is decreased.

2 Plasma bicarbonates would be decreased.

3 In acidosis the respiratory center in the medulla is stimulated to increase respiration and blow off CO_2, which is carried to the lung as carbonic acid (H_2CO_3); lowering carbonic acid raises serum pH.

106. 2 The client is hyperventilating and blowing off excessive carbon dioxide, which leads to these symptoms; if uninterrupted this could lead to respiratory alkalosis. (3) (ME; AS; PA; FE)

1 Eupnea is normal, quiet breathing; the client has shallow, rapid breathing.

3 Kussmaul respirations are deep, gasping respirations associated with diabetic acidosis and coma, not hyperventilation associated with anxiety.

4 These symptoms are related to a decreased carbon dioxide level in the body.

107. 3 Reassurance decreases anxiety and slows respirations; the bag is used so that exhaled carbon dioxide can be rebreathed to resolve respiratory alkalosis and return the client to acid-base balance. (3) (ME; IM; PA; FE)

1 This is not necessary because there is no evidence of hypoxia.

2 This is not necessary; this is used to prevent atelectasis.

4 The client is already alkalotic; bicarbonate ions would increase the problem.

108. 3 Normal plasma pH is 7.35 to 7.45; the client is in alkalosis; normal plasma bicarbonate is 23 to 25 mEq/L; the client has an excess of base bicarbonate indicating a metabolic cause for the alkalosis. (1) (SU; AS; PA; FE)

1 Normal plasma potassium is 3.5 to 5.0 mEq/L; the potassium is within normal limits.

2 Normal plasma chloride is 95 to 105 mEq/L; the client has hypochloremia because of vomiting of gastric secretions.

4 To be acidotic the plasma pH would have to be below 7.35.

109. 4 Hyperventilation results in the increased elimination of carbon dioxide from the blood. (2) (SU; AN; PA; FE)

1 The PO_2 would not be affected.

2 The pH will be increased.

3 The carbonic acid will be decreased.

110. 3 Decreased O_2 increases the conversion of pyruvic acid to lactic acid, resulting in metabolic acidosis. (3) (SU; AN; PA; FE)

1 Hyperkalemia would occur because of renal shutdown; hypokalemia could occur in early shock.

2 The PCO_2 would be increased in profound shock.

4 Respiratory alkalosis could occur in early shock because of rapid, shallow breathing, but in late shock metabolic or respiratory acidosis occurs.

111. 3 In respiratory alkalosis the pH is elevated because of loss of hydrogen ions; PCO_2 is low because carbon dioxide is lost by hyperventilating. (3) (ME; AS; PA; FE)

1 This is partially compensated metabolic alkalosis.

2 This is respiratory acidosis.

4 This is metabolic acidosis with some compensation.

112. 2 The urinary system compensates by retaining H^+ ions, which become part of the bicarbonate ions; the bicarbonate becomes elevated and raises the pH to near normal; the normal HCO_3 is 22 to 26 mEq/L, and the normal pH is 7.35 to 7.45. (3) (SU; AS; PA; FE)

1 The normal PO_2 is 80 to 95 mmHg; this is within the normal range.

3 The normal PCO_2 is 35 to 45 mmHg; although in compensated respiratory acidosis the PCO_2 may be elevated, it is the elevated HCO_3 level that indicates compensation.

4 This K^+ level is within the normal range, which is 3.5 to 5.0 mEq/L; serum potassium is not significant in identifying compensated respiratory acidosis.

113. 3 The client is in respiratory acidosis probably caused by the depressant effects of anesthesia or a plugged airway; coughing clears the airway and deep breaths blow off CO_2. (3) (SU; IM; ED; FE)

1 This will not correct respiratory acidosis and may aggravate hypokalemia if present.

2 This is the treatment for respiratory alkalosis; the client is in respiratory acidosis.

4 This is not necessary if clearing of the airway rectifies the problem.

114. 1 This is the correct flow rate; multiply the amount to be infused (50 ml) by the drop factor (10) and divide the result by the amount of time in minutes (20). (2) (SU; AN; TC; FE)

2 This is an inaccurate calculation; this would deliver the solution too rapidly and would irritate the vein.

3 Same as answer 2.

4 Same as answer 2.

115. 2   This is the correct flow rate; multiply the amount to be infused (2000 ml) by the drop factor (10) and divide the result by the amount of time in minutes (12 hours × 60 min). (2) (SU; AN; TC; FE)

1   This is an incorrect calculation; this flow rate is too slow to administer the ordered solution in the 12 hour time frame.

3   This is an incorrect calculation; this flow is too fast to administer the ordered solution over 12 hours.

4   Same as answer 3.

116. 3   This is the correct flow rate; to determine amount of fluid, take the sum of all IV fluid for the period (2750 ml), multiply this by the drop factor (15), and divide the result by the time in minutes (24 hr × 60 min). (2) (SU; AN; TC; FE)

1   This is too slow a drip rate to infuse the required amount of fluid.

2   Same as answer 1.

4   This is too rapid a drip rate and the required fluid will be infused in too short a period.

117. 3   Different infusion sets deliver different preset numbers of drops per ml; knowing this is a necessity for calculating the drip rate. (1) (SU; AN; TC; FE)

1   This does not determine the drip rate.

2   Same as answer 1.

4   This determines the size of the drop, not the drip rate.

118. 2   Amount to be infused (850 ml) multiplied by the drop factor (10) divided by total time in minutes (480) equals 18 gtt/min. (2) (SU; AN; TC; FE)

1   This is less than the desired flow rate; it would take longer to infuse than the time ordered.

3   This is more than the desired flow rate; the fluid would be infused in less than the time ordered.

4   Same as answer 3.

119. 2   Total volume (1250 ml) multiplied by the drop factor (15) divided by the total time in minutes (480) equals 39 gtt/min. (2) (SU; AN; TC; FE)

1   This is too slow; it would not deliver the ordered amount of fluid in the ordered time period.

3   This is too fast; it would deliver too much fluid too quickly.

4   Same as answer 3.

120. 3   Air in the secondary line will not enter the vein; fluid from the primary bottle is under pressure and will flow before air from the secondary line could reach the port in the primary line. (1) (SU; IM; TC; FE)

1   This is possibly true, but this answer would increase anxiety.

2   Gentamicin bypasses the large IV bottle because it is piggybacked into the primary line below the drip chamber and check-valve.

4   This is contraindicated; this stops the infusion, which can clog the lumen of the catheter that is inserted into the vein.

121. 2   When calculated:
90 ml per hour = 1.5 ml per minute (90 ÷ 60); 1.5 ml × drop factor of 15 gtt/ml = 22.5 or 23 gtt per minute. (2) (SU; AN; TC; FE)

1   This drip rate would infuse too slowly to deliver the amount ordered in the specified time.

3   This drip rate would infuse too rapidly and would deliver the ordered amount too quickly.

4   Same as answer 3.

BLOOD AND IMMUNITY

122. 4   Drains are usually inserted into the splenic bed to facilitate removal of fluid that could lead to abscess formation. (2) (SU; IM; ED; BI)

1   Splenectomy has a low mortality (5%) except when multiple injuries are present (15% to 40%).

2   Bleeding occurs more frequently with splenic repair than with removal.

3   There is no need to frighten the client unnecessarily, but the operative risk increases with multiple injuries.

123. 3 With shock the heart rate accelerates to increase blood flow and oxygen to body tissues. (1) (SU; AS; PA; BI)

1 With shock there would be a decreased urinary output because of the lowered glomerular filtration rate.

2 With shock the respirations would be increased and shallow.

4 With shock there would be hypotension.

124. 1 A decreased blood volume leads to decreased glomerular filtration; compensatory ADH and aldosterone secretion cause sodium and water retention. (2) (SU; AS; TC; BI)

2 The respirations become rapid and shallow to compensate for decreased oxygenation.

3 The peripheral pulse rate may be rapid and thready but it is the same rate as the apical rate.

4 Hypokalemia occurs because as sodium is retained, potassium is excreted.

125. 4 Hypovolemia results in a decreased cardiac output and a decreased arterial pressure which are reflected by a feeble, weak peripheral pulse. (3) (ME; AS; TC; BI)

1 The skin would be cool and pale because of vasoconstriction.

2 These are late signs of shock.

3 The pulse pressure narrows with decreased cardiac pressure associated with hypovolemic shock.

126. 3 In shock, arteriolar vasoconstriction occurs raising the total peripheral vascular resistance and shifting blood to the major organs. (2) (ME; AN; PA; BI)

1 With shock more antidiuretic hormone (ADH) is produced to promote fluid retention, which will elevate the blood pressure.

2 Although this is a response to hypoxia, peripheral vasoconstriction is a more effective compensatory mechanism.

4 With shock the mineralocorticoids increase to promote fluid retention, which will elevate the blood pressure.

127. 1 A decreased intravascular volume results in hypovolemia and hypotension, which is evidenced by a decreased blood pressure and a decreased pulse pressure. (3) (ME; AN; PA; BI)

2 Vasomotor stimulation to the arterial walls is increased with shock.

3 This is a description of neurogenic shock, which is unlikely in this situation.

4 Although electrolyte imbalances can precipitate cardiac decompensation, cardiogenic shock is unlikely in this situation.

128. 4 When an abdominal aneurysm ruptures, shock ensues because fluid volume depletion occurs as the heart continues to pump blood out of the ruptured vessel. (2) (SU; AN; PA; FE)

1 This type of shock results from humoral or toxic substances acting directly on the blood vessels, causing vasodilation.

2 This type of shock results from decreased neuromuscular tone, causing decreased vasoconstriction.

3 This type of shock results from a decrease in cardiac output.

129. 2 Peritonitis and shock are potentially life-threatening complications following abdominal surgery; prompt, rigorous treatment is necessary. (1) (SU; IM; TC; BI)

1 Fluids, not blood, would be needed to expand and maintain the circulating blood volume.

3 The head of the bed should be flat to increase tissue perfusion and oxygenation to the vital organs.

4 The physician should be notified; the oxygen was prescribed and the client should already be receiving it.

130. 1   This occurs during the progressive stage of shock as a result of accumulated lactic acid. (3) (ME; AN; TC; BI)

2   Metabolic alkalosis cannot occur with the buildup of lactic acid associated with the progressive stage of shock.

3   This can result from decreased respiratory function in late shock, further compounding metabolic acidosis.

4   This occurs as a result of hyperventilation during early shock.

131. 3   Blood replacement is needed to increase the O_2 carrying capacity of the blood; the normal hematocrit for women is 37% to 47% and for men 45% to 52%. (1) (SU; PL; TC; BI)

1   Serum albumin helps maintain volume but does not affect hemoglobin.

2   Ringer's lactate does not increase the O_2 carrying capacity of the blood.

4   Dextran does expand blood volume, but it causes cell aggregation, which aggravates the existing decreased tissue perfusion.

132. 4   This is absolutely necessary to prevent an acute immunologic reaction if the donated blood is not compatible with the client's blood. (1) (SU; AN; TC; BI)

1   Although important, this is not the highest priority.

2   Blood must be kept cold until ready to use; if blood is at room temperature for 30 minutes prior to administration it should be returned to the blood bank; after it is started, blood must be administered within 4 hours.

3   This is not the highest priority; these laboratory results were part of the data used to determine the need for the blood.

133. 3   Transfusion reactions from mismatched blood will usually occur early during the transfusion (first 30 ml of blood); initially keeping the infusion at a slow rate decreases the amount of blood infused, so that the nurse has an opportunity to assess the recipient's response. (2) (SU; PL; TC; BI)

1   Blood must be administered within 4 hours to prevent hemolysis from occurring before infusion.

2   Blood should be administered via gravity; volume control and peristaltic infusion devices cause hemolysis.

4   For monitoring the client's response, blood would not be drawn until several hours after the infusion.

134. 2   This results from a recipient's antibodies that are incompatible with transfused red blood cells; also called a type II hypersensitivity; these signs result from RBC hemolysis, agglutination, and capillary plugging. (3) (ME; AS; PA; BI)

1   This results from an immune sensitivity to foreign serum protein; also called a type I hypersensitivity; signs include urticaria, wheezing, dyspnea, and shock.

3   Bacterial pyrogens are present in contaminated blood and can cause a febrile transfusion reaction; signs include fever and chills.

4   There is no transfusion reaction called by this name, although anaphylaxis occurs with an allergic transfusion reaction.

135. 2   This is a sign of an acute hemolytic transfusion reaction indicating the recipient's blood is incompatible with the transfused blood; pain is caused by hemolysis, agglutination, and capillary plugging in the kidneys. (2) (SU; IM; TC; BI)

1   This is unsafe; this is a classic sign of a transfusion reaction, and the blood must be immediately stopped; while the assessment was being made, more incompatible blood would be infused, increasing the severity of the reaction.

3   Same as answer 1.

4   This is unsafe; blood must be stopped first and then normal saline should be infused to keep the line patent and maintain blood volume.

136. 4   The length of time a low-grade temperature is present, together with a history of night sweats and other physical findings, is valuable in making a diagnosis. (2) (ME; AS; PA; BI)

1   This is not immediately relevant to presenting signs and symptoms; more should be explored about the temperature itself

before investigating causes of the temperature.
2 Same as answer 1.
3 Same as answer 1.

137. 2 Equipment used is disposable; the donor does not come into contact with anyone else's blood. (2) (ME; AN; PA; BI)
1 The risk would depend on the spouse's prior behavior.
3 An individual may be infected for many weeks before testing positive for the antibody; the individual could still transmit the virus.
4 Condoms offer some protection but are subject to failure because of condom rupture or improper use; risks of infection are present with any sexual contact.

138. 2 These tests confirm the presence of HIV antibodies that occur in response to the presence of the human immunodeficiency virus. (1) (ME; AN; PA; BI)
1 This places someone at risk but does not constitute a positive diagnosis.
3 These do not confirm the presence of HIV; these adaptations are related to many disorders.
4 HIV infection is confirmed with the ELISA and Western blot tests; an opportunistic infection (included in the CDC surveillance case definition for AIDS) in the presence of HIV antibodies and T_4/CD_4 lymphocyte counts below 200 cells/μL indicate that the individual has AIDS.

139. 1 The HIV selectively infects helper T-cell lymphocytes; therefore, 300 or fewer CD_4/T_4 cells per cubic millimeter of blood or T_4/CD_4 cells accounting for less than 20% of lymphocytes is suggestive of AIDS. (1) (ME; AS; PA; BI)
2 The thymic hormones necessary for T-cell growth are decreased.
3 This finding is associated with allergies and parasitic infections.
4 This finding is associated with drug-induced hemolytic anemia and hemolytic disease of the newborn.

140. 4 Blood and body fluid precautions require that hands be washed before and after client care to minimize risk of transmission; since this procedure normally does not involve contact with blood or secretions, additional protection is not indicated. (1) (ME; IM; TC; BI)
1 These are necessary only when there is risk of contact with blood or body fluid.
2 Same as answer 1.
3 A mask and gown would be indicated only if there were danger of secretions or blood splattering on the nurse (for example, during suctioning).

141. 2 These items prevent contact with feces, sputum, or other body fluids during intimate body care. (2) (ME; AN; TC; BI)
1 Goggles and a mask would be required because the client is producing copious sputum.
3 Gloves are not necessary, because touching body fluids when giving oral medication is not likely.
4 Only gloves are necessary when assisting the client with a bed pan.

142. 3 *Pneumocystis carinii* is a protozoan that causes pneumonia in immunosuppressed hosts, which can cause death in 60% of the clients; the client's respiratory status is the priority. (3) (ME; PL; TC; BI)
1 Although this is a concern, the client's respiratory status is the priority.
2 Same as answer 1.
4 There are no data to support this diagnosis.

143. 3 Palliative measures are aimed at relieving discomfort without curing the problem. (1) (ME; PL; TC; BI)
1 A cure or recovery is not part of palliative care; with a terminal disease these goals are unrealistic.
2 Same as answer 1.
4 Support of significant others is indicated, but it is not a palliative measure because it is not aimed at relieving the client's discomfort.

144. 3 Pernicious anemia is caused by the inability to absorb vitamin B_{12} due to a lack of intrinsic factor in gastric juices; for the Schilling test, radioactive vitamin B_{12} is administered and its absorption and excretion can be ascertained. (3) (ME; AS; PA; BI)
  1 Not measured by this test.
  2 Same as answer 1.
  4 Vitamin B_{12} is not produced in the body.

145. 3 IM injections bypass the B_{12} absorption defect (lack of intrinsic factor, the transport carrier component of gastric juices); a monthly dose is usually sufficient since it is stored in active body tissues such as the liver, kidney, heart, muscles, blood, and bone marrow. (3) (ME; IM; PA; BI)
  1 The Z-track method need not be used as for iron dextran injections; injections once a month are usually sufficient.
  2 Since it is stored and only slowly depleted, it is not necessary to give injections this frequently.
  4 It cannot be taken by mouth because of the lack of intrinsic factor.

146. 3 Since the intrinsic factor does not return to gastric secretions even with therapy, B_{12} injections will be required for the remainder of the client's life. (2) (ME; EV; ED; BI)
  1 It must be taken on a regular basis for the rest of the client's life.
  2 Same as answer 1.
  4 Same as answer 1.

147. 2 A protocol consisting of three or four chemotherapeutic agents that attack the dividing cells at various phases of development is the therapy of choice at this stage; alternating courses of different protocols may be used. (3) (ME; AN; TC; BI)
  1 Radiation, alone or in combination with chemotherapy, is used in stages IA, IB, IIA, IIB, and IIIA.
  3 This is recommended for use in stage IIIA.
  4 This is not a therapy for Hodgkin's disease at any stage; nodes may be removed for biopsy; nodes may be irradiated as part of therapy.

148. 1 Women in the childbearing years should be informed of all options available to preserve ovarian function. (3) (SU; AN; TC; BI)
  2 This is an incorrect statement; always is too absolute.
  3 This is an incorrect statement because radiation can influence or destroy ovarian functioning.
  4 Once the ovaries have been destroyed, they cannot regenerate.

149. 2 Reduced platelets increase the likelihood of uncontrolled bleeding; reduced lymphocytes increase susceptibility to infection. (2) (ME; PL; ED; BI)
  1 This would be helpful for stomatitis, not pancytopenia; aggressive oral hygiene could precipitate bleeding from the gums.
  3 Although fluids may be increased to flush out the toxic byproducts of chemotherapy, this would have no effect on pancytopenia.
  4 This is a sign of hypocalcemia that would not apply to pancytopenia.

150. 4 Thrombocytopenia occurs with most chemotherapy; using a soft toothbrush helps prevent bleeding gums. (1) (ME; IM; TC; BI)
  1 While alopecia does occur, it is not related to bone marrow depression.
  2 Increasing fluids will neither reverse bone marrow depression nor stimulate hematopoiesis.
  3 This is not related to bone marrow depression.

151. 1 Suppression of bone marrow increases bleeding susceptibility associated with decreased platelets. (1) (ME; IM; TC; BI)
  2 This will not affect the bone marrow; citrus juices should be avoided by the client receiving chemotherapy because of the side effects of stomatitis.
  3 With bone marrow suppression the red blood cells are decreased in number and there is a decreased O_2 carrying capacity of the blood; this position will not increase the number of red blood cells.
  4 With bone marrow depression there

would be a decrease in red blood cells; rest should be encouraged.

152. 1 Brief pressure is generally enough to prevent bleeding. (2) (ME; IM; TC; BI)
2 Complications are rare; no special positions are required.
3 The site is cleaned prior to aspiration.
4 Complications are rare; frequent monitoring is unnecessary.

153. 3 Anemia with petechiae occurs because of bone marrow depression and rapidly proliferating leukocytes; anorexia is a general response to many illnesses. (3) (ME; AS; PA; BI)
1 There is no change in hair growth in the absence of chemotherapy.
2 While anorexia occurs, the client would more likely be sleeping excessively.
4 Same as answer 2.

154. 2 Splenomegaly usually accompanies chronic myelogenous leukemia (CML); it is usually gross, palpable, and tender and necessitates removal; the spleen is located high in the abdomen on the left side and is not usually palpable unless it is enlarged. (3) (ME; AS; PA; BI)
1 The urinary output is not affected.
3 These signs and symptoms are not associated with leukemia or splenomegaly but rather diabetes mellitus.
4 With leukemia and splenomegaly there is increased destruction of blood cells; the count will be low.

155. 2 This protein (globulin) is thought to be the result of tumor cell metabolites; it is often present in clients with multiple myeloma. (2) (ME; AS; PA; BI)
1 Hypercalcemia occurs with multiple myeloma because of bone erosion.
3 Although this can be a late complication of multiple myeloma because of coagulation defects, it is not specific to multiple myeloma.
4 Multiple myeloma is not caused by a bacterial infection.

156. 4 Because of bone erosion, pathological fractures are a frequent complication of multiple myeloma. (2) (ME; PL; TC; BI)
1 Although this would be done, the priority is to prevent injury.
2 Although this is an adaptation to the associated anemia, it is not life-threatening.
3 Although this is important, preventing pathological fractures is the priority.

157. 4 This is the treatment of choice; a variety of drugs affect rapidly dividing cells at different stages of cell division. (3) (ME; AN; TC; BI)
1 Although this may be done, it is not the primary treatment.
2 Although this may be used to alleviate pain and treat acute vertebral lesions, it is not the primary approach.
3 Multiple myeloma is a diffuse disorder of the bone and no single lesion can be removed.

158. 4 This is the schedule for active immunization recommended by the American Academy of Pediatrics. (2) (ME; PL; PA; BI)
1 This regimen does not follow the schedule for active immunization recommended by the American Academy of Pediatrics.
2 Same as answer 1.
3 Same as answer 1.

159. 1 Tetanus antitoxin provides antibodies, which confer immediate passive immunity. (3) (ME; IM; PA; BI)
2 Antitoxin does not stimulate production of antibodies.
3 Passive, not active, immunity occurs.
4 Passive immunity, by definition, is not long lasting.

160. 1   It takes this length of time for antibodies to respond to the antigen and form an indurated area. (1) (ME; AS; PA; BI)

2   This is longer than necessary; the site will reveal induration in 2 to 3 days.

3   Same as answer 2.

4   Same as answer 2.

161. 1   Drug hypersensitivity and anaphylaxis are most common with antimicrobial agents. (1) (ME; IM; TC; BI)

2   This is a dependent function; it is not crucial to starting antibiotic therapy.

3   This is an important assessment, but it is not crucial to starting antibiotic therapy.

4   Withholding treatment until culture results are available may extend the infection.

162. 2   Hypersensitivity to a foreign substance can cause an anaphylactic reaction; histamine is released, causing bronchial constriction, increased capillary permeability, and dilation of arterioles; this decreased peripheral resistance is associated with hypotension and inadequate circulation to major organs. (3) (ME; AN; PA; BI)

1   These are the problems that result from bronchial constriction and vascular collapse.

3   Dilation of arterioles occurs.

4   Arterioles dilate, capillary permeability increases, and eventually vascular collapse occurs.

INTEGUMENTARY

163. 1   Shearing force occurs when two surfaces move against each other; when the bed is at an angle greater than 30 degrees, the torso tends to slide and cause this phenomenon. (1) (ME; PL; TC; IT)

2   This would raise the head of the bed too high to prevent the client from sliding in bed.

3   Same as answer 2.

4   Same as answer 2.

164. 4   The client who is confined to bed should be encouraged to move in the bed to prevent prolonged pressure on any one skin surface. (2) (SU; PL; PA; IT)

1   This will help promote peripheral circulation, but prolonged presssure must be avoided.

2   This does not prevent prolonged pressure although it can help decrease skin breakdown by allowing air to circulate beneath the client.

3   Range-of-motion exercises move joints to prevent contractures; they do not relieve prolonged pressure.

165. 4   Exercise would promote extension of the local infection from the leg into the circulation, causing septicemia. (3) (ME; AN; TC; IT)

1   This is not accomplished by bedrest.

2   Although bedrest does this, it is not the purpose for it in this situation.

3   Same as answer 2.

166. 1   Surgical asepsis means that the defined area will contain no microorganisms. (2) (SU; AN; PA; IT)

2   This would be true of isolation procedures.

3   This would apply to isolation and medical asepsis.

4   This would apply to medical asepsis.

167. 2   A mask and sterile gloves protect the infusion site against contamination with airborne and other pathogenic organisms. (2) (SU; PL; TC; IT)

1   Sterile gloves will not protect against airborne pathogens.

3   A gown and gloves will not protect against airborne pathogens.

4   A gown would serve no useful purpose during site care.

168. 4   In the obese individual this helps to inject the medication into subcutaneous tissue rather than adipose tissue, where its absorption would be poor. (2) (ME; IM; ED; IT)

1   This will result in the drug being injected into adipose tissue, where it will be poorly absorbed.

2   Same as answer 1.

3   Same as answer 1.

169. 2 An iatrogenic infection is one that is caused by medical personnel, procedures, or the environment of the health care facility. (1) (SU; AN; PA; IT)
  1 This is not the cause of an iatrogenic infection.
  3 Same as answer 1.
  4 Same as answer 1.

170. 2 A nosocomial infection, by definition, is acquired during hospitalization. (1) (SU; IM; ED; IT)
  1 Exposure to the pathogen must have occurred after admission to the hospital for classification as a nosocomial infection.
  3 It may or may not be highly contagious; in this situation, others need to be protected from the client.
  4 This nosocomial infection is a primary, not a secondary, infection.

171. 1 Teaching for the postoperative period should begin as soon as the client is admitted; knowledge of what to expect decreases anxiety and may improve compliance with the treatment regimen. (1) (SU; PL; ED; IT)
  2 This is too late; the client must have time to ask questions and demonstrate the ability to care for the wound; teaching begins preoperatively.
  3 This is too late; at this time the client may be in too much discomfort to concentrate on learning.
  4 Same as answer 3.

172. 4 Delayed wound healing is often caused by a lack of nutrients, such as protein and vitamin C, in the diet. (1) (SU; AS; TC; IT)
  1 This usually occurs with severe protein deficiency and congestive heart failure.
  2 This usually occurs with iron-deficiency anemia.
  3 This usually indicates prolonged malnutrition.

173. 3 The nurse epidemiologist acts as a consultant to help devise an infection control strategy. (1) (ME; IM; ED; IT)
  1 This the role of the physician.

2 This is the role of the laboratory technician or technologist.
4 This is usually done by the primary nurse.

174. 3 Barriers reduce the contact of bile with skin and limit excoriation. (2) (SU; PL; TC; IT)
  1 Dressings should be changed when wet, not reinforced; usually the T-tube drainage empties into a pouch.
  2 Antiseptics are drying and irritating to excoriated skin, and they sting when applied; this would require a physician's order.
  4 This action may help, but the excoriation is probably caused by bile, not adhesive tape.

175. 3 Lubricating the skin with a moisturizer effectively relieves the dryness and thus the pruritus. (1) (ME; IM; PA; IT)
  1 Warm or cool, not hot, tub baths would decrease the itching.
  2 This would do nothing to lubricate the skin or relieve the pruritus.
  4 Exposing the skin to air causes further drying and would not relieve the pruritus.

176. 3 Bicarbonate solution is soothing and prevents scratching, which can cause abrasions and lead to infection. (1) (ME; PL; PA; IT)
  1 This is irritating and drying to the skin; also, alcohol can be absorbed through the skin and should be avoided.
  2 This would have no effect on the pruritus.
  4 Same as answer 2.

177. 3 Increased venous pressure alters the permeability of the veins, allowing extravasation of RBCs; lysis of RBCs causes brownish discoloration of the skin. (3) (ME; IM; ED; IT)
  1 The arterial circulation is not affected by varicose veins.
  2 Although tissue healing may be delayed, the brownish discoloration results from lysis of RBCs, not trauma.
  4 There is no increase in melanocyte activity with varicose veins.

178. 3   To make effective decisions, baseline information on the client's condition, extent of injury, and significant past health history is needed. (3) (ME; AS; TC; IT)

1   This would be unnecessary; hyperimmune antirabies serum is not a preferred treatment because many people are sensitive to horse serum.

2   Notification of authorities is done after the injured person has received care.

4   Inoculation for establishment of short-term, passive immunity to rabies would be done after the initial assessment and treatment of the wound.

179. 4   This is a viral infection that enters the body through a break in the skin and is characterized by convulsions and choking. (3) (ME; AN; PA; IT)

1   Rabies is not bacterially caused; its outstanding symptoms are convulsions and choking.

2   Rabies is not associated with a bacterial septicemia; it is caused by a virus.

3   This is not true; the virus specifically attacks nervous tissue and is carried in the saliva of infected animals.

180. 2   Radiodermatitis occurs 3 to 6 weeks after the start of treatment. (2) (ME; IM; ED; IT)

1   The word burn should be avoided because it may increase anxiety.

3   This response does not address the client's concern.

4   Emollients are contraindicated; they may alter the calculated x-ray route and injure normal tissue.

181. 2   These contain alcohol and metals that can increase the skin reaction. (1) (ME; IM; ED; IT)

1   This is contraindicated; compresses can precipitate skin breakdown.

3   This is contraindicated; gauze and tape may irritate the skin.

4   This is not necessary and controlling movement while sleeping is usually not possible.

182. 3   The skin is the first line of defense; keeping it dry and safe from injury promotes skin integrity. (1) (ME; PL; PA; IT)

1   This is unsafe because irradiated skin is fragile; if soap is used, a film left after rinsing can change the angle and intensity of radiation.

2   This is unsafe; irradiated skin is fragile and subject to blistering and sloughing.

4   This is unsafe; the skin should be free of emollients because they change the angle or degree of radiation.

183. 2   Scleroderma causes chronic hardening and shrinking of the connective tissues of any organ of the body including the esophagus and face; pureed foods limit the need to chew and this facilitates swallowing. (2) (ME; IM; TC; IT)

1   Liquefied foods are difficult to swallow; there is decreased esophageal peristalsis, and they are easily aspirated.

3   This will not help; it is equally difficult to swallow solids and liquids and aspiration may result.

4   This is not necessary; no oral pain is associated with scleroderma.

184. 2   Raynaud's phenomenon is caused by vasospasm, precipitated by exposure to cold or emotional stress; Raynaud's is commonly associated with scleroderma, a connective tissue disorder. (1) (ME; PL; PA; IT)

1   Decreased blood flow would interfere with perception of temperature and increase the risk of burns.

3   Trauma to the hands must be avoided; nerve endings are affected by the diminished blood supply.

4   Vasodilators, not anticoagulants, are prescribed to counteract vasospasm and increase blood flow.

185. 2   With scleroderma the skin becomes dry because of interference with the underlying sweat glands. (3) (ME; PL; PA; IT)

1   Pruritis is not associated with scleroderma.

3   There are no inflamed areas associated with scleroderma.

4   There are no scaly lesions associated with scleroderma.

186. 1 The changes in connective tissue associated with scleroderma lead to muscle weakness; optimal function must be preserved. (1) (ME; AN; PA; IT)
  2 Tissue regeneration will not occur; this is a progressive degenerative disorder.
  3 Prevention of spread is not possible in this systemic disease, which involves a number of organs.
  4 Exercise of stiff and painful joints causes pain, not a sense of well-being.

187. 3 This action effectively extinguishes the flames; avoiding additional intervention until the person receives medical attention prevents further injury. (2) (SU; EV; TC; IT)
  1 This may protect the person from further burns but it could further injure the burned tissue.
  2 This action does not deny the necessary oxygen and may, in fact, fan the flames.
  4 This may extinguish the flames but it is not as effective as rolling in the grass.

188. 2 A patent airway is most vital; if the person is not breathing CPR should be begun. (1) (SU; AS; TC; IT)
  1 The person should be kept npo because large burns decrease intestinal peristalsis and the person may vomit and aspirate.
  3 This is not done until the assessment for breathing has been completed.
  4 This is not the priority; this assessment will be done after transfer to a medical facility.

189. 3 A tablecloth is nonfuzzy and nonadhering and will keep the burned person warm. (2) (SU; IM; TC; IT)
  1 This is unsafe; body heat should be conserved with a nonadhering covering.
  2 Cream is difficult to remove and may result in additional damage.
  4 This is contraindicated because ice can result in additional tissue damage.

190. 3 In deep partial-thickness burns, destruction of the epidermis and upper layers of the dermis and injury to deeper portions of the dermis occur. (3) (SU; AS; PA; IT)
  1 Eschar, a dry leathery covering of denatured protein, occurs with full-thickness burns.
  2 In full-thickness burns, total destruction of the epidermis, dermis, and some underlying tissue occurs.
  4 In superficial partial-thickness burns, the epidermis is destroyed or injured and a portion of the dermis may be injured.

191. 2 The anterior part of the lower legs are 4.5% each which equals 9%. (2) (SU; AS; PA; IT)
  1 4.5% would only represent the anterior part of one leg from the knee to the foot.
  3 This would represent more than the anterior part of both legs from the knees to the feet.
  4 Same as answer 3.

192. 4 The entire right lower extremity is 18%; the anterior portion of the right upper extremity is 4.5%. (2) (SU; AS; PA; IT)
  1 This is less than the total percent of body surface burned.
  2 Same as answer 1.
  3 Same as answer 1.

193. 2 Heat inhalation can cause edema of the respiratory lumens, interfering with oxygenation; evaluation of respiratory status is a priority assessment. (3) (SU; AS; TC; IT)
  1 This would be done after the client's respiratory status has been evaluated.
  3 Burns should be evaluated by the physician, and then the ordered medical therapy should be implemented; the airway has priority.
  4 Same as answer 1.

194. 3   Hoarseness is a sign of potential respiratory insufficiency as a result of inhalation burns, which cause edema in the surrounding tissues, including the vocal cords. (3) (SU; AS; PA; IT)

1   This would indicate metabolic acidosis, not respiratory insufficiency.

2   Sputum would be sooty, not frothy; pink tinged, frothy sputum is associated with pulmonary edema.

4   Same as answer 1.

195. 2   Massive amounts of potassium are released from the injured cells into the extracellular fluid; large amounts of sodium are lost in edema. (3) (SU; AS; TC; IT)

1   The serum potassium will rise.

3   The serum potassium will rise; the serum sodium will fall.

4   The serum sodium will fall.

196. 3   Extreme restlessness in a severely burned client usually indicates cerebral hypoxia. (3) (SU; AS; PA; IT)

1   With renal failure the client would become progressively confused and lethargic, not restless.

2   At this stage the client would be hypovolemic rather than hypervolemic.

4   With metabolic acidosis the client would be lethargic.

197. 2   Pain is from the loss of the protective covering of the nerve endings; blisters and redness occur because of the injury to the dermis and epidermis. (1) (SU; AS; PA; IT)

1   Because some epithelial cells remain, grafting is not needed with a partial-thickness burn unless it becomes infected and further tissue damage occurs.

3   Partial-thickness burns involve only the superficial layers of skin, unless they become infected.

4   Recovery from partial-thickness burns with no infection occurs in 2 to 3 weeks.

198. 2   Topical antibiotics are directly applied to the wound and are effective against many gram positive and gram negative organisms that are found on the skin. (2) (SU; PL; PA; IT)

1   Although these may be administered, they are most effective for systemic rather than local infections; the vasculature in and around a burn is impaired and the medication may not reach the organisms in the wound.

3   Same as answer 1.

4   Same as answer 1.

199. 4   Care of burns is a painful procedure; pain medication should be administered before care to limit discomfort. (1) (SU; PL; TC; IT)

1   Surgical asepsis should be used.

2   No dressings are applied when the exposure method is used.

3   This is unnecessary; Sulfamylon is not hepatotoxic.

200. 2   The first step is to determine what the physician has told the client. (3) (SU; IM; ED; IT)

1   This statement would be inappropriate; grafting begins when the granulation bed is formed.

3   Same as answer 1.

4   Grafting will not be done until the wound is clean and granulation tissue has formed; there are no data to indicate the client has an infection.

201. 1   Clients with burns are sensitive to environmental changes; loss of the skin's microcirculation in the burned areas decreases the ability to retain body heat. (3) (SU; PL; TC; IT)

2   The room temperature should be kept at approximately 85° F or 24.4° C to limit loss of body heat.

3   This is too low; higher humidity (40% to 50% usually) is needed to maximize the warmth of the room.

4   A sterile sheet is not necessary; some clients may be treated by the open method and have burns exposed.

202. 3   The graft covers nerve endings which reduces pain and provides a framework for granulation. (3) (SU; AN; PA; IT)

1 The graft promotes epithelialization; enzymatic preparations or surgery debride wounds.

2 This is untrue; pig skin grafts are not sutured.

4 This is contraindicated; topical antimicrobials would soften the graft and impede healing.

203. 2 Range of motion should be instituted as soon as it will not compromise the individual's cardiorespiratory status. (2) (SU; PL; TC; IT)

1 Pain will continue for some time, and if ROM is delayed until it subsides, contractures will have already developed.

3 If ROM is delayed until skin grafts heal, contractures will have already developed.

4 Pain and inability to cope may be prolonged; if ROM is delayed, contractures will have already developed.

204. 2 Well-differentiated cells are associated with a positive prognosis, whereas undifferentiated cells are ominous. (1) (SU; PL; PS; IT)

1 The client's pathology report provides specific data that are more significant than general statistics.

3 Although the cancer could recur, a primary lesion in another location would not be expected.

4 This is inappropriate because the prognosis is fairly positive.

205. 4 The negative pressure of a portable wound drainage system exerts a sucking force that pulls fluid toward the collection chamber. (1) (SU; AN; PA; IT)

1 Gravity is the environmental force that pulls weight toward the center of the earth; an indwelling urinary catheter allows urine to flow by gravity from the bladder to a collection bag placed below the level of the bladder.

2 Osmosis occurs when solvent moves from a solution of lesser concentration to one of greater solute concentration when the two solutions are separated by a semipermeable membrane; fluid moving from the interstitial compartment into the intracellular compartment uses osmosis.

3 Active transport occurs when ions move across a cell membrane against a concentration gradient with the assistance of metabolic energy; the sodium-potassium pump uses active transport.

206. 2 Once the drugs that interfere with cell division are stopped, the hair will grow back; sometimes the hair will be a different color or texture. (1) (SU; IM; PA; IT)

1 Alopecia is a common side effect of chemotherapy.

3 Hair loss persists while the drugs are being received; once the drugs are withdrawn, the hair grows back.

4 Although ice caps on the head and rubber bands around the scalp have been used to try to limit alopecia, they have not been particularly effective.

SKELETAL

207. 3 These symptoms are consistent with a torn cartilage, which is also a common injury with basketball. (1) (SU; AS; PA; SK)

1 A fractured patella would cause pain and usually manifests itself at the time of injury.

2 A ruptured Achilles tendon is painful and prevents plantar flexion of the foot; symptoms are usually manifested immediately upon injury.

4 A stress fracture is associated with pain, not with a clicking or locking of the knee.

208. 2 This is a truthful description of arthroscopy; the physician uses a scope to visualize the knee structures to determine the extent of injury. (1) (SU; IM; ED; SK)

1 While this is true, it evades the client's concern and does not describe the procedure.

3 Arthroscopy is not a radiologic procedure.

4 Same as answer 1.

209. 4   A bone scan reflects the uptake of a bone-seeking radioactive isotope; an increased uptake is seen in metastatic bone disease, osteosarcoma, osteomyelitis, and certain fractures. (2) (ME; EV; ED; SK)

1   A bone scan measures the uptake of radioactive material, not the absence of calcium, which would be seen in an x-ray examination of bone.

2   This is a bone marrow aspiration when a small amount of marrow is examined to determine the presence of abnormal cells in diseases such as leukemia.

3   A bone scan involves a small diagnostic dosage of a radioactive substance; it is not therapeutic.

210. 2   Numbness is a neurologic sign that should be reported immediately because it indicates pressure on the nerves and blood vessels. (2) (SU; EV; TC; SK)

1   Warmth is a normal reaction to a new cast.

3   This results from inadequate skin care but can be easily managed with lotion or oil.

4   Some degree of discomfort is expected following cast application.

211. 3   Damage to the blood vessels may decrease the circulatory perfusion of the foot; the absence of the pedal pulse would indicate a lack of blood supply to the lower extremity. (2) (SU; EV; PA; SK)

1   The break is between the knee and the ankle, not the thigh.

2   Damage to the major blood vessels would more likely cause a decrease in blood pressure from shock.

4   Decreased circulatory perfusion of the foot would cause the skin temperature to decrease, but the foot could also feel cool because of shock.

212. 3   This indicates tissue hypoxia or breakdown and should be reported to the physician. (1) (SU; IM; TC; SK)

1   Other data, such as elevated temperature or increased white cells, are not present to support the presence of an infection.

2   This is not a typical response to a cast and may indicate a complication.

4   The priority is to notify the physician; this could be done to provide relief to the client after the physician is notified.

213. 3   Elevation will help control the swelling that normally occurs. (3) (SU; IM; ED; SK)

1   Because the ankle has been at rest, discomfort and stiffness are expected after the cast is removed.

2   Because the skin has not been exposed, it needs gentle washing to prevent breaking the skin.

4   The leg should be put through full range of motion more than once daily.

214. 4   These movements include all possible range of motion for the ankle joint. (1) (ME; IM; PA; SK)

1   Although the ankle can be moved in a circular motion, flexion and extension are more specifically called dorsiflexion and plantar flexion in relation to the ankle; also, eversion and inversion should be done when manipulating the ankle.

2   Flexion and extension are more specifically called dorsiflexion and plantar flexion in relation to the ankle; the ankle cannot be abducted or adducted; the ankle can be inverted and everted.

3   These motions refer to the upper extremities.

215. 3   These sets of muscles will be used in crutch walking and, therefore, need strengthening. (2) (SU; AN; TC; SK)

1   Although these muscles keep the person erect, the most important muscles for walking with crutches are the triceps, elbow extensors, and finger flexors of the arms, and the muscles in the unaffected leg.

2   This will do nothing to strengthen the weight-bearing leg.

4   A pushing, not a pulling, motion is used with crutches; the triceps, not the biceps, are used.

216. 2   The palms should bear the client's weight to avoid damage to the nerves in the axilla (brachial plexus). (1) (SU; EV; ED; SK)

1 This would be unsafe; pressure on the axillary region could injure the nerves in the brachial plexus.
3 The physician ordered non-weight bearing on the affected leg.
4 Same as answer 1.

217. 3 In a comminuted fracture, the bone is splintered or crushed. (2) (SU; AN; PA; SK)
1 This is a compound fracture.
2 This is a green-stick fracture.
4 This is a complete fracture.

218. 3 The infected bone is placed at rest in a cast, splint, or traction to reduce pain and limit the spread of infection. (2) (SU; PL; TC; SK)
1 This is contraindicated; this would increase pain and spread the infection.
2 Osteomyelitis is usually caused by a microorganism traveling through the bloodstream to the bone, not the reverse; the client is already septic.
4 This is contraindicated; ambulation may facilitate the spread of infection.

219. 3 The antibody called rheumatoid factor is present in 90% of clients with advanced arthritic changes; it is not found in the early stages of the disease process. (2) (ME; IM; ED; SK)
1 This denies the client's discomfort and does not deal with the stated confusion.
2 This denies the client's immediate feelings and blocks communication of them.
4 This response reinforces the client's felt discomfort and confusion over negative test results.

220. 3 Moist heat increases circulation and decreases muscle tension, which helps relieve chronic stiffness. (1) (ME; IM; PA; SK)
1 While this is advisable for someone with arthritis, it will not relieve morning stiffness.
2 This is related to preventing muscle fatigue, not to stiffness of joints.
4 Inactivity promotes stiffness.

221. 2 This is caused by inflammation of the synovium, resulting in vascular congestion, fibrin exudate, and cellular infiltrate. (1) (ME; AN; PA; SK)
1 Urate crystals occur with gouty arthritis, not rheumatoid arthritis.
3 This is unrelated to rheumatoid arthritis.
4 Increased interstitial fluid (edema) is only one aspect of the inflammatory response.

222. 1 Palpation will elicit tenderness because pressure stimulates nerve endings and causes pain. (1) (ME; AN; PA; SK)
2 It is already swollen, and the pressure causes pain.
3 Nodules associated with rheumatoid arthritis are not caused by pressure; they occur spontaneously in about 25% of individuals with rheumatoid arthritis and are composed of collagen fibers, exudate, and cellular debris.
4 These are present in gout, not arthritis; they are composed of sodium urate.

223. 2 This position provides for extension of joints. (1) (ME; PL; PA; SK)
1 The side-lying position supports flexion of joints.
3 This creates continued flexion of joints.
4 This position does not influence position of joints.

224. 2 The hips and shoulders should be against the back of the chair; the thighs should be fully supported, with the knees and ankles at 90°; this provides support and limits contractures. (2) (ME; IM; PA; SK)
1 In a low chair the hips will be flexed less than 90°; the client needs a high-backed chair.
3 In this position the thighs and knees are not fully supported because they extend beyond the depth of the seat.
4 This would encourage flexion contractures.

225. 4 Some pain is to be expected, but the activity should not be continued when the pain becomes severe because it can further traumatize the inflamed synovial membrane. (2) (ME; EV; TC; SK)
  1 Some discomfort is expected; inactivity will promote the development of muscle atrophy and joint contracture.
  2 This is unrealistic because some discomfort is expected.
  3 This is unsafe; activity should be curtailed when pain becomes severe.

226. 3 The Valsalva maneuver raises cerebrospinal fluid pressure thereby causing pain. (1) (ME; AS; PA; SK)
  1 Calf tenderness is associated with thrombophlebitis, not disc problems.
  2 Dysuria is associated with urinary problems, not disc problems.
  4 This type of pain is not associated with intervertebral disc problems; it may occur with renal calculi.

227. 3 Pain results because herniation of a disc into the spinal column irritates the spinal cord or the roots of spinal nerves. (1) (ME; AN; PA; SK)
  1 This is not involved; the lamina is that portion of the vertebrae which is removed during surgery to gain access to the disc.
  2 The vertebral bodies themselves are not shifting.
  4 Circulation of cerebrospinal fluid is not affected.

228. 3 Coughing places strain on the lumbar area, increasing the herniation of the disc. (2) (SU; IM; ED; SK)
  1 This does not increase intervertebral pressure.
  2 This will not increase pressure or cause pain; flexed knees are usually a more comfortable position.
  4 This will not increase pressure or increase pain.

229. 2 Putting the upper arm and leg toward the side to which the client is turning uses body weight to facilitate turning; the spine is kept straight. (3) (SU; AN; ED; SK)

  1 This is unsafe; this would result in twisting the spinal column.
  3 This could be done if another person were turning the client; when turning alone in this position, the client would have no leverage and turning would probably result in twisting the spinal column.
  4 This would interfere with turning because the bent leg becomes an obstacle and provides a force opposite to the leverage needed to turn.

230. 4 This maintains vertebral alignment, decreasing trauma to the operative site. (2) (SU; IM; TC; SK)
  1 This is contraindicated; it does not maintain vertebral alignment and may raise cerebrospinal fluid pressure.
  2 This is contraindicated; the contour position flexes the vertebral column.
  3 Traction is not used with this surgery.

231. 2 Alteration in circulation and sensation indicates damage to the spinal cord and must be monitored. (2) (SU; AS; TC; SK)
  1 Logrolling from side to side is preferred; the prone position may hyperextend the vertebral column.
  3 Although observation is part of assessment, these assessments are not a priority.
  4 Fluid intake is not a problem with these clients postoperatively.

232. 2 Sitting maintains alignment of the back and allows the nurses to support the client until orthostatic hypotension subsides. (2) (SU; IM; TC; SK)
  1 This would permit flexion of the vertebrae, which could traumatize the spinal cord.
  3 Same as answer 1.
  4 Rapid movement could flex the vertebrae, which would traumatize the spinal cord; safety is the priority; if the blood pressure were taken it would probably reveal orthostatic hypotension.

233. 2 This is contraindicated; maintaining the sitting position for a prolonged period of time places excessive body weight and stress on the surgical area. (2) (SU; EV; ED; SK)

1 This maintains lordosis of the small of the back and provides proper support.

3 This prevents excessive pressure on the musculature and vertebral column.

4 This relieves pressure on the back and promotes comfort in bed.

234. 2 This is done while in the supine position before the body is subjected to the force of gravity in a vertical position; anatomic landmarks are easier to locate for correct application of the brace, and intraabdominal organs have not shifted toward the pelvic floor by gravity. (2) (SU; PL; PA; SK)

1 This is unsafe; it should be applied while in the supine position before getting out of bed and should be worn the entire day for support.

3 The brace should be applied while in the supine position, not the sitting position.

4 Twisting exercises are contraindicated because they exert excessive pressure on the operative site.

235. 2 Phantom limb pain is a real experience with no known cause or cure. (1) (SU; AN; TC; SK)

1 This may be an appropriate diagnosis for the client with an amputation, but it is not the diagnosis related to phantom limb pain.

3 This is not an appropriate diagnosis for the individual with an amputation.

4 Same as answer 1.

236. 1 The wrapping of the stump is implemented to reduce swelling and shape the stump for fitting a prosthesis in the future. (3) (SU; AN; TC; SK)

2 The stump sock, not the bandage, is used to protect the stump from irritation and injury.

3 Infection is not prevented in this manner; surgical asepsis should be maintained.

4 Secretion drainage is not promoted by wrapping the limb; portable drainage systems are used for this purpose.

237. 4 Pressure supports tissue, promotes venous return, and limits edema, thus promoting shrinkage. (2) (SU; IM; PA; SK)

1 Activity, not bandaging, usually decreases the occurrence of phantom-limb pain.

2 Although it may, its primary purpose is to promote venous return, prevent edema, and shrink the stump.

3 While pressure may prevent hemorrhage, its primary purpose is to prevent edema and shrink the stump.

238. 3 This stretches the flexor muscle and prevents a flexion contracture of the hip. (2) (SU; IM; ED; SK)

1 This flexes the hip and may result in a hip flexion contracture; the stump is usually elevated for only 24 to 48 hours.

2 This may result in an abduction deformity; the stump should be kept in functional alignment.

4 This should be started on a soft surface with a physician's order approximately 5 days postoperatively.

239. 2 Preparation for crutch walking includes exercises to strengthen the arm and shoulder muscles. (1) (SU; IM; PA; SK)

1 This is important in healing and preparation for the prosthesis, not for crutch walking.

3 Position changes are to prevent hip flexion contractures, not to prepare for crutch walking.

4 Phantom-limb phenomenon is a sensation that the absent limb is present; there are no such exercises.

240. 2 Without the prosthesis, a walker or crutches would be necessary and require the readjustment of weight bearing on one leg. (3) (SU; AN; PA; SK)

1 Early use of a prosthesis does not affect the development or presence of phantom limb pain, which occurs in about 10% of clients with an amputation.

3 Early use of a prosthesis has no effect on wound infection.

4 While this is true, it is not the major purpose; a prosthesis can easily be fitted after discharge when the stump is completely healed and no longer edematous.

241. 3   The even distribution of hemosiderin (iron-rich pigment) in the tissue in response to pressure of the prosthesis indicates proper fit. (2) (SU; AS; PA; SK)
  1   This would result in an improper fit.
  2   This has nothing to do with a proper fit.
  4   This indicates that the prosthesis is too long or too short.

242. 2   Gentle intervention reduces pain and shock and inhibits release of bone marrow into the system preventing an embolus. (2) (SU; IM; PA; SK)
  1   This will not prevent fat emboli; it may limit edema and pain, a local effect.
  3   Maintaining alignment will not prevent fat emboli; immobility may result in other complications.
  4   This will not prevent fat emboli; it may prevent hypostatic pneumonia and atelectasis.

243. 2   Weight greater than 8 pounds causes excessive tension on the skin, leading to damage. (2) (SU; AN; TC; SK)
  1   The spreader bar should be wide enough to keep materials away from the malleoli.
  3   If moleskin is used it is placed on the medial and lateral portions of the leg.
  4   Covering the malleoli causes skin breakdown; tape is unnecessary if a Buck's traction splint with Velcro is used.

244. 1   The client probably has a fat embolus; oxygen reduces surface tension of the fat globules and reduces hypoxia. (3) (SU; IM; PA; SK)
  2   Oxygen should be administered and the client placed in semi-Fowler's position before the physician is called.
  3   The client is not in shock resulting from hemorrhage, but has a fat embolus; oxygen takes priority.
  4   This will cause hip flexion, putting stress on the fractured femur; the semi-Fowler's position is preferred.

245. 4   A complete assessment must be performed to determine the location, characteristics, intensity and duration of the pain; the pain could be incisional, result from a pulmonary embolus, or be caused by neurovascular trauma to the affected leg, and the intervention for each would be different. (1) (SU; EV; TC; SK)
  1   This may be done after a complete assessment reveals that this would be the appropriate intervention; assessment is the priority.
  2   Same as answer 1.
  3   Same as answer 1.

246. 2   Compressed air inflates the plastic stockings systematically from ankle to calf to thigh and then deflates; this promotes venous return and prevents venous stasis and thromboembolism. (1) (SU; PL; PA; SK)
  1   Turning on the operative side is contraindicated because it places tension on the hip joint and may traumatize the incision.
  3   Although this may be ordered to promote muscle strength, the major complication, preventing thromboembolism, is the priority.
  4   This is contraindicated without a specific physician's order.

247. 1   After surgery, abduction is maintained to reduce the chance of dislocation of the femoral head. (1) (SU; PL; ED; SK)
  2   This can lead to dislocation of the femoral head.
  3   This causes adduction, which can lead to dislocation of the femoral head and is contraindicated.
  4   Same as answer 2.

248. 4   The pelvis is elevated by actions involving the unaffected upper extremities and unoperative leg. (2) (SU; IM; TC; SK)
  1   This is not permitted because it causes adduction of the leg and can lead to dislocation of the femoral head.
  2   No pressure is permitted on the operative hip because it can cause dislocation of the femoral head.
  3   Lifting only with the arms requires strength; the use of both heels puts pressure on the operative hip.

249. 3   At the time of a fracture or orthopaedic surgery fat globules may move from the bone marrow into the blood stream; also elevated catecholamines cause mobilization of fatty acids and the development of fat globules; in addition to obstruction of vessels in the lung, brain, and kidneys by systemic embolization from fat globules, petechiae are noted in the buccal membranes, conjunctival sacs, the hard palate and over the chest and anterior axillary folds; petechiae only occur with a fat embolism. (3) (SU; AS; TC; SK)

1 This is a sign of an embolus, but it is not specific to a fat embolus.

2 Same as answer 1.

4 Same as answer 1.

250. 3 This puts the least strain on the prosthesis and the hip may be flexed to 90 degrees ten days after surgery. (2) (SU; PL; TC; SK)

1 A soft chair would permit hip flexion greater than 90 degrees.

2 Elevation of the leg places increased strain on the prosthesis.

4 Same as answer 1.

251. 4 Avoidance of strain is essential to provide time for the prosthesis to sit adequately in the socket and not become dislodged; this usually takes two months. (2) (SU; PL; TC; SK)

1 This is an inadequate time for healing to take place.

2 This is too long; it is usually up to 2 months for partial weight-bearing, although positional restrictions may go beyond 2 months.

3 Same as answer 1.

NEUROMUSCULAR

252. 1 The afferent sensory branch of the trigeminal nerve (cranial nerve V) innervates the cornea. (3) (ME; AS; PA; NM)

2 This would test the function of cranial nerve VII.

3 This would test the function of cranial nerves III, IV, and VI.

4 This would test the function of cranial nerve XI.

253. 2 These are used to observe the pharynx and larynx, assess the symmetry of the soft palate, and determine the presence of the gag reflex; it provides data about cranial nerve X (vagus nerve). (3) (ME; AS; TC; NM)

1 This is used to assess cranial nerve VIII (auditory).

3 This is used to assess cranial nerve II (optic).

4 These are used to assess sensory function; that is, light touch and pain.

254. 1 Staying flat for 6 to 12 hours helps prevent spinal fluid leakage. (1) (SU; PL; PA; NM)

2. This may predispose to spinal fluid leakage; the client should be kept flat for 6 to 12 hours.

3. This position may increase intracranial pressure and is not appropriate.

4. Same as answer 2.

255. 3 This is done to assess electrical activity and determine whether symptoms are primarily musculoskeletal or neurologic. (1) (ME; IM; ED; NM)

1 No special preparation for an electromyography is required.

2 No special care is required during the procedure.

4 No special care is required after the procedure.

256. 3 This drug is a cholinergic and an anticholinesterase; it blocks the action of cholinesterase at the myoneural junction and inhibits the destruction of acetylcholine; its action of increasing muscle strength is immediate. (2) (ME; AS; PA; NM)

1 The results will be added to the data base, but they are non-specific.

2 This is a slower-acting anticholinesterase drug that is frequently ordered to treat myasthenia gravis; Tensilon is used, instead of this drug, to diagnose myasthenia gravis because when injected IV it immediately increases muscle strength.

4 Same as answer 1.

257. 2   Use reduces strength, and rest increases strength; eyelid movement, chewing, swallowing, speech, facial expression, and breathing are often affected. (3) (ME; AS; TC; NM)

1   Muscle strength increases with rest and decreases with activity.

3   Anticholinesterase drugs improve muscle strength.

4   Same as answer 3.

258. 4   Increased activity and stress precipitate exacerbation of symptoms because nerve impulses fail to pass to muscles at the myoneural junction; theories include inadequate acetylcholine, excessive cholinesterase, or a nonresponse of the muscle fibers to acetylcholine. (2) (ME; AS; PA; NM)

1   Muscle weakness and fatigue come on quickly and disappear rapidly with rest in the initial stages of the disease.

2   Rest promotes a decrease in symptoms because the demand for muscle contraction is reduced.

3   Strength decreases with progressive activity.

259. 2   Facial muscles innervated by the cranial nerves are often affected; dysphagia, ptosis, and diplopia are most common. (2) (ME; AS; PA; NM)

1   Myasthenia gravis is a neuromuscular disease with lower motor neuron characteristics, not CNS symptoms.

3   This is associated with multiple sclerosis.

4   This is associated with Parkinson's disease.

260. 3   Excessive weakness and impaired diaphragmatic innervation result in a depressed ability to breathe; airway clearance and effective gas exchange are the priority. (3) (ME; AN; TC; NM)

1   This is not the priority nursing diagnosis at this time.

2   Same as answer 1.

4   Same as answer 1.

261. 4   Because of myoneural junction defects, repeated use depletes acetylcholine, ele-

vates cholinesterase, or exhausts acetylcholine receptor sites. (3) (ME; PL; PA; NM)

1   Hot baths tend to increase muscle weakness.

2   With myasthenia gravis, muscle weakness increases with muscle use.

3   There is no evidence that eating meals will bring about improvement.

262. 2   Rest will decrease the demands at the synoptic membrane of the neuromuscular junction reducing fatigue; activity should be paced to prevent fatigue before it begins. (1) (ME; IM; PA; NM)

1   This will aggravate the fatigue; activity and rest should be delicately balanced to prevent fatigue

3   Same as answer 1.

4   This cannot be done without a physician's order; rest will usually alleviate the fatigue.

263. 3   Mestinon is a vital drug that must be taken on time; missed or late doses can result in severe respiratory and neuromuscular consequences or even death. (3) (ME; EV; TC; NM)

1   This is unnecessary because it is not a gastric irritant.

2   This is unnecessary because food does not impair absorption of the drug.

4   This is unnecessary.

264. 3   Remissions and exacerbations are common; a decrease in symptoms is related to rest and adequate blood levels of an anticholinesterase drug; an increase in symptoms is related to physical activity, stress, and inadequate blood levels of an anticholinesterase drug. (3) (ME; AS; PA; NM)

1   Intention tremors are associated with multiple sclerosis.

2   Exercise decreases muscle strength.

4   The proximal muscles are more involved than the distal muscles.

265. 2   Respiratory infections place people with myasthenia gravis at high risk because they do not cough effectively and may develop pneumonia or airway obstruction. (1) (ME; EV; ED; NM)

1 Activity should be done earlier in the day before the energy reserve is depleted; periods of activity should be alternated with periods of rest.

3 This is unsafe; the client should eat sitting up to prevent aspiration.

4 This is contraindicated; these potentiate weakness because of their effect on the myoneural junction.

266. 3 Tensilon acts systemically to increase muscle strength with a peak effect in 30 seconds; it lasts several minutes. (3) (ME; IM; ED; NM)

1 Tensilon produces a brief increase in muscle strength; with a negative response the client would demonstrate no change in symptoms.

2 The duration of Tensilon's action is about 3 minutes.

4 Tensilon acts systemically on all muscles, rather than selectively on the eyelids.

267. 3 Until the diagnosis is confirmed, the primary goal should be to maintain adequate activity and prevent muscle atrophy. (3) (ME; AN; TC; NM)

1 It is too early to develop a teaching plan; the diagnosis is not yet established.

2 This is too early; the client cannot adjust if diagnosis is not yet confirmed.

4 This is not a goal.

268. 4 Respiratory failure will require emergency intervention, and inability to swallow may lead to aspiration. (3) (ME; AS; PA; NM)

1 These are symptoms of myasthenia that may occur but are not life threatening.

2 This is a long-term problem that needs attention but is not life threatening.

3 Same as answer 1.

269. 4 Dysphagia should be minimized during peak effect of pyridostigmine bromide (Mestinon), thereby decreasing probability of aspiration. (2) (ME; IM; TC; NM)

1 There are insufficient data to know whether this is appropriate because liquids can also be aspirated.

2 This will not prevent aspiration.

3 This action will not prevent aspiration, although it is vital that the respiratory function be monitored.

270. 2 Spacing activities will encourage maximum functioning within the limits of client's strength and fatigue. (2) (ME; PL; PA; NM)

1 This is probably unnecessary if client is closely observed by the nursing staff; it should be permitted if requested by the client or family.

3 Bedrest and limited activity may lead to muscle atrophy and calcium depletion.

4 This is necessary for lifelong psychologic adjustment but more appropriate as the client is moving toward discharge.

271. 3 Results are unpredictable and symptoms may gradually return over several years. (3) (SU; IM; ED; NM)

1 This may increase the client's anxiety, and details of the actual surgery are not required with informed consent.

2 Thymectomy is a well-established treatment and is not considered experimental.

4 This may actually increase the client's anxiety; although complications should be mentioned, they should not be emphasized.

272. 3 Steps are short and dragging; this is seen with basal ganglia defects. (2) (ME; AS; PA; NM)

1 This is a staggering gait often associated with cerebellar disease.

2 This is associated with unilateral upper motor neuron disease.

4 This is associated with bilateral spastic paresis of the legs.

273. 3   Amplitude of the voice is reduced by neuromuscular involvement. (1) (ME; AS; PA; NM)
  1   Constipation is a common problem because of a weakness of muscles used in defecation.
  2   The tendency is for the head and neck to be drawn forward by loss of basal ganglia control.
  4   Usually loss of weight occurs because of the embarrassment caused by slowness and untidiness in eating.

274. 2   There is a lack of neural control of individual muscle fibers, resulting in a characteristic mask-like facies. (1) (ME; AS; PA; NM)
  1   This is unrelated to Parkinson's disease; this is often associated with a CVA.
  3   Movement usually abolishes tremors which are known as nonintention tremors.
  4   This does not occur; both arms fall rigidly to the sides and do not swing with a normal rhythm when walking.

275. 4   Visual disturbances such as diplopia and blurred vision are common initial symptoms of optic nerve lesions. (1) (ME; AS; PA; NM)
  1   Constipation may occur late in the disease because of immobility.
  2   Although this is a neuromuscular disorder, headaches are not a common symptom.
  3   Decubiti may become infected if they occur late in the disease because of immobility.

276. 4   This is a truthful answer that provides hope for the client. (3) (ME; IM; ED; NM)
  1   This response avoids the client's question and could increase anxiety.
  2   Analgesics are not commonly prescribed unless pain results from some other condition.
  3   This avoids the client's question by suggesting a task to complete.

277. 1   An increase in intraocular pressure (IOP) results from a resistance of aqueous humor outflow; open-angle glaucoma, the most common type of glaucoma, results from increased resistance to aqueous humor outflow through the trabecular meshwork, Schlemm's canal, and the episcleral venous system. (1) (ME; AN; PA; NM)
  2   This is the description of a cataract.
  3   This is the description of astigmatism.
  4   This is the description of a detached retina.

278. 4   Increased intraocular pressure damages the optic nerve, interfering with peripheral vision. (1) (ME; AS; PA; NM)
  1   These may be associated with detached retina.
  2   There is difficulty in adjusting to darkness.
  3   Same as answer 1.

279. 2   A major goal of early postoperative care is to prevent increased intraocular pressure; lying on the unaffected side or in the supine position will minimize intraocular pressure. (1) (SU; EV; ED; NM)
  1   This is contraindicated; this increases intraocular pressure.
  3   Same as answer 1.
  4   Same as answer 1.

280. 3   Bending increases intraocular pressure and must be avoided. (2) (SU; IM; ED; NM)
  1   Activities do not have to be restricted this long.
  2   This should be avoided because it raises intraocular pressure.
  4   Same as answer 1.

281. 1   Safety is a priority; this will keep the client from falling out of bed and will provide a sense of security. (1) (SU; PL; TC; NM)
  2   The affected eye is patched; therefore, the level of light is insignificant.
  3   This may increase anxiety and reduce the client's feeling of being in control.
  4   It is not necessary to immobilize the head so rigidly; also, this may increase anxiety.

282. 2   An antiemetic would prevent vomiting; vomiting increases intraocular pressure and should be avoided. (2) (SU; IM; TC; NM)

1   This is unsafe; vomiting increases intraocular pressure and aggressive intervention is required.

3   Same as answer 1.

4   Same as answer 1.

283. 4   Postoperatively the client must check daily for signs of rejection, which include redness, irritation, discomfort, or vision loss; the surgeon should be notified if any of these appear; pain following a cataract extraction may indicate infection or hemorrhage and should be reported to the physician immediately. (3) (SU; EV; ED; NM)

1   Driving should be avoided until given specific permission to do so by the physician.

2   Soap may irritate the eye and showers or shampooing the hair should be avoided as instructed, usually from several days to two weeks.

3   This is a symptom of retinal detachment and would not be expected.

284. 1   To protect against physical injury and infection, the dropper tip should not touch the eye. (1) (SU; EV; ED; NM)

2   This is incorrect technique; drops should be placed within the lower lid.

3   This is incorrect technique; the lower lid should be retracted for placement of eyedrops.

4   This is incorrect technique; it would squeeze medication out of the eye.

285. 3   This subjective symptom is caused by stimulation of retinal cells by ocular movement. (3) (SU; AS; PA; NM)

1   This is a disease of the connective tissue, not of the eye.

2   Glaucoma causes the individual to see halos around lights, not flashes of light.

4   Cerebral concussions do not result in this ocular symptom.

286. 4   The thermal inflammatory response, caused by a laser beam, results in a chorioretinal scar that holds the retina in place. (2) (SU; IM; ED; NM)

1   Radiation is not used because it destroys retinal tissue.

2   Burr holes are used in brain surgery.

3   Dermabrasion is used in acne vulgaris.

287. 3   Bleeding from the ears occurs only with basal skull fractures; bleeding from the ears is an assessment that assists in diagnosing the location of the injury. (2) (ME; AS; TC; NM)

1   This would be a positive response; pupils should react to light.

2   This would occur only in an infant in the presence of dehydration.

4   This occurs with increased intracranial pressure and pressure on the brain stem; it would be an expected response but not an immediate one.

288. 2   Controlled ventilation induces hypocapnea; subsequently it causes vasoconstriction and reduced cerebral blood flow. (3) (SU; EV; PA; NM)

1   The fluid may be cerebrospinal fluid; clearing the ear may cause further damage.

3   Because of manipulation during a craniotomy, anticonvulsants are given prophylactically to prevent seizures.

4   This would not increase cerebral blood flow and is inappropriate.

289. 4   This lessens the possibility of hemorrhage, provides for better circulation of cerebral spinal fluid, and promotes venous return. (3) (SU; IM; TC; NM)

1   Gatching the knees is contraindicated because it raises intracranial pressure.

2   This position is appropriate for infratentorial surgery.

3   A low Fowler's position and turning the head impedes venous return, which increases intracranial pressure.

290. 2 An inability to completely extend the legs is the classic sign of meningeal irritation. (3) (SU; AS; TC; NM)

1 Sunset eyes occur when the eyelid falls above the iris, allowing the sclera to show; this is often associated with hydrocephalus in children.

3 Homan's sign is pain caused by vascular irritability when the foot is flexed; this indicates thrombophlebitis.

4 The plantar reflex is a normal spinal cord reflex; not altered with meningeal irritation.

291. 2 Recognition of effort is motivating. (3) (SU; PL; ED; NM)

1 This may decrease both self esteem and motivation.

3 Constantly focusing on the problem may decrease both self esteem and motivation.

4 The problem is a motor, not a sensory (receptive), problem.

292. 2 Emboli, occurring from atrial fibrillation, cause complete occlusion of vessels; usually middle cerebral arteries are involved; the infarct may cause hemiplegia, aphasia, or spatial perceptual deficits. (3) (ME; AN; PA; NM)

1 Hypertension is a disease that may cause spasm of the arteries, but does not cause anatomic occlusion.

3 Developmental defects of the arterial wall are associated with sacular aneurysms.

4 Seizures are caused by inappropriate paroxysmal discharge.

293. 1 Narrowing of arteries supplying the brain causes temporary neurologic deficits that last for a short period of time; between attacks the neurologic examination is normal. (2) (ME; AN; PA; NM)

2 This is not the description of a TIA; remissions and exacerbations occur with progressive degenerative neurologic disorders.

3 Emboli result in a CVA; the damage is usually permanent.

4 This occurs with multiple small cerebrovascular accidents; TIAs do not result in permanent damage.

294. 3 The cause of the hypotension must be evaluated by the physician. (3) (SU; IM; TC; CV)

1 This is a dependent function, and the physician must be notified first.

2 This is contraindicated; it would further decrease blood flow to the brain.

4 This is contraindicated; the physician must be notified first.

295. 3 Muscles used for swallowing are innervated by the 9th (glossopharyngeal) and 10th (vagus) cranial nerves. (3) (SU; EV; PA; NM)

1 This is unrelated to cranial nerves; this is associated with neck edema and potential compromise of the airway.

2 This is unrelated to cranial nerves; some edema is expected because of the inflammatory process at the site of surgery.

4 Alterations in blood pressure may occur but are not caused by cranial nerve dysfunction.

296. 2 This assessment would indicate if there is a progression of symptoms or improvement and assist the physician in determining the diagnosis. (2) (ME; AS; PA; NM)

1 An elevation in temperature is not an early sign of an extension of a cerebral vascular accident.

3 The data indicate the vital signs were normal and do not reflect hypertension; while vital signs would be monitored, the client's motor status in this instance is most significant.

4 This is not the priority assessment.

297. 3 This position will neither raise intracranial pressure nor interfere with respirations and will permit oral secretions to drain from the mouth by gravity. (2) (ME; IM; TC; NM)

1 This could compromise the airway by permitting the tongue to fall to the posterior pharynx and obstruct the airway.

2 Elevating the head of the bed could compromise vital functions by compressing the brain stem.

4 This is contraindicated because it may increase intracranial pressure.

298. 4 Increased intracranial pressure is manifested by sluggish pupils and elevation of the systolic blood pressure. (1) (ME; AN; PA; NM)

1 Spinal shock is manifested by a lowered systolic blood pressure with no pupillary changes.

2 Hypovolemic shock is indicated by a decrease in systolic pressure and tachycardia with no changes in pupillary reaction.

3 Transtentorial herniation is manifested by dilated pupils and severe posturing.

299. 2 Shortening and eventual atrophy of muscles occurs, resulting in contractures. (3) (ME; AN; PA; NM)

1 Muscles will atrophy, not hypertrophy, from disuse.

3 Flexion abnormalities, not extension rigidity, occur resulting in contractures.

4 It does not predispose to infection, but to atrophy and contractures.

300. 2 The client has lost vision from the right visual field; scanning compensates for loss. (3) (ME; IM; ED; NM)

1 This is the approach to be used for apraxia.

3 This is the approach to be used for denial of the right side (unilateral neglect).

4 This alleviates neglect of the affected side.

301. 4 If the client exhibits emotional instability, it is usually caused by lesions affecting the thalamic area; the part of the neural system most responsible for emotions. (1) (ME; IM; ED; NM)

1 The client may have remote memory, but there is no selective process of what events are remembered.

2 This is associated with consistent behavior and cognitive thinking, of which the client is incapable at this time.

3 Same as answer 2.

302. 3 Recovery from aphasia is a continuous process; the amount of recovery cannot be predicted. (1) (ME; IM; ED; NM)

1 This response abdicates the nurse's responsibility; the physician cannot predict return of function.

2 This gives false reassurance; it may take a year or longer or may never return.

4 Speech return is a continuous process; it may take a year or longer or may never return.

303. 4 In addition to the extent of injury, a factor in relearning speech is the client's motivation and effort; the more the client attempts to talk, the more likely speech will progress to its optimal level; relearning is a slow process. (1) (ME; IM; ED; NM)

1 Clients with aphasia are not deaf.

2 This will cause frustration and anger in the client.

3 Although the nurse should instruct the family to approve and support every effort by the client to communicate, their action would provide external rather than internal motivation and is therefore not as effective.

304. 3 A weak grasp, pain, and uncoordinated movements could result in the dropping of tools which could be dangerous. (3) (SU; AN; TC; NM)

1 Although this could be a problem, safety is the priority.

2 Same as answer 1.

4 Although in the future this could become an issue if the client can no longer work, at this time safety is the priority.

305. 2 The tonic-clonic contractions which occur during a seizure place the client at risk for developing a head injury; safety of the client takes precedence. (1) (ME; IM; TC; NM)

1 Safety must be established first.

3 During a seizure changes in the pupils are not likely to occur.

4 This should be done but only after the client's safety is secured.

306. 2 The nerves for arm innervation are above the injury level at C4. (3) (SU; AS; PA; NM)
1 Innervation of muscles used to move the lower arm is not affected by this injury; they are innervated above C7.
3 Innervation for pain sensation of the hands is not affected by this injury; they are innervated above C7.
4 Diaphragm innervation is not affected by this injury; it is innervated above C4.

307. 2 The T6 level is the sympathetic visceral outflow level, and any injury above this level results in autonomic dysreflexia. (3) (SU; AN; PA; NM)
1 The reflex arc remains after spinal cord injury.
3 The important point is not that the cord is totally transected but the level at which the injury occurs.
4 This is not related to autonomic dysreflexia; all cord injuries result in flaccid paralysis during the period of spinal shock; as the inflammation subsides spasticity gradually increases.

308. 4 These symptoms occur as a result of exaggerated autonomic responses, and if autonomic dysreflexia is identified, immediate intervention is necessary to prevent serious complications. (3) (SU; AS; PA; NM)
1 Paralysis is related to transection, not dysreflexia; the client will have no sensation below the injury.
2 Profuse diaphoresis occurs.
3 Bradycardia occurs.

309. 4 The client has the capability; this maintains a positive identity and is necessary for progression to long-term goals. (2) (SU; AN; PA; NM)
1 This is a long-term goal.
2 Same as answer 1.
3 Same as answer 1.

310. 2 Arm strength is necessary for transfers and activities of daily living and for the use of crutches or a wheelchair. (2) (SU; IM; ED; NM)
1 The client has no neurologic control of this activity.

3 Equilibrium is not a problem.
4 Same as answer 1.

ENDOCRINE

311. 3 Excessive thirst, excessive hunger, and frequent urination are caused by the body's inability to correctly metabolize glucose. (1) (ME; AS; PA; EN)
1 Lethargy, not irritability, results because of a lack of metabolized glucose for energy.
2 Confusion is related to both severe hypoglycemia and hyperglycemia.
4 Frequent urination occurs throughout a 24-hour period because glucose in the urine pulls fluid with it; weight loss occurs with insulin dependent diabetes mellitus, not with non-insulin dependent diabetes mellitus.

312. 3 The actual reason for the lack of ketonuria in NIDDM is unknown; one theory is that extremely high hyperglycemia and hyperosmolarity block the formation of ketones, stimulating lipogenesis, rather than lipolysis (2) (ME; AS; PA; EN)
1 This does not occur with either type of diabetes mellitus.
2 This is impossible; if glycosuria is present, there must first be a level of glucose in the blood above the renal threshold of 160 to 180 mg/dl.
4 This is expected in insulin dependent diabetes mellitus.

313. 1 Blood glucose testing is a more direct and accurate measure; urine testing provides an indirect measure that can be influenced by kidney function and the amount of time the urine is retained in the bladder. (1) (ME; IM; ED; EN)
2 While both blood and urine testing are relatively simple, testing the blood involves additional knowledge of surgical aseptic technique.
3 Both procedures can be done by the client.
4 This would not be a factor; while some urine tests are influenced by drugs, there are methods to test urine to bypass this effect.

314. 4 Knowledge of the signs and treatment for hypoglycemia or hyperglycemia is critical to client health and well-being and essential for survival. (3) (ME; AN; ED; EN)
1 Although this is important, it is not the priority.
2 The client has non-insulin dependent diabetes mellitus; insulin injections are not necessary.
3 A finger stick with serum glucose monitoring is more accurate than urine S & A measurements to identify present serum glucose levels.

315. 4 Controlling the diabetes decreases the risk of infection; this is the best prevention. (1) (ME; EV; TC; EN)
1 If not completely absorbed, these may provide a warm, moist environment for bacterial growth.
2 Coexisting neuropathy may result in injury from heat application.
3 Protein, carbohydrates, and fats must be in an appropriate balance; high carbohydrate intake could provide too many calories.

316. 4 Exercise improves glucose metabolism; with exercise there is a risk of developing hypoglycemia, not hyperglycemia. (2) (ME; IM; ED; EN)
1 Exercise should not be decreased because it improves glucose metabolism.
2 An extra tablet would probably result in hypoglycemia because exercise alone improves glucose metabolism.
3 Control of glucose metabolism is achieved through a balance of diet, exercise, and pharmacologic therapy.

317. 4 Physiologic stress increases gluconeogenesis, requiring continued pharmacologic therapy despite an inability to eat; fluids prevent dehydration; monitoring serum glucose permits early intervention if necessary. (1) (ME; IM; ED; EN)
1 Skipping the oral hypoglycemic could precipitate hyperglycemia; serum glucose must be monitored.
2 Food intake should be attempted to prevent acidosis; oral hypoglycemics should

be taken, and serum glucose should be monitored.
3 These are incomplete instructions; oral hypoglycemics should be taken, and serum glucose should be monitored; eating as much as possible could precipitate hyperglycemia.

318. 1 In individuals with NIDDM, occasional alcohol can be used with caloric substitution for equivalent fat exchanges in the diet because it is metabolized like fat. (2) (ME; IM; ED; EN)
2 Moderation is vital; these may not be used in unlimited quantities; they must be accounted for in the dietary calculations.
3 Alcohol can be used as long as it is accounted for in the diet.
4 This is untrue; regular foods can be used in the ADA diet.

319. 3 According to the individual's needs, consistency and regularity in the basic food plan should be maintained; this is a basic principle of dietary management of diabetes mellitus. (2) (ME; IM; ED; EN)
1 This is not necessary; the client can use the ADA food plan to make selections.
2 This is unrealistic; it cannot always be done; it is unnecessary because choices can be made within the ADA diet.
4 This is unnecessary because the client is not taking insulin.

320. 1 These vegetables are under the vegetable exchange, as are asparagus, broccoli, and mushrooms. (1) (ME; EV; PA; EN)
2 These are starchy vegetables and are listed as bread exchanges.
3 These food items are from the bread exchange.
4 Same as answer 2.

321. 4 Improper foot care can lead to skin break-down, poor healing, and subsequent infection. (1) (ME; IM; ED; EN)

1 This potentially increases anxiety and reduces the client's ability to learn.

2 This is only one aspect of proper foot care; foot care must be more comprehensive.

3 Same as answer 2.

322. 3 Blood glucose needs to be reduced; regular insulin begins to act in 30 to 60 minutes. (1) (SU; PL; PA; EN)

1 Oral hypoglycemics are long acting and begin to act about 1 hour after administration; in addition, the client has Type I, not Type II, diabetes mellitus and an oral hypoglycemic would be ineffective.

2 Blood glucose levels are far more accurate than urine glucose levels.

4 The rate may be increased because polyuria often accompanies hyperglycemia.

323. 3 Emotional and physical stress may cause insulin requirements to remain elevated in the postoperative period. (1) (SU; PL; PA; EN)

1 Fluctuating insulin requirements indicate less than adequate control.

2 An increase in the client's insulin requirements could indicate sepsis, but this is not expected.

4 Insulin requirements would remain elevated, rather than decrease.

324. 1 Incomplete oxidation of fat results in fatty acids that further breakdown to ketones. (3) (ME; AN; PA; EN)

2 Protein metabolism results in nitrogenous waste production, causing an elevated blood urea nitrogen (BUN).

3 Potassium is not oxidized; in hypokalemia or hyperkalemia no ketones are formed.

4 Carbohydrates do not contain fatty acids that are broken down into ketones.

325. 2 Potassium is the principal intracellular cation, and during ketoacidosis it moves out of cells into the extracellular compartment to replace K^+ lost due to glucose-induced osmotic diuresis; overstimulation of the cardiac muscle results. (3) (ME; AS; PA; EN)

1 P waves are abnormal because the PR interval may be prolonged and the P wave may be lost; however, the T wave is peaked, not depressed; the T wave is depressed in hypokalemia.

3 Initially, the QT segment is short and as K^+ level rises, QRS complex widens; the ST segment becomes depressed.

4 The PR interval is prolonged and the P wave may be lost; QRS complexes and thus T waves become irregular, and the rate does not necessarily change.

326. 3 This is a short-term goal, client oriented, necessary for client to control the diabetes and measurable when the client performs a return demonstration for the nurse. (2) (ME; AN; ED; EN)

1 This is not a short term goal.

2 This is measurable, but it is a long-term goal.

4 While this is measurable and is a short-term goal, it is not the one with the greatest priority when a client has an insulin pump that must be mastered prior to discharge.

327. 3 The basal infusion rate mimics the low rate of insulin secretion during fasting, and the bolus before meals mimics the high output after meals. (2) (ME; PL; PA; EN)

1 The subcutaneous needle may be left in place for as long as 3 days.

2 Blood glucose monitoring is done a minimum of four or more times a day.

4 Most insulin pumps are battery-driven syringes external to the body, which access the body via a subcutaneous needle.

328. 2 Wearing shoes protects the feet; they should fit well and be worn over socks that are wool or cotton to cushion the foot and absorb perspiration. (3) (ME; IM; ED; EN)

1 While smoking should be avoided, self removal of corns can result in injury to the feet.

3 Nylon is not a natural fiber and it promotes perspiration.

4 Shoes that do not fit well will create friction and cause sores, blisters, and callouses; corn removers should be avoided.

329. 1 The client with liver disease has a decreased ability to metabolize CHO because of a decreased ability to form glycogen (glycogenesis) and to form glucose from glycogen (glycogenolysis). (3) (ME; AN; PA; EN)

2 Hypertension is not related to decreased serum glucose.

3 Clients with Type II diabetes do not depend on exogneous insulin, nor are they prone to ketosis; the blood glucose levels fall much more slowly, and there is ample time to monitor signs and symptoms before hypoglycemia can develop.

4 Hyperthyroidism is not related to decreased serum glucose.

330. 3 The dose of exogenous insulin causes a rapid drop in blood glucose, especially if food is not eaten; the oral hypoglycemic acts slowly, and there is time to take evasive measures if a hypoglycemic reaction begins to develop. (3) (ME; AN; PA; EN)

1 Stress usually contributes to hyperglycemia; the primary reason for this client's precipitous fall in blood glucose was because insulin had been taken and the client had not eaten at all.

2 This would lead to hyperglycemia.

4 The use of insulin over long periods does not build up tolerance or cause blood glucose levels to fluctuate dramatically.

331. 2 This is the point at which a client is generally hypoglycemic, resulting in increased sympathetic nervous system activity and deprivation of CNS glucose supply. (2) (ME; AS; PA; EN)

1 This is within the norm of 90 to 120 mg/dl.

3 Same as answer 1.

4 This is not a sufficient drop to cause hypoglycemia; hypoglycemia usually occurs at 50 to 70 mg/dl.

332. 2 This occurs with low serum glucose levels because of sympathetic nervous system activity. (2) (ME; AS; PA; EN)

1 This is a sign of hyperglycemia and is related to metabolic acidosis and inadequate energy production.

3 This is a sign of hyperglycemia; it is caused by dehydration associated with osmotic diuresis related to glycosuria.

4 This is a sign of hyperglycemia and is related to metabolic acidosis; it is a compensatory response in an attempt to blow off CO_2 and raise the pH.

333. 1 These are classic signs of hypokalemia that occur when potassium levels are reduced as potassium reenters cells with glucose. (3) (ME; EV; PA; EN)

2 Symptoms of hyponatremia are nausea, malaise, and changes in mental status.

3 Symptoms of hypoglycemia are weakness, nervousness, tachycardia, diaphoresis, irritability, and pallor.

4 Symptoms of hypercalcemia are lethargy, nausea, vomiting, paresthesias, and personality changes.

334. 2 The suggested treatment of hypoglycemia in a conscious client is a simple sugar (such as 2 packets of sugar), followed by a complex CHO (such as a slice of bread) and lastly a protein (such as milk); the simple sugar elevates blood glucose rapidly; the complex CHO and protein produce a more sustained response. (2) (ME; EV; ED; EN)

1 These are fast-acting sugars, and neither of them will provide a sustained response.

3 The fat content of chocolate candy decreases the rate of absorption of glucose.

4 Neither of these are fast-acting sugars; peanut butter crackers and milk can be used to maintain the glucose level after it has been raised.

335. 4 An aldosteronoma is an aldosterone-secreting adenoma of the adrenal cortex. (2) (ME; AN; PA; EN)

1 An aldosteronoma is a tumor of an adrenal gland, not the thyroid.

2 An aldosteronoma is a tumor of an adrenal gland, not the kidneys.

3 An aldosteronoma is a tumor of an adrenal gland, not the pituitary.

336. 1 Renal and cardiac complications will occur if the hypertension caused by the tumor is not arrested. (3) (SU; IM; ED; EN)

2 An aldosteronoma is a benign tumor; metastasis is not possible.

3 This is not true; surgery is required to remove the tumor.

4 Drugs are not used; the tumor must be removed.

337. 1 Once the excessive secretion of aldosterone is stopped, the BP gradually drops to a near normal level. (3) (SU; PL; PA; EN)

2 The BP drops gradually; it does not rise.

3 The BP will only fluctuate if the hypervolemia is over corrected causing hypovolemia; this is not expected.

4 The BP drops gradually in response to decreasing serum corticosteroid levels; a rapid drop immediately following surgery may indicate hemorrhage.

338. 2 The body has two adrenal glands; an aldosteronoma is unilateral. (2) (SU; IM; PS; EN)

1 The prognosis is usually excellent; this is unnecessarily alarming.

3 This is unnecessary; the prognosis is usually excellent.

4 No hormones are necessary; there is another adrenal gland.

339. 3 The x-ray contrast media for a cholecystogram contain iodides that can alter test results; although ultrasonography has replaced oral cholecystography as the diagnostic procedure of choice, it is still performed when the ultrasonography is not conclusive. (3) (ME; IM; TC; EN)

1 No iodide-containing dyes are used with roentgenographic diagnostic procedures.

2 Same as answer 1.

4 No iodide-containing dyes are used with this test; oral or parenteral glucose is administered.

340. 1 These tests provide a measure of thyroxine production, a disturbance of which is associated with the client's symptoms. (1) (ME; AS; PA; EN)

2 Prothrombin time (PT) and partial thromboplastin time (PTT) assess blood coagulation.

3 The VDRL test is for syphilis; the CBC assesses the hematopoietic system.

4 This measures the kind and amount of circulating barbiturates; the client's symptoms are not associated with barbiturate intake.

341. 3 These are the classic signs associated with hyperthyroidism; weight loss and restlessness occur because of an increased basal metabolic rate; exophthalmos occurs because of edema behind the eye. (2) (ME; AS; PA; EN)

1 These are all associated with hypothyroidism because of the decreased metabolic rate.

2 Lethargy and weight gain are associated with hypothyroidism as a result of a decreased metabolic rate; forgetfulness is not related.

4 Although weight loss and exophthalmos occur with hyperthyroidism, the client would be hyperactive, not hypoactive.

342. 1 Increased basal metabolic rate, increased circulation, and vasodilation result in warm moist skin. (3) (ME; AS; PA; EN)

2 This symptom is associated with hypothyroidism.

3 Same as answer 2.

4 Same as answer 2.

343. 4 The mask may irritate or scratch the eye if the client turns and lies on it during the night. (3) (ME; EV; ED; EN)

1 Blinking of the eyes will bathe the eyes and prevent corneal ulceration.

2 This will do nothing to relieve edema or prevent ulceration of the eye.

3 Although this will help reduce periorbital edema, it will not prevent ulceration of the cornea.

344. 3 This relieves tension on the incision and limits the risk of dehiscence. (2) (SU; IM; ED; EN)

1 Coughing should be avoided during the early postoperative period to prevent trauma to the operative site.

2   This should be avoided until advised by the physician, usually after the sutures or skin clips are removed.

4   Pressure against the operative area is not necessary to promote the integrity of the incision, and it may act to inhibit swallowing.

345. 2   The remaining thyroid tissue may provide enough hormone for normal function. (1) (SU; AN; PA; EN)

1   This would be a total, not a subtotal, thyroidectomy.

3   No parathyroid glands should be removed in a thyroidectomy.

4   Same as answer 3.

346. 2   Acute respiratory obstruction can result from edema, nerve damage, or tetany. (1) (SU; PL; TC; EN)

1   A cardiac arrest is not an expected response following thyroid surgery.

3   If the airway were obstructed by postoperative edema, the use of a mechanical airway would be ineffective because it would not bypass the point of obstruction; a rebreathing mask would be used for clients with COPD, not a thyroidectomy.

4   Acidosis or cardiac arrest are not expected responses after a thyroidectomy.

347. 3   If the pharyngeal nerve is damaged during surgery the client will be hoarse and have difficulty speaking. (3) (SU; EV; TC; EN)

1   This would not indicate injury to the pharyngeal nerve; this is part of the assessment for a compromised airway.

2   This would be an assessment for hypocalcemia resulting from inadvertent removal of the parathyroid glands.

4   This assesses for bleeding and possible hemorrhage, not pharyngeal nerve injury.

348. 4   This detects complications such as thyroid storm, hemorrhage, and respiratory obstruction which occur early in the postoperative period. (3) (SU; EV; TC; EN)

1   This is contraindicated; humidifiers contribute to the spread of bacteria and infection.

2   This should not be begun until 2 to 4 days postoperatively because it can disrupt the suture line.

3   Hoarseness and voice weakness are usually temporary and not life-threatening; the priority is to observe for thyroid storm, hemorrhage, and respiratory obstruction.

349. 1   Bleeding may occur, and blood will pool in back of the neck because the blood will flow via gravity. (1) (SU; EV; TC; EN)

2   This is contraindicated; this would increase pain and would put tension on the suture line.

3   Talking should be avoided in the immediate postoperative period except to assess for a change in pitch or tone, which may indicate laryngeal nerve damage.

4   Activity should be gradually resumed and frequent rest periods encouraged.

350. 2   Injury to the parathyroid gland results in a deficiency of parathormone, which decreases calcium levels in the blood. (3) (SU; EV; PA; EN)

1   This is characterized by generalized weakness, a decrease in reflexes, shallow respirations, and cardiac dysrythmias.

3   This is characterized by tachycardia, hyperpyrexia, and an exacerbation of thyroid symptoms.

4   This is characterized by a weak, thready pulse and hypotension.

351. 2   The client is exhibiting signs and symptoms of hypocalcemia which occurs with accidental removal of the parathyroids; calcium gluconate is the treatment of choice. (3) (SU; PL; TC; EN)

1   This is prescribed for hyperthyroidism because it inhibits the release of thyroid hormones.

3   This is prescribed for hypomagnesemia or to prevent convulsions in eclampsia or preeclampsia.

4   This is prescribed for hypokalemia.

352. 4 Thyroid crisis is severe hyperthyroidism; excessive amounts of thyroxine increase the metabolic rate, thereby raising the pulse and temperature. (2) (SU; AS; PA; EN)

1 During thyroid crisis there is usually no increase in the difference between the apical and peripheral pulse rates (pulse deficit).

2 The blood pressure will rise to meet the oxygen demand caused by the increased metabolic rate during thyroid crisis.

3 Because of the increased metabolic rate the pulse and respiratory rates increase to meet the body's oxygen needs.

353. 2 The radioactive material will be excreted in urine, feces, perspiration, and other body discharges; disposal should be made according to hospital procedure to contain the radioactive discharges. (1) (SU; IM; TC; EN)

1 Universal precautions protect the staff from microorganisms not radioactivity; these precautions would be used for this client as well as every other client; visitors would be limited when radioactive material is involved.

3 The purpose of isolation is not for protection of the client but for containment of the radioactivity and protection of staff, family, and friends.

4 Contact should be avoided, except to meet necessary needs; distance should be maintained.

354. 1 Dry, thickened skin and cold intolerance are characteristic adaptations to low serum thyroxine. (1) (SU; EV; ED; EN)

2 Muscle cramping is associated with hypocalcemia.

3 Low thyroxine levels reduce the metabolic rate, resulting in fatigue, and should not increase the pulse rate.

4 Low thyroxine levels reduce the metabolic rate, resulting in weight gain and bradycardia, not tachycardia.

355. 3 After thyroidectomy the thyroxine output is usually inadequate to maintain an appropriate metabolic rate. (1) (SU; AN; PA; EN)

1 Hypothyroidism is a decrease in thyroid functioning, not a slowing of the entire body's functions.

2 With hypothyroidism the level of thyroid-stimulating hormone (TSH) from the pituitary is usually increased.

4 Atrophy of the thyroid tissue remaining after surgery does not occur.

356. 1 Dry skin is most likely caused by decreased glandular function and fatigue is caused by a decreased metabolic rate. (2) (SU; EV; ED; EN)

2 This is associated with hyperthyroidism, not hypothyroidism.

3 Same as answer 2.

4 Same as answer 2.

RESPIRATORY

357. 3 These are normal respiratory sounds heard on auscultation as inspired air enters and leaves the alveoli. (1) (ME; AS; PA; RE)

1 These are fine crackling sounds heard at the end of an inspiration; they are associated with pulmonary edema.

2 Adventitious is the general term for all abnormal breath sounds.

4 This is evidence of a reduction in the amount of air entering the alveoli, usually caused by obstruction or consolidation.

358. 3 Rhonchi are coarse sounds heard over the larger airways; including rhonchi in the notation makes it inaccurate. (2) (ME; AS; TC; RE)

1 Crackles and rhonchi are client adaptations, not a nursing diagnosis.

2 It would be incorrect to use the term rhonchi to refer to crackling sounds in the lower lung.

4 Crepitus, which indicates subcutaneous emphysema, is a condition unrelated to the breath sounds heard on auscultation.

359. 4 This position promotes lung expansion and gas exchange; it also decreases venous return and cardiac work load. (2) (ME; IM; PA; RE)

1 This may be done but positioning should be done first because it will have an

immediate effect and time will be used in preparing for the delivery of the oxygen.

2 A friction rub is not related to congestive heart failure but to inflammation of the pleura.

3 Maintaining adequate oxygen exchange is the priority; an x-ray film will be obtained, but after breathing is supported.

360. 4 These are top priorities in trauma management; basic life functions must be maintained or reestablished. (2) (SU; AS; TC; RE)

1 This is an assessment for head injury that follows determination of respiratory and circulatory status.

2 This is an assessment for abdominal injury that follows determination of respiratory and circulatory status.

3 Pain assessment would follow the appraisal of airway, breathing, and circulation.

361. 3 This is secondary to cerebral hypoxia, which accompanies ARDS; cognition and level of consciousness are reduced. (3) (ME; AS; PA; RE)

1 Hypotension occurs because of hypoxia of the heart.

2 The sputum is not tenacious, but it may be frothy if pulmonary edema is present.

4 Breathing will be fast and shallow.

362. 3 Nothing is achieved if the equipment is working and the client is not responding. (3) (SU; EV; TC; RE)

1 This is presumptive; the data base is incomplete for the assessment that surgery is necessary.

2 Endotracheal intubation does not permit verbal communication.

4 This is important but not the priority.

363. 4 Increased rate and depth of breathing result in excessive elimination of CO_2 and respiratory alkalosis results. (1) (ME; EV; TC; RE)

1 Hypoxia is associated with respiratory acidosis, not respiratory alkalosis which is related to hyperventilation.

2 With hyperventilation, CO_2 levels will be decreased (hypocapnea), not elevated.

3 This results from excess hydrogen ions caused by a metabolic problem, not a respiratory problem.

364. 2 This is necessary to prevent flooding of the trachea with fluid; some systems have receptacles attached to the tubing to collect the fluid and others have to be temporarily disconnected while emptying the fluid. (3) (ME; IM; TC; RE)

1 This circumstance does not require assistance from a respiratory therapist.

3 This is unsafe; humidity is necessary to preserve moistness of the respiratory tract and liquefy secretions.

4 The amount of condensation is irrelevant in terms of recording the intake and output.

365. 4 This position promotes respirations by removing the pressure of abdominal organs on the diaphragm; it requires the least amount of energy to maintain, and it helps reduce edema at the tracheostomy site. (2) (SU; IM; TC; RE)

1 This position promotes collection of fluid around the operative site, which impedes healing; it also impedes respirations because of the pressure of the abdominal organs against the diaphragm.

2 It requires too much energy to maintain this position.

3 Same as answer 2.

366. 3 These cuffs do not compress the capillary beds and thus do not cause tracheal damage. (2) (SU; AN; TC; RE)

1 Surgical asepsis, not the use of these cuffs, prevents infection.

2 A minimal air leak is desirable to ensure the lowest possible pressure in the cuff while still maintaining placement of the tube.

4 Secretions will be increased because the cuff is a foreign body in the trachea.

367. 4 Emphysema involves destructive changes in the alveolar walls, leading to dilation of the air sacs; there is subsequent air trapping and difficulty with expiration. (1) (ME; AN; PA; RE)
1 Bronchospasm is characteristic of asthma and it causes narrowing of the airways.
2 The vital capacity is increased to compensate for inefficient gaseous exchange; however, this is a secondary adaptation.
3 Although slow expiration tends to keep the airways open so there is less air trapping, rapid expulsion of air is not the primary problem.

368. 3 Restlessness is an early sign of cerebral hypoxia. (2) (SU; AS; PA; RE)
1 Tachypnea, not bradypnea, would occur.
2 Tachycardia, not bradycardia, would occur.
4 Light-headedness is a sign of respiratory alkalosis.

369. 3 Clients with chronic obstructive pulmonary disease (COPD) must be given only low concentrations of oxygen; a decreased oxygen blood level is the only stimulus for breathing for these clients. (2) (ME; AN; TC; RE)
1 Prolonged hypoxia will stimulate erythrocyte production; the goal of therapy is to relieve hypoxia.
2 The pressure, rather than the concentration, at which oxygen is administered increases this risk.
4 To prevent its drying effects on secretions and the mucosa, oxygen should be humidified.

370. 3 The orthopneic position lowers the diaphragm and provides for maximum thoracic expansion. (1) (SU; PL; PA; RE)
1 This would not facilitate thoracic expansion because it still permits abdominal organs to press against the diaphragm.
2 Same as answer 1.
4 Although this could help, it would not be as beneficial as the orthopneic position.

371. 4 With COPD the diaphragm is flattened and weakened; strengthening the diaphragm is desirable. (2) (ME; PL; PA; RE)

1 The opposite is more desirable; clients with COPD retain too much carbon dioxide which eventually causes a barrel chest.
2 The abdominal muscles are accessory muscles of respiration and their contraction and relaxation are involved in diaphragmatic breathing.
3 Sit-ups are too strenuous for clients with emphysema.

372. 3 This pause allows added time for gaseous exchange at the alveolar capillary beds. (3) (SU; EV; ED; RE)
1 Inhalation should be through the nose to moisten, filter, and warm the air.
2 This decreases the effectiveness of respirations.
4 The expiratory phase should be lengthened, and exhalation should be through pursed lips.

373. 4 The enlarged liver is caused by long-term respiratory acidosis with increased pulmonary pressures that eventually cause right heart enlargement and failure (cor pulmonale); the elevated pressures cause backup pressure in the hepatic circulation. (3) (SU; AN; PA; RE)
1 Liver hypoxia would cause atrophy and necrosis of cells, not enlargement.
2 Right ventricular heart failure with increased pressure in the ascending vena cava causes increased pressure in the hepatoportal system, resulting in an enlarged liver, not hepatic acidosis.
3 These are the result of hepatic portal hypertension, not the cause of an enlarged liver.

374. 2 An initial symptom of right ventricular heart failure because of COPD (cor pulmonale) is sudden weight gain. (3) (ME; AN; PA; RE)
1 This is associated with polycythemia vera, not COPD.
3 A sudden weight gain is not associated with this condition.
4 Right, not left, ventricular heart failure occurs with COPD.

375. 1 Eating small meals will decrease the amount of O_2 necessary for digestion at any one time. (2) (ME; PL; PA; RE)

2 Lying down increases intraabdominal pressure, pushing a full stomach against the diaphragm and limiting respiratory excursion.

3 While fluids do help liquefy secretions, they should not be encouraged in a client with right ventricular heart failure.

4 Protein maintains or increases hydrostatic pressure; it does not decrease it.

376. 2 There is air in the tissues, and palpation results in a crackling sound referred to as crepitus. (2) (SU; EV; TC; RE)

1 This is a harsh, vibrating sound usually produced on inspiration because of airway obstruction.

3 This is excessive accumulation of fluid in tissue spaces.

4 The size of the chest is determined by the bony structure; a barrel chest with an increase in the AP diameter is associated with COPD, not cancer of the lung.

377. 2 A mediastinal shift with airway obstruction may occur because pressure builds up on the operative side, causing the trachea to deviate toward the unoperative side; assessment of the airway takes priority. (3) (SU; AS; TC; RE)

1 The situation needs immediate verification before the physician is called.

3 Same as answer 1.

4 There is no need for a chest tube when a pneumonectomy is performed.

378. 3 These positions permit ventilation of the remaining lung and prevent fluid from draining into the sutured bronchial stump. (3) (SU; PL; TC; RE)

1 Lying on the unoperative side restricts left lung excursion and may allow fluid to drain into the right bronchial stump.

2 Although the high Fowler's position promotes ventilation, it is extremely tiring.

4 Same as answer 1.

379. 1 Loss of the large vascular lung and/or the presence of a mediastinal shift can result in cardiac overload. (3) (SU; AS; TC; RE)

2 These signs are associated with hypoxia, which is a common complication of surgery and not unique to a pneumonectomy.

3 These are common complications of all thoracic surgery and are not unique to a pneumonectomy.

4 An elevated BP may be associated with cardiac overload, but the other symptoms are not unique to a pneumonectomy.

380. 3 A plugged chest tube increases intrathoracic pressure, which pushes the heart to the opposite side, thereby reducing venous return and cardiac output. (3) (SU; AS; TC; RE)

1 A hemothorax would not necessarily be life threatening.

2 Dyspnea may develop but it would not necessarily be life threatening.

4 A pneumothorax would not necessarily be life threatening and is unrelated to abdominal pressure.

381. 3 A productive cough indicates mucus is being raised from the lungs. (2) (ME; EV; PA; RE)

1 Crackles (rales) are unaffected by postural drainage or coughing.

2 The depth of respirations may not be altered by postural drainage.

4 Saliva comes from the mouth and does not indicate clearance of lungs.

382. 3 To prevent aspiration during the procedure, clients are required to be npo for at least 8 to 12 hours prior to the procedure. (2) (SU; IM; TC; RE)

1 Chest tubes are not required unless the lungs are accidentally punctured; the client will have a small incision near the clavicle.

2 A mediastinoscopy permits visualization of the anterior mediastinum or hilum extrapleurally; a bronchoscopy permits visualization of the main stem bronchus.

4 Fluid is removed from the pleural space during a thoracentesis.

383. 3 The mechanism is unclear, but this is probably caused by fluid shifts. (2) (SU; AN; TC; RE)

1 This is untrue; this is done only occasionally to slow development of new effusion in clients with recurrent effusions.

2 This is untrue; it can provide dramatic relief and improvement.

4 This is untrue; dyspnea should be immediately relieved; if dyspnea increases, pneumothorax should be suspected.

384. 3 Compression of the lung by fluid that accumulates at the base of the lungs reduces expansion and air exchange. (3) (SU; AS; PA; RE)

1 There is no fluid in the alveoli, so no crackles are produced.

2 If there is tracheal deviation, it is away from the involved side.

4 Dullness is produced on percussion of the involved area.

385. 1 Clients with pleuritic disease are prone to develop pneumonia because of impaired expansion, air exchange, and lung drainage. (2) (SU; PL; TC; RE)

2 Sedation is not therapeutic because the client must be alert for deep breathing and coughing.

3 Coughing should not be suppressed; it enhances expansion, air exchange, and lung drainage.

4 Oral fluids are encouraged; pulmonary edema does not develop unless the client has severe cardiovascular disease.

386. 3 Tension is placed on the pleura at the height of inspiration and causes pain. (3) (SU; AS; PA; RE)

1 This is typical of congestive heart failure.

2 This may indicate pulmonary infection.

4 Same as answer 2.

387. 4 Increased negative pressure on inspiration causes the fluid to rise; a decrease in the negative intrapleural pressure on expiration causes the fluid to fall. (2) (SU; EV; PA; RE)

1 This would indicate an air leak.

2 This would indicate that there is an obstruction in the drainage tubing or the suction is too low; there should be a slight increase in fluid in this chamber postoperatively.

3 The suction is too high; bubbling should be gentle.

388. 4 After general anesthesia, these activities expand alveoli and prevent atelectasis. (1) (SU; IM; TC; RE)

1 This is not necessary; the abdomen has not been entered, and there should be no interference with peristalsis.

2 This is not necessary.

3 This is not necessary; clients can ambulate after recovery from anesthesia.

389. 3 General anesthesia is delivered via an endotracheal tube that irritates the posterior pharynx and larynx and causes discomfort when swallowing. (2) (SU; EV; PA; RE)

1 Occasionally this may occur; however, it is a systemic, not a local, effect.

2 This is not an effect of general anesthesia.

4 Same as answer 2.

390. 1 Both sides of the posterior pharynx should be touched to elicit the gag reflex; absence of the reflex indicates the client is at risk for aspiration of secretions or fluid. (1) (SU; IM; TC; RE)

2 This is unsafe; if the gag reflex is absent, the client would aspirate.

3 This is unsafe; this could happen even in the absence of a gag reflex.

4 This is unsafe; the client might be able to breathe deeply and cough without an adequate gag reflex.

391. 4 There is no respiratory movement in stage 4 of anesthesia; before this stage, respirations are depressed but present. (3) (SU; AN; PA; RE)

1 The gag reflex is lost in the first phase of stage 3 of anesthesia.

2 The corneal reflex is lost in the second phase of stage 3 of anesthesia.

3 Consciousness is lost in stage 2.

392. 1 The respiratory process is essential to life and therefore is the first priority. (1) (SU; AS; TC; RE)

2 This may eventually be done, but respiratory assessment is the priority.

3 Same as answer 2.

4 The Trendelenburg position decreases respiratory functioning and should be avoided.

393. 1 To allow for the insertion of the bronchoscope, throat muscles are anesthetized, diminishing the protective gag reflex. (1) (SU; PL; TC; RE)

2 This does not occur after a bronchoscopy.

3 General anesthesia is not usually used; therefore paralytic ileus is not a complication.

4 Dysphasia is difficulty in talking and does not occur with a bronchoscopy; dyspepsia is disturbed digestion and is not the reason for withholding food or fluids.

394. 3 This is a safe and reliable method of testing the gag reflex. (1) (SU; AS; TC; RE)

1 Talking can occur without the gag reflex.

2 This could cause choking if the gag reflex has not returned.

4 Coughing can occur without the gag reflex.

395. 4 These are correct techniques; deep inhalation promotes alveolar expansion, and exhalation promotes lung recoil. (2) (SU; EV; ED; RE)

1 Coughing is done after deep breathing.

2 The breaths should not be in succession; they should be spaced by several normal breaths to avoid fatigue.

3 These are incorrect techniques; inhalation should be through the mouthpiece.

396. 3 During chest surgery, the negative pressure around the lung is disrupted and the lungs do not fill normally during inspiration; chest tubes are inserted to reestablish negative intrapleural pressure. (3) (SU; IM; ED; RE)

1 Chest tubes are inserted into the intrapleural space not the pericardial sac.

2 Atelectasis refers to the collapse of alveoli or a lobule caused by a blockage of small airways; chest tubes do not cause or correct atelectasis.

4 Although the amount of drainage from chest tubes is measured, the reason for chest tubes is to reestablish negative intrapleural pressure.

397. 2 Fluid in the water seal chamber should rise and fall as the client breathes in and out (tidaling) until the lungs have expanded completely; a lack of tidaling on the first postoperative day would indicate that the tube is obstructed. (1) (SU; IM; TC; RE)

1 This is contraindicated without a physician's order because it could traumatize pleural tissue.

3 The level of the fluid, as long as it covers the tube in the water seal chamber, does not affect tidaling.

4 While full expansion of the lung will eliminate tidaling this is unlikely on the first postoperative day; an obstruction of the tube should be ruled out.

398. 4 This allows for measuring the output without interrupting the closed drainage system. (1) (SU; IM; TC; RE)

1 This is only done to obtain a specimen for diagnostic procedures.

2 Clamping the chest tube is contraindicated because it can precipitate a pneumothorax; opening the system destroys the sterility of the closed drainage system.

3 This is only done when the drainage collection chamber is full and the closed chest drainage must continue.

399. 1 Excessive bubbling indicates an air leak, which must be eliminated to prevent a pneumothorax. (3) (SU; IM; TC; RE)

2 Excessive suction pressure results in excessive bubbling in the suction control bottle.

3 Excessive bubbling is not expected; it indicates a leak in the system.

4 Stasis or clots in the tubing will not result in excessive bubbling; "milking" or "stripping" the tubing is generally contraindicated because it can cause a pneumothorax.

400. 4 This is ineffective; this exercises the elbow rather than the shoulder joint and muscles. (2) (SU; EV; ED; RE)
1 This is effective; this exercises the trapezius muscle and shoulder joint.
2 Same as answer 1.
3 This is effective; this provides circular range of motion to the shoulder joint.

401. 1 The chest tube normalizes intrathoracic pressure, drains fluid and air from the pleural space, and improves pulmonary function. (2) (SU; EV; PA; RE)
2 This may be a sign of pain, respiratory obstruction, or bleeding.
3 This indicates that air has entered the subcutaneous tissue (subcutaneous emphysema).
4 This indicates a probable leak in the drainage system.

402. 3 During inspiration negative pressure in the pleural space increases, causing fluid to rise in the chamber; during expiration negative pressure in the pleural space decreases, causing fluid to drop in the chamber. (3) (SU; EV; TC; RE)
1 If the system is closed to the atmosphere, as it should be, no bubbles will be present.
2 If the system is closed to the atmosphere, as it should be, no bubbling will occur.
4 Changes in intrapleural pressure cause fluid to rise on inspiration and fall on expiration (tidaling).

403. 1 This is sufficient to move blood, fluid, or air, which may be obstructing drainage; "stripping" or "milking" is avoided because it raises pressure significantly beyond the 15 to 20 cm of water used to suction and may cause injury. (2) (SU; IM; TC; RE)
2 This is contraindicated unless there is a break in the system.
3 This is a medical decision and would not be done unless the tube could not be made patent.
4 This is not indicated unless other symptoms, such as dyspnea, are present.

404. 4 This is an emergency situation and atmospheric air must be prevented from entering the thoracic cavity; the client's respiratory status takes priority over the potential for infection. (3) (SU; IM; TC; RE)
1 This action is useless in this situation and would further impair the client's breathing.
2 This is unsafe because it would allow atmospheric air to enter the thoracic cavity.
3 Although an occlusive dressing, such as Vaseline gauze, is desirable, atmospheric air will enter the thoracic cavity while time is taken to obtain the occlusive dressing.

405. 3 To prevent further possibility of pneumothorax, the nurse should immediately reconnect the tube. (3) (SU; IM; PA; RE)
1 This is unnecessary.
2 Clamping is appropriate for changing a broken drainage system or to check for an air leak; it should not be done needlessly.
4 The high Fowler's position is appropriate for a client in respiratory distress but this does not remedy this problem.

406. 2 This prevents atelectasis and collection of secretions and promotes respiratory exchange. (2) (SU; IM; PA; RE)
1 Observing for dyspnea remains important, but crepitus is unlikely to occur with stabilization of respiratory status.
3 This is important but not as conducive to improving respiratory status as are coughing and deep breathing.
4 Activity should be promoted within limits of physical ability; bedrest is unnecessary.

407. 4 The client's chronic illness and advanced age increase vulnerability; the daughter's condition should be explored in greater detail. (3) (ME; AN; PA; RE)
1 Children before puberty and adolescence have the least incidence of tuberculosis.
2 The morbidity and mortality due to tuberculosis are increasing, not decreasing.
3 Although the incidence of tuberculosis has increased some in the general population, it is increasing at an alarming rate in those who are HIV positive.

408. 3 Blood-tinged sputum in the absence of pronounced coughing may be the presenting symptom; diaphoresis at night is a later symptom. (2) (ME; AS; PA; RE)

1   Recurrent fever is present; however, frothy sputum is present with pulmonary edema, not tuberculosis.

2   The cough would be productive, not dry.

4   A productive cough may occur, but engorged neck veins are symptomatic of congestive heart failure.

409. 4   The Mantoux is the most accurate skin test because of the testing material used and the intradermal method; no other skin test would be appropriate as a follow-up; further tests are now warranted, including a chest x-ray. (1) (ME; EV; PA; RE)

1   The test result was positive, not negative; further testing is necessary.

2   The Tine test is less accurate than the Mantoux and would not be used as a follow-up test.

3   Above 10 mm induration is a positive test result, not a doubtful test result.

410. 4   The tubercle bacilli can be stained with carbolfuchsin, an acid, when the stain is applied with heat; the bacilli resist discoloration when an acid-alcohol wash is applied. (1) (ME; AS; PA; RE)

1   This reflects pulmonary status but does not identify the organism.

2   This indicates the presence of antibodies but is not diagnostic for the presence of the disease.

3   Same as answer 1.

411. 2   Clients with tuberculosis tend to lose weight and have anorexia; this will encourage food intake and provide calories for weight gain. (1) (ME; PL; TC; RE)

1   This is not necessary; protein can be obtained through natural foods.

3   This is not possible; carbohydrates contain calories.

4   Proteins are needed for tissue building.

412. 3   Fresh airflow into the house changes the air and lowers the concentration of microorganisms. (3) (ME; IM; ED; RE)

1   This is not necesssary.

2   This is not necessary; only articles contaminated with infected sputum, such as used tissues, should be contained.

4   It is permissible to do this because the extreme heat used to process the dishes kills the mycobacterium.

413. 1   The specimen must represent phlegm containing the mycobacterium, which is in the lung, not the oronasopharynx. (1) (ME; IM; ED; RE)

2   This is not necessary.

3   Same as answer 2.

4   Same as answer 2.

414. 3   Tubercle bacilli are transmitted through airborne droplets; therefore, respiratory isolation with an Ultra-Filter mask is necessary. (1) (ME; IM; TC; RE)

1   This is unnecessary as long as appropriate isolation precautions are followed.

2   This would not be necessary unless objects are contaminated by respiratory secretions.

4   This is not necessary; tuberculosis is spread by airborne droplets; gloves are only necessary when touching articles contaminated by respiratory secretions.

415. 4   Tubercle bacilli are particularly resistant to treatment and can remain dormant for prolonged periods of time; medication must be taken consistently as ordered for prolonged periods. (1) (ME; AN; TC; RE)

1   Although this is important, the microorganisms must be eliminated by the use of medication.

2   Same as answer 1.

3   Same as answer 1.

CARDIOVASCULAR

416. 3 The carotid artery is located along the anterior edge of the sternocleidomastoid muscle at the level of the lower margin of the thyroid cartilage. (1) (ME; AS; PA; CV)
1 This is not the anatomic landmark for locating the carotid artery.
2 Same as answer 1.
4 Same as answer 1.

417. 1 The first heart sound is produced by closure of the mitral and tricuspid valves; it is best heard at the apex of the heart. (2) (ME; AS; PA; CV)
2 This is where the second heart sound (S_2) is best heard; S_2 is produced by closure of the aortic and pulmonic valves.
3 This border covers a large area; the auscultatory areas that lie near it are the pulmonic and mitral areas.
4 This border covers a large area; the only auscultatory area near it is the aortic area.

418. 1 Closure of the atrioventricular valves, the mitral and tricuspid, produces the first heart sound (S_1). (3) (ME; AN; PA; CV)
2 These valves do not close simultaneously.
3 Same as answer 2.
4 These are the semilunar valves; closure of these valves produces the second heart sound (S_2).

419. 3 Inactivity causes venous stasis, hypercoagulability, and external pressure against the veins, all of which lead to thrombus formation; early ambulation or exercise of the lower extremities reduces the occurrence of this phenomenon. (1) (SU; IM; TC; CV)
1 This will be helpful, but it is not an independent activity; elastic stockings require a physician's order.
2 Massaging would be contraindicated because any developing clot could be dislodged.
4 Although this may help, the primary intervention is to provide exercise of the extremities until ambulation is permitted.

420. 2 Oxygen is necessary for the production of fire. (1) (ME; PL; TC; CV)
1 Oxygen does not burn itself; it supports combustion.
3 This is irrelevant to the need for safety precautions.
4 Same as answer 3.

421. 3 This is an early typical finding after a myocardial infarct because of the altered contractility of the heart. (3) (ME; AS; PA; CV)
1 Flattened or depressed T waves indicate hypokalemia.
2 This occurs in atrial and ventricular fibrillation.
4 Q waves may become distorted with conduction or rhythm problems, but they do not disappear unless there is cardiac standstill.

422. 4 The Valsalva maneuver produces an increased central venous pressure that will lessen the risk of air entering the circulation. (2) (SU; IM; TC; CV)
1 This is irrelevant to the procedure; it is required for a paracentesis.
2 This is not necessary; a local rather than a general anesthetic is given.
3 These are inappropriate instructions; this would create a negative central venous pressure.

423. 4 Pulmonary capillary wedge pressure is an indirect measure of left ventricular end diastolic pressure, an indication of ventricular contractility. (2) (ME; AN; PA; CV)
1 Right atrial pressure measures only the function of the right heart and indirectly its ability to receive blood.
2 Cardiac output by thermodilution does not measure intracardiac pressures.
3 Pulmonary artery diastolic pressure may not be as accurate an indicator of left ventricular pressure if COPD or pulmonary hypertension exist.

424. 2 This is a radionuclear study that determines viability of myocardial tissue; necrotic or scar tissue does not extract thallium isotope. (2) (ME; AN; TC; CV)

1   This information is available from a cardiac catheterization with an angiography.

3   This is determined by cardiac angiography.

4   This is determined by a 12-lead ECG.

425. 3   Chocolate has a high caffeine content, which may stimulate catecholamine release and act as a cardiac stimulant. (2) (ME; PL; ED; CV)

1   Yogurt is not a cardiac stimulant; it aids digestion if lactose intolerance is present.

2   Club soda contains sodium chloride but does not stimulate the myocardium.

4   Red meats do not stimulate the myocardium; red meats may be decreased or eliminated if serum cholesterol levels are elevated.

426. 3   The Prudent Diet contains reduced fat with less saturated animal fat, increased carbohydrate with more of it in complex forms, and moderate protein with emphasis on lean forms. (2) (ME; AN; TC; CV)

1   This caloric distribution does not represent the Prudent Diet proposed by the American Heart Association.

2   Same as answer 1.

4   Same as answer 1.

427. 3   The essential fatty acid, linoleic acid, is necessary for muscle tissue integrity, especially of the myocardium. (2) (ME; IM; ED; CV)

1   All fats cannot and should not be eliminated from the diet.

2   Proteins and carbohydrates do not contain the essential fatty acid called linoleic acid.

4   The body does manufacture cholesterol.

428. 4   The fiber component of complex carbohydrates helps bind and eliminate dietary cholesterol and foster growth of intestinal microorganisms to break down bile salts and release the cholesterol component for excretion. (3) (ME; IM; ED; CV)

1   It is what the client eats, not when the client eats, that is most important.

2   Of the fats in the diet, saturated fats should be decreased.

3   Fat-binding fiber should be increased.

429. 2   Food and fluids are usually withheld for approximately 6 to 8 hours to prevent vomiting and aspiration. (1) (SU; IM; TC; CV)

1   The procedure takes approximately 2 hours.

3   Bedrest with legs extended and a weight applied to the femoral site is suggested for several hours after the femoral method of entry.

4   A mild sedative is used because the client must be alert enough during the procedure to follow directions.

430. 1   The presence and specific location of pedal pulses are identified as a frame of reference for future readings. (1) (SU; AS; PA; CV)

2   The femoral artery, not a small artery in the foot, is used for cannulation.

3   Pedal pulses reflect the functioning of the arterial system; edema reflects the inadequacy of the venous system or decreased cardiac output.

4   Pedal pulses reflect the functioning of the arterial system, not the venous system.

431. 3   Immobilization of the left leg and pressure over the groin promote coagulation and healing at the puncture site of the femoral artery. (1) (SU; AN; TC; CV)

1   The catheterization does not decrease blood pressure in the presence of adequate fluid replacement.

2   These interventions cannot prevent or limit these symptoms; these symptoms are not usual.

4   A small amount of radiopaque dye is injected (via the catheter) directly into the heart, where it is diluted by the blood; it does not create a problem at the puncture site.

432. 2   An apical pulse is taken to detect dysrhythmias related to cardiac irritability; blood pressure is monitored to detect hypotension, which may indicate bleeding or shock. (1) (SU; EV; TC; CV)
1   This is contraindicated; flexion of the groin may compromise the clot at the femoral insertion site.
3   This is not necessary; the client did not undergo a general anesthetic and will soon be ambulatory.
4   A temperature may indicate a bacterial invasion, but this will not be evident during the first few hours after the catheterization.

433. 4   A sustained diastolic pressure above 90 mmHg reflects pathology and indicates hypertension. (1) (ME; AS; PA; CV)
1   This is unrelated to hypertension.
2   This reflects the heart rate, not the pressures within the artery.
3   This is not the most significant indicator; an elevated diastolic pressure is more important because it reflects the pressure while the heart is at rest.

434. 2   Headache is the most common symptom because of the increased pressure within the arterial circulation. (1) (ME; AS; PA; CV)
1   Fatigue can be associated with hypertension in the elderly, but this is not common.
3   Nosebleeds are possible when the blood pressure does reach extremely elevated levels; however, this is not a common indication.
4   A flushed face may occur because of increased pressure, but it is not the most common symptom.

435. 3   Muscle contraction associated with walking prevents edema and pooling of blood in the extremities. (1) (ME; IM; ED; CV)
1   This is inactivity, and movement is required.
2   This is an inactive position, and no exercise is involved; this will not prevent thrombus formation.
4   This does not include movement, which is essential to prevent thrombus formation.

436. 2   The failing left ventricle cannot accept blood returning from the lungs; this results in increased vascular pressure in the lungs. (3) (ME; AN; PA; CV)
1   This is associated with right ventricular failure.
3   This is the result of left, not right, ventricular failure.
4   Wheezing and coughing are associated with paroxysmal nocturnal dyspnea and right ventricular heart failure.

437. 1   Morphine is a narcotic analgesic that acts on the central nervous system by a sympathetic mechanism; it decreases systemic vascular resistance, which decreases left ventricular afterload, thus decreasing myocardial oxygen consumption. (2) (ME; IM; TC; CV)
2   Oxygen administration elevates arterial oxygen tension with the potential for improving tissue oxygenation; however, oxygen administration usually does not deliver enough oxygen to the myocardium to reverse the infarction and thus relieve the pain.
3   Nitroglycerin sublingually is effective in relieving anginal pain but not myocardial infarction pain.
4   Lidocaine is an antidysrhythmic, not an analgesic.

438. 3   Cessation of blood flow to the myocardium results in pain because of ischemia of the tissue, as in angina. (1) (ME; AN; PA; CV)
1   Neither myocardial infarction nor angina involve compression of the heart.
2   These are not related to pain or relief of pain; isoenzymes are indicators of myocardial damage.
4   Vasodilation would increase perfusion and contribute to pain relief.

439. 2   Morphine is a specific central nervous system depressant used to relieve the pain associated with myocardial infarction; it also decreases apprehension and prevents cardiogenic shock. (2) (ME; IM; PA; CV)
1   This is not the reason for the use of morphine.

3 This is not the primary reason for the use of morphine; diazepam (Valium) will be prescribed for this purpose as necessary.

4 Lidocaine is given intravenously to accomplish this.

440. 4 Creatine phosphokinase (CPK) isoenzyme levels, especially the MB sub-unit, begin to rise in 3 to 6 hours, peak in 12 to 18 hours, and are elevated for 48 hours after the occurrence of the infarct; they are therefore most reliable in assisting with early diagnosis. (2) (ME; AS; PA; CV)

1 Serum aspartate aminotransferase (AST) levels begin to rise later and do not peak until 24 to 36 hours, so they are not as early an indicator.

2 Lactic dehyrogenase (LDH) isoenzyme levels, especially LDH_1, do not begin to rise until 12 hours after the infarct and peak in 48 hours, so they are a much later indicator.

3 Serum glutamic oxaloacetic transaminase (SGOT) isoenzyme is another name for AST.

441. 3 Fever causes an increase in the body's metabolism which results in an increase in oxygen consumption; this need for oxygen is met by increasing the heart rate, which is reflected in the increased pulse rate. (1) (ME; AS; PA; CV)

1 Although the respiratory rate may increase slightly, fever will not cause dyspnea.

2 Chest pain is not related to the fever unless its cause is respiratory in nature.

4 Blood pressure elevation will not accompany a fever.

442. 4 A direct relationship exists between the strength of cardiac contractions and the electrical conductions through the myocardium. (3) (ME; AN; PA; CV)

1 The heart rate is related to factors such as SA node function, partial pressures of oxygen and carbon dioxide, and emotions.

2 This is the period when the heart is at rest, not when it is contracting.

3 Pulmonary pressure does not influence action potential; it becomes elevated in the presence of left ventricular failure.

443. 3 Dyspnea at night, which usually requires the assumption of the orthopneic position, is a symptom of left ventricular failure; orthopnea, a compensatory mechanism, limits venous return, which decreases pulmonary congestion and promotes ventilation, easing the dyspnea. (2) (ME; AS; PA; CV)

1 This occurs with right ventricular failure because of hypervolemia.

2 Anorexia and nausea occur with right ventricular failure because of venous stasis and venous engorgement of abdominal viscera; weight gain would occur because of fluid retention.

4 This occurs with right ventricular failure because of portal hypertension and liver congestion.

444. 4 A direct relationship exists between the systolic blood pressure and the force of left ventricular contraction. (2) (ME; AN; PA; CV)

1 An increased blood volume would be indicated by hypertension, not a decreased pulse pressure.

2 Hyperactivity of the heart would be indicated by dysrhythmias and tachycardia.

3 A decreased pulse pressure would indicate decreased cardiac sufficiency.

445. 2 This is the cardinal reason for PVBs. (2) (ME; AS; PA; CV)

1 This is a type of dysrhythmia, not the cause of PVBs; the source of atrial fibrillation is the atrium not the ventricles.

3 This type of dysrhythmia is associated with interference with the conduction system, not cardiac irritability.

4 This is a type of dysrhythmia, not the cause of PVBs.

446. 3 The greater saphenous vein from the leg is often removed and used to bypass the diseased coronary artery because one surgical team can obtain the vein while another team performs the chest surgery; this shortens the surgical time and lessens the risks of surgery; the internal mammary arteries are the grafts of choice but the surgery is usually longer because of the procedure of dissecting the arteries from the chest wall. (1) (SU; IM; ED; CV)
  1 Cardiopulmonary bypass (extracorporeal circulation) is accomplished by placement of a cannula in the right atrium, vena cava, or femoral vein to withdraw blood from the body; blood is returned to the body via a cannula in the aorta or the femoral artery.
  2 This is not done during a coronary artery bypass graft (CABG).
  4 Same as answer 2.

447. 2 This type pacemaker synchronizes impulses to the atria and ventricles to more closely simulate the normal action of the heart; it may be a fixed-rate or, most usually, a demand mode pacemaker and may stimulate the atria, the ventricles, or both. (2) (SU; IM; ED; CV)
  1 The physiologic pacemaker stimulates both the atria and ventricles to contract.
  3 It affects the electrical conduction system of the heart, not the anatomic structures.
  4 It will increase the heart beat to a more normal rate.

448. 3 This is the primary indication for a pacemaker because there is an interference with the electrical conduction system of the heart. (1) (SU; AN; TC; CV)
  1 The primary treatment for this disorder is medication; this is not an indication for a pacemaker.
  2 Same as answer 1.
  4 Same as answer 1.

449. 4 Milliamps are used, not volts of electricity; higher voltages are needed to electrocute. (1) (SU; IM; ED; CV)
  1 This is a patronizing response and minimizes the stated concern.

  2 The voltage used in pacemakers can never cause electrocution; technology is not related.
  3 The voltage used can never cause electrocution; all pacemakers are pretested for accuracy.

450. 1 Shoes that become too tight indicate pedal edema which is a sign of fluid retention; 2.2 pounds is equal to 1 liter of fluid. (3) (ME; AS; PA; CV)
  2 Eventually the physician will be notified, but the nurse should have more data before calling.
  3 With fluid retention the rate is not as significant as a bounding characteristic to the pulse.
  4 Although left ventricular failure can proceed to right ventricular failure the client has given no indication that pulmonary edema may be developing.

451. 2 Pulmonary congestion and edema occur because of fluid extravasation from the pulmonary capillary bed, resulting in difficult breathing. (1) (ME; AS; PA; CV)
  1 This is a hallmark of myocardial infarction; it is caused by inadequate oxygen supply to the myocardium.
  3 This results from increased venous pressure associated with right ventricular heart failure.
  4 This is a sign of right ventricular, not left ventricular, heart failure; a weakened right ventricle causes venous congestion in the systemic circulation.

452. 2 Rest decreases demand on the heart and will also prevent fatigue. (1) (ME; PL; PA; CV)
  1 Client should sleep with the head slightly elevated to facilitate respiration.
  3 The client needs potassium; a low-potassium diet when the client is taking digoxin predisposes to toxicity and dangerous dysrhythmias.
  4 To avoid becoming obsessed with the pulse rate, the client should not be taught to take pulse so often; once daily is adequate.

453. 1 Restriction of sodium reduces the amount of water retention, thus reducing cardiac workload. (1) (ME; PL; TC; CV)

2 This is not true for a client with CHF; calcium is restricted in individuals who develop renal calculi with a calcium phosphate base and are placed on an acid-ash diet.

3 Potassium would not be restricted, especially if a diuretic and cardiac glycoside are ordered.

4 Magnesium is not restricted.

454. 4 Crackles are the sound of air passing through fluid in the alveolar spaces; in pulmonary edema, fluid moves from the intravascular compartment into the alveoli. (1) (ME; AS; PA; CV)

1 The blood pressure is usually increased with hypervolemia.

2 This would occur with angina or a myocardial infarction.

3 The pulse would be bounding with hypervolemia.

455. 3 A client's knowledge about the treatment program enhances conformity and reduces stress. (1) (ME; IM; PS; CV)

1 This response does not answer the client's question and might produce frustration.

2 This is a general statement that does not focus on the specific client.

4 This does not support the treatment regimen; it may cause more stress if the client interprets it as a conflict between the physician and nurse.

456. 3 This is caused by hypervolemia and pulmonary hypertension. (1) (ME; AS; PA; CV)

1 The pulse would most likely be rapid and bounding, not slowed.

2 This is present in pleurisy, not heart failure.

4 Hypertension, not hypotension, would occur because of hypervolemia.

457. 3 Stressful situations will increase the body's oxygen demands. (2) (ME; IM; ED; CV)

1 Clients with low cardiac reserve cannot tolerate extremes of temperature; a hot bath will increase the body's oxygen demands.

2 Hot, humid weather is not good for those with chronic heart disease; these individuals should use an air conditioner.

4 The heart of a client with low cardiac reserve cannot tolerate a pulse rate this high.

458. 2 This pulse rate increase indicates activity tolerance is exceeded; rest brings the heart rate back to normal. (2) (ME; IM; PA; CV)

1 Activity should be stopped, not continued.

3 Though descending the stairs requires less energy than climbing, rest is essential to permit the heart rate to return quickly to normal.

4 This still constitutes activity, which aggravates the cardiac work load.

459. 4 As the heart contracts, an expanding midline mass can be palpated to the left of the umbilicus. (2) (SU; AS; PA; CV)

1 This is not definitive for abdominal aortic aneurysm.

2 These are not definitive for abdominal aortic aneurysm; pallor is associated with shock.

3 There is no disease in the intestinal tract; this finding is associated with intestinal obstruction.

460. 2 Immediate surgical intervention to clamp the aorta is necessary for survival; the aneurysm has ruptured. (2) (SU; IM; TC; CV)

1 This may eventually be done, but notifying the physician is the priority.

3 Same as answer 1.

4 Sedatives mask important signs and symptoms.

461. 4 Ambulation is essential to promote venous return and prevent thrombus formation. (1) (SU; PL; TC; CV)

1 This causes increased popliteal pressure and impairs venous return.

2 Same as answer 1.

3 This helps prevent atelectasis, not thrombi.

462. 4   When the legs are dependent, gravity and incompetent valves promote increased hydrostatic pressure in leg veins and, as a result, fluid moves into the interstitial spaces. (2) (ME; AS; PA; CV)
1   This reflects inadequate arterial blood supply; arterial circulation is not affected by varicose veins.
2   Same as answer 1.
3   This pain is referred to as Homan's sign and is most often associated with thrombophlebitis.

463. 1   Incompetent valves result in retrograde venous flow and subsequent dilation of veins. (1) (SU; IM; ED; CV)
2   Pressure is increased, not decreased.
3   Plaque formation is considered an arterial, rather than a venous problem.
4   These are considered a result of, rather than a cause of, varicose veins.

464. 1   To prevent distention of the veins, the stockings should be applied before the legs are placed in a dependent position. (2) (ME; IM; ED; CV)
2   Knee-high stockings should end 2 inches below the knee to avoid popliteal pressure, which limits venous return.
3   The stockings should be used preventively before the discomfort associated with venous pressure and edema occurs.
4   The stockings apply uniform pressure; elastic bandages may slip, creating uneven pressure and constriction; edema may also result.

465. 1   Impaired venous return causes increased pressure, with subjective symptoms of fatigue and heaviness. (2) (SU; AS; PA; CV)
2   Homan's sign is indicative of thrombophlebitis.
3   Symptoms of hypoxia are related to impaired arterial, rather than venous, circulation.
4   Ecchymosis may occur in some individuals, but there is insufficient bleeding into tissue to cause hematomas.

466. 2   This results from venous pooling with increased hydrostatic pressure; fluid moves from intravascular to interstitial spaces. (2) (SU; AS; PA; CV)
1   Pigmentation, not pallor, occurs.
3   This occurs with arterial, not venous, insufficiency.
4   Same as answer 3.

467. 1   After ligation, the saphenous vein is removed. (1) (SU; IM; ED; CV)
2   Plaque is considered an arterial, rather than a venous, problem.
3   They are normally attached by communicating veins; surgery involves ligation to isolate the saphenous vein.
4   This prevents emboli from traveling to the lung; it is not a vein ligation and stripping.

468. 4   Because of the client's history and the site of the surgery, thrombi are likely to develop; activity is a preventive measure. (2) (SU; PL; TC; CV)
1   This alone will not prevent thrombi; activity is necessary.
2   Getting out of bed will provide little exercise if the client only sits in a chair; also, an order is needed.
3   Although body alignment is important for all clients, it will not discourage thrombus formation.

469. 1   Seeing the exercises demonstrated will reinforce the verbal explanations. (2) (SU; IM; ED; CV)
2   This statement is too vague; it does not explain how to move them.
3   This statement is too vague and thus may be ineffective; the time period should be stipulated.
4   This response is vague and open to interpretation; nonspecific instructions may be ineffective.

470. 4   This provides support and promotes venous return; applying stockings while legs are horizontal before arising ensures that stockings are applied before dependent edema occurs. (2) (ME; IM; ED; CV)
1   Although helpful, it will not provide continuous support for the veins, which is mandatory.

2   These need to be ordered by the physician.

3   Warm soaks resolve inflammation; they do not prevent development of thrombophlebitis.

471. 1   Swelling of the extremity is indicative of thrombophlebitis. (2) (ME; AS; TC; CV)

2   Difficulty with mobility would occur with musculoskeletal or neuromuscular problems.

3   This is associated with neurologic deficits in the corticospinal tracts.

4   This assessment would be made to determine the status of the arterial, not venous, system.

472. 3   Nicotine causes vasoconstriction and spasm of peripheral arteries. (1) (ME; AN; TC; CV)

1   Alcohol is useful as a drug to stimulate dilation of blood vessels.

2   Lowering the limb enhances flow of blood into the foot by gravity.

4   This decreases the viscosity of blood, possibly preventing thrombus formation.

473. 2   This is a truthful answer that explains how nicotine is detrimental to physical status; nicotine also promotes platelet aggregation and clot formation. (3) (ME; IM; TC; CV)

1   This may be true, but it is not an appropriate explanation of why the client should not smoke.

3   Intermittent claudication is caused by impaired arterial, not venous, circulation.

4   The physician will probably advise against smoking because resuming smoking will continue to decrease oxygen to the lower extremities.

474. 3   An altered quality of a variety of pulses in the extremity is the earliest indication of limited circulation. (1) (ME; AS; TC; CV)

1   This would interfere with gravity that facilitates the flow of arterial blood to the legs and feet.

2   This could release an embolus into the circulation; it may also cause tissue trauma.

4   Altered sensation may limit sensitivity to heat, which could result in burns.

475. 3   Intermittent claudication is the pain that occurs during exercise because of a lack of O_2 to muscles in the involved extremities. (2) (ME; AN; PA; CV)

1   It is the exercise, not the lack of it, that precipitates the pain.

2   This is related to a venous problem, not an arterial one.

4   Same as answer 2.

476. 2   Decreasing the demand for oxygen by resting will relieve the pain. (1) (ME; IM; ED; CV)

1   Pain will not resolve as long as exercise and, thus muscle hypoxia, is continued, regardless of whether ASA is taken or not.

3   This is appropriate for venous insufficiency, not arterial insufficiency.

4   Nitroglycerin is a coronary artery dilator, not a peripheral vascular dilator.

477. 1   Arterial ulcers are painful because of the depth and interruption of the blood supply. (3) (ME; AN; PA; CV)

2   This is characteristic of venous ulcers.

3   Same as answer 2.

4   Same as answer 2.

478. 4   Pressure promotes coagulation and prevents the complication of bleeding. (2) (SU; IM; TC; CV)

1   Bending the operative leg may cause decreased perfusion to the leg or bleeding at the catheter insertion site.

2   Elevation would resist gravity flow of arterial blood, reducing O_2 to distal tissue.

3   Bedrest is required for 6 to 12 hours after the procedure.

479. 4 Because of the trauma associated with the insertion of the catheter during the procedure, the involved extremity should be assessed for sensation, motor ability, and arterial perfusion; hemorrhage or an arterial embolus could occur. (2) (SU; IM; TC; CV)

1 The client has an arterial problem, and perfusion is promoted by keeping the legs at the level of the heart.

2 General anesthesia is not used; therefore voiding is really not a concern.

3 This is unsafe; this position increases pressure in the groin area which could dislodge the clot at the catheter insertion site resulting in bleeding; it also impedes arterial perfusion and venous return.

480. 3 The client is hypertensive, and the intra-arterial pressure is elevated; this increased pressure could cause the arterial suture line to rupture. (2) (SU; AN; TC; CV)

1 This is unlikely because the blood pressure is elevated and the client is at risk for bleeding.

2 Hypervolemia would be an assumption; other causes, such as arterial constriction, can precipitate hypertension.

4 Although this could occur, the priority for this client is protecting the graft.

481. 1 Hypertension increases pressure on the suture lines of the graft. (3) (SU; AN; TC; CV)

2 Signs of shock, including a drop in the BP, would be associated with a severe allergic reaction.

3 An increased BP does not necessarily mean the client is hypervolemic.

4 This would be indicated by absent pedal pulses.

482. 3 Mobility will reduce venous stasis and edema as well as promote arterial perfusion and healing. (3) (SU; IM; PA; CV)

1 Bedrest is contraindicated because it promotes the development of thrombophlebitis and pulmonary emboli.

2 This is contraindicated; it constricts circulation at the hips and knees.

4 This would limit arterial perfusion.

483. 4 Presence of pulses and a normal skin color indicate adequate arterial perfusion and graft viability. (1) (SU; EV; ED; CV)

1 This is contraindicated in peripheral vascular disease because it may traumatize vessels; it could cause a thrombus to become an embolus.

2 This is appropriate for venous, not arterial, problems.

3 Clients with arterial insufficiency usually have paresthesias and may perceive water as cool when it is actually hot enough to cause tissue damage; the peripheral dilation produced by a hot bath would increase the work load on the heart, which is undesirable in a client with hypertension.

REPRODUCTIVE AND GENITOURINARY

484. 3 It is a fact that *E. coli* is commonly found in the bowel and, because of close anatomic proximity and improper hygiene after bowel movements, may spread to the urethra. (1) (ME; AN; PA; RG)

1 *E. coli* is no more virulent than other infective agents.

2 *E. coli* is not commonly found in the kidneys.

4 *E. coli* does not compete with *Candida* organisms for host sites.

485. 4 Laxatives remove feces and flatus, providing better visualization. (2) (SU; PL; ED; RG)

1 A light supper may be indicated; however, there is no restriction as to fat content.

2 Large amounts of water may dilute the dye, impairing visualization.

3 A light dinner and beverage are permitted.

486. 1 Assessment is the priority; the nurse should determine if symptoms are caused by a full bladder. (2) (ME; AS; TC; RG)

2 This may eventually be necessary, but is not the initial action.

3 This may be done to reduce urinary bacterial count and stone formation, but it is not the initial action.

4 This could be done, but it would not be the initial action.

487. 4   This uses gravity to allow urine to exert pressure on the area of the trigone, initiating relaxation of the urinary sphincter and facilitating micturition. (1) (ME; IM; ED; RG)

1   Although this may be important so that urine may be collected to be strained, it will not facilitate micturition.

2   An acid ash diet may be used to prevent urinary infection and the formation of calcium stones; it will do nothing to facilitate micturition.

3   This is important after urination but will not help facilitate micturition.

488. 2   Promoting hydration maintains urine production at a higher rate, which flushes the bladder and prevents urinary stasis and possible infection. (2) (ME; PL; TC; RG)

1   Although this could help identify a urinary tract infection, it would not prevent it.

3   Same as answer 1.

4   The drainage bag is emptied once every shift unless it fills before then; changing the bag periodically, not emptying it, would help prevent infection.

489. 2   The glomerulus is not permeable to large proteins like albumin or to red blood cells. (1) (SU; EV; PA; RG)

1   The proximal tubules are responsible for regulating water, electrolytes including sodium and potassium, urea nitrogen, and pH; the byproducts of this regulation will appear in normal urine.

3   Same as answer 1.

4   Same as answer 1.

490. 3   More than 90% of pulmonary emboli originate in the deep veins of the pelvis and thighs because of the extensive vascular network. (2) (SU; AN; PA; CV)

1   This is untrue; most pulmonary emboli originate in the pelvis or thighs.

2   Same as answer 1.

4   Same as answer 1.

491. 1   Muscle contraction during ambulation improves venous return which prevents venous stasis and thrombus formation. (2) (SU; PL; TC; CV)

2   Gatching the bed places pressure on the popliteal spaces, limiting venous return and increasing the risk of thrombus formation.

3   Dangling the legs places pressure on the popliteal spaces, limiting venous return and increasing the risk of thrombus formation.

4   Bedrest is associated with venous stasis, which increases the risk of thrombus formation.

492. 2   Cholinergics intensify and prolong the action of acetylcholine, which increases the tone in the genitourinary tract, preventing urinary retention. (3) (ME; AN; PA; RG)

1   Cholinergics will not prevent renal calculi.

3   Anticholinergics are prescribed for the frequency and urgency associated with a spastic bladder.

4   This would be a secondary gain because cholinergics help prevent urinary retention that can lead to a urinary tract infection, but this is not the primary purpose for administering these drugs.

493. 3   This increases lymphatic drainage, reducing edema and pain. (2) (SU; IM; TC; RG)

1   This increases circulation to the area, intensifying edema and pain.

2   Same as answer 1.

4   This is not indicated; scrotal swelling is caused by the trauma of surgery, not infection.

494. 3   This method obtains a specimen uncontaminated by environmental organisms. (3) (ME; IM; TC; RG)

1   This is not as accurate as obtaining the purulent discharge from the site of origin.

2   This would contaminate the specimen with organisms external to the body.

4   This would dilute and possibly contaminate the specimen.

495. 2   Anal itching and irritation result from erythema and edema of the anal crypts from the gonococcus. (3) (ME; AS; PA; RG)

1   Frank, rectal bleeding, not upper GI bleeding, occurs.

3   Diarrhea, not constipation, occurs.

4   Shape of formed stool does not change; however, diarrhea does occur.

496. 4   Secondary syphilis, occurring 1 to 3 months after healing of the primary lesion and lasting for several weeks to as long as a year, is the stage at which the individual is most infectious. (2) (ME; AN; PA; RG)

1   This is the fourth or final stage of syphilis.

2   This is the third stage of syphilis.

3   Primary syphilis is the stage of initial infection; it precedes secondary syphilis.

497. 4   The client is in the secondary stage, which begins from 6 weeks to 6 months after primary contact; therefore, a 6-month history is needed to ensure that all possible contacts and original contacts are located. (3) (ME; IM; TC; RG)

1   Any time less than 6 months may miss contacts who could have become infected.

2   Same as answer 1.

3   Same as answer 1.

498. 4   Neurotoxicity, as manifested by ataxia, is evidence of tertiary syphilis, which may involve the CNS; other CNS signs include confusion, paralysis, delusions, impaired judgment, and slurred speech. (2) (ME; AS; PA; RG)

1   This occurs in the secondary stage.

2   Same as answer 1.

3   This is not a sign of late-stage syphilis.

499. 2   The headaches are the result of the retention of fluid and hypertension. (3) (ME; AS; PA; RG)

1   The client would have oliguria, not nocturia.

3   The client would have a weight gain because of the retention of fluid.

4   The client would have anorexia related to elevated toxic substances in the blood.

500. 2   Sucking on a hard candy will relieve thirst and increase carbohydrates, but does not supply extra fluid. (2) (ME; IM; TC; RG)

1   Carbonated beverages are high in sodium and provide additional fluid, which must be restricted.

3   A milk shake contains both fluid and protein, which must be restricted.

4   Broth contains sodium, which can compound the fluid retention problem.

501. 4   Streptococci, common in throat infections, initiate an antibody formation that damages the glomerulus. (2) (ME; IM; ED; RG)

1   The alkalinity of bubble baths has been linked to urethritis, not glomerulonephritis.

2   Moderate activity is helpful in preventing urinary stasis, which could precipitate an infection.

3   Any fluid restriction is moderated as the client improves; fluid is permitted to prevent urinary stasis.

502. 2   Infection is responsible for $\frac{1}{3}$ of the traumatic or surgically induced deaths of clients with renal failure, as well as for medically induced acute renal failure (ARF); resistance is reduced in clients with renal failure because of decreased phagocytosis which makes them very susceptible to microorganisms. (3) (ME; AS; TC; RG)

1   Anemia occurs frequently with ARF, but it is not the most serious complication and should be treated in relation to the client's symptoms; erythropoietin and iron supplements are usually used.

3   Weight loss is not life-threatening in and of itself.

4   Platelet dysfunction does occur because of decreased cell surface adhesiveness, but it is not as serious as infection.

503. 2   An excessive use of antacids may result in hypercalciuria; most calculi contain calcium combined with phosphate or other substances. (3) (ME; AS; PA; RG)

1   Cholesterol is unrelated to the formation of renal calculi; cholesterol stones in the

gallbladder are the result of increased cholesterol synthesis in the liver.

3 Immobility with the associated demineralization of bone, not exercise, may cause renal calculi.

4 Alcohol intake is unrelated to renal calculi formation.

504. 4 The pain of renal colic is excruciating; unless relief is obtained the client is unable to cooperate with other therapy. (3) (SU; AN; TC; RG)

1 Any urine can be saved and strained after the client's priority needs are met.

2 Increasing fluid intake helps mobilize the stone, but a client who has severe pain may be nauseated and unable to drink.

3 Although a culture is generally ordered, it is not a priority when a client has severe pain.

505. 4 Pain with ureteral stones is caused by spasm and is excruciating and intermittent; it follows the path of the ureter to the bladder. (2) (SU; AS; PA; RG)

1 Pain is spasmodic and excruciating, not boring.

2 This is untrue; pain intensifies as the stone is caught in the ureter and spasms occur in an attempt to dislodge it.

3 This is typical of pain caused by a stone in the renal pelvis.

506. 4 Purines are precursors of uric acid. (3) (ME; AN; PA; RG)

1 Cystine stones are caused by a rare hereditary defect resulting in inadequate renal tubular reabsorption of cystine (inborn error of cystine metabolism).

2 A struvite stone is sometimes called a magnesium ammonium phosphate stone and is precipitated by recurrent urinary tract infections with coliform bacteria.

3 An oxalate stone would be composed of calcium oxalate.

507. 2 A calculus may obstruct the flow of urine to the bladder, allowing the urine to distend the ureter, causing hydroureter. (3) (SU; AN; PA; RG)

1 There is insufficient information to come to this conclusion even though output is less than intake; oliguria is present when the output is between 100 and 500 ml in a 24-hour period.

3 Calculi do not cause renal shutdown directly; they may obstruct the urinary tract and cause damage indirectly as a result of pressure from urine buildup.

4 If the urethra was obstructed, the bladder would be distended.

508. 4 If the calculus is in the renal pelvis a percutaneous pyelolithotomy is performed; the stone is removed via a small flank incision. (2) (SU; AN; TC; RG)

1 This is not necessary.

2 This is usually unnecessary.

3 This route is used for stones in the distal portion of the ureters.

509. 1 These occur with a urinary tract infection because of bladder irritability; burning on urination and fever are additional signs of a UTI. (1) (SU; EV; PA; RG)

2 This is not related to a urinary tract infection.

3 This is a symptom of urinary calculus, not infection.

4 This is not a sign of a urinary tract infection; this may be caused by altering the diet to include foods that form acid ash or alkaline ash.

510. 1 Cancer of the prostate is rare before the age of 50, but increases with each decade; Black men develop it twice as frequently as Caucasian men and at an earlier age. (3) (ME; AN; PA; RG)

2 This group of men have a lower incidence of prostatic cancer than Caucasians, as well as a lower mortality rate.

3 Same as answer 2.

4 Caucasian men develop prostatic cancer half as frequently as Black men, but more frequently than Asian or Hispanic men.

511. 4   These are routine postoperative expectations following a transurethral prostatectomy (TURP) to provide for hemostasis and excretion. (1) (SU; IM; ED; RG)

1   These will be present with a suprapubic prostatectomy.

2   Following a TURP the client can initially expect hematuria and some blood clots; the continuous bladder irrigation keeps the bladder free of clots and catheter patent.

3   This is true of a perineal prostatectomy.

512. 3   An indwelling urethral catheter is used, because surgical trauma can cause urinary retention leading to further complications such as bleeding. (2) (SU; IM; EV; RG)

1   Urinary control is not lost in most cases; loss of control is temporary if it does occur.

2   This is usually not affected; sexual ability is maintained if the client was able to perform before the surgery.

4   A cystostomy tube is not used if the client has a transurethral resection; however, it is used if a suprapubic resection is done.

513. 3   Patency promotes bladder decompression, which prevents distention and bleeding; continuous flow of fluid through bladder limits clot formation and promotes hemostasis. (2) (SU; PL; TC; RG)

1   There is no abdominal dressing with a TURP; surgery is performed via the urethra.

2   There is no cystostomy tube; a cystostomy tube is used when a suprapubic resection is performed.

4   There is no external wound because there is no abdominal incision.

514. 2   The pressure of the balloon against the small blood vessels of the prostatic fossa causes them to constrict, thereby preventing bleeding. (2) (SU; AN; TC; RG)

1   It may actually cause spasms and discomfort but it is necessary to limit bleeding.

3   Same as answer 1.

4   It is not the balloon but the Foley catheter that promotes urinary drainage.

515. 4   The amount of irrigant instilled into the bladder must be deducted from the total output to determine the amount of urine voided. (1) (SU; IM; TC; RG)

1   Unless irrigant is subtracted from the output, the total would be inaccurate.

2   Specific gravity measures the concentration of urine; this measurement would be inaccurate because the urine is diluted with GU irrigant.

3   This is unnecessary; the bladder is constantly being irrigated with GU irrigant.

516. 2   After transurethral surgery, hemorrhage is common because of venous oozing and bleeding from many small arteries in the area. (1) (SU; EV; TC; RG)

1   Sepsis is unusual and occurs later in the postoperative course.

3   Leaking around the catheter is not a major complication.

4   Urinary retention is highly unlikely with an indwelling catheter in place.

517. 3   Milking the tubing will usually dislodge the plug and will not harm the client; no physician's order is necessary to check patency. (2) (SU; IM; TC; RG)

1   The nurse should call the physician after trying measures to restore patency of catheter.

2   The nurse should not remove a catheter without specific instructions from a physician.

4   The catheter may be irrigated after milking it and only with a physician's order.

518. 4   Traction on the Foley catheter pulls the balloon tight against the prostatic fossa, which promotes hemostasis. (2) (SU; IM; TC; RG)

1   This is unsafe; the tension on the catheter must be maintained until the physician determines that there is no longer a risk of bleeding.

2   Same as answer 1.

3   It is unnecessary to call the physician; pressure at the site is expected.

519. 4   Because of the trauma to the mucous membranes of the urinary tract, burning on urination is an expected response which should gradually subside. (2) (SU; EV; ED; RG)

1   The urine may have a slight pink tinge because of the trauma from the surgery and the presence of the catheter but it should no longer be dilute once the continuous bladder irrigation is removed.

2   This is a sign of hemorrhage which should not occur.

3   This should not occur unless the Foley is removed too soon and there is still edema of the urethra.

520. 3   The urethral mucosa in the prostatic area is destroyed during surgery, and strictures may form with healing. (3) (SU; EV; ED; RG)

1   The client should void as the need arises; straining can cause pressure in the operative area, precipitating hemorrhage.

2   The client should be out of bed ambulating; sitting for several hours is contraindicated because it promotes venous stasis and thrombus formation.

4   Although vigorous exercise should be avoided, six months is too long a period for this restriction.

521. 3   In a suprapubic prostatectomy an incision is made into the bladder via the abdomen so that the bladder abnormalities can be corrected concurrently with prostatic resection. (1) (SU; AN; ED; RG)

1   This is untrue; resection via the transurethral route would necessitate a shorter convalescence.

2   An indwelling catheter is required following surgery to provide for drainage of urine until postoperative edema subsides.

4   Radical perineal prostatectomy, when perineal nerves are severed, can result in impotence.

522. 2   Because venous stasis is the major predisposing factor of pulmonary emboli, venous flow velocity should be increased. (2) (SU; PL; TC; RG)

1   Increasing the coagulability of the blood would lead to the development of deep vein thrombosis.

3   This would not affect the development of deep vein thrombosis.

4   Same as answer 3.

523. 2   The kidney, an extremely vascular organ, receives a large percentage of the blood flow. (3) (SU; PL; TC; RG)

1   This may occur, but it would be later in the postoperative period.

3   This can occur but is not acute and develops later.

4   This can occur but is not life threatening.

524. 3   Turning facilitates drainage from the operative site. (3) (SU; PL; TC; RG)

1   Because clients are prone to develop paralytic ileus, they are kept npo or on clear fluid for at least 24 to 48 hours.

2   A nephrostomy tube should never be clamped unless specifically ordered by the physician.

4   The dressing should be changed frequently because the wound generally drains large amounts.

525. 4   The wound will drain urine until healing takes place, sometimes up to several weeks. (3) (SU; AS; PA; RG)

1   The hourly urine output must be 30 ml or more to be adequate.

2   A specific gravity this low indicates that the kidneys have lost their ability to concentrate urine.

3   Urine begins to clear within about 24 hours; urine that remains dark red and contains clots indicates abnormal bleeding.

526. 4   The dressing will need to be changed at home because drainage can persist for several weeks. (1) (SU; IM; ED; RG)

1   The client should be encouraged to take fluids.

2   The client should be up and about at home.

3   A nephrostomy tube is generally not irrigated unless specifically ordered by the physician.

527. 2 High biologic value (HBV) protein contains essential amino acids needed by the body for tissue building and repair. (1) (ME; EV; ED; RG)

   1 A high caloric diet would provide for weight gain.

   3 Low biologic value (LBV) proteins avoid the accumulation of urea in the body.

   4 This is not the purpose of high biologic value proteins; sodium restrictions would decrease blood pressure.

528. 3 One cup of cottage cheese is approximately 225 calories, 27 grams of protein, 9 grams of fat, 30 milligrams of cholesterol, and 6 grams of carbohydrate; proteins of high biologic value (HBV) contain optimal levels of the amino acids essential for life. (1) (ME; EV; PA; RG)

   1 Apple juice is a source of vitamin 3, not protein.

   2 Raw carrots are a carbohydrate source and contain beta carotene.

   4 Whole wheat bread is a source of carbohydrates and fiber.

529. 2 The accumulation of metabolic wastes in the blood (uremia) can cause pruritus; edema results from fluid overload caused by impaired renal excretion. (1) (SU; AS; PA; RG)

   1 Pallor occurs with chronic renal failure as a result of the related anemia.

   3 This is a urinary pattern that is not caused by chronic renal failure; this often occurs after prostate surgery.

   4 This occurs with an enlarged prostate, not renal insufficiency.

530. 3 An elevation in uremic waste products causes irritation of the nerves, resulting in flapping hand tremors (asterixis, liver flap). (3) (ME; AS; PA; RG)

   1 Hypertension results from kidney failure because of sodium and water retention.

   2 The diseased kidney is unable to excrete potassium ions, resulting in hyperkalemia, not hypokalemia.

   4 The hematocrit will be low because of a decreased production of erythropoietin, a hormone synthesized in the kidney; erythropoietin regulates the production of erythrocytes.

531. 1 Lack of motivation is the most serious impediment to successful continuous ambulatory peritoneal dialysis (CAPD); CAPD may be contraindicated for some clients such as those who are blind or have a colostomy, a psychosis, or PVD. (3) (SU; AS; ED; RG)

   2 This is not a contraindication if the client is receiving medical supervision.

   3 Same as answer 2.

   4 Same as answer 2.

532. 3 Dialysate is introduced into the peritoneal cavity where fluids, electrolytes, and wastes are exchanged through the peritoneal membrane. (2) (SU; IM; ED; RG)

   1 The client can dialyze alone in any location without need for machinery and continuous technical supervision.

   2 Hemodialysis is not necessary with this procedure.

   4 Between 1 and 2 L of dialysate is maintained intraperitoneally and exchanged by the client.

533. 2 While proteins may be restricted, those eaten should be high quality proteins to replace proteins lost during the dialysis. (3) (SU; IM; ED; RG)

   1 This client would be encouraged to eat a high caloric diet.

   3 This is inappropriate; there is usually a modest restriction of fluids when the client is on dialysis.

   4 This is inappropriate; there is usually a restriction of high potassium foods when the client is on dialysis.

534. 4 Warming of the dialysate before use or during infusion decreases discomfort. (2) (SU; IM; TC; RG)

   1 A low fiber diet may impede emptying of the bowel, which could then interfere with outflow of the dialysate.

   2 It may take up to two weeks to tolerate a full two liters of exchange without leakage around the catheter; too quick an exchange may cause disequilibrium phenomenon.

3   The outflow bag should be lower than the abdomen to allow gravity flow of the return dialysate.

535. 4   A cleansing enema is given and the bladder emptied to lessen the possibility of bladder perforation; invasive procedures require consent. (2) (SU; PL; TC; RG)
1   An IV pyelogram is not required.
2   None of these is required.
3   Local anesthesia is used.

536. 2   The infusion should be at room temperature to lessen abdominal discomfort and allow for dilation of peritoneal vessels. (3) (SU; IM; TC; RG)
1   The infusion should be unrestricted, taking approximately 5 to 10 minutes.
3   The side-lying position may restrict fluid inflow and prevent maximum urea clearance; usually the client is in the semi-Fowler's position.
4   Medications are administered before the infusion.

537. 3   Pressure from the fluid may cause upward displacement of the diaphragm. (3) (SU; IM; PA; RG)
1   Additional fluid would aggravate the problem.
2   Auscultation is important, but it does not alleviate the problem.
4   The client is already in semi-Fowler's position, which would normally relieve dyspnea; however, intraabdominal pressure must be reduced by draining the fluid.

538. 4   These symptoms may indicate peritonitis. (3) (SU; EV; TC; RG)
1   Oliguria is not a complication of this therapy; these are symptoms of illness, not complications of therapy.
2   Pruritus may be present as a result of the illness, not the therapy.
3   Same as answer 2.

539. 2   The external shunt may come apart; external temperatures make clotting a potential hazard; frequent handling increases risk of infection. (3) (SU; EV; TC; RG)

1   Neither the shunt nor the fistula will affect the blood pressure reading; obtaining a blood pressure in an arm with a fistula or shunt is contraindicated; blood pressures using the thighs should be obtained.
3   An infusion should not be in the extremity with the shunt or fistula to avoid pressure from the tourniquet used during catheter insertion and lessen the chance of phlebitis.
4   The ends of the shunt cannula should be left exposed for rapid reconnection in the event of disruption.

540. 3   These are signs and symptoms of the disequilibrium phenomenon, which results from rapid changes in composition of the extracellular fluid and cerebral edema; the rate of exchange should be decreased. (3) (SU; EV; TC; RG)
1   This will not alleviate or reverse the cause of the symptoms, although it will provide relief from the nausea.
2   The cause of the confusion must be reversed and this intervention will not accomplish this.
4   While these would be assessed, this action would do nothing to alleviate the symptoms.

541. 1   The recipient's own kidneys are not removed unless a chronic infection is present. (3) (SU; IM; ED; RG)
2   Both kidneys are left in place unless a chronic infection is present; the new kidney is placed in the right lower quadrant.
3   Same as answer 2.
4   Same as answer 2.

542. 2 An appendectomy is performed to avoid appendicitis in the future, which might be confused with rejection of the renal transplant which is usually placed in the right lower quadrant. (3) (SU; IM; ED; RG)

1 The intestines are not involved in a kidney transplant; therefore an examination of the colon is not necessary.

3 The stomach is not involved with renal function or with a kidney transplant.

4 There is usually no problem with the bladder, but only with the kidneys.

543. 3 Hourly output is critical in assessing kidney function; decreasing urinary output is a sign of rejection. (2) (SU; EV; TC; RG)

1 It is not necessary to monitor this frequently.

2 Same as answer 1.

4 This is too infrequent to monitor output immediately after a transplant; it is essential to monitor output more frequently to evaluate if the new kidney is working or if it is being rejected.

544. 2 Serum creatinine, a test of renal function, measures the kidneys' ability to excrete metabolic wastes; creatinine, a nitrogenous product of protein breakdown, is elevated in renal insufficiency. (2) (SU; EV; TC; RG)

1 This would not provide any information about the filtering ability of the new kidney.

3 Although intake and output would be monitored, these would not provide information about the constituents of the urine.

4 A WBC count would not reflect functioning of the new kidney.

545. 3 Hypertension is caused by a return of hypervolemia because of the failure of the new kidney. (2) (SU; EV; ED; RG)

1 There will be a weight gain because of fluid retention, which is indicative of failure of the transplanted kidney.

2 The client will have an elevated temperature above 100°F.

4 Urine output will be decreased or absent, depending on the degree of failure.

546. 4 The WBC count can drop precipitously; if leukocytes are below 3,000/mm³, the drug should be stopped to prevent irreversible bone marrow depression. (2) (SU; EV; PA; RG)

1 Leukocytosis, not leukopenia, would occur with an infection.

2 High creatinine levels are related to kidney failure, but do not cause leukopenia.

3 The WBC count would be elevated, not decreased, if the kidney were being rejected.

GASTROINTESTINAL

547. 3 Complementary mixtures of essential amino acids in plant proteins provide complete dietary protein equivalents. (3) (ME; IM; PA; GI)

1 A total vegetarian does not consume flesh, milk, milk products, or eggs.

2 Same as answer 1.

4 Same as answer 1.

548. 2 A new dietary regimen, with a balance of foods from the food pyramid, must be established and continued for weight reduction to occur and be maintained. (3) (ME; AN; PA; GI)

1 Although this would be true in a weight reduction diet, this response does not address this nutrient's relationship to the other food groups.

3 Same as answer 1.

4 This is only one part of a weight reduction regimen; usually in obese individuals caloric intake exceeds energy expenditure.

549. 4 Increased exercise builds skeletal muscle mass and reduces excess fatty tissue. (3) (ME; EV; PA; GI)

1 This is unrelated to weight loss; during the aerobic exercise the heart rate will increase, but between periods of exercise the heart rate will decrease because of the development of collateral circulation.

2 Appetite is usually increased.

3 The metabolic rate will increase.

550. 3 With an inflammatory response the body increases its production of WBCs and fibrinogen, which increases the WBC count

and blood sedimentation rate, respectively. (1) (ME; AN; PA; GI)
1 This is untrue; this would not affect the white blood cell count or the sedimentation rate.
2 Same as answer 1.
4 Same as answer 1.

551. 2 The stomach is located within the sternal angle; thus the area is known as the epigastric area. (1) (ME; AS; PA; GI)
1 This is in the area of the iliac bones.
3 This is the lowest middle abdominal area.
4 This is the area above the sternum.

552. 3 Abdominal distention, which may be associated with pain, may indicate perforation, a complication that can lead to peritonitis. (3) (SU; EV; TC; GI)
1 A local inflammatory response to insertion of the fiberoptic tube may result in a sore throat and dysphagia once the anesthesia wears off.
2 This, together with cramping, is considered a normal response.
4 These are not indicative of any particular problem in this situation.

553. 2 Barium will harden and may create an impaction; a laxative and increased fluids promote elimination of barium. (2) (ME; PL; TC; GI)
1 Iodine is not used in a GI series with barium.
3 The client must be kept npo.
4 This is not part of the preparation; feces in the lower GI tract would not interfere with visualization of the upper GI tract.

554. 2 Carbohydrates provide 4 kcal per gram; therefore 3 L × 50 g/L × 4 kcal/g = 600 kcal, only about a third of the basal energy need. (1) (SU; AN; TC; GI)
1 This is less than the calories provided by the ordered IV fluid.
3 This is more than the calories provided by the ordered IV fluid.
4 Same as answer 3.

555. 3 This series of diets progresses from the one which makes the least metabolic demand on the client (clear liquid) to a regular diet, requiring the capability of unimpaired digestion. (1) (SU; AN; PA; GI)
1 The caloric content is not the focus in a progressive post-surgical diet.
2 Initially, a progressive diet has very little nutritional value; the focus is to rest the gastrointestinal tract immediately after surgery.
4 Initially, a limited variety of fluids is presented to rest the gastrointestinal tract; food is not included until later.

556. 2 There are 9 calories in each gram of fat and 4 calories in each gram of carbohydrate and protein; this diet contains 1970 calories. (3) (ME; AN; TC; GI)
1 This is too high for the diet prescribed.
3 This is too low for the diet prescribed.
4 Same as answer 3.

557. 2 This serum albumin indicates severe depletion of visceral protein stores; the normal range for serum albumin is 3.5 to 5.5 g /dl; white meat turkey (2 slices 4 × 2 × 1/4 inch) contains approximately 28 g protein. (3) (ME; EV; ED; GI)
1 A 6 oz serving of mixed fruit contains approximately 0.5 g of protein.
3 A 3 cup serving of raw spinach contains approximately 2 g of protein.
4 A 4 oz serving of beef broth contains approximately 2.4 g of protein.

558. 3 Smoking accelerates oxidation of tissue vitamin C, so smokers need 100 mg /day, whereas adult RDA is 60 mg /day. (3) (ME; IM; TC; GI)
1 This is not oxidized more rapidly in the smoker.
2 Same as answer 1.
4 Same as answer 1.

559. 1 Tofu products increase protein without increasing vitamin D because unlike milk products, tofu does not contain vitamin D. (2) (ME; EV; ED; GI)
2 Eggnog contains milk and should be avoided.
3 This contains vitamin D and should be avoided.
4 This contains milk, which has vitamin D, and should be avoided.

560. 3 Vitamin C (ascorbic acid), an antioxidant, is found in vegetables such as broccoli, tomatoes, and potatoes; one cup of broccoli has 140 mg of vitamin C. (2) (ME; AN; PA; GI)
1 Apples, depending on their size, contain only 6 to 8 mg of vitamin C.
2 An entire head of lettuce contains only 13 mg of vitamin C.
4 Apricots contain only 11 mg of vitamin C; they are a source of beta carotene.

561. 1 The antioxidants, vitamin E and beta carotene, that help inhibit oxidation and therefore tissue breakdown, are found in these foods. (3) (ME; AN; PA; GI)
2 These are excellent sources of vitamin E, but not beta carotene.
3 These are excellent sources of vitamin C, not vitamin E and beta carotene.
4 These are excellent sources of beta carotene, but not vitamin E.

562. 4 According to the ADA diet, green beans and broccoli are equivalent vegetable substitutes. (2) (ME; IM; ED; GI)
1 This is a bread exchange.
2 Same as answer 1.
3 Same as answer 1.

563. 4 Stress ulcers are asymptomatic until they produce massive hematemesis and rectal bleeding. (2) (ME; AS; PA; GI)
1 Shock is the outcome of massive hemorrhage; it would not be unexplained because the sudden gastrointestinal bleeding would be seen.
2 Sudden massive bleeding occurs; not the slow oozing that causes melena.
3 A gradual drop in hematocrit indicates slow blood loss.

564. 3 Green vegetables contain fiber, which promotes defecation. (1) (SU; EV; ED; GI)
1 This has a binding effect and would cause constipation with resultant straining at stool.
2 Same as answer 1.
4 Same as answer 1.

565. 4 This produces bulk, which is a stimulant to defecation; the muscles used in defecation are weak in clients with Parkinson's disease which often causes constipation. (2) (ME; IM; PA; GI)
1 Bananas are binding and will intensify the problem of constipation.
2 This will intensify the problem; fluids need to be increased.
3 Cathartics are irritating to the intestinal mucosa, and their regular administration promotes dependence.

566. 1 Red meat can react with reagents used in the test to cause false-positive results. (2) (ME; AS; ED; GI)
2 This may apply for testing for ova and parasites, but not for occult blood.
3 If the correct procedure is followed, discarding the first specimen is unnecessary.
4 Random stool testing can be done, but must be on three different bowel movements during the screening period.

567. 3 These characteristics describe steatorrhea which results from impaired fat digestion. (3) (ME; AS; PA; GI)
1 This is descriptive of stools resulting from constipation.
2 This is descriptive of acholic stools occurring with biliary obstruction and resulting from an absence of urobilin.
4 This would be descriptive of upper and lower gastrointestinal bleeding.

568. 4 Nutrition by intravenous route eliminates pancreatic stimulation, therefore reducing the pain experienced in pancreatitis. (1) (SU; IM; ED; GI)

1 TPN meets the client's needs not the nurses' needs.
2 TPN creates many safety risks for the client.
3 Hunger can be experienced with total parenteral nutrition therapy.

569. 3 The solution is hyperosmolar and a very concentrated source of glucose; too rapid infusion can cause a shift of fluid into the intravascular compartment resulting in overload; an infusion pump should be used as an added precaution. (3) (SU; PL; TC; GI)
1 Although important, it is not the priority.
2 Same as answer 1.
4 Same as answer 1.

570. 1 Rapid infusion of concentrated glucose into the vascular system does not allow time for adequate insulin release to transport glucose to the cells. (3) (SU; AN; TC; GI)
2 A hyperconcentrated solution usually results in hypervolemia, rather than hyperglycemia.
3 This finding is not an expected response, and it will not subside without intervention.
4 If this were true, the blood glucose would not be 240 mg/dl.

571. 4 The less disruptive the procedure, the greater the acceptance by the client. (2) (SU; PL; ED; GI)
1 Most frequently, total parenteral nutrition is set up to run during sleeping hours.
2 Depending on the type of circulatory access used, it may not need to be changed for weeks .
3 The client or a significant other can be taught the principles of administration.

572. 2 The *Salmonella* organism thrives in warm, moist environments; washing, cooking, and refrigeration of food limits the growth of or eliminates the organism. (1) (ME; AS; PA; GI)
1 Salmonellosis is unrelated to cancer.

3 Salmonellosis is caused by the *Salmonella* organism, not stress.
4 The *Salmonella* organism is ingested; it is not an airborne or blood borne infection.

573. 2 This medical aseptic technique reduces the possibility of transmitting the organisms to others. (2) (ME; PL; TC; GI)
1 Enteric precautions for adults can be handled in a semi-private room as long as fecally contaminated articles are disposed of appropriately.
3 The type of exposure, not the length of exposure, increases the risk of transmission; visitors are allowed, as long as those having close contact wear gowns and gloves.
4 The organism is not transmitted via the airborne route.

574. 3 The *Salmonella* bacilli can be visualized via microscopic examination. (1) (ME; AS; PA; GI)
1 Although this test might be done, it is not definitive for the diagnosis of salmonellosis.
2 Same as answer 1.
4 Same as answer 1.

575. 2 Fluids of dextrose and normal saline and electrolytes are administered to prevent profound dehydration caused by an excessive loss of water and electrolytes through diarrheal output. (3) (ME; PL; PA; GI)
1 These are not necessary; salmonellosis is an infection, not a condition caused by hyperacidity.
3 These are not used when there is a possibility of bacterial infection because slowed peristalsis decreases excretion of the *Salmonella* organism.
4 Same as answer 3.

576. 1 A cold environment limits growth of microorganisms. (1) (ME; EV; TC; GI)
2 All food should be refrigerated before and after it is cooked to limit the growth of microorganisms.
3 This promotes the growth of microorganisms because the stuffing would still be warm for a period of time before the refrigerator's cold environment cooled the center of the bird; poultry should be stuffed immediately before being cooked.
4 This promotes the growth of microorganisms because they thrive in warm, moist environments.

577. 1 The decreased hemoglobin, hematocrit, and RBC count may be due to malnutrition; also, cancer of the esophagus can cause dysphagia and anorexia. (3) (ME; AN; PA; GI)
2 There are no data given related to airway obstruction or metastasis.
3 There are no data given related to pressure on surrounding structures producing pain.
4 There are no data given related to airway obstruction or injury.

578. 2 Because of the trauma of surgery and the close proximity of the esophagus to the trachea, respiratory assessments become the priority. (1) (SU; EV; TC; GI)
1 Although this is important, an adequate airway is the priority.
3 Same as answer 1.
4 Same as answer 1.

579. 3 An increased heart rate is related to an autonomic nervous system response; pain is related to the trauma of the perforation and possibly gastric reflux. (3) (SU; EV; TC; GI)
1 These are signs of the dumping syndrome.
2 Same as answer 1.
4 An increased blood pressure may occur but frequent burping has no relationship to esophageal perforation.

580. 3 Weight reduction decreases intraabdominal pressure, thereby decreasing the tendency to reflux into the esophagus. (3) (ME; IM; ED; GI)
1 Fats decrease emptying of the stomach extending the time period that reflux can occur; fats should be decreased.
2 This increases the pressure against the diaphragmatic hernia, increasing symptoms.
4 This would increase pressure; fluid should be discouraged with meals.

581. 1 Classic symptoms include gnawing, boring, or dull pain located in the mid-epigastrium or back; pain is caused by irritability and erosion of the mucosal lining. (2) (ME; AS; PA; GI)
2 This type of pain is more characteristic of the complication of a perforated ulcer.
3 This type of pain is more characteristic of a hiatal hernia.
4 This type of pain is more characteristic of cholecystitis.

582. 4 Some medications, such as aspirin and prednisone, irritate the stomach lining and may cause bleeding with prolonged use. (2) (ME; AS; PA; GI)
1 This may be related to intestinal irritation causing diarrhea and intestinal bleeding, not gastric bleeding.
2 This is not the cause of gastric bleeding; it is important to ascertain dietary habits when teaching about dietary therapy.
3 Although stress may play a part, the use of some medications has a more direct relationship.

583. 3 Presence of food in the stomach at regular intervals interacts with HCl, limiting acid mucosal irritation. (1) (ME; PL; TC; GI)
1 The plan should be specific to try to keep food in the stomach at close intervals to limit mucosal irritation.
2 Food will relieve the pain.
4 Small frequent meals or meals with planned snacks would be most appropriate; limiting intake to 3 large meals would leave the stomach empty for long periods of time.

584. 2 These are classic indicators of perforated ulcer, for which immediate surgery is indicated; this should be anticipated. (2) (SU; PL; TC; GI)

1 Tachycardia and tachypnea are related to pain and possible blood loss, not to oxygen; keeping the client npo is the priority.

3 Black, tarry stools or red stools indicate bleeding, not perforation.

4 The symptoms are more indicative of perforation than shock.

585. 3 Without an adequate stomach reservoir, the hypertonic concentrated food mass "dumps" into the small intestine, drawing fluid from surrounding vessels and tissue and causing hypovolemia and typical shock symptoms. (2) (SU; AN; PA; GI)

1 The opposite is true; the food passes too quickly into the small intestine.

2 The opposite is true; the food mass is more concentrated (hypertonic).

4 Same as answer 2.

586. 1 Statistics demonstrate that these are the most likely sites for metastasis of this tumor. (2) (SU; AN; PA; GI)

2 It is less likely that the tumor will spread to these areas.

3 Same as answer 2.

4 These are routes of metastasis, not sites.

587. 3 Large amounts of blood or excessive bloody drainage 12 hours postoperatively must be reported immediately because the client is hemorrhaging. (2) (SU; IM; TC; GI)

1 This must be ordered by the physician; this is not an independent function of the nurse; although ice might constrict vessels, 30 ml would not be effective; many physicians now order room temperature normal saline lavages to prevent lowering core body temperature.

2 This is contraindicated; accumulation of secretions would cause pressure on the suture line; this prevents further observation of drainage.

4 This is an unsafe intervention at this time; the physician should be notified.

588. 1 Intrinsic factor is lost with removal of the stomach, and vitamin B_{12} is needed to maintain the hemoglobin level. (2) (SU; PL; PA; GI)

2 Adequate diet, fluid intake, and exercise should prevent constipation.

3 This would not be a routine expectation.

4 Pancreatic enzymes should be normal because surgery has not altered this function.

589. 1 The stomach's capacity is reduced because of surgery; smaller, frequent feedings with controlled bulk prevent the dumping syndrome. (1) (SU; EV; ED; GI)

2 This is not usually necessary; a diet of unblenderized foods is the goal.

3 This is not realistic.

4 The diet should be high in protein, low in carbohydrates, and normal in fats.

590. 4 This cancer is usually asymptomatic in the early stages; the stomach accommodates the mass. (1) (SU; AN; PA; GI)

1 This is untrue; it can be accurately diagnosed by gastric washings or biopsy.

2 This is untrue; this cancer is painless in its early stages.

3 This is untrue; this is typical of Hodgkin's disease, not gastric carcinoma.

591. 1 The thoracic cavity is usually entered for a complete resection, necessitating a chest tube. (2) (SU; PL; ED; GI)

2 Fluids are contraindicated until the suture line has healed and nasogastric suction is no longer being used.

3 The client would ambulate early to minimize the hazards of immobility.

4 There would be no physiologic necessity for this position.

592. 2 Taking fluids with meals causes rapid emptying of the food from the stomach into the jejunum before it has been adequately subjected to the digestive process; the hyperosmolar mixture causes a fluid shift to the jejunum. (1) (SU; IM; ED; GI)

1 Rest, not activity, after meals will assist in relieving dumping syndrome.

3 Small meals, with low carbohydrate, moderate fat, and high protein are recommended; these are more readily digested and prevent rapid stomach emptying.

4 Low carbohydrate meals are recommended to reduce the osmolarity of chyme as it empties into the jejunum.

593. 2 As a result of the trauma of surgery, some bleeding can be expected for 4 to 5 hours. (3) (SU; EV; PA; GI)

1 Clamping the tube would cause increased pressure on the gastric sutures from a buildup of gas and fluid.

3 Iced saline is rarely used because it causes vasoconstriction, local ischemia, and a reduction in body temperature.

4 This is not necessary; this is a normal occurrence.

594. 2 Rigidity and pain are hallmarks of bleeding from the suture line and/or of peritonitis; vital signs provide supporting data. (1) (SU; AS; TC; GI)

1 Ambulation would be indicated if pain were the result of flatulence; however, rigidity is clearly associated with bleeding or peritonitis and more data are needed.

3 An analgesic may mask the symptoms delaying diagnosis.

4 This is unrelated to the symptoms presented.

595. 1 Bowel sounds and flatulence indicate the return of intestinal peristalsis; peristalsis is necessary for movement of nutrients through the GI tract. (1) (SU; EV; PA; GI)

2 Incisional pain is unrelated to intestinal peristalsis.

3 Hematocrit levels indicate blood loss; they are unaffected by GI functioning.

4 Dumping syndrome occurs after, not before, the ingestion of food and would not be an indication that the client was ready to ingest food.

596. 4 Over-the-counter antacid preparations are taken to neutralize gastric acid and relieve pain. (2) (SU; EV; TC; GI)

1 Although eating food initially prevents the gastric acids from irritating the gastric walls, it can precipitate acid production and weight gain.

2 This is contraindicated; aspirin irritates gastric mucosa and promotes bleeding by preventing platelet aggregation.

3 Reduction of fluids with meals does not affect pain; it does help control symptoms of dumping syndrome.

597. 4 Dark brown or black stools (melena) could indicate gastrointestinal bleeding. (1) (ME; AS; PA; GI)

1 Frothy stools are indicative of poor fat absorption and are associated with sprue.

2 Ribbon-shaped stools indicate a bowel mass or obstruction.

3 Clay-colored stools are usually related to problems causing a decrease in bile.

598. 3 Nausea with a nasogastric tube in place could mean tube displacement or obstruction; checking placement can determine if it is in the stomach; once placement is verified then it can be irrigated to ensure patency. (3) (SU; IM; TC; GI)

1 The nurse should always assess a situation carefully before notifying the physician.

2 This may relieve the discomfort but will not determine the cause.

4 The tube should never be irrigated before checking tube placement; if the tube is displaced it could be in the trachea or bronchi and instillation of fluid would cause respiratory impairment.

599. 1 Abdominal distention, nausea, and abdominal pain can be signs of nasogastric tube blockage. (2) (SU; IM; TC; GI)

2 Although narcotics are usually ordered postoperatively, they tend to decrease

peristalsis and may increase abdominal distention and nausea.

3 There will be no stools for several days; gastric drainage may contain some blood from surgery.

4 No bowel sounds are expected for several days after stomach or intestinal surgery.

600. 3 Some bright blood at this point would be a normal finding that should be monitored; large amounts of blood or bleeding should be reported immediately. (2) (SU; EV; PA; GI)

1 If the tube is draining, there is no need to irrigate; also, irrigations should be ordered by the physician.

2 This is contraindicated; secretions would accumulate and cause pressure on suture line; this prevents observation of drainage.

4 Reducing suction would allow secretions to accumulate and cause pressure on the suture line.

601. 4 Symptoms characteristic of the dumping syndrome can be lessened with small, frequent meals that are low in carbohydrates and, therefore, not as hyperosmolar. (2) (SU; EV; TC; GI)

1 Fluids during meals should be limited; increased fluid intake speeds the emptying time of the stomach.

2 The client may need to avoid these foods to minimize irritating the gastric mucosa, but they are not the cause of the dumping syndrome.

3 Resting after meals might mitigate the symptoms of dumping syndrome, but resting before meals will not prevent them; resting is non-specific; the client should be lying down to slow the emptying of the stomach.

602. 4 The rapid absorption of sugars from the food mass causes elevation of blood sugar, and the insulin response often causes transient hypoglycemic symptoms. (2) (SU; AN; PA; GI)

1 The response is a rebound hypoglycemia, not hyperglycemia.

2 This is unrelated; usually a bland diet is prescribed following a gastrectomy.

3 The insulin-adjusting mechanism is not overwhelmed but responds vigorously, causing rebound hypoglycemia.

603. 1 All these characteristics are well-established risk factors for gallbladder disease (female, obese, and over 40). (1) (ME; AS; PA; GI)

2 None of these factors are correctly associated with cholecystitis.

3 The age is correct, but clients are usually female and have elevated serum cholesterol.

4 Risk factors include being a female and having a family history of gallstones, but clients are usually over 40.

604. 1 Pain is a cardinal symptom; it is helpful to have as much specific information about it as possible, particularly its description and its relationship to foods ingested. (2) (ME; AS; ED; GI)

2 It is not necessary to save all urine and stools, although changes in color should be reported.

3 The client should be free to question orders that are not understood or agreed with.

4 This would not add any valuable information.

605. 4 Cholecystitis is frequently accompanied by intolerance to fatty foods, including fried foods and butter. (2) (ME; AS; PA; GI)

1 These cause flatulence and pain for clients with lower intestinal problems such as diverticulosis.

2 These foods contain less fat than do fried foods or butter.

3 Neither chocolate nor boiled seafood has as much fat as fried chicken or butter.

606. 3 Local fat-stimulated duodenal glands dispatch the hormone, cholecystokinin, that signals the gallbladder to contract and release bile. (1) (ME; AN; PA; GI)
1 Soft-textured foods are unnecessary.
2 This would only be necessary if the cholecystitis was percipitated by cholelithiasis and the stones were composed of cholesterol.
4 Although this would be desirable before surgery, it is not the priority.

607. 4 During the procedure, a sedative is administered as required intravenously to help the client stay calm. (3) (SU; IM; ED; GI)
1 This is not used during this procedure.
2 Same as answer 1.
3 Same as answer 1.

608. 1 Bile promotes the absorption of the fat soluble vitamins A, D, E, and K; an obstruction of the common bile duct limits the flow of bile to the duodenum. (3) (SU; AS; PA; GI)
2 This is not relevant to the situation.
3 This is unnecessary; protein would be desirable for wound healing.
4 These would be unexpected.

609. 3 Self-splinting results in shallow breathing, which does not aerate the lungs adequately, particularly the lower right lobe. (1) (SU; AN; TC; GI)
1 The T-tube is never irrigated; it drains by gravity until the edema in the operative area subsides; the tube is then removed by the physician.
2 The dressing is not changed by the nurse in the immediate postoperative period; the client's respiratory status takes first priority.
4 The client would be npo for the first 48 hours after surgery.

610. 4 The inflammatory response occurs because of trauma of surgery; the T-tube maintains patency of the common bile duct until edema subsides. (2) (SU; AN; TC; GI)
1 It diverts the bile out of the body into a collection bag.

2 This is the purpose of the portable wound drainage system, not of a T-tube.
3 Surgical asepsis prevents infection at the site of the incision; the T-tube is a portal of entry for microorganisms and places the client at risk for infection.

611. 4 Slight hip flexion reduces tension on the abdominal musculature and the operative site. (1) (SU; PL; TC; GI)
1 This position places pressure on the abdominal wall, causing pain.
2 This position causes tension on the abdominal musculature and operative site.
3 Same as answer 1.

612. 1 Vitamin K, a precursor for prothrombin, cannot be absorbed without bile. (2) (SU; AS; PA; GI)
2 This is frequently related to electrolyte imbalances, not fat-soluble vitamin deficiency.
3 Jaundice results from a backup of bile, not a deficiency of fat-soluble vitamins.
4 This may be related to electrolyte imbalances or deficiency of B vitamins, which are water-soluble.

613. 1 Biliary colic may occur in the postoperative period as a result of the passage of pulverized fragments of the calculi; this may occur 3 or more days after the lithotripsy. (3) (SU; IM; ED; GI)
2 Fever would indicate pancreatitis, which is a rare occurrence.
3 The delivery of shock waves during the procedure is synchronized with the heart beat to avoid initiation of dysrhythmias.
4 Light sedation may be used to keep the client comfortable and as still as possible.

614. 4 Mild shoulder pain is common up to one week after surgery because of diaphragmatic irritation secondary to abdominal stretching or residual carbon dioxide that was used to inflate the abdominal cavity during surgery. (3) (SU; EV; ED; GI)
1 This is not necessary; the bandages are removed the second day postoperatively.
2 This is not necessary; clients generally tolerate food after 24 to 48 hours.

3 This is not necessary; the client may bathe and shower as usual.

615. 3 It may take 4 to 6 months, but ultimately most people can eat anything they want. (2) (SU; EV; ED; GI)
1 Although fats may have to be gradually reintroduced, most people can tolerate them after a cholecystectomy.
2 Foods that caused gastric distress before surgery are usually tolerated after surgery.
4 Increased protein is only needed until healing has occurred.

616. 3 This surgery involves the stomach, duodenum, pancreas, and common bile duct; a nasogastric tube removes gastric secretions and prevents distention. (1) (SU; PL; TC; GI)
1 A chest tube is used to remove air or blood from the chest cavity, which is not entered in the Whipple procedure.
2 Intestinal tubes are used for small bowel obstructions; except for the duodenum, the small bowel is not included in the Whipple procedure.
4 This tube is used to deliver nutrients into the stomach of a client who cannot swallow; this is unnecessary for this client.

617. 2 A patent nasogastric tube prevents distention and compression in the surgical area. (2) (SU; IM; TC; GI)
1 A low Fowler's position is preferred to limit tension on the abdominal wall; movement should be encouraged.
3 Replacement of vitamins is a dependent function; vitamins must be ordered by the physician.
4 Tube feedings are contraindicated because peristalsis is absent, and the feeding would place pressure on the suture line.

618. 4 The Whipple procedure leads to malabsorption because of impaired delivery of bile to the intestine; fat metabolism is interfered with, causing dyspepsia. (3) (SU; IM; ED; GI)
1 These clients are anorexic, require small frequent meals, and should eat high-calorie, high-protein, low-fat diets.

2 High-calorie meals are needed for energy and to promote use of protein for tissue repair.
3 High protein is required for tissue building; there is no problem with the liver in cancer of the pancreas unless direct extension occurs.

619. 4 Polydipsia is characteristic of hypoinsulinism (diabetes mellitus) because of impaired carbohydrate metabolism. (2) (SU; EV; PA; GI)
1 Polyuria, not oliguria, is characteristic of diabetes mellitus because excess fluid is excreted with the glucose by the kidneys.
2 Increased appetite is characteristic of diabetes mellitus because of impaired metabolism.
3 Weight loss characterizes diabetes mellitus because of the use of body mass as a source of energy.

620. 2 Rapid administration can cause glucose overload, leading to osmotic diuresis and dehydration; slowing the infusion decreases glucose overload. (2) (SU; IM; TC; GI)
1 Stopping the flow would jeopardize the central line; slowing the infusion will give the client's body a chance to handle the excess glucose.
3 Signs of bowel obstruction are not present.
4 The client's headache should disappear with oral fluid replacement; analgesics are not indicated.

621. 4 Professional assistance would ensure correct administration which may limit complications such as intravascular overload and sepsis. (3) (SU; IM; TC; GI)
1 This is usually done by the physician.
2 TPN is usually administered every day.
3 A TPN solution of 1000 to 2000 ml per day is usually administered at a prescribed rate of 50 to 125 ml/hour; the infusion usually runs continuously, not intermittently.

622. 4 Formation of lipase necessary for digestion of fats is an exocrine function; the endocrine function is to secrete insulin, which is a hormone essential in carbohydrate metabolism. (3) (SU; IM; TC; GI)

1 Although it is necessary to avoid alcohol, this is not related to the exocrine functioning of the pancreas.

2 Deficiencies of both may occur because of poor intake, but these deficiencies are not specifically related to exocrine or endocrine pancreatic functioning.

3 Fluid and electrolyte problems are not related specifically to exocrine or endocrine pancreatic functioning.

623. 1 A client's vital signs, especially the pulse and temperature, will rise before the client demonstrates any of the more severe symptoms of withdrawal from alcohol. (3) (ME; AS; PA; GI)

2 This is contraindicated initially because it may cause cerebral edema.

3 This becomes a priority after the problems of the withdrawal period have subsided.

4 This is not a priority until after the detoxification process.

624. 3 Scar tissue that forms as cirrhosis progresses causes the liver tissue to contract, making the liver small with a rough surface; little lumps are formed as scar tissue pulls the liver at certain points. (3) (ME; AS; PA; GI)

1 The client has cirrhosis, not hepatitis.

2 The liver converts ammonia to urea; therefore the blood ammonia level increases when the liver fails.

4 This is a manifestation of liver infection.

625. 4 Petechiae are evidence of capillary bleeding; the diseased liver is no longer able to metabolize vitamin K, which is necessary to activate blood clotting factors. (1) (ME; PL; PA; GI)

1 Although bile is synthesized and secreted in the liver, bile salts are not involved in the clotting process.

2 Folic acid is stored in the liver but not involved in the clotting process.

3 Vitamin A is not involved in clotting,

even though the transformation of carotene to vitamin A takes place in the liver.

626. 4 This keeps the bladder in the pelvic area and prevents puncture when the abdominal cavity is entered. (1) (SU; IM; ED; GI)

1 This is not necessary.

2 This is unsafe; the bladder will rise into the abdominal cavity and may be punctured.

3 Same as answer 1.

627. 1 Hepatitis A is primarily spread via a fecal-oral route; sewage-polluted water may harbor the virus. (3) (ME; AS; PA; GI)

2 This does not increase the risk of developing the disease but will increase the risk of an infected individual spreading the disease to others.

3 Hepatitis types 2, 3, and 4 are more often spread via the blood-borne route; using disposable equipment and proper handling of syringes decrease the risk of spreading the virus.

4 Exposure to arsenic or carbon tetrachloride can cause toxic hepatitis, which is not communicable.

628. 2 Damage to liver cells affects the ability to remove bilirubin from the blood, with resulting deposition in the skin and sclera. (2) (ME; AN; PA; GI)

1 With hepatitis, the liver does not secrete excess bile.

3 There is no increased destruction of red blood cells in hepatitis.

4 This is unrelated; decreased prothrombin levels cause spontaneous bleeding, not jaundice.

629. 4 High carbohydrates provide calories for energy, high proteins provide for tissue repair, and fats are permitted as tolerated. (2) (ME; PL; PA; GI)

1 High carbohydrates are needed for body fuel, otherwise proteins will have to be used for metabolism rather than tissue repair; proteins will be high and fats permitted as tolerated.

2 This diet does not offer adequate proteins,

which are required for tissue repair in the client with hepatitis; carbohydrates will be high, and fats are permitted as tolerated.

3 Same as answer 2.

630. 4 Hepatitis A is spread via the fecal-oral route; transmission is interfered with by proper hand washing. (2) (ME; IM; TC; GI)

1 This may increase transmission because no provision is made for the cleaning of equipment or disposal of contaminated wastes.

2 This is untrue; hepatitis can be transmitted via the fecal-oral route and precautions, such as hand washing, must be taken.

3 This is inadequate; transmission is still possible via the roll of toilet tissue unless hand washing is done.

631. 4 Hepatitis A is transmitted via the fecal-oral route; enteric precautions must be used when there are articles that have potential fecal and/or urine contamination. (2) (ME; PL; TC; GI)

1 Neither a private room nor a closed door is required; these are necessary only for respiratory (airborne) infections.

2 Hepatitis A is not transferred via the airborne route and therefore a mask is not necessary; a gown and gloves are required only when handling articles that may have fecal and/or urine contamination.

3 This is too limited; a gown and gloves should also be worn when handling other fecally contaminated articles, such as a bedpan or rectal thermometer.

632. 4 This is a vascular lesion associated with cirrhosis; it is thought to be related to elevated estrogen levels. (3) (ME; AS; PA; GI)

1 This refers to patches of depigmentation resulting from destruction of melanocytes.

2 This is excessive growth of hair; in cirrhosis, endocrine disturbances result in loss of axillary and pubic hair.

3 Black pigments do not occur with liver disease.

633. 1 Pressure applied to the puncture site compresses blood vessels, thereby preventing bleeding. (1) (SU; IM; ED; GI)

2 The right side-lying position will not restore circulating blood volume.

3 The semi- or high-Fowler's positions would be more comfortable, because they decrease pressure on the diaphragm.

4 This position will have little or no effect on biliary ducts.

634. 3 The flow of bile through the puncture site indicates a biliary vessel was punctured; this is a common complication following a liver biopsy. (2) (SU; AN; TC; GI)

1 Fluid would leak through the puncture site or into the peritoneum, not the intestine.

2 The pancreas does not contain bile; also it is in the upper left quadrant, not the upper right quadrant.

4 This is a complication, not an expected outcome.

635. 2 An increased serum ammonia level impairs the CNS, causing an altered level of consciousness. (2) (ME; PL; TC; GI)

1 Rising ammonia levels are not related to weight; client safety is the priority.

3 The priority is to protect the client; rising ammonia levels will precipitate hepatic encephalopathy.

4 An alteration in the fluid intake will not affect the serum ammonia level.

636. 3 One lumen inflates the esophageal balloon, the second inflates the gastric balloon, and the third decompresses the stomach. (1) (ME; AN; PA; GI)

1 It is a triple-lumen tube.

2 It is a triple-lumen tube; the stomach is decompressed, not the intestine.

4 The intestine is not decompressed.

637. 3 With increased intraabdominal pressure, the abdominal wall will become rigid and tender. (2) (SU; AS; PA; GI)

1 The pulse rate will increase in an effort to compensate for impending septic shock.

2 Hypovolemia, and therefore hypotension, results because of a loss of fluid, electrolytes, and protein into the peritoneal cavity.

4 Peristalsis and associated bowel sounds will decrease or be absent in the presence of increased intraabdominal pressure.

638. 3 This position promotes localization of purulent material and inflammation and prevents an ascending infection. (1) (SU; IM; TC; GI)

1 The risk of an ascending infection may be increased in this position, because it allows fluid in the abdominal cavity to bathe the entire peritoneum.

2 Same as answer 1.

4 The client would probably prefer a Sims' position, which increases risk of an ascending infection.

639. 2 Medical treatment is directed toward reducing motility of the inflamed bowel, restoring nutrition, and treating and preventing infection; surgery is used selectively for those who are acutely ill or have excessive exacerbations. (2) (SU; PL; ED; GI)

1 This is untrue; medical treatment is symptomatic, not curative.

3 It is usually performed as a last resort.

4 Although there is an emotional component, the physiologic adaptations determine whether surgery will be necessary.

640. 2 The client's feelings, knowledge, and skills concerning the ileostomy must be assessed before discharge. (1) (SU; EV; ED; GI)

1 People should not be pressured into performing self-care before they are physically and emotionally ready.

3 After an ileostomy the client is usually encouraged to eat a high-protein diet or a regular diet with supplemental protein; a high fluid intake should be maintained.

4 Frequently the client no longer needs a dressing on the incision at the time of discharge; a collection pouch is used over the stoma.

641. 3 Constipation, diarrhea, and/or constipation alternating with diarrhea are the most common symptoms of colorectal cancer. (3) (SU; AS; PA; GI)

1 Pain is reported as a symptom in less than 25% of clients; also it is a late sign after other organs are invaded, intestinal obstruction occurs, or tissue necrosis develops.

2 This is the second most common complaint that results from destruction of the epithelial lining of the intestine.

4 This is a later sign that only becomes evident when the lumen of the intestine narrows as a result of the enlarging mass.

642. 4 This diet is low in fiber; after digestion and absorption there is only a small amount of residue to be eliminated. (1) (SU; AN; TC; GI)

1 This diet does not influence the bacterial flora of the intestine; antimicrobials, such as neomycin, are given to do this.

2 This diet does not promote peristalsis; the products of digestion remain in the intestine longer, and flatus is increased.

3 Although a low-residue diet is less irritating, this is not the primary reason for its use before surgery.

643. 1 When intestinal continuity cannot be restored after removal of the anus, rectum, and adjacent colon, a permanent colostomy is formed. (2) (SU; PL; ED; GI)

2 This segment of colon lies on the right side of the abdomen and has no anatomic proximity to the rectum.

3 This procedure is performed to allow a segment of colon to heal; intestinal continuity can be restored.

4 This procedure is commonly performed for inflammation of the colon when intestinal continuity can be restored.

644. 2 Irrigations regulate the bowel to function at a specific time for the convenience of the client. (2) (SU; AN; PA; GI)

1 Although irrigations will prevent straining, this is not the purpose of the irrigation.

3 Irrigations will facilitate expulsion of flatus but will not decrease the amount; avoidance of gas-forming foods will accomplish this.

4 This is not the function of the irrigation; most ingested fluid already has been absorbed in the large intestine by the time it reaches the sigmoid.

645. 4 Left or right side-lying position puts the least strain or pressure on the perineal suture line. (2) (SU; IM; TC; GI)

1 This position is difficult to maintain and would place stress on the suture line.

2 Flexion of one hip and knee would increase tension on the perineal suture line; depending on placement of the stoma one of the Sims' positions would result in the client lying on the new colostomy, which would be traumatic.

3 This position places undue stress on the suture line and is the most uncomfortable position.

646. 2 There is no need to irrigate before the stool is formed. (2) (SU; IM; ED; GI)

1 If proper technique is used, fecal elimination should flow through the sleeve of the colostomy bag to the commode.

3 This is premature; the stool is not yet formed.

4 The perineal wound may take weeks to heal, and irrigations must be started when the stool is formed.

647. 2 This would indicate stenosis of the stoma and should be reported to the physician. (2) (SU; IM; ED; GI)

1 This is a common response that can be remedied by clamping the tubing until the discomfort subsides.

3 Flatus is always present in the bowel to some degree, and a colostomy irrigation will facilitate its expulsion.

4 This is not indicative of a medical problem; a colostomy irrigation usually can be completed in 1 hour, but some individuals may need a little more time.

648. 3 This is caused by the trauma of intestinal manipulation and the depressive effects of anesthesia and analgesics. (1) (SU; AN; PA; GI)

1 Edema would not totally interfere with peristalsis, which may be less effective but would still result in some output.

2 Any ingested food or fluid initiates the gastrocolic reflex and would therefore result in some output.

4 A nasogastric tube decompresses the stomach; it does not influence intestinal motility at this time.

649. 4 Irrigation should be performed at the time the client normally defecated before the colostomy to maintain continuity in lifestyle. (2) (SU; PL; ED; GI)

1 This may be true for some people; however, irrigations usually can be completed in 1 hour.

2 Most people defecate after breakfast because the ingestion of food on an empty stomach initiates the gastrocolic reflex.

3 An irrigation cannot be postponed until the client accepts the altered body image because this may take weeks or months.

650. 4 The irrigation bag should be hung no higher than 12 to 18 inches above the level of the stoma, and a clothes hook is too high. (1) (SU; EV; ED; GI)

1 Fluid flowing into the intestines can cause distention and discomfort; clamping the tubing is an appropriate intervention.

2 The tip of the catheter should be lubricated to prevent trauma to mucosal tissue and to facilitate insertion.

3 There is not enough information provided to choose this response; the amount of fluid ordered is not included.

651. 4 This occurs with stenosis of the stoma; forcing insertion of the tube could cause injury. (2) (SU; EV; ED; GI)

1 This is an expected response.

2 Same as answer 1.

3 This is expected; feces and flatus accompany fluid expulsion.

652. 3   These clients can eat a regular diet; only gas-forming foods that cause distention and discomfort should be avoided. (1) (SU; EV; ED; GI)

1   The amount of stool does not have to be limited; therefore a low-residue diet is not necessary.

2   The affected tissue has been removed, and normal mucosal tissue lines the intestine and forms the stoma; therefore bland foods are not necessary.

4   Nutrients are absorbed by the small, not the large, intestine; a regular diet is usually easily digested and absorbed.

653. 3   Pain is wavelike, colicky, and sharp because of obstruction and localized bowel ischemia. (2) (SU; AS; PA; GI)

1   Flatus would be impeded by strangulation.

2   Vomiting is persistent, not projectile.

4   This is not an early sign of obstruction; decreased bowel sounds occur after gas and fluid accumulate.

654. 3   Because of pain and the proximity of the operative site to the lower urinary tract, voiding problems are common. (3) (SU; EV; PA; GI)

1   This is not a complication of herniorrhaphy.

2   The abdomen was not entered and there should be no interference with peristalsis.

4   This should not be a complication of herniorrhaphy because early ambulation is permitted.

DRUG RELATED RESPONSES

655. 3   Using ratio and proportion:
8 mg /10 mg = X minims /15 minims
10 X = 120
X = 12 minims
(2) (ME; IM; TC; DR)

1   This is an inaccurate calculation; this is less than the desired dose.

2   Same as answer 1.

4   This is an inaccurate calculation; this is more than the desired dose.

656. 4   Vistaril potentiates the CNS effects of narcotics. (1) (SU; AN; PA; DR)

1   General anesthesia and manipulation of the bowel during surgery inhibit peristalsis.

2   General anesthesia produces this effect.

3   Antidysrhythmic drugs such as quinidine and lidocaine limit dysrhythmias.

657. 4   First convert milligrams to micrograms and then use ratio and proportion:
(0.2 mg = 200 mcg)
200 mcg /100 mcg = X ml/1 ml
100 X = 200
X = 2 ml
(2) (ME; IM; TC; DR)

1   This is an inaccurate calculation; this is less than the desired dose.

2   Same as answer 1.

3   Same as answer 1.

658. 4   This is the correct flow rate; 500 mg of the drug added to 100 ml of IV fluid produces a solution in which 1 ml contains 5 mg of the drug; the required amount of the drug is contained in 0.3 ml of fluid; to calculate the dosage to be delivered, multiply the amount to be delivered (0.3 ml) by the drop factor (60) and divide the result by the amount of time in minutes (1 min). (2) (ME; AN; TC; DR)

1   This is too slow; this would not deliver the ordered amount of lidocaine HCl.

2   Same as answer 1.

3   Same as answer 1.

659. 4   Use ratio and proportion to calculate:
375 mg /225 mg = X ml /1 ml
225 X = 375
X = 1.6 ml or 25 minims
(3) (SU; AN; TC; DR)

1   This is too little; it would not provide enough drug.

2   This is too much; it would provide an excess of drug.

3   Same as answer 1.

660. 1   250 mg is equal to 0.25 g; therefore,
4 g/0.25 g = X ml/1 ml
0.25 X = 4
X = 16 ml. (2)
(ME; AN; PA; DR)

2   This is an inaccurate calculation; too little to provide the ordered amount.

3   Same as answer 2.

4   Same as answer 2.

661. 3   Use ratio and proportion:

250 mg is equal to 0.25 g;

0.25 g /1g = X ml /3ml

X = 0.75 ml

0.75 ml = 12 minims.

(2) (SU; AN; TC; DR)

1   This is an incorrect calculation; too little medication will be administered.

2   Same as answer 1.

4   This is an incorrect calculation; too much medication will be administered.

662. 2   Use ratio and proportion:

30 U /100 U = X ml /1 ml

100 X = 30 ml

X = 1/3 ml or 5 minims.

(2) (ME; AN; TC; DR)

1   This is an inaccurate calculation; this would deliver too small a dose.

3   This is an inaccurate calculation; this exceeds the ordered dose.

4   Same as answer 3.

663. 2   Use ratio and proportion:

2,450,000 U /300,000 U = X ml /1 ml

300,000 X = 2,450,000

X = 8.2 ml

(2) (ME; AN; TC; DR)

1   This would deliver more than the ordered amount.

3   This would deliver less than the ordered amount.

4   Same as answer 3.

664. 2   1000 mcg = 1 mg; 500 mg of the drug added to 500 ml of IV fluid results in a solution where 1 ml contains 1 mg of the drug; the physician's order is for 1 mg/minute, therefore, multiply total solution (1 ml) times the drop factor (60) and divide by total time in minutes (1). (2) (SU; AN; TC; DR)

1   This is an incorrect calculation; this would deliver half the desired dose.

3   This is an incorrect calculation; this would deliver 50% more than the desired dose.

4   This is an incorrect calculation; this would deliver twice the desired dose.

665. 4   Use ratio and proportion:

1200 mg = 1.2 g

1.2 g /1 g = X ml /3 ml

X = 3.6 ml.

(2) (SU; AN; TC; DR)

1   This is an incorrect calculation; this amount is too small to deliver the desired dose.

2   Same as answer 1.

3   Same as answer 1.

666. 2   Organism mutation commonly results in drug resistance when treatment is inadequate. (2) (ME; IM; ED; DR)

1   Rifampin decreases tubercle bacillus' replication; pyridoxine (B_6) is used to prevent neuropathy associated with INH.

3   High concentrations of at least two antitubercular drugs are necessary for an extended period.

4   This may raise anxiety and may not be true; combination drug therapy is always used for tuberculosis.

667. 4   Rifampin causes the body fluids, such as sweat, tears, and urine, to turn orange. (2) (ME; EV; ED; DR)

1   Damage to the 8th cranial nerve is not a side effect of rifampin; it is a side effect of another drug sometimes used to treat tuberculosis, streptomycin sulfate.

2   It is not necessary to drink large amounts of fluid with this drug; it is not nephrotoxic.

3   This is not a side effect of rifampin.

668. 4   One of the most common side effects of INH is peripheral neuritis, and vitamin B_6 will counteract this problem. (2) (ME; IM; ED; DR)

1   It does help nutrition, but that is not the specific reason it is given.

2   It counters the side effects of INH; it does not act to enhance its action.

3   It does not speed the destruction of the causative organism.

669. 1 Hepatitis is a toxic effect of isoniazid. (1) (ME; EV; TC; DR)
2 Rifampin can produce orange coloration of excretions, which is not harmful.
3 This temperature is within acceptable limits.
4 Weight gain would indicate improvement in the client's health status.

670. 1 This medication causes hyperuricemia, leading to joint swelling and pain; fluids dilute the urine and help remove the uric acid. (2) (ME; EV; ED; DR)
2 This medication causes GI irritation and should be taken with food.
3 This is not a side effect of this medication.
4 This is a side effect of rifampin (Rifadin), not pyrazinamide.

671. 1 Antitubercular drugs such as isoniazid (INH), ethionamide (Trecator SC), rifampin (Rifadin), and para-aminosalicylate sodium (Parasal Sodium) are hepatotoxic. (3) (ME; IM; PA; DR)
2 These are not related to the administration of antitubercular drugs or to their side effects.
3 Same as answer 2.
4 The white blood cell count is expected to be higher in the presence of infection, but with AIDS the WBC count will be less than 2500/cm^3 and helper T cells will be about 400/mm^3; the T4/T8 ratio will be 1:2; these tests will not provide information relative to starting antitubercular therapy or to its side effects.

672. 4 AZT can cause anemia, leukopenia, and granulocytopenia; these blood dyscrasias can be life threatening, so the CBC is monitored. (2) (ME; EV; PA; DR)
1 These are not directly affected by the drug.
2 Same as answer 1.
3 Once infected, the client will continue to test positive for the antibody.

673. 4 Pentamidine can cause either hypoglycemia or hyperglycemia even after therapy is discontinued and therefore blood glucose levels should be monitored. (3) (ME; IM; TC; DR)
1 Pentamidine should be mixed with Injectable Sterile Water or 5% Dextrose Injection and then further diluted before IV administration.
2 Clients should be monitored closely for sudden, severe hypotension; clients should lie flat when receiving the drug.
3 This is too quick; the drug should be given over at least 60 minutes.

674. 4 This drug relaxes the respiratory muscles; it inhibits transmission of nerve impulses by binding with cholinergic receptor sites and antagonizing the action of acetylcholine; the client will die without mechanical ventilation. (2) (ME; IM; TC; DR)
1 This is not the priority.
2 Same as answer 1.
3 Same as answer 1.

675. 3 Regular insulin is the only insulin that acts rapidly and is compatible with intravenous solutions. (1) (SU; AN; TC; DR)
1 This insulin is not compatible with intravenous solutions; it is an intermediate acting insulin.
2 Same as answer 1.
4 Ultralente insulin is not compatible with intravenous solutions; it is a long acting insulin.

676. 1 Oral hypoglycemics stimulate endogenous insulin production by the beta cells of the pancreas. (1) (ME; AN; PA; DR)
2 This occurs when serum glucose drops below normal levels.
3 This occurs in the presence of insulin and potassium.
4 Beta cells must have some function to enable this drug to be effective.

677. 4 Oral hypoglycemic agents decrease serum glucose levels. (1) (ME; IM; ED; DR)
1 Ketoacidosis occurs with insulin dependent diabetes.
2 Weight gain is usually present in adult onset diabetes.
3 Same as answer 1.

678. 3 NPH insulin's onset of action is 1 to 2 hours, peak action is 8 to 12 hours, and duration of action is 18 to 24 hours; if hypoglycemia were to occur it would happen between 4 PM and 8 PM. (1) (ME; EV; PA; DR)

1 Regular insulin peaks in 2 to 4 hours.

2 Semilente insulin peaks in 4 to 7 hours.

4 No insulin peaks in 12 to 14 hours; however, protamine zinc insulin and Ultralente insulin peak in 16 to 18 hours.

679. 1 These are the most commonly reported signs of hypoglycemia and are related to increased sympathetic nervous system activity. (2) (ME; EV; PA; DR)

2 These are signs of hyperglycemia.

3 Same as answer 2.

4 Same as answer 2.

680. 2 This drug does not interfere with thyroxine already stored in the gland; symptoms remain until the hormone is depleted. (3) (ME; PL; ED; DR)

1 Duration of therapy varies depending on the severity of the disease and the client's response to therapy.

3 This drug is not irritating to mucosal tissue, and no special precautions are necessary.

4 Absorption is not affected by the presence of food in the stomach.

681. 2 Zyloprim may prolong the half-life of Diabinese, producing signs of hypoglycemia. (3) (ME; EV; TC; DR)

1 This is not necessary; the dosage of Diabinese needs to be decreased.

3 Same as answer 1.

4 Same as answer 1.

682. 3 ASA may damage the eighth cranial (acoustic) nerve causing ringing in the ears and impairing hearing. (3) (ME; EV; PA; DR)

1 Pain, not ringing in the ears, is a sign of otitis media; ASA toxicity affects the eighth cranial nerve, not the middle ear.

2 Aging may cause decreasing acuity in the extremes of pitch, but would not cause ringing in the ears.

4 Diminished hearing, not ringing, occurs because of mechanical obstruction of the outer ear.

683. 1 This is necessary because ibuprofen is nephrotoxic and hepatotoxic and prolongs the bleeding time. (2) (ME; EV; ED; DR)

2 This is important for all clients with arthritis; it is not related to ibuprofen.

3 Ibuprofen does not cause postural hypotension.

4 Ibuprofen causes epigastic distress and occult bleeding; it should be taken with meals or milk to reduce these adverse reactions.

684. 1 Excessive ASA ingestion can influence the vestibulocochlear nerve (cranial nerve VIII) causing tinnitus and dizziness. (2) (ME; EV; TC; DR)

2 These are signs of toxicity, not an allergic response.

3 These are signs of toxicity, not withdrawal.

4 Buffered aspirin contains ASA, not acetaminophen.

685. 3 Pain is most effectively relieved when analgesia is administered at its onset, before the pain becomes intense; this prevents a pain cycle from occurring. (1) (SU; IM; ED; DR)

1 Analgesia is least effective when it is administered as pain is at its peak.

2 This may or may not be necessary; the medication should be taken when the client begins to feel uncomfortable within the parameters specified by the physician's order.

4 Same as answer 1.

686. 3 These drugs tend to irritate the gastric mucosa and should be taken with food or milk. (2) (SU; EV; TC; DR)

1 This is an expected side effect; safety precautions are indicated, but the drug should not be discontinued.

2 These drugs should be taken with food or milk to limit GI irritation.

4 This could result in toxicity; the dosage should be prescribed by the physician.

687. 3 This provides for the quickest use of the narcotic, so that relief of pain can occur immediately. (3) (SU; PL; TC; DR)
1 Nausea, vomiting, and paralytic ileus may occur post-burn, making oral medication impractical.
2 This route does not provide a uniform absorption; also, relief of pain would be delayed.
4 The medication may be sequestered in the tissues and, with fluid shifts, it is unknown when the medication will take effect.

688. 2 Anabolic agents are synthetic androgenic steroids, which may produce masculinizing effects in women. (3) (SU; EV; PA; DR)
1 With an increase in muscle mass and stimulation of erythropoiesis, the client should have an increase in energy.
3 The client may become hypernatremic, not hyponatremic; the client may become hypercalcemic as well.
4 This drug will not cause hyperglycemia; it may cause hypoglycemia in clients with diabetes mellitus.

689. 1 Sulfamylon is effective against a wide variety of gram-positive and gram-negative organisms including anaerobes. (1) (SU; AN; PA; DR)
2 This is an antimicrobial not an analgesic; topical application causes pain.
3 It promotes healing and decreases the need for grafting.
4 This medication is an antimicrobial; it does not provide chemical debridement.

690. 3 Sorbitrate dilates the coronary vasculature, improving the supply of oxygen to the hypoxic myocardium. (2) (ME; IM; ED; DR)
1 This is the action of anticoagulants.
2 This is the action of antidysrhythmics.
4 This is the action of cardiac glycosides.

691. 4 Sorbitrate may produce vasodilation, resulting in postural hypotension from sudden changes in position. (2) (ME; PL; ED; DR)

1 This drug may cause tachycardia, not bradycardia.
2 The only gastrointestinal complications may be nausea and vomiting.
3 This drug results in a more efficient cardiac output; therefore the lungs will not have to compensate for inadequate cardiac output by increasing the respiratory rate.

692. 4 Lasix may cause hypovolemia, which can result in orthostatic hypotension with sudden position changes. (1) (ME; EV; PA; DR)
1 Lasix does not cause photophobia.
2 This has no relationship to Lasix.
3 Citrus fruits, particularly oranges, are high in potassium and should be encouraged when the client is taking Lasix because this medication can cause hypokalemia.

693. 3 Lasix enhances the excretion of potassium, producing symptoms of hypokalemia, such as hyporeflexia. (3) (ME; EV; PA; DR)
1 This is not a side effect of Lasix.
2 Same as answer 1.
4 Same as answer 1.

694. 4 Nipride decreases blood pressure by both of these mechanisms. (2) (ME; AN; PA; DR)
1 It decreases cardiac workload by decreasing preload and afterload.
2 Actually, Nipride may increase the heart rate as a response to the vasodilation.
3 It should decrease peripheral resistance by dilating peripheral vessels.

695. 1 Pruritus is a frequent side effect of clonidine (Catapres). (3) (ME; EV; ED; DR)
2 This drug causes constipation, not diarrhea.
3 This drug may cause depression, anxiety, fatigue, and drowsiness, not euphoria.
4 This is not a side effect of this medication; photosensitivity occurs with chlorpromazine.

696. 2 Inderal and Lanoxin both exert a negative chronotropic effect. (2) (ME; AN; PA; DR)

1 Inderal reduces headache associated with hypertension.
3 These drugs may cause hypotension.
4 These drugs may depress nodal conduction.

697. 1 Coumadin inhibits vitamin K; therefore, vitamin K is the antidote for Coumadin (2) (ME; PL; TC; DR)
2 This is a blood clotting factor, not the antidote for Coumadin.
3 Same as answer 2.
4 This is the antidote for heparin.

698. 3 This is necessary for monitoring cardiac function; the drug slows and strengthens the heart rate. (1) (ME; EV; PA; DR)
1 This is not appropriate; it is not related to digoxin.
2 Hypokalemia increases the potential for digitalis toxicity; potassium intake should be increased.
4 This is not an appropriate decision for the client; the physician makes this decision.

699. 4 This is the site of action of Lasix. (3) (ME; AN; PA; DR)
1 Thiazides act here.
2 Potassium-sparing diuretics act here.
3 Plasma expanders and xanthines act here.

700. 4 A cardiac glycoside such as digitalis decreases the conduction speed within the myocardium and slows the heart rate. (2) (ME; EV; PA; DR)
1 The primary effect of a diuretic is on the kidneys, not the heart.
2 A vasodilator could cause tachycardia, not bradycardia, which is an adverse effect.
3 This does not drastically reduce the heart rate.

701. 4 The most common adverse effect of a tissue plasminogen activator is bleeding because of the thrombolytic action of the drug. (3) (SU; EV; TC; DR)
1 Although this is important for any client with a decreased cardiac output, it is not specific to the administration of a tissue plasminogen activator.
2 Same as answer 1.
3 Same as answer 1.

702. 4 Nitroglycerin does this by its vasodilating effect; it dilates coronary arteries, reduces myocardial ischemia, strengthens contractility, and increases efficiency of cardiac output. (3) (ME; AN; PA; DR)
1 Peripheral resistance is not affected by dilating the coronary arteries but by dilating the peripheral arteries.
2 Cardiac output is increased, not decreased.
3 Decreasing the pulse rate does not strengthen cardiac contractility.

703. 2 The speed of conduction is decreased when digoxin is given and this can result in premature beats, atrial fibrillation, and first degree heart block. (1) (ME; EV; PA; DR)
1 Digoxin does not deplete potassium and therefore orange juice does not need to be given; the orange juice is high in calories and would need to be calculated in the diet.
3 The purpose of the drug is to reduce this fast rate; the drug should be withheld if the rate is below 60.
4 Insulin and digoxin can be given at the same time.

704. 4 This drug suppresses ventricular activity; therefore it is used for the treatment of PVBs. (2) (ME; PL; PA; DR)
1 This drug increases myocardial contractility and heart rate; therefore it is contraindicated in the treatment of PVBs.
2 This drug blocks vagal stimulation; therefore it increases the heart rate; it is used for bradycardia.
3 This drug raises the serum pH level; therefore it combats metabolic acidosis.

705. 1 Tremors are a precursor to the major adverse effect of seizures or convulsions. (3) (ME; EV; PA; DR)
2 Although this can occur, it is not a serious side effect.
3 Bradycardia, which can lead to heart block, occurs, not tachycardia.
4 Hypotension, not hypertension, occurs.

706. 4 Lasix promotes potassium excretion; hypokalemia increases cardiac excitability; digitalis in the presence of low extracellular potassium produces ectopic pacemaker activity. (1) (ME; AN; PA; DR)
   1 Digitalis does not affect potassium excretion; Lasix causes potassium excretion.
   2 Potassium is excreted by the kidneys, not destroyed by the liver.
   3 Lasix causes diuresis and consequent potassium loss regardless of the serum potassium level.

707. 4 Generalized weakness is a sign of significant hypokalemia, which may be a sequela to diuretic therapy. (1) (ME; EV; ED; DR)
   1 Insomnia is not known to be related to hypokalemia or HydroDIURIL therapy.
   2 Although this is unrelated to HydroDIURIL therapy, it can occur with other antihypertensive drugs.
   3 Increased thirst is associated with hypernatremia; because this drug increases excretion of water and sodium in addition to potassium and chloride, hyponatremia, not hypernatremia, may occur.

708. 2 Potassium supplements can cause gastrointestinal ulceration and bleeding. (2) (ME; EV; ED; DR)
   1 Most salt substitutes contain potassium, and their use with potassium supplements can cause hyperkalemia.
   3 Because they can be irritating to the stomach, potassium supplements should not be taken on an empty stomach.
   4 Although muscle cramps can indicate hypokalemia, clients should not adjust their own dosage.

709. 2 Nausea is the most frequent and immediate side effect of Mustargen therapy. (2) (ME; EV; PA; DR)
   1 This is not a side effect of Mustargen therapy.
   3 Mustargen is more likely to cause urinary retention than urinary incontinence.
   4 Same as answer 1.

710. 2 Congestive heart failure and dysrhythmias are the only life threatening toxic effects unique to Adriamycin. (2) (ME; EV; PA; DR)
   1 When bone marrow is depressed to precarious levels, the dose is altered and/or blood components administered.
   3 This is not a side effect of Adriamycin nor of any of the other antineoplastic agents.
   4 This is a very uncomfortable side effect but is not life threatening.

711. 1 Stomatitis and hyperuricemia are possible complications of therapy; therefore oral care and hydration are very important. (1) (ME; PL; PA; DR)
   2 Hot substances are avoided because of the frequent occurrence of stomatitis.
   3 Abnormal bleeding is a common problem and thus injections are contraindicated; rest is important for increased fatigability.
   4 This is false reassurance; although complete remission occurs in 50% to 75% of treated clients, the median survival time is 2 to 3 years.

712. 1 Chemotherapy destroys normal erythrocytes, white blood cells, and platelets indiscriminately along with the neoplastic cells. (1) (ME; IM; ED; DR)
   2 This is not a true description of the side effects of steroids.
   3 Although true, this does not explain pancytopenia.
   4 This is not the cause for fewer erythrocytes, white blood cells, and platelets.

713. 4 Alkylating drugs frequently cause severe bone marrow depression because they affect rapidly dividing cells. (3) (ME; EV; PA; DR)
   1 These are complications that are more common with antimetabolites.
   2 These are complications associated with hormonal therapy.
   3 These are common side effects with the administration of steroids.

714. 2 Aspirin is contraindicated in the presence of bleeding tendencies, which often occur with ALL, because of its inhibitory effect on platelet aggregation. (2) (ME; IM; TC; DR)

1 An antacid will reduce the gastric irritation common with aspirin but will not alter its effect on platelets.

3 The dosage is within acceptable limits.

4 Action needs to be taken before the temperature is 102°F.

715. 2 Leucovorin calcium limits toxicity of folic acid antagonists, such as methotrexate sodium, by competing for transport into cells. (3) (ME; AN; TC; DR)

1 This is not the action of leucovorin calcium.

3 This is the purpose of antiemetics such as prochlorperazine maleate (Compazine).

4 Leucovorin calcium does not interfere with cell division; this is the purpose of a multiple drug protocol.

716. 1 This helps flush the kidneys and prevent nephrotoxicity, especially during the early phase of treatment. (3) (ME; EV; TC; IT)

2 Reconstituted solution can be stored in the refrigerator for 1 month.

3 Confusion, dizziness, and hallucinations are side effects of this drug; the client should avoid hazardous tasks, such as driving or using machinery.

4 Activity may have to be altered because fatigue and other flu-like symptoms are common with this drug.

717. 2 Antacids may interfere with complete absorption of Tagamet; therefore they should be administered at least one hour apart. (2) (ME; PL; TC; DR)

1 This would interfere with absorption of Tagamet.

3 Same as answer 1.

4 Maalox would interfere with absorption of Tagamet, and orange juice may be irritating and slow the client's recovery; milk may be used with Tagamet because it may enhance effectiveness of the medication.

718. 3 Morphine sulfate increases spasm of smooth muscle and is contraindicated in all conditions in which there is obstruction of smooth muscle ducts. (3) (SU; AN; PA; DR)

1 Morphine sulfate and meperidine hydrochloride cause respiratory depression.

2 Ingestion of food stimulates pancreatic function; drugs do not have this effect.

4 Morphine sulfate and meperidine hydrochloride are central nervous system depressants.

719. 2 The pancreatic enzymes (amylase, trypsin, and lipase) must be present when food is ingested for digestion to take place. (2) (ME; EV; ED; DR)

1 At this time the food eaten for dinner has already passed beyond the duodenum; the enzyme would be given too late to aid in digestion.

3 The client would have no chyme in the duodenum for the enzyme to act on.

4 Same as answer 3.

720. 3 Morphine sulfate should be avoided because it causes spasms at the sphincter of Oddi, thereby increasing pain. (3) (ME; EV; TC; DR)

1 Cimetidine (Tagamet) is useful in reducing gastric acid stimulation of pancreatic enzymes.

2 Promethazine HCl (Phenergan) is useful as an antiemetic for clients with pancreatitis.

4 Meperidine HCl (Demerol) would be useful for pain relief for clients with pancreatitis.

721. 3 It is necessary to clarify the route of administration because medication can be given po, IV, or IM. (2) (ME; IM; TC; DR)

1 This is the usual dose of ranitidine when given twice a day.

2 Ranitidine is used to decrease gastric acid and is helpful to clients with peptic ulcer.

4 Ranitidine is usually given with meals.

722. 3 Prednisone inhibits phagocytosis and suppresses other clinical phenomena of inflammation; this is a symptomatic treatment that is not curative. (1) (ME; IM; ED; DR)

1 The drug supresses the immune response and increases the potential for infection.

2 The appetite is increased; weight gain may result from this or from fluid retention.

4 Generally, the response is rapid.

723. 2 Oral corticosteroids should be taken with food or antacids to prevent gastric irritation and gastric hemorrhage. (3) (SU; EV; ED; DR)

1 The client understands; this will have to be done because long-term administration of steroids leads to elevated blood glucose and possible steroid-caused diabetes.

3 The client understands; usually a larger dose is given at 8 AM and the second dose is given prior to 4 PM to mimic the normal hormonal secretion and prevent insomnia.

4 The client understands; neurological and emotional side effects include euphoria, mood swings, sleeplessness, and excitement.

724. 4 This reduces bacterial activity on blood and wastes in the GI tract, thereby reducing the level of blood ammonia, a by-product of protein metabolism. (2) (ME; AN; PA; DR)

1 Neomycin interferes with bacterial protein synthesis but has little or no effect on intestinal edema.

2 Neomycin reduces bacterial action in the GI tract but does not reduce abdominal distention.

3 Neomycin is an aminoglycoside antimicrobial used specifically against intestinal bacteria such as *Escherichia coli.*

725. 1 Demerol is an effective narcotic analgesic; it alleviates pain by binding with opiate receptors in the brain and, thus, altering the perception of and response to pain. (1) (SU; IM; ED; DR)

2 Narcotics do not affect oxygen utilization;

with this drug, the respiratory rate is decreased and should be monitored.

3 This drug is not given to dilate coronary blood vessels; antianginal medications are used for this purpose.

4 This is not an antianxiety medication; the anxiety resulting from surgical pain will diminish when the prescribed analgesic relieves the pain.

726. 3 This detergent action promotes addition of fluid into stool to soften feces. (2) (ME; AN; PA; DR)

1 This is the action of lubricant laxatives such as mineral oil.

2 This is the action of saline laxatives such as milk of magnesia.

4 This is the action of peristaltic stimulants such as cascara and castor oil.

727. 2 Increased acidity caused by the stress occurring with burns and crushing injuries contributes to the formation of Curling's ulcer; Tagamet, a histamine H_2 antagonist, decreases the formation of gastric acid, and Maalox, an antacid, neutralizes it once it is formed. (1) (ME; IM; ED; DR)

1 These drugs do not decrease irritability of the bowel; their purpose is to decrease gastrointestinal acidity, not irritation.

3 This does not explain how these drugs work and why they are prescribed for this client.

4 Same as answer 3.

728. 2 Maalox can cause diarrhea and sometimes needs to be given alternately with another more constipating antacid. (2) (SU; EV; PA; DR)

1 Immobility causes constipation, not diarrhea.

3 Cimetidine causes constipation, not diarrhea.

4 Although diet can affect elimination, no data support this conclusion.

729. 4 Atropine can increase intraocular pressure because of its cycloplegic action, which paralyzes the ciliary muscles and causes pain and blindness. (1) (SU; AN; PA; DR)

1 It does not affect extrinsic ocular muscles that support the orb.

2 Although this is a side effect of the drug, it is not related to glaucoma.

3 It causes pupillary dilation, not constriction.

730. 4 This is a miotic that constricts the pupil, permitting fluid drainage, which reduces intraocular pressure. (2) (ME; PL; PA; DR)

1 This is a topical anesthetic; it will not reduce the increased intraocular pressure associated with glaucoma.

2 This is contraindicated; this dilates the pupil and paralyzes ciliary muscles.

3 This is contraindicated; this is a mydriatic that dilates the pupil, obstructing drainage, which increases intraocular pressure.

731. 3 Tachycardia and palpitations, not bradycardia, occur. (3) (ME; EV; PA; DR)

1 Nausea may occur; it reflects a central emetic reaction to levodopa.

2 Anorexia may occur; decreased appetite results because of nausea and vomiting.

4 Changes in affect, mood, and behavior are related to toxic effects of the drug.

732. 2 Abnormal involuntary movements (dyskinesias) such as muscle twitching, rapid eye blinking, facial grimacing, head bobbing, and an exaggerated protrusion of the tongue are signs of toxicity probably due to the body's failure to readjust properly to the disappearance of dopamine. (3) (ME; EV; TC; DR)

1 This is a side effect of therapy, not toxicity.

3 Same as answer 1.

4 This is unrelated to Levodopa toxicity.

733. 1 These are signs of a MAOI-induced hypertensive crisis and should be reported to the physician immediately. (3) (ME; EV; TC; DR)

2 The opposite is true because increased amounts of dopamine react with supersensitive post-synaptic receptors.

3 This is unsafe; the recommended daily dose of 10 mg should not be exceeded.

4 This is unnecessary; routine medical evaluations of the client should be done.

734. 3 Corticosteroids act to decrease inflammation, which decreases edema. (2) (ME; AN; PA; DR)

1 This is an antiinflammatory agent, not a diuretic; it does not cause diuresis by action on the kidney.

2 Resistance to infection is decreased, but this is not pertinent in this situation.

4 The problem is not with increased cerebrospinal fluid.

735. 3 Corticosteroids, such as Decadron, have a hyperglycemic effect. (2) (ME; EV; PA; DR)

1 Corticosteroids are not known to precipitate cessation of gastrointestinal activity.

2 Corticosteroids would not increase bacterial growth in the lungs.

4 This is unnecessary; this is required when administering magnesium sulfate.

736. 3 Administration of an anticoagulant to a client who is bleeding would interfere with clotting and increase hemorrhage. (2) (ME; IM; ED; NM)

1 This is unsafe; it would not be used in this situation because it would increase bleeding; anticoagulants may be used with cerebral thrombosis.

2 Same as answer 1.

4 Although contraindicated, if given, it would increase signs and symptoms.

737. 1 This site should not be rubbed to avoid dispersion of the heparin around the site and subsequent bleeding into the area. (1) (ME; IM; TC; DR)

2 This is not a routine practice; the extra volume would not be advantageous.

3 The drug should be injected deep into the subcutaneous tissue slowly, not quickly.

4 This technique and the intramuscular route are not used with heparin; subcutaneous injection or intravenous administration is used.

738. 4 This drug binds with heparin sodium to form a physiologically inert complex; it corrects clotting deficits. (3) (ME; PL; TC; DR)

1 Vitamin K counteracts the effects of warfarin sodium (Coumadin) type drugs.

2 This is an alternate name for heparin sodium.

3 This is an oral anticoagulant that interferes with the synthesis of prothrombin.

739. 1 Acetylsalicylic acid (aspirin) should be avoided because it interferes with platelet aggregation; acetaminophen (Tylenol) should be used instead. (2) (ME; EV; PA; DR)

2 This causes venous pooling and could predispose the client to deep vein thrombosis.

3 Prothrombin times, not complete blood counts, need to be done periodically.

4 This is not necessary; this is done when clients have had rheumatic fever, prosthetic heart valve replacements or other cardiac problems.

740. 2 The client must increase the dietary intake of potassium because of potassium loss associated with Diuril. (3) (ME; IM; ED; DR)

1 Protein should be obtained from food.

3 These are part of the food pyramid and should be included in the diet.

4 The client should be taught about medication induced deficiencies.

741. 2 Aspirin interferes with platelet aggregation and will impede the formation of thrombi. (2) (ME; EV; PA; DR)

1 Although aspirin has antiinflammatory properties, one month after the surgery the edema has already subsided.

3 This is not an expected response following surgery, and it would indicate infection; a prescription for antibiotics would be more appropriate.

4 At this point, there should no longer be discomfort at the surgical site.

742. 4 Peak response occurs 1 hour after administration and lasts up to 8 hours; the response will influence dosage levels. (3) (ME; EV; PA; DR)

1 This medication must be administered on time whether the dosage is already established or is being adjusted.

2 This reduces gastrointestinal upset whether the dosage is established or is being adjusted.

3 There are no psychologic side effects associated with Mestinon.

743. 4 A positive response to the administration of Tensilon indicates myasthenic crisis, while an increase in the severity of symptoms indicates cholinergic crisis. (3) (ME; PL; TC; DR)

1 This is the treatment for cholinergic crisis.

2 This is the antidote for heparin.

3 This is a narcotic antagonist.

744. 4 Exacerbation of myasthenia may occur within 2 weeks of steroid therapy, causing respiratory embarrassment and dysphagia. (3) (ME; EV; PA; DR)

1 Steroids increase sodium retention and this would be contraindicated.

2 Although clients should avoid contact with persons having upper respiratory infections, protective isolation is not required.

3 This is unnecessary; adequate fluid intake should be maintained.

745. 2 The drug should be taken as ordered, usually before meals, to limit dysphagia and possible aspiration. (1) (ME; EV; TC; DR)

1 This is not necessary; it may be kept at room temperature.

3 The action of the drug will begin within 30 minutes and start to peak in an hour.

4 This is unsafe; the drug should be taken with milk to prevent GI irritation; it is usually taken about 30 to 60 minutes before meals.

746. 4 Oxacillin is a form of penicillin and should be given on an empty stomach; food delays absorption. (2) (ME; EV; ED; DR)

1 This is incorrect; food or milk delays absorption of this drug.

2 Same as answer 1.

3 This is not necessary; however, it is appropriate with sulfonamides.

747. 3 Gentamicin can cause ototoxicity, resulting in vertigo, tinnitus, and hearing loss. (3) (ME; EV; PA; DR)

1 This is unlikely; the client has not been on prolonged bedrest.

2 A liquid diet and IV therapy may cause weakness because of a low calorie intake, but dizziness does not occur.

4 This is unrelated; over 24 hours have passed since anesthesia was administered.

748. 1 Because the drug was just administered, the blood level of the drug would be at its highest level. (2) (SU; IM; TC; DR)

2 The result would reveal a drug blood level halfway between the peak and trough levels.

3 This would be done for a trough level when the drug level would be at its lowest.

4 This would result in inaccurate results; peak and trough levels are measured in relation to the time a drug is administered.

749. 4 These are the drugs of choice for suppression of normal immunologic response to prevent rejection of the donor kidney. (1) (SU; IM; ED; DR)

1 None of these drugs are used for immunosuppression.

2 Only cyclosporine (Sandimmune) is used for immunosuppression; this drug is frequently used in the elderly and those with diabetes mellitus.

3 Methylprednisolone (Solu-Medrol) in large doses is the only drug in this option that is used to prevent kidney rejection.

750. 2 Epogen stimulates red blood cell production thereby elevating hematocrit levels. (3) (ME; EV; PA; DR)

1 An elevated liver panel may signify liver disease; it is not affected by Epogen.

3 WBC counts are not affected by Epogen.

4 Increased Kaposi sarcoma lesions are significant of AIDS progression and are not affected by Epogen.

Medical–Surgical Nursing Quiz

1. A client with cancer of the prostate has an extremely elevated serum alkaline phosphatase level. This finding should prompt the nurse to plan to:
   1. Institute seizure precautions
   2. Measure his intake and output
   3. Monitor his plasma pH for acidosis
   4. Handle him gently when turning him

2. When preparing a client for a liver biopsy the nurse should instruct the client to:
   1. Turn on the left side after the procedure
   2. Breathe normally throughout the procedure
   3. Hold the breath at the moment of the actual biopsy
   4. Bear down (Valsalva maneuver) during the insertion of the biopsy needle

3. A 40-year-old visits a neurologist with complaints of blurred or double vision and muscular weakness. After multiple sclerosis is diagnosed the client, visibly upset, reports this diagnosis to a friend who is a nurse. The nurse could best respond:
   1. "Don't worry; early treatment often alleviates symptoms of the disease."
   2. "See another physician. I've heard of several treatments that aid recovery."
   3. "You should see a psychiatrist who will help you cope with this shocking news."
   4. "That must have really floored you. Tell me what the physician told you about it."

4. A client with a history of heavy alcohol use develops portal hypertension and an elevated serum aldosterone level. The nurse should carefully observe the client for:
   1. Chloride depletion and hypovolemia
   2. Potassium retention and dysrhythmias
   3. Sodium retention and fluid accumulation
   4. Calcium depletion and pathologic fractures

5. When removing an elderly client's meal tray the nurse notices that the client did not eat any of the chicken. When asked why the chicken was not eaten the client states, "I only eat meat once a week because old people don't need protein every day." Based on this statement the nurse knows that the client should be taught about the:
   1. Need for home-delivered meals
   2. Effect of aging on the need for some foods
   3. Foods included in the Food Guide Pyramid
   4. Need for meat at least once per day throughout life

6. The nurse notes that two weeks after severe burns, a client is losing 2 pounds of weight per day. The nurse's best action would be to adjust the client's diet by adding:
   1. Low-sodium milk
   2. High-protein drinks
   3. Fruit juices low in potassium
   4. 10% more calories in the form of fats

7. A client with the tentative diagnosis of Hodgkin's disease asks how the surgeon will know that it is definitely this disease. The nurse explains that the diagnosis is routinely confirmed by:
   1. Bone scan
   2. Lymph node biopsy
   3. Computerized tomography (CT) scan
   4. Radioactive iodine (^{131}I) uptake studies

8. The diet regimen that would be appropriate for a client with a gastric ulcer would be:
   1. A mechanical soft diet
   2. A low-fat, high-protein liquid diet
   3. Hourly feedings of cream and milk
   4. Regular meals that can be tolerated

9. A client, who has been diagnosed as having peripheral vascular disease, tells the nurse that before hospitalization exercise resulted in severe cramplike pain in both legs. The nurse should include in the teaching plan specific measures the client can use to increase arterial blood flow to the extremities. These measures should include:
   1. Exercises that promote muscular activity
   2. Meticulous care of minor skin breakdown
   3. Elevation of legs above the level of the heart
   4. Daily cleansing of feet by soaking in hot water

10. The nurse should teach a male client with angina pectoris that he will know the prescribed nitroglycerin sublingual tablet is effective when his:
    1. Pain subsides because his arterioles and venules dilate
    2. Pulse rate increases because the cardiac output is stimulated
    3. Sublingual area tingles because sensory nerves are being triggered
    4. Capacity for activity escalates because of increased collateral circulation

11. When reviewing the laboratory results for a client in acute renal failure, the nurse notes that the serum potassium level is 6.2 mEq. The nurse should first:
    1. Call the cardiac arrest team to alert them
    2. Call the laboratory to schedule a repeat test
    3. Obtain an ECG strip and have lidocaine available
    4. Take the client's vital signs and notify the physician

12. One week after an above-the-knee amputation a client refuses to go to physical therapy and tells the nurse, "I'll never be a whole person again!" The nurse's best response would be:
    1. "Relax, you're still the same person you've always been."
    2. "You've lost a part of yourself. That must be very difficult for you."

3. "You may feel that way but I'm sure your family considers you a whole person."
4. "You must go to physical therapy every day or you will develop muscle contractures."

13. A 67-year-old client is diagnosed as having a right-sided cerebrovascular accident (CVA) and is admitted to the hospital. When preparing to care for this client, the nurse should plan to:
    1. Use a bed cradle to prevent dorsiflexion of the feet
    2. Apply elastic stockings to prevent flaccid leg muscles
    3. Do passive range-of-motion exercises to prevent muscle atrophy
    4. Use a hand roll and extend the left upper extremity on a pillow to prevent contractures

14. The nurse would expect a client with jaundice to also complain of:
    1. Pruritus
    2. Diarrhea
    3. Blurred vision
    4. Bleeding tendencies

15. A common early sign of laryngeal cancer for which the nurse should assess a client is:
    1. Aphasia
    2. Dyspnea
    3. Dysphagia
    4. Hoarseness

16. At the accident scene, emergency treatment for a client who has sustained partial- and full-thickness burns to the chest, right arm, and upper legs should include:
    1. Wrapping the client in a clean dry sheet
    2. Removing clothing from the burned areas
    3. Applying sterile dressings to the burned areas
    4. Standing the client under a gentle-spray shower

17. During a teaching session about insulin injections, a client asks the nurse, "Why can't I take the insulin in pills instead of taking shots?" The nurse should respond:
    1. "Insulin cannot be manufactured in pill form."

2. "Your doctor will order oral hypo-glycemics when you are ready."
3. "The route of administration is decided on by the physician."
4. "Insulin is destroyed by gastric juices, rendering it ineffective."

18. A 50-year-old client is admitted to the hospital with a suspected brain tumor. Based on the history of loss of equilibrium and coordination, the nurse suspects the tumor is located in the:
   1. Cerebellum
   2. Parietal lobe
   3. Basal ganglia
   4. Occipital lobe

19. A client with cancer of the larynx is to have a total laryngectomy with a radical neck dissection. When reinforcing the physician's explanation about what the surgery entails and what abilities will be lost, the nurse's discussion should also focus on what abilities the client will retain, such as the ability to:
   1. Blow the nose
   2. Sip through a straw
   3. Chew and swallow food
   4. Smell and differentiate odors

20. The nurse checks for hypocalcemia by placing a blood pressure cuff on a client's arm and inflating it. After about 3 minutes the client develops carpopedal spasm. The nurse records this finding as a positive:
   1. Homan's sign
   2. Romberg sign
   3. Chvostek's sign
   4. Trousseau's sign

21. A client undergoes removal of a pituitary tumor through a transsphenoidal approach. Postoperatively the nurse should plan to:
   1. Keep the client npo until nasal packing is removed
   2. Provide vigorous oral hygiene, including toothbrushing
   3. Raise the head of the bed to a 30 degree angle at all times
   4. Encourage the client to deep breathe and cough frequently

22. During preoperative teaching before a transurethral prostatectomy, the nurse tells the client that after the surgery:
   1. His urine will be bright red for at least 24 to 48 hours
   2. He can expect spasms of the bladder during the first 24 to 48 hours
   3. Oral fluids should be avoided because of continuous urinary irrigation
   4. He should use the Valsalva maneuver to decrease bladder contractions

23. A client develops acute respiratory distress, and a tracheostomy is performed. An important intervention that should be included in the care plan is:
   1. Encouraging a fluid intake of 3000 ml daily
   2. Suctioning via the tracheostomy tube every hour
   3. Applying an occlusive dressing over the wound site
   4. Cleansing the stoma with peroxide and cotton balls

24. A 52-year-old engineer is admitted to the hospital with Laennec's cirrhosis and chronic pancreatitis. Bile salts are ordered and the client asks why they are needed. The nurse replies that they:
   1. Stimulate prothrombin production
   2. Aid absorption of vitamins A, D, and K
   3. Promote bilirubin secretion in the urine
   4. Stimulate contraction of the common bile duct

25. A client is admitted to the hospital with a diagnosis of insulin dependent diabetes mellitus. The nurse understands that insulin dependent diabetes mellitus is classified as:
   1. Gestational diabetes
   2. Type I diabetes mellitus
   3. Type II diabetes mellitus
   4. Impaired glucose tolerance diabetes

26. A client with chronic obstructive pulmonary disease (COPD) has been receiving low-flow oxygen by nasal cannula for 4 hours. The nurse notes that the client has increased restlessness and confusion followed by a decreased respiratory rate and lethargy. The nurse should:
   1. Percuss and vibrate the chest wall
   2. Increase the oxygen by 2% increments
   3. Decrease or discontinue the oxygen flow
   4. Quietly ask the client about the confusion

27. In a three-chamber underwater drainage system, the main purpose of the third chamber is to:
   1. Act as a drainage container
   2. Control the amount of suction
   3. Provide for an air-tight water seal
   4. Allow for escape of any air bubbles

28. A client has surgery to remove a stone from the common bile duct. The nurse is aware that the bile flow into the duodenum has been reestablished after biliary surgery when:
   1. The liver is no longer tender
   2. Stools are normal brown in color
   3. Colic is absent after ingestion of fats
   4. The serum bilirubin returns to normal

29. After a thyroidectomy the client should be placed in the:
   1. Prone position
   2. Supine position
   3. Left Sims' position
   4. Semi-Fowler's position

30. A 59-year-old diabetic client is admitted in diabetic ketoacidosis. Under medical supervision, the client has been adjusting insulin dosage based on blood glucose levels at home. Of the statements made by the client during the health history, the nurse realizes that the best explanation of the etiology of the ketoacidosis is that the client:
   1. Has a chronic postnasal drip
   2. Is going to turn 60 next week
   3. Is planning to retire next year
   4. Has been taking steroids for a rash

31. When receiving chemotherapy for non-Hodgkin's lymphoma a client states, "I get so sick to my stomach. The medication is use-less." The response by the nurse that employs the technique of paraphrasing is:
   1. "You get sick to your stomach?"
   2. "I'll get an order for an antiemetic."
   3. "Tell me more about how you are feeling."
   4. "You don't think the medication is helping you?"

32. After 1 week a client with acute renal failure moves into the diuretic phase. During this phase the client must be carefully assessed for signs of:
   1. Hypovolemia
   2. Hyperkalemia
   3. Metabolic acidosis
   4. Chronic renal failure

33. A client with a rigid and painful abdomen is determined to have a perforated peptic ulcer. A nasogastric tube is inserted and surgery is scheduled. Before surgery the nurse should place the client in the:
   1. Sims' position
   2. Supine position
   3. Semi-Fowler's position
   4. Dorsal recumbent position

34. A client is scheduled for a cardiac catheterization, which is to be done via the femoral approach. When planning preoperative preparation for this client, the nurse should include information that:
   1. The physician will immediately tell the client about the results of the procedure
   2. The client will be permitted to get up and walk around after returning to the room
   3. The client will be on bedrest, with the affected leg extended for several hours
   4. A general anesthetic will be given, and the client will be asleep during the procedure

35. A client with Crohn's disease is admitted to the hospital with a history of chronic, bloody, diarrhea; weight loss; and signs of general malnutrition. The client also has edema, anemia, low serum albumin, and symptoms of negative nitrogen balance. The client's health status is related to a major deficiency of:
   1. Iron

2. Protein
3. Potassium
4. Linoleic acid

36. The physician orders IV Ringer's lactate to infuse at the rate of 150 ml/hr. The nurse calculates that a liter bottle of this solution will infuse in:
1. 6 hours and 40 minutes
2. 6 hours and 50 minutes
3. 7 hours and 10 minutes
4. 7 hours and 30 minutes

37. A client with cancer of the pancreas is scheduled for surgery. When arranging for the next appointment the client says to the nurse, "Wouldn't I be better off with some other treatment instead of surgery?" The nurse's best response would be:
1. "Why don't you explore the other acceptable treatments for your cancer with the doctor?"
2. "Surgery is the recommended approach, but why don't you discuss this further with the doctor?"
3. "Maybe you would be more confident with a second opinion. Would you like a referral to another doctor?"
4. "With your disease your prognosis will improve if you follow the doctor's suggestion and have the recommended surgery."

38. When teaching how to use a nebulizer, the nurse should instruct the client to:
1. Hold the breath while spraying the medication carefully into each nostril
2. Instill the medication from the nebulizer while exhaling through the nostrils
3. Seal the lips around the mouthpiece taking rapid, shallow breaths through the nose
4. Loosely place the lips around the mouthpiece taking a slow, deep breath through the mouth

39. The nurse would expect that the diagnostic work up for a client with a suspected brain tumor would include:
1. Myelography
2. Lumbar puncture
3. Electromyography
4. Computerized tomography

40. During the immediate postoperative period following a total laryngectomy for cancer of the larynx, a priority nursing intervention would be to:
1. Provide emotional support
2. Observe for signs of infection
3. Keep the trachea free of secretions
4. Promote a means of communication

41. A client with Hodgkin's disease, Stage III is started on a MOPP regimen of nitrogen mustard, vincristine (Oncovin), procarbazine, and prednisone. The client wonders why so many drugs have to be used at once. The nurse should explain that:
1. Using groups of drugs reduces the likelihood of serious side effects
2. Each drug destroys the cancer cell at a different time in the cell cycle
3. The drugs are used to destroy cells that are not susceptible to radiation therapy
4. As there are stages of Hodgkin's disease, if one drug is ineffective another will work

42. A client develops a thrombophlebitis in the right calf. Bedrest is prescribed and heparin sodium IV is started. When describing the purpose of this drug to the client, the nurse should explain that it:
1. Reduces the size of the thrombus
2. Dissolves the blood clot in the vein
3. Prevents extension of the blood clot
4. Promotes absorption of red blood cells

43. The nurse is preparing a client, who has had a transurethral prostatectomy for cancer of the prostate, for discharge. The nurse is aware that the client understands the teaching when he states:
1. "I will drink 8 cups of fluid daily, but none after 9 PM."
2. "I will use stool softeners regularly for 1 to 2 months after I get home."
3. "I am so glad this is over. Now I don't have to keep going to the doctor."
4. "I was so worried and now I can hardly wait to get home and have sex with my wife."

44. A client has ear surgery. An early response that may be associated with possible damage to the motor branch of the facial nerve is:
1. A bitter metallic taste
2. Dryness of the lips and mouth
3. A sensation of pain behind the ear
4. An inability to wrinkle the forehead

45. During the first 36 hours after surgery for cancer of the pancreas, a client complains of severe pain and is medicated every four hours with meperidine (Demerol) 75 mg IM. Because the client rests or sleeps between injections the nurse can conclude that:
1. Pain management is effective
2. The dosage of the drug is excessive
3. Another narcotic should be substituted
4. The Demerol can probably be given orally

46. One week after beginning antithyroid medication for the treatment of hyperthyroidism, a client reports that diarrhea, abdominal pain, and fever have developed. The client is admitted for thyrotoxicosis. The most important goal of immediate treatment for this condition is:
1. Rapid reduction of body temperature and heart rate
2. Prevention of fluid overload by limiting client's intake
3. Observation for an exaggerated response to the sedatives
4. Treatment of associated hyperglycemia and ketoacidosis

47. The nurse teaches a client how to use a nebulizer. The nurse would recognize that the nebulizer is not being used correctly and that additional instruction is needed when the client:
1. Holds the inspired breath for at least 3 seconds
2. Positions the tip of the nebulizer beyond the lips
3. Inhales with the lips tightly sealed around the mouthpiece
4. Exhales slowly through the mouth with lips pursed slightly

48. A client, who has been admitted to the hospital with a possible small bowel obstruction, is to have an intestinal tube inserted. Before assisting the physician with this procedure, the nurse should:
1. Place the client flat in bed, lying on the right side
2. Instruct the client in the techniques of mouth breathing
3. Spray the client's oropharynx with a local anesthetic solution
4. Reassure the client that the procedure will not cause discomfort

49. After emptying a portable wound suction device, the nurse creates negative pressure by:
1. Attaching it to a wall suction unit
2. Compressing the device and then closing the air plug
3. Periodically milking the tubing toward the suction device
4. Keeping the device in a position lower than the site of insertion

50. An obese client has an abdominal cholecystectomy and returns from surgery with a nasogastric tube to low continuous suction, a T-tube, and a Foley catheter. The nurse should first:
1. Irrigate each tube with normal saline
2. Fasten each of the tubes to the bed sheets
3. Empty the drainage from collection devices
4. Check the drainage tubes and collection devices

51. After surgery to create an ileal conduit, a client is admitted to the recovery room. During the first hour of the postoperative period, the nurse should notify the physician if:
1. Vomiting occurs
2. The stoma is swollen
3. No urine output is noted
4. Bowel sounds are diminished

52. A client is admitted to the trauma unit with multiple injuries including a crushed chest, abdominal trauma, probable head injury, and multiple fractures. In order of priority, the initial emergency care interventions for this client are to:
1. Start an IV, get blood for typing and crossmatching, obtain a history
2. Assess vital signs, obtain a history, arrange for emergency x-ray films

3. Conduct a thorough physical assessment, assess vital signs, cover open wounds
4. Assess vital signs, control accessible bleeding, determine the presence of critical injuries

53. Elderly individuals with non-insulin dependent diabetes mellitus (NIDDM):
1. Seldom develop ketoacidosis
2. Secrete no endogenous insulin
3. Have a lower incidence of chronic complications
4. Have a sudden and dramatic onset of symptoms

54. An elderly female admitted with an acute episode of rheumatoid arthritis asks why her roommate, who also has arthritis, goes to physical therapy every day and she does not. The most appropriate response by the nurse would be:
1. "It usually depends on who your physician is."
2. "Her condition is much more advanced than yours."
3. "Your joints are still inflamed and it would be harmful."
4. "Physical therapy is an important aspect of rheumatology care."

55. A client's spouse asks how coronary artery bypass surgery will help the client. The nurse bases a response on the knowledge that:
1. This surgery significantly decreases symptoms in a large percentage of clients
2. Studies have consistently shown that this surgery increases an individual's life span
3. The surgery will permit the client to return to gainful employment after healing occurs
4. Evidence substantiates that surgery can prevent progression of coronary artery disease

56. A female client with a history of rheumatic fever and a heart murmur has gained weight even though she has nausea and a loss of appetite. She wakes up short of breath several times nightly and notices that she gets tired

and has trouble breathing while doing normal daily tasks. When hearing the client's symptoms the nurse should immediately seek additional critical data such as:
1. A retrospective 24-hour calorie count
2. Her elimination pattern over the last month
3. A complete gynecologic and sexual history
4. The presence of a recent cough and pulmonary secretions

57. To assess an elderly client for a fracture of the hip the nurse should:
1. Observe for bruising over the affected hip
2. Observe for shortening of the affected leg
3. Move the affected leg to see if it causes pain
4. Move the affected leg to feel and hear crepitus

58. A client with chronic obstructive pulmonary disease has an elevated hemoglobin and hematocrit. The nurse should recognize that this is due to the fact that chronic:
1. Hypoxia stimulates red blood cell production
2. Infection stimulates white blood cell production
3. Hypercapnia stimulates red blood cell production
4. Infection promotes loss of extracellular fluid volume

59. A client with chronic obstructive pulmonary disease is admitted to the hospital with pneumonia. On the third day the client complains of a sharp pain on the left side of the chest. The nurse suspects a left pneumothorax. When assessing breath sounds on the affected side, the nurse would expect to hear:
1. Crackling sounds
2. Wheezing sounds
3. Adventitious sounds
4. Decreased breath sounds

60. A client is receiving MOPP therapy for Hodgkin's disease. About halfway through the first 6-month course of treatment, the client complains of burning and tingling in the feet. The nurse should recognize that these complaints are symptoms of the:
    1. Side effects of prednisone therapy
    2. Neurotoxicity caused by vincristine
    3. Peripheral vasoconstriction caused by nitrogen mustard
    4. Electrolyte imbalances resulting from the anorexia and vomiting

61. A 56-year-old client is brought to the emergency room after experiencing a sudden onset of retrosternal chest pain while shoveling snow. The pain had stopped before arrival at the hospital but the client is admitted. The nurse explains to the client that the physician will diagnose the pain on the basis of the findings from:
    1. A stress test
    2. A detailed history
    3. Physical examination
    4. X-ray films of the heart

62. The nurse encourages a postoperative client who had an abdominal cholecystectomy and choledochostomy with a T-tube in place to perform deep breathing and coughing every hour. The client resists doing these exercises primarily because the:
    1. Nasogastric tube is irritating
    2. Pain at the incision site increases
    3. T-tube moves and produces cramps
    4. Bandage on the abdomen is constricting

63. After a prostatectomy a client complains of painful bladder spasms. To limit these spasms the nurse should:
    1. Administer a narcotic every 4 hours
    2. Irrigate the Foley catheter with 60 ml of normal saline
    3. Encourage the client not to contract his muscles as if he were voiding
    4. Advance the catheter to relieve the pressure against the prostatic fossa

64. The physician schedules a paracentesis for a client with ascites. Immediately before the paracentesis the nurse should:
    1. Instruct the client to void
    2. Position the client on the side
    3. Measure the client's abdominal girth
    4. Have the client drink a glass of water

65. The physician orders a stationary (nonrolling) walker for a client to aid in ambulation. The nurse plans to teach the client to:
    1. Place the back legs of the walker about 10 inches in front of the feet, shift the body weight to the walker, and step forward
    2. Move the walker about 8 inches forward while stepping forward to the walker with body weight on the walker and both legs
    3. Place the walker flat on the floor with the front legs about 12 inches in front of the feet, shift the body weight to the walker, and step forward
    4. Move the walker about 10 inches in front of the feet with only the front legs of the walker on the floor, then step forward and put the walker flat

66. A 58-year-old client is admitted to the emergency room with a blood pressure of 240/150. The client is complaining of a severe headache, blurred vision, and swelling of the ankles. At this time it would be most appropriate for the nurse to:
    1. Assess the other vital signs
    2. Obtain a glucometer reading
    3. Obtain urine and blood samples
    4. Place the client in the supine position

67. While setting up a male client's dinner tray, the nurse notices that he has a tremor of the right hand when it is lying in his lap but the tremor disappears when he reaches for his fork. The nurse recognizes that this is:
    1. A resting tremor
    2. A voluntary tremor
    3. An intention tremor
    4. An idiopathic tremor

68. A 30-year-old steamfitter, who weighs 143 pounds and has 40% of the body surface area burned, is admitted to the burn unit. The physician orders fluid replacement of 7200 ml during the first 24 hours. The hourly IV fluid intake will be approximately:

1. 125 ml/hr
2. 200 ml/hr
3. 300 ml/hr
4. 425 ml/hr

69. A client who has inoperable cancer of the head of the pancreas involving the common bile duct has a T-tube inserted. During the first 48 hours after surgery the nurse should:
1. Maintain T-tube patency via gravity drainage
2. Prevent the client from turning onto the right side
3. Irrigate the T-tube with 30 ml of normal saline q2h
4. Connect and maintain the T-tube to low intermittent suction

70. A client with hypertension is placed on a low-sodium diet. When teaching the client about a low-sodium diet, the nurse provides a list of foods to avoid. This list of foods includes:
1. Ground beef
2. Fresh salmon
3. Luncheon meat
4. Cooked broccoli

71. A couple, aged 82 and 80, live alone. During a home visit, the nurse finds that the husband has a prostate condition and at times is incontinent of urine. He is alert and cooperative but forgetful. The wife has diabetes that is controlled by oral medication and diet. She is severely arthritic and walks with difficulty. They both need some help with dressing, bathing, and meal preparation. The plan that appears most suitable for this couple would be to:
1. Place them together in a health-related facility
2. Place them together in a skilled nursing facility
3. Keep them in their home with a long-term health care program
4. Move them in with one of their children but allow them to choose which one

72. A client with non-insulin dependent diabetes mellitus (NIDDM) has gangrene of the foot and ulcerations of the ankle. In addition to the lesions on the lower extremities, the nurse might expect to find:
1. Arthritic changes in the hands
2. Increased vascularization of the retina
3. Hyperactive knee- and ankle-jerk reflexes
4. Dependent pallor of the lower legs and feet

73. Outcome criteria on discharge from the clinic after a bacterial cystitis should include a statement that the client will:
1. Understand the need for 7 to 8 liters of fluid per day
2. Be able to plan menus to include any dietary restrictions
3. Have relief of symptoms and show no loss of kidney function
4. Be able to state activities to be avoided because of possible bleeding

74. During peritoneal dialysis the nurse observes that drainage of dialysate from the peritoneal cavity has ceased before the required amount has drained out. The nurse should assist the client to:
1. Turn from side to side
2. Drink 8 ounces of water
3. Deep breathe and cough
4. Periodically rotate the catheter

75. The physician orders bedrest for a client who is admitted with a left-sided cerebrovascular accident (CVA). To avoid potential problems, the nurse should:
1. Place the client on an air mattress
2. Insert an indwelling urinary catheter
3. Develop an appropriate activity schedule with the client
4. Encourage the intake of high-protein fluid supplements between meals

76. A client has a basal cell epithelioma that is to be removed. The client tells the nurse about concerns that the cancer has spread. To best reduce the client's anxiety the nurse should respond:
1. "You are a good surgical risk."
2. "I can understand how you must feel."
3. "Basal cell tumors usually do not spread."
4. "The physician probably caught it just in time."

77. A client with Lyme disease is to self-administer ceftriaxone sodium (Rocephin) 200,000 mg via IV at home. The drug is to be diluted in 100 ml of D5W and infused over a period of 35 minutes. The drop factor of the tubing the client will be using is 10 gtt/ml. The nurse should teach the client to set the flow at:
    1. 17 gtt/min
    2. 22 gtt/min
    3. 29 gtt/min
    4. 35 gtt/min

78. A client with the diagnosis of multiple sclerosis develops increased visual problems, progressive muscular weakness, and frequent episodes of emotional lability, which are very distressing to the client. During a visit to the clinic, while having a discussion with the nurse, the client bursts into tears for no apparent reason. The nurse should:
    1. Ascertain why the client is upset
    2. Tell the client there is no reason to cry
    3. Let the client cry; then resume the discussion
    4. Tell the client it is perfectly normal to be crying and upset

79. A client, who was hospitalized with severe cirrhosis of the liver, improves and is to be discharged. When planning the discharge with family members, the nurse tells them about:
    1. The need for a high-protein diet
    2. The use of chlorpromazine for relaxation
    3. The need for increased fluids to promote kidney output
    4. The importance of reporting personality changes to the physician

80. One of the medical orders the nurse would expect for a client who is to have a hemicolectomy would be:
    1. Give oil retention enemas daily for 2 days preoperatively
    2. Administer Neomycin 1 gram q6h orally for 2 days preoperatively
    3. Have a Sengstaken-Blakemore tube at the client's bedside preoperatively
    4. Provide a high-protein, high-carbohydrate regular diet for 2 days preoperatively

81. A client visits the primary health care center because of persistent pyrexia, abdominal pain, and neuritis symptoms that the physician believes are suggestive of polyarteritis nodosa. When assessing the client the nurse should expect to find:
    1. An elevated blood pressure
    2. Enlarged cervical lymph nodes
    3. An unexplained excessive gain in weight
    4. A hypersensitivity of the fifth cranial nerve

82. A client with a cardiac dysrhythmia is placed on Lanoxin (digoxin) and Pronestyl (procainamide hydrochloride). Because of the combined effect of Lanoxin and Pronestyl, the nurse should monitor the client for signs of increased:
    1. CNS depression
    2. Reflex stimulation
    3. Myocardial depression
    4. Respiratory stimulation

83. Measured intake and output is ordered for a postoperative client. The client requests permission to keep the intake and output record. The nurse should:
    1. Determine the client's willingness to really help
    2. Explain that this job is the responsibility of the nurse
    3. Identify the client's reason for wanting to assume this task
    4. Assess the client's ability to measure the intake and output

84. A client with full-thickness burns on the chest has a skin graft. During the first 24 hours after a skin graft, care of the donor site includes immediately reporting:
    1. A small amount of yellowish green oozing
    2. A moderate area of serosanguinous oozing
    3. Epithelialization under the non-adherent dressing
    4. Separation of the edges of the non-adherent dressing

85. A client who has had a myocardial infarction receives 15 mg of morphine sulfate for chest pain. Fifteen minutes later, the client complains of feeling dizzy. The nurse should:

1. Ask if the client feels this is an allergic reaction
2. Elevate the client's head and keep the extremities warm
3. Place the client in the supine position and take the vital signs
4. Tell the client this is a normal sensation after receiving morphine

86. After a diagnostic workup the physician informs a client with hypertension that it is probably related to atherosclerosis. Later while talking with the nurse the client wants to know more about atherosclerosis. The nurse bases the response on the fact that atherosclerosis is characterized by:
   1. Lipid plaque formation within the arterial vessels
   2. Mobilization of free fatty acid from adipose tissue
   3. Development of atheromas within the myocardium
   4. Gradual decrease in arterial pressure as a result of renin

87. During the early postoperative period following open heart surgery adequate oxygenation is essential because:
   1. All clients have a chest tube in place
   2. Hypoxia can precipitate respiratory alkalosis
   3. Hypoxia can stimulate dangerous dysrhythmias
   4. An increased respiratory rate adds to postoperative pain

88. A client who has had a colostomy is to be discharged in several days. A primary nursing goal should be to:
   1. Determine the client's ability to care for the colostomy
   2. Cajole the client into caring for the colostomy without assistance
   3. Teach the client about the special precautions concerning the diet
   4. Show the client how to change the dry sterile dressing on the incision

89. A client is to be discharged with prescriptions for lanoxin (Digoxin), furosemide (Lasix), and a low sodium diet. The nurse identifies that the discharge teaching was not understood when the client states:
   1. "I must check my pulse for its rate and rhythm every day."
   2. "I can gradually increase my exercise as long as I take rest periods."
   3. "I should call my physician if I have difficulty breathing when I am lying down."
   4. "I will use a little table salt on my food only when I do not use it when cooking."

90. A client with an intestinal obstruction has an intestinal tube (Miller-Abbott) inserted. The nurse is to maintain patency of the tube by instilling 30 ml of normal saline prn. When instilling this normal saline the nurse should:
   1. Subtract the 30 ml from the gastric output
   2. Record the 30 ml on the intake and output record
   3. Consider the amount too small to record on the I&O
   4. Recognize that it will equal insensible losses and therefore is insignificant

Medical–Surgical Nursing Quiz Rationales

1. 4 This finding suggests metastasis to the bone, which results in pain and risk of pathologic fractures. (2) (SU; PL; TC; SK)

1 Seizure precautions are not necessary; a serum alkaline phosphatase elevation indicates bone, not brain, involvement.

2 Measuring intake and output is necessary for any client with prostatic cancer because of the high risk of obstruction, not just because of this test result.

3 An elevated serum alkaline phosphatase does not significantly affect the pH.

2. 4 This ensures that the liver does not move as it does with normal respiratory excursions. (2) (SU; IM; TC; GI)

1 Lying on the right side, not the left side, after the procedure applies pressure at the insertion site, preventing hemorrhage.

2 Movement or breathing increases the danger of damage to the liver.

3 There is no rationale for this, and it is difficult to carry out.

3. 4 This acknowledges the impact of this diagnosis on the client and should explore what is really known. (1) (ME; IM; PS; EH)

1 This statement is untrue and gives false reassurance.

2 Same as answer 1.

3 There is no evidence of ineffective coping.

4. 3 Aldosterone, a corticosteroid, causes sodium and water retention and potassium excretion by the kidneys. (2) (ME; AS; PA; FE)

1 Hypovolemia would not occur with increased aldosterone levels because sodium and water are retained.

2 Potassium is excreted in the presence of aldosterone and therefore would not accumulate and cause dysrhythmias.

4 Calcium is unaffected by aldosterone.

5. 3 The need for the six basic food groups in the Food Guide Pyramid continues throughout life. (1) (ME; PL; ED; GD)

1 The priority is to educate the client, although home-delivered meals may be one way to provide adequate nutrition.

2 Aging per se has no effect on the specific nutrients needed; however, it may influence digestion and/or absorption of food.

4. Protein is needed every day, but it need not be in the form of meat.

6. 2 High-protein drinks have twice the calories per volume of other fluids and provide protein for wound healing. (2) (SU; PL; PA; IT)

1 Low-sodium milk does not contain adequate calories to help meet the high metabolic rate associated with burns.

3 Fruit juices are comparably low in calories; potassium need not be restricted at this time; potassium is restricted during the hypovolemic stage (first 48 to 72 hours after burn injury).

4 More fats are not indicated; increased calories in the form of protein and carbohydrates are needed.

7. 2 The diagnosis depends on the identification of characteristic histologic features of an excised lymph node. (1) (SU; IM; ED; BI)

1 This is a diagnostic device to assess bony metastasis of cancers other than Hodgkin's disease.

3 This is not used to diagnose Hodgkin's disease; it can identify the extent of the disease by locating abdominal or chest lesions.

4 These are not indicated for Hodgkin's disease; they are usually used for radiotherapy or diagnosis of thyroid diseases.

8. 4 No specific diet is recommended; the client is encouraged to avoid meals that overdistend the stomach and foods that cause GI distress. (3) (ME; PL; PA; GI)

    1 There is no need for a mechanical soft diet, which would be appropriate for those who have difficulty with chewing and swallowing.

    2 The client does not have to be restricted to a liquid diet.

    3 High-fat dairy products increase GI secretion and should be avoided.

9. 1 Exercise causes muscle contractions, which require an increase in arterial circulation to supply oxygen and nutrients for energy being expended. (1) (ME; PL; ED; CV)

    2 This is important for the person with diabetes, but it does not improve arterial blood flow.

    3 This would reduce arterial blood flow; the legs should be kept dependent.

    4 Hot water is contraindicated because it can burn the skin and/or cause drying; also, individuals with peripheral vascular disease have an altered perception of temperature.

10. 1 Nitroglycerin causes vasodilation, increasing the flow of blood and oxygen to the myocardium and reducing anginal pain. (1) (ME; EV; TC; DR)

    2 An increased pulse rate does not indicate effectiveness; it is a side effect of nitroglycerin.

    3 The tingling indicates that the medication is fresh; relief of pain is the only indicator of effectiveness.

    4 Nitroglycerin does not promote the formation of new blood vessels.

11. 4 Vital signs monitor the cardiorespiratory status; hyperkalemia can cause serious cardiac dysrhythmias that must be treated. (3) (ME; EV; TC; FE)

    1 The cardiac arrest team is always on alert and will respond when called for a cardiac arrest.

    2 A repeat laboratory test would take time and probably reaffirm the original results.

    3 The priority is medical attention, and the physician should be notified immediately.

12. 2 This response acknowledges and reflects the client's feelings and encourages further communication. (2) (SU; IM; PS; EH)

    1 This response negates the client's feelings.

    3 The nurse does not know how the client's family feels; this response takes the focus off the client.

    4 This is true, but telling the client this serves no therapeutic purpose at this time.

13. 4 These interventions maintain the affected left arm in functional alignment; the left side of the body will be affected with a right-sided CVA. (2) (ME; PL; PA; NM)

    1 Plantar flexion (footdrop), not dorsiflexion, may occur with a CVA; high top sneakers or splints more appropriately prevent plantar flexion contractures.

    2 Elastic stockings promote venous return rather than prevent flaccid muscles; also, this requires a physician's order.

    3 Passive range-of-motion exercises prevent contractures rather than muscle atrophy; the institution of ROM should be discussed with the physician because activity during the acute phase can increase intracranial pressure; ROM may not be started until after the first 24 hours following the CVA.

14. 1 Itching associated with jaundice is believed to be caused by an accumulation of bile salts in the skin. (1) (ME; AS; PA; IT)

    2 This symptom is not related to jaundice.

    3 Same as answer 2.

    4 Same as answer 2.

15. 4 Hoarseness is caused by the inability of the vocal cords to come close during speech when a tumor exists. (2) (SU; AS; PA; RE)

    1 Aphasia refers to an expressive or receptive communication deficit as a result of cerebral disease; it is not related to laryngeal cancer.

    2 Dyspnea is a late sign, occurring when the tumor is large enough to obstruct air flow.

    3 Dysphagia is a late sign, occurring when the tumor is large enough to compress the esophagus.

16. 1 Covering exposed burned surfaces limits contamination by microorganisms and prevents exposure to air, which increases pain. (2) (SU; IM; TC; IT)

2 This is unsafe; this would traumatize the skin.

3 Same as answer 2.

4 Same as answer 2.

17. 4 Insulin in tablet form would be inactivated by gastric juices; insulin given by injection bypasses the destructive gastric juices. (2) (ME; IM; ED; EN)

1 Oral insulin would be inactivated in the stomach; oral hypoglycemics contain substances such as sulfonylurea that stimulate beta cells to produce insulin.

2 This is incorrect information for a client who is currently insulin-dependent; this provides false reassurance.

3 This does not answer the client's question; insulin is administered IV or subcutaneously and the route depends on the client's needs.

18. 1 The cerebellum is involved in synergistic control of the skeletal muscles and the coordination of voluntary movement. (1) (SU; AN; PA; NM)

2 The parietal lobe is concerned with localization and two-point discrimination; tumors here cause motor seizures and sensory function loss.

3 Basal ganglia are concerned with large subconscious movements and muscle tone; damage here may cause paralysis as in stroke or involuntary movements and uncontrollable shaking as in Parkinson's disease.

4 Occipital lobe is concerned with special sense perception; tumors here cause visual disturbances, visual agnosia, or hallucinations.

19. 3 Normal eating patterns are not lost when a laryngectomy is performed. (3) (SU; IM; ED; RE)

1 There is no passage of air from the lungs to the nose, and the ability to blow the nose is lost.

2 There is no passage of air from the lungs to the mouth, and the ability to sip through a straw is lost.

4 Air goes directly to the trachea, bypassing the nose and olfactory organs.

20. 4 Peripheral muscular hypoxia precipitates carpopedal spasm in the presence of hypocalcemia. (2) (ME; AS; PA; FE)

1 This indicates thrombophlebitis when pain results from dorsiflexing the foot.

2 This indicates the loss of position sense; swaying results when the client stands still with the feet close together and the eyes closed.

3 Although this sign indicates hypocalcemia, it is elicited by tapping over the facial nerve.

21. 3 This decreases pressure on the sella turcica, as well as promoting venous return, thus limiting cerebral edema. (2) (SU; PL; TC; NM)

1 There is no need to limit oral fluids because of the presence of nasal packing.

2 Gentle oral hygiene is performed, excluding brushing of teeth to prevent trauma to the surgical site.

4 Although deep breathing is encouraged, initially coughing is discouraged to prevent increasing intracranial pressure.

22. 2 Spasms result from irritation of the bladder during surgery; they decrease in intensity and frequency as healing occurs. (3) (SU; IM; ED; RG)

1 This is too long; it would indicate hemorrhage; after the first few hours, drainage should be dark red and then gradually turn pink.

3 The presence of a continuous bladder irrigation is unrelated to the amount of oral fluids that should be consumed; oral fluids should be encouraged.

4 The Valsalva maneuver should be avoided because it may initiate prostatic bleeding.

23. 1 Forcing fluids helps to liquefy secretions, enabling the client to clear the respiratory tract by coughing. (2) (SU; PL; PA; RE)
2 Excessive suctioning will irritate the mucosal lining of the respiratory tract and can actually result in more secretions.
3 An occlusive dressing would totally block air exchange.
4 The use of cotton balls around a tracheostomy introduces the risk of aspiration of one of the cotton fibers.

24. 2 Bile salts are used to aid digestion of fats and absorption of the fat-soluble vitamins A, D, and K. (2) (ME; IM; ED; DR)
1 Bile salts play no role in prothrombin production.
3 Bile salts are not necessary to stimulate the secretion of bilirubin.
4 Bile salts do not initiate the contraction of the common bile duct.

25. 2 Type 1 diabetes is classified as insulin dependent diabetes mellitus (IDDM) because the person needs exogenous insulin to maintain carbohydrate, fat, and protein metabolism. (2) (ME; AN; PA; EN)
1 Gestational diabetes (GDM) occurs only during pregnancy; this client is not pregnant.
3 Type II diabetes is classified as non-insulin dependent diabetes mellitus (NIDDM) because the condition can be controlled with diet, exercise, and/or oral hypoglycemics, without insulin.
4 Impaired glucose tolerance diabetes (IGT) describes glucose levels higher than normal but lower than those diagnostic for diabetes mellitus.

26. 3 The decreased respiratory drive resulting from excessive O_2 administration indicates CO_2 narcosis. (3) (ME; IM; TC; RE)
1 This is unnecessary; there are no indications that secretions have increased.
2 Increasing O_2 administration will further diminish respiratory drive until respiratory arrest occurs.
4 This is inappropriate; a confused client cannot answer questions about the confusion.

27. 2 The first chamber collects drainage; the second chamber provides for the underwater seal; the third chamber controls the amount of suction by the depth of the tube under water. (3) (SU; AN; TC; RE)
1 The first chamber, not the third chamber, collects drainage.
3 The second chamber, not the third chamber, provides an underwater seal.
4 Although this occurs in a three-chamber system, the main purpose of the third chamber is to control suction.

28. 2 The return of brown color to the stool indicates that bile is entering the duodenum and being converted to urobilinogen by bacteria. (2) (SU; AN; PA; GI)
1 Liver tenderness is unrelated to bile flow.
3 The absence of biliary colic is unrelated to the removal of the stone, not the flow of bile.
4 The serum bilirubin is not affected.

29. 4 This limits edema in the operative area and promotes respirations. (2) (SU; IM; PA; EN)
1 This would promote edema in the operative area, and the edema could compromise respirations.
2 Same as answer 1.
3 Same as answer 1.

30. 4 Steroids cause gluconeogenesis and glycogenolysis, both of which raise blood glucose levels. (3) (ME; AN; PA; EN)
1 This is a chronic condition that has probably been incorporated into the client's coping patterns; it would not cause sufficient stress to elevate the serum glucose level to this degree.
2 There are no data to indicate that this is a stressful event for the client.
3 This event is in the future and would not cause sufficient stress to elevate the serum glucose level to this degree at this time; retirement may be welcomed and may not cause stress.

31. 4 Rewording of the client's statement is paraphrasing that promotes further verbalization. (2) (ME; IM; PS; EH)

1   This is not paraphrasing; this merely re-peats the client's exact words.

2   This is not an interviewing technique; immediate movement to intervention cuts off communication.

3   This encourages clarification, a therapeutic technique; it is not paraphrasing.

32. 1   In the diuretic phase, fluid retained during the oliguric phase is excreted and hypovolemia may occur. (3) (ME; AS; PA; RG)

2   This develops in the oliguric phase when glomerulofiltration is inadequate.

3   Same as answer 2.

4   Diuresing is an indication of improved renal functioning, not progression into chronic failure.

33. 3   Semi-Fowler's position will localize the spilled stomach contents in the lower part of the abdominal cavity. (2) (SU; IM; TC; GI)

1   This position will exert pressure on the abdomen, which may be uncomfortable for the client.

2   This position exerts pressure against the diaphragm, inhibits breathing, and intensifies discomfort.

4   Same as answer 2.

34. 3   Bedrest with the leg extended prevents trauma caused by hip flexion and provides time for the insertion site to heal. (2) (SU; PL; ED; CV)

1   The physician will thoroughly review test results and may consult other physicians before talking with the client.

2   With the femoral approach, bedrest is maintained for several hours.

4   Mild sedation and local infiltration are used for adults; the client is conscious.

35. 2   Protein deficiency causes a low serum albumin, which permits fluid shifts from the intravascular to the interstitial compartment, causing edema; decreased protein also causes anemia; protein intake must be increased. (2) (ME; AN; PA; GI)

1   Although a deficiency of iron would result in anemia, it would not cause the other symptoms.

3   Hypokalemia would not cause these symptoms; it causes cramps and weakness.

4   This is unrelated to these symptoms; it is an essential fatty acid.

36. 1   The amount of solution (1000) is divided by the hourly amount to be infused (150) which equals 6.66; the decimal portion of the result must be converted to minutes (0.66 × 60 min), which equals 40 minutes plus the 6 hours. (2) (SU; AN; TC; FE)

2   The solution should be infused before this time.

3   Same as answer 2.

4   Same as answer 2.

37. 2   This response provides needed information and establishes the opportunity for further discussion of surgery. (2) (SU; IM; PS; EH)

1   This implies the other approaches are as effective as surgery; this places doubt in the client's mind that surgery is the most effective option.

3   This is an inappropriate response; the competence of the physician was not questioned, but there exists a need for a further discussion of the treatment; making this type of referral is not the nurse's role.

4   This is false reassurance; it cuts off communication and does not address the need for further discussion.

38. 4   This permits air to enter through the mouth along with the medication from the nebulizer; slow deep breaths deliver medication deep into the lung. (1) (ME; IM; ED; RE)

1   This is a nasal spray that does not deliver medication to the lung.

2   This would not deliver the medication to the lungs but would deposit it in the oral cavity.

3   It is impossible to breathe through the mouth with the lips sealed around the mouthpiece; shallow breaths are ineffective in delivering medication into the lung.

39. 4 Computerized tomography provides a three-dimensional view of cranial contents and defines outlines of masses and other abnormalities. (1) (SU; AS; TC; NM)
    1 Myelography is an x-ray examination of the spinal cord and vertebral canal, not the cranium.
    2 This is not done; removal of CSF in the presence of increased intracranial pressure may cause compression of the brain stem.
    3 Electromyography measures electrical currents produced by skeletal muscles, not the cranium.

40. 3 A patent airway is always a priority concern; therefore removal of secretions is imperative. (1) (SU; AN; TC; RE)
    1 This is an important postoperative intervention but is not the priority immediately after surgery.
    2 This is an important postoperative concern but infection does not occur immediately.
    4 Same as answer 1.

41. 2 Cells are vulnerable to specific drugs through the stages of mitosis, and a combination bombards the malignant cells at various stages. (1) (ME; IM; ED; DR)
    1 This is not true; the side effects of a drug are not ameliorated by a combination with others.
    3 This is true, but it is not the reason for using a combination of drugs.
    4 There is more than one stage of Hodgkin's, but this is not the reason for using a combination of drugs.

42. 3 Heparin interferes with activation of prothrombin to thrombin and inhibits aggregation of platelets. (2) (SU; AN; PA; DR)
    1 This is not the action of Heparin.
    2 Same as answer 1.
    4 Same as answer 1.

43. 2 Straining at stool should be avoided for 4 to 6 weeks after surgery to permit healing and avoid initiating bleeding. (1) (SU; EV; ED; RG)
    1 This is insufficient fluid; at least 2500 ml/day should be consumed.

3 The client has carcinoma and needs continued medical supervision.
4 Sexual intercourse should be avoided for 3 to 4 weeks after surgery.

44. 4 The motor fibers of the facial nerve innervate the superficial muscles of the face and scalp. (2) (SU; AS; PA; NM)
    1 This response is usually not related to damage to the facial nerve but may indicate infection.
    2 This is a sensory response that may be manifested when the injury is to the sensory branch of the facial nerve.
    3 Same as answer 2.

45. 1 This behavior indicates that the client is comfortable; therefore the medication regimen is effective. (2) (SU; EV; TC; NM)
    2 This is the accepted dose; no data exists to indicate it is excessive for this client.
    3 This is not necessary; the medication regimen is effective.
    4 The efficacy of Demerol decreases when the drug is given orally; this is too soon after surgery to alter the route.

46. 1 Immediate treatment in this emergency focuses on reduction of oxygen demands and thus cardiac workload to prevent cardiac decompensation. (2) (ME; AN; TC; EN)
    2 The need is for an increase in fluid intake to compensate for that lost because of the very high metabolic rate.
    3 This is not likely because drugs are metabolized more rapidly in this condition; there is a danger of exaggerated effects with hypothyroidism.
    4 Clients with thyrotoxicosis are more apt to develop hypoglycemia from the high metabolic rate.

47. 3 This technique promotes nasal breathing, which negates the effects of aerosol medication; a loose seal around the mouthpiece allows for inhalation through the mouth. (3) (ME; EV; ED; RE)
    1 This is a correct technique; it promotes contact of medication with the bronchial mucosa.

2 This is a correct technique; the nebulizer tip must be past the lips to deliver medication.

4 This is a correct technique; it prolongs and improves delivery of the medication to the respiratory mucosa.

48. 2 This helps to decrease the gag reflex, therefore easing the passage of the tube. (2) (SU; IM; TC; GI)

1 This does not take advantage of gravity; the side-lying position makes naso-oral cavities less accessible to the individual passing the tube.

3 This will make it more comfortable but will interfere with swallowing, which is necessary during the procedure.

4 This is false reassurance; the procedure is not painful, but it is uncomfortable.

49. 2 Compressing the device expels air in the unit, and closing the plug while it is compressed reestablishes the closed system and its negative pressure. (1) (SU; IM; TC; IT)

1 A portable suction device is not attached to a mechanical suction unit.

3 Milking the tubing promotes patency but will not create negative pressure.

4 This facilitates drainage by gravity not negative pressure.

50. 4 All tubes should be immediately attached to appropriate collection devices to permit drainage; T-tube and nasogastric tube drainage lessens tension on the operative site. (2) (SU; IM; TC; GI)

1 A T-tube drains by gravity and is never irrigated by the nurse.

2 A T-tube should not be fastened to the bed sheets; a T-tube is surgically positioned in the common bile duct, and tension on the tube must be avoided to prevent accidental removal; it is best to avoid fastening any tubes to the bed sheets

3 This is not the priority at this time; this would be done later at the change of shift or when the collection devices get too full.

51. 3 Urine should drain continually from the conduit because there is no sphincter control unless a continent conduit is created. (2) (SU; EV; TC; RG)

1 Vomiting is a common occurrence after anesthesia.

2 This is expected; the stoma may be swollen for several weeks after surgery.

4 This is expected; bowel sounds should be diminished because of anesthesia and intestinal manipulation during surgery.

52. 4 Initial rapid assessment will determine priorities of care and subsequent actions. (3) (ME; PL; TC; CV)

1 Intravenous therapy and transfusions will be ordered, but baseline data are needed to assess the client's present condition and significance of future responses.

2 Although important, obtaining a history and x-ray films can be postponed until bleeding is controlled and injuries are assessed.

3 A thorough physical assessment is too time consuming initially; open wounds can be covered at a later time.

53. 1 Lipolysis is not a common response to meeting the metabolic needs of those with NIDDM; therefore, ketones are not present in large enough amounts to cause ketoacidosis. (2) (ME; AN; PA; EN)

2 Adults with non-insulin dependent diabetes mellitus do secrete endogenous insulin, but secretion is slow and subnormal.

3 The incidence of chronic complications is higher in those with non-insulin dependent diabetes mellitus than those with insulin dependent diabetes mellitus.

4 The onset of non-insulin dependent diabetes mellitus is usually slow, whereas in insulin dependent diabetes mellitus it is sudden and dramatic.

54. 3 Rest is required during active inflammation of the joints to prevent injury; once active inflammation has receded, an activity and exercise regimen can begin. (1) (ME; AN; TC; SK)

1 This is untrue; physical therapy would not be prescribed during a period of exacerbation.

2 The extent of the arthritis is not the determinant; whether the process is in exacerbation or remission is the deciding factor.

4 Although this is true, physical therapy is not performed during acute exacerbation of the arthritis.

55. 1 More than 80% of those who have this surgery have marked relief of their symptoms. (3) (SU; AN; ED; CV)

2 So far, studies have failed to show that coronary artery bypass surgery affects life span.

3 This depends on the client's presurgical condition and occupation, not the surgery itself.

4 The surgery itself does not affect the disease process; clients must also reduce risk factors (obesity, smoking, and poor diet).

56. 4 These symptoms, in addition to a history of rheumatic fever, would require an assessment for other cardiopulmonary symptoms. (2) (ME; AS; PA; CV)

1 Anorexia and weight gain do not indicate a nutritional problem but a fluid balance problem.

2 Loss of appetite in conjunction with shortness of breath and the history of rheumatic fever make gastrointestinal symptoms secondary in importance.

3 There is no reason to investigate the gynecologic and sexual history in relation to the current problem.

57. 2 Shortening of the affected leg occurs because of the overriding of bone fragments. (1) (SU; AS; PA; SK)

1 Although bruising may be present with a fracture, it also may be present from soft tissue injury.

3 The affected leg should not be moved because it can cause further damage to nerves and blood vessels.

4 Same as answer 3.

58. 1 Hypoxia stimulates production of large quantities of erythrocytes in an attempt to compensate for the lack of oxygen. (2) (ME; AN; PA; BI)

2 White blood cell production increases with infection, but hemoglobin and hematocrit are not measures of white blood cell counts.

3 Hypercapnia is an increase in P_{CO_2} in extracellular fluid; this has no direct effect on blood cell counts.

4 There is a loss of extracellular fluid in acute infections with a fever, but in a chronic condition this fluid is replenished.

59. 4 Because the affected lung will not expand, aeration of the lung will not be complete and breath sounds will be diminished. (1) (SU; AS; PA; RE)

1 This occurs with congestive heart failure, not with a pneumothorax; with a pneumothorax there is no air in the alveoli to produce crackles.

2 This occurs with asthma, not with a pneumothorax.

3 This is a broad term that includes all abnormal breath sounds; it is not specific to pneumothorax.

60. 2 This is a common and expected side effect of vincristine. (3) (ME; EV; TC; DR)

1 Prednisone is not known to cause neurotoxicity.

3 Burning and tingling are not related to vasoconstriction, but rather to neurotoxicity.

4 Tingling is associated with hypocalcemia, which is not induced by nausea and vomiting.

61. 2 The presenting clinical symptoms must be evaluated in light of a complete and detailed history of present and past episodes, life-style practices, and family history. (2) (ME; AS; PA; CV)

1 A stress test would be dangerous at this point.

3 This is insufficient by itself for diagnosis.

4 Same as answer 3.

62. 2 The incision is just below the diaphragm; deep breathing causes tension and pain. (2) (SU; EV; PA; GI)
1 Clients with nasogastric tubes mouth breathe, limiting nasal irritation.
3 It would not move because it is sutured in place; it is unlikely to cause cramps because it is not in the intestine.
4 Dressings do not encircle the abdomen; they should not be tight enough to restrict respirations.

63. 3 This action causes the bladder muscle to contract, initiating painful bladder spasms. (1) (SU; IM; ED; RG)
1 Narcotics may dull the pain, but they will not necessarily limit muscle spasms.
2 Instillation of fluid will not decrease bladder spasms and may be irritating and precipitate additional spasms.
4 Manipulating the catheter may precipitate additional spasms.

64. 1 The bladder should be empty to avoid injury during insertion of the abdominal trocar. (2) (SU; IM; TC; GI)
2 The upright position is used to allow accumulation of fluid in the lower abdomen by gravity.
3 Although regular monitoring of girth is important, it is not necessary immediately before this procedure.
4 This is unrelated to the procedure; however, it would be preferable to offer fluids after the procedure if allowed.

65. 3 Placing the walker flat on the floor provides stability; putting weight on the walker equalizes weight bearing on the upper and lower extremities. (2) (ME; IM; ED; SK)
1 This is unsafe; this places the walker too far in front of the client for safe transfer of body weight.
2 It is not possible to move the walker and have it bear weight at the same time; the walker should be flat on the ground when stepping forward.
4 This is unsafe; all four points of the walker should be flat on the ground when the client is stepping forward.

66. 1 Baseline pulse and respiratory rates will aid in monitoring treatment efficacy and identifying concurrent problems such as CHF and bradydysrhythmias. (1) (ME; IM; PA; CV)
2 This is unnecessary; it is unrelated to hypertension.
3 This is not the priority at this time; this may be done later.
4 This could precipitate respiratory distress; a semi- to high Fowler's position should be maintained.

67. 1 A resting tremor is typically present when the hand is not involved in a purposeful activity; also known as nonintention tremor; the tremor is caused by decreased neurotransmitter substance. (1) (ME; AS; PA; NM)
2 This implies the tremor is under the client's control, which is not true.
3 An intention tremor is exhibited or intensified when purposeful movements are attempted.
4 The cause of the disease may be idiopathic, but the tremor is known as a resting or nonintention tremor.

68. 3 7200 ml ÷ 24 hours = 300 ml/hour. (1) (SU; AN; PA; FE)
1 This is an inadequate hourly rate; the rate should be 300 ml/hr.
2 Same as answer 1.
4 This is an excessive hourly rate; the rate should be 300 ml/hr.

69. 1 A T-tube drains by gravity into a small collection bag; gravity drainage is enhanced by the right side-lying or semi-Fowler's position. (2) (SU; PL; TC; EN)
2 The right side-lying position facilitates drainage and should be encouraged.
3 A T-tube is never irrigated by the nurse; it drains by gravity.
4 A T-tube drains by gravity, not intermittent suction.

70. 3   Luncheon meat is processed and has high sodium levels to help in preservation. (1) (ME; PL; ED; CV)
    1   Beef is lower in sodium than are preserved meats; however, beef is high in saturated fat.
    2   Canned salmon is high in sodium, but fresh salmon is not.
    4   Broccoli does not have significant sodium levels.

71. 3   A home-care program would be more efficient and cost effective; this couple can manage with proper assistance. (2) (ME; PL; TC; GD)
    1   Because the couple appear to be functioning, as long as some assistance at home is provided, it is not necessary to move them at this time.
    2   There is nothing in the history to demonstrate that a skilled nursing facility is necessary.
    4   Same as answer 1.

72. 2   Diabetic retinopathy is characterized by neovascularization. (2) (ME; AS; PA; EN)
    1   Arthritic changes of the hands are not a usual complication associated with diabetes mellitus.
    3   Clients who are diabetic have peripheral neuropathy, which is characterized by hypoactive reflexes.
    4   Peripheral vascular disease is indicated by dependent rubor and pallor on elevation.

73. 3   These are measurable responses to therapy and are the desired outcomes. (2) (ME; EV; TC; RG)
    1   This is too much; it is approximately double the amount that is necessary.
    2   No dietary restrictions are necessary.
    4   There is no need to limit activities.

74. 1   Turning from side to side will change the position of the catheter, thereby freeing its drainage holes, which may be obstructed. (2) (SU; IM; TC; RG)
    2   Taking fluids into the gastrointestinal tract does not influence the drainage of dialysate from the peritoneal cavity; the client could also be on restricted fluids.
    3   This improves pulmonary ventilation and helps in maintaining comfort but does not significantly improve the flow of dialysate from the catheter.
    4   The position of the catheter should be changed only by the physician.

75. 3   This encourages involvement in care and promotes activity that will decrease potential problems related to immobility. (1) (ME; PL; TC; NM)
    1   There are no data to indicate how long the client will be on bedrest; this addresses only the potential for impaired skin integrity and does not take other client needs into consideration.
    2   There are no data to indicate that the client is incontinent or has urinary retention; this intervention could promote rather than prevent problems; also, it requires a physician's order.
    4   There are no data to indicate that the client cannot chew or swallow or has any extraordinary nutritional needs; this is a dependent function of the nurse and requires a physician's order.

76. 3   This provides factual information and addresses the client's concern. (2) (ME; IM; PS; EH)
    1   This does not speak to the client's concern and may increase anxiety.
    2   This may provide reassurance but does not permit further exploration of concern.
    4   This reinforces the client's fears instead of pointing out reality.

77. 3   This is the correct flow rate; the drug is dissolved in 100 ml of D5W so the amount to be infused (100) multiplied by the drop factor (10) =1000; this result divided by the amount of time in minutes (35) = 28.57 which should be rounded off to 29 gtt/min. (2) (ME; AN; ED; DR)
    1   This rate is too slow; the IV with the drug would not be infused in 35 minutes.
    2   Same as answer 1.
    4   This rate is too fast; the IV with the drug would be infused in less than 35 minutes.

78. 3 Emotional outbursts are common and fleeting in these clients; it is best not to emphasize them. (2) (ME; IM; PA; EH)
1 The client may be unaware of the reason; inappropriate responses and emotional outbursts are common.
2 The client is unable to control this emotion, and focusing on it may exaggerate the outburst.
4 The client is probably unaware of the cause of the crying, and saying it is normal is not reassuring.

79. 4 The damaged liver causes rising ammonia levels resulting in CNS irritation producing behavioral changes. (3) (ME; PL; ED; GI)
1 The liver cannot metabolize protein, and a low-protein diet is indicated.
2 Chlorpromazine is detoxified by the liver and is therefore contraindicated in severe hepatic disease.
3 Kidney function is usually not affected.

80. 2 This is an antibiotic given to decrease gram negative bacteria in the colon, which should limit postoperative infection. (3) (SU; PL; TC; GI)
1 These are used for constipation; oil retention enemas would not be ordered before surgery; tap water enemas until clear might be ordered.
3 This would be used for a client with ruptured esophageal varices, not for one having a hemicolectomy.
4 This is contraindicated; a diet to decrease bulk and empty the colon would be ordered.

81. 1 This is a very common manifestation caused by vascular disease, particularly renal vascular disease (renin/angiotensin mechanism). (3) (ME; AS; PA; CV)
2 Lymphadenopathy does not generally occur.
3 Weight loss is common.
4 Peripheral nerves, not cranial nerves, can be involved.

82. 3 Both Lanoxin and Pronestyl decrease cardiac conduction, with resultant depression of the myocardium. (2) (ME; EV; TC; DR)
1 These drugs do not influence the CNS.
2 These drugs do not influence the body's reflexes.
4 These drugs do not influence respirations.

83. 4 Clients should be allowed to maintain some control, depending on their ability to perform a given task. (2) (SU; AS; TC; FE)
1 The client has indicated willingness by the request.
2 Able clients should be supported to perform self-care.
3 This is immaterial.

84. 1 This indicates infection and should immediately be reported. (1) (SU; EV; PA; IT)
2 Serosanguinous oozing is to be expected.
3 This indicates healing and is desirable.
4 This is not a problem.

85. 3 Vertigo may be a symptom of hypotension. (2) (ME; EV; TC; DR)
1 Hypotension is a side effect, not an allergic response to morphine.
2 Raising the client's head may aggravate symptoms.
4 Dizziness is not a normal sensation after morphine.

86. 1 The term atherosclerosis means a thickening of the arterial lining by lipid plaques, which become atheromas. (1) (ME; AN; PA; CV)
2 Mobilization of free fatty acids will produce an acid-base imbalance.
3 Atheromas develop within the lining of the artery, not within the muscle tissue.
4 Arterial pressure is increased as a result of renin.

87. 3 Inadequate oxygenation can cause premature ventricular beats. (3) (SU; AN; PA; CV)

1 Although this may be true, it does not explain why adequate oxygenation is important.

2 Hypoxia can precipitate respiratory acidosis; hyperventilation causes respiratory alkalosis.

4 The reverse is true; postoperative pain can increase the respiratory rate.

88. 1 The client's feelings, knowledge, and skills concerning the colostomy must be assessed before discharge. (2) (SU; AN; ED; EH)

2 Individuals should not be coaxed into doing something they are not ready to do, particularly on a long-term basis.

3 After a colostomy the client is usually placed on a regular diet and told only to eliminate gas-producing foods.

4 Frequently the client no longer needs a dressing on the incision at this time.

89. 4 This is unsafe which demonstrates that the client did not understand the discharge teaching; sodium helps retain fluid which could cause a fluid volume excess which in turn could precipitate congestive heart failure. (1) (ME; EV; TC; CV)

1 Digoxin should be held if the client's pulse is below 60 or above 120 beats per minute because these dysrhythmias are signs of digitalis toxicity; the risk of digitalis toxicity is increased if the client develops hypokalemia as a result of receiving Lasix.

2 Slowly increasing activities and rest periods limit the stress on the heart and are desirable.

3 Orthopnea is a sign of pulmonary edema related to congestive heart failure and the physician should be notified.

90. 2 All fluid taken in by the client regardless of the route should be recorded on the intake and output record; documentation implies that the action was carried out. (2) (SU; IM; TC; GI)

1 Fluid instilled must be added to the intake, not subtracted from the output; the tube is an intestinal tube, not a gastric tube.

3 The instillation is to be repeated as necessary and the total amount instilled may be significant.

4 No amount of fluid should be considered insignificant; insensible losses through the skin and lungs generally equal approximately 800 ml daily.

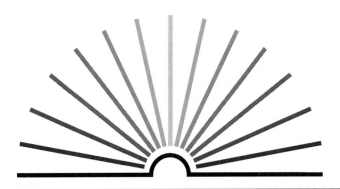

CHAPTER 3

Childbearing and Women's Health Nursing Review Questions

REPRODUCTIVE CHOICES

1. A client asks the nurse for contraceptive information. The nurse, as part of the teaching plan on contraception, tells the client that:
   1. The rim of the condom must be held in place while withdrawing the penis from the vagina
   2. Diaphragms are equally effective whether or not the partners choose to use spermicidal creams
   3. No sperm can reach the ovum if the man uses coitus interruptus and withdraws before ejaculation
   4. Individuals using periodic abstinence should have intercourse on days when the woman has a rise in temperature

2. When obtaining the health history from a client who is seeking contraceptive information, the nurse should consider that oral contraceptives are contraindicated in a client who:
   1. Is over 30 years of age
   2. Smokes a pack of cigarettes per day
   3. Has a history of borderline hypertension
   4. Has had at least one multiple pregnancy

3. A client is taking oral contraceptives. The nurse should inform the client to stop taking the contraceptive and report to the physician immediately if she experiences:
   1. Vertigo and nausea
   2. Weight loss and breast pain
   3. Hypotension and amenorrhea
   4. Headaches and visual disturbances

4. When counseling the client with diabetes mellitus who requests contraceptive information, it would be most therapeutic for the nurse to focus on:
   1. Rhythm
   2. The IUD
   3. A diaphragm
   4. Oral contraceptives

5. When teaching a client to use a diaphragm to prevent pregnancy, the nurse should tell the client that the diaphragm:
   1. May or may not be used with a spermicidal lubricant to be effective
   2. Must be inserted with the dome facing down to be maximally effective
   3. Often appears puckered but this will not interfere with its effectiveness
   4. Can be inserted as much as 6 hours before intercourse and still be effective

6. A couple tell the nurse that they wish to use the rhythm method of birth control. The wife tells the nurse that she menstruates every 32 days for 2 days. The nurse should teach the couple that based on this cycle, ovulation probably occurs:
1. On the fourteenth day of the cycle
2. 10 days after the first day of bleeding
3. 14 days before the start of the next menses
4. 2 to 3 days after the last day of menstrual bleeding

7. A client has stated she wishes to use the calendar method of birth control. The nurse is aware that the client understands how to calculate the beginning of the fertile period when she states, "I will:
1. Subtract 11 days from the length of my longest cycle."
2. Subtract 18 days from the length of my shortest cycle."
3. Abstain from sexual intercourse after the 10th day of my cycle."
4. Abstain from intercourse from the 10th day prior to the middle of my average cycle."

8. A client asks the nurse about the use of an intrauterine device (IUD) for contraception. When discussing this method with the client, the nurse includes that a common problem with IUDs is:
1. Expulsion of the device
2. Occasional dyspareunia
3. Perforation of the uterus
4. Frequent vaginal infections

9. The nurse informs a client contemplating implantable Progestin (Norplant) as a means of contraception that the most common side effect is:
1. Vertigo
2. Dyspareunia
3. An increase in breast size
4. Irregular menstrual bleeding

10. A female client, undergoing infertility testing, is taught how to examine her cervical mucus. After listening to the instructions the client says, "That sounds gross. I don't think I can do it." The nurse is aware that:

1. Having a baby is not that important to this client
2. It is possible that the client is being unduly fastidious
3. The client is afraid of finding out that the problem is her fault
4. Some women are uncomfortable touching their genitals and discharges

HEALTHY CHILDBEARING

11. A client comes to the antepartal clinic and states that her last menstrual period (LMP) was May 31. Using Nägele's rule the nurse would estimate the expected date of delivery (EDD) to be:
1. March 7
2. March 30
3. February 24
4. February 27

12. When discussing fetal development with a pregnant client the nurse explains that:
1. If a baby is to be left-handed after birth, the structures on the left side of the embryo's body develop before those on the right side
2. Development proceeds from head to tail, so the embryo's brain, central nervous system, and heart are formed and start functioning before limb buds appear
3. Development of structures in the embryo proceeds from external to internal structures so the heart is formed and starts functioning after the limb buds appear
4. The brain and central nervous system are formed early in the embryonic period, and the right side of the brain starts functioning much earlier than the left side

13. A positive early diagnosis of pregnancy is based on the presence of:
1. Quickening
2. Chadwick's sign
3. A fetal heart rate
4. Chorionic gonadotropin

14. A pregnant client is experiencing nausea and vomiting. The nurse is aware that this discomfort:

1. Is always present in early pregnancy
2. Will disappear when lightening occurs
3. Is a frequent response to an unwanted pregnancy
4. May be related to the HCG (chorionic gonadotropin) level

15. The nurse is aware that absorption of drugs taken orally during pregnancy may be diminished as the result of:
1. Decreased glomerular filtration rates
2. Developing fetal-placental circulation
3. Delayed emptying of gastric contents
4. Increased secretion of hydrochloric acid

16. The nurse instructs a pregnant client to increase her daily protein intake by at least:
1. 15 grams
2. 30 grams
3. 45 grams
4. 60 grams

17. A client who is 8 weeks pregnant tells the nurse that she does not feel like making love to her husband and is concerned that her husband may not understand. The nurse could most appropriately respond:
1. "How long have you had this problem?"
2. "Why don't you feel like having intercourse?"
3. "A decrease in libido is a normal occurrence in pregnant women during the first trimester."
4. "I'm sure your husband eventually will understand your feelings are related to pregnancy."

18. A primigravida complains of morning sickness. The nurse should plan to teach her to:
1. Increase fluid intake
2. Increase calcium in her diet
3. Eat three small meals a day
4. Avoid long periods without food

19. The nurse discusses with a newly pregnant client, who is 5 feet 3 inches tall and weighs 125 pounds, the recommended weight gain during pregnancy. The nurse is aware that, to fall within the recommended weight gain during pregnancy, at term, the client should weigh about:

1. 130 pounds
2. 135 pounds
3. 140 pounds
4. 150 pounds

20. The nurse should explain to the newly pregnant primigravida that the fetal heartbeat will first be heard with:
1. A fetoscope around 8 weeks
2. A fetoscope at 12 to 14 weeks
3. An electronic doppler after 17 weeks
4. An electronic doppler at 10 to 12 weeks

21. A client tells the nurse that her mother told her she should not take tub baths during pregnancy because she will get an infection. The nurse should tell the client that tub bathing:
1. Makes one prone to infections
2. Is not recommended during pregnancy
3. Is permitted only during the first trimester
4. Usually is permitted through late pregnancy

22. A client, 10 weeks gestation, tells the nurse that she voids frequently without dysuria and would like to know what to do. The nurse is aware that this client will have to:
1. Decrease her fluid intake during the day
2. Contact her physician as soon as possible
3. Maintain increased fluid intake during the day
4. Try to resist the urge to void as long as possible

23. Between 12 and 24 weeks gestation, applicable prenatal teaching for a pregnant client should include information about:
1. Preparation for the baby, travel to the hospital, signs of labor
2. Growth of the fetus, personal hygiene, and nutritional guidance
3. Growth of the fetus, interventions for nausea and vomiting, expectations for care
4. Danger signs of preeclampsia, relaxation breathing techniques, and signs of labor

24. The nurse determines the fundal height of a client at sixteen weeks gestation to be one finger above the umbilicus. The nurse should:
1. Assess for two distinct fetal heart rates
2. Ascertain the birth weights of children of any siblings
3. Inform the client that she is mistaken about her dates
4. Instruct the client on appropriate weight gain during pregnancy

25. A client is now in her second trimester. While listening to the fetal heart, the nurse hears a heart beat at the rate of 136 in the right upper quadrant and also at the midline below the umbilicus. The sources of these sounds are:
1. Heart rates of two fetuses
2. Maternal and fetal heart rates
3. Fetal heart rate and funic souffle
4. Uterine souffle and fetal heart rate

26. A client, 28 weeks pregnant, has gained 13 pounds and tells the nurse in the antepartum clinic that she is glad she has not gained as much weight as her sister during pregnancy. An appropriate response by the nurse to the client's comment would be:
1. "Do you think you are getting fat?"
2. "Are you trying to watch your figure?"
3. "You have to eat right during pregnancy."
4. "Tell me what you have been eating lately."

27. A client, 28 weeks gestation, experiences low back pain and asks the nurse to teach her exercises which will provide some relief. The nurse would consider the teaching effective if the client performs:
1. Leg lifts
2. Tailor sitting
3. Pelvic rocking
4. Kegel exercises

28. A pregnant client is told by the nurse that fetal weight gain during pregnancy is:
1. Begun in the second trimester
2. Greatest during the first trimester
3. Most marked in the third trimester
4. Equally distributed throughout pregnancy

29. A client who has missed two periods comes to the clinic. The home pregnancy test was positive. Her last menstrual period was June 18. Using Nägele's rule, her estimated date of delivery (EDD) would be:
1. February 25
2. March 18
3. March 25
4. April 18

30. The nurse explains to a pregnant couple that in childbirth classes the emphasis is on:
1. Birth as a family experience
2. Labor without using analgesics
3. Nutrition, relaxation, and breathing
4. Education, breathing, and exercise

31. A pregnant client, interested in childbirth education, asks how the Lamaze method differs from the Read method. The nurse explains that the Lamaze method:
1. Is a much easier method to teach and learn
2. Requires a good deal of prenatal preparation
3. Forbids the use of pain-relieving drugs during labor
4. Is a calm, relaxed approach based on "childbirth without pain"

32. During a childbirth class the nurse evaluates that the clients understand how to use effleurage correctly when the clients are observed:
1. Rocking gently back and forth on their knees
2. Practicing panting to avoid pushing during labor
3. Taking deep breaths before simulated contractions
4. Massaging their abdomens gently with their fingertips

33. The need to improve pubococcygeal muscle tone is explored during a childbirth class. The nurse recognizes that a client understands the instructions on how to strengthen the muscle when she states she should do:
1. Tailor sitting
2. Pelvic rocking
3. Forward tilting
4. Kegel exercises

34. When teaching about normal childbearing and contraceptive options, the nurse explains that fertilization of the ovum by the sperm occurs when:
1. The male sperm count is high
2. The ovum reaches the endometrium of the uterus
3. One sperm successfully penetrates the wall of the ovum
4. The sperm prevents the ovum from moving along the tube

35. The nurse would know that a pregnant client does not understand the teaching about fetal growth and development when the client states:
1. "The mother must observe proper nutrition."
2. "The fetus gets food from the amniotic fluid."
3. "There are two umbilical arteries and one vein."
4. "The baby's oxygen needs are provided for by the mother."

36. During a class for prepared childbirth, the nurse discusses the importance of the "spurt of energy" that occurs prior to labor. The nurse teaches the women to conserve this energy because:
1. Fatigue may influence the need for pain medication
2. Energy helps to increase the woman's progesterone level
3. This energy decreases the intensity of uterine contractions
4. Extra energy is needed to push during the first stage of labor

37. A pregnant couple attend Lamaze preparation-for-childbirth classes. The exercise the nurse teaches for toning the pelvic floor is:
1. Pelvic tilt
2. Half sit-ups
3. Pelvic rocking
4. Kegel exercises

38. To ensure proper nutrition during pregnancy for a client who is a vegetarian, the nurse should:
1. Advise the client to include meat in her diet at least once daily
2. Help the client plan meals that use foods that she is willing to eat
3. Encourage the client to join a diet group to teach her good nutrition
4. Tell the client to discontinue the vegetarian practice entirely until she delivers

39. To evaluate if a short-term goal for a low-income pregnant client with iron deficiency anemia is being met, the nurse asks the client:
1. "Do you try to have beef liver twice a week?"
2. "Do you have red meat at least once a week?"
3. "Have you increased lean meat in your diet to four meals a week?"
4. "Did you like the three bean casserole for which I gave you the recipe?"

40. A young client asks the nurse if she needs to change her diet during pregnancy. After teaching her about nutrition in relation to pregnancy, the nurse would know that the client understands the teaching when she says, "I should:
1. Drink only skim milk."
2. Restrict my salt intake."
3. Include 6 to 7 ounces of protein daily."
4. Increase my caloric intake by 1500 calories."

41. The nurse knows that clients need a well balanced diet daily and possibly vitamin and iron supplements during pregnancy to maintain their own and fetal needs during gestation. Folic acid may also need to be supplemented. To obtain this nutrient the nurse should tell pregnant clients to eat:
1. Celery
2. Bananas
3. Cooked beef liver
4. Broiled turkey breast

42. Folic acid supplements are prescribed for a prenatal client. The nurse is aware that these are necessary to:
1. Treat pernicious anemia
2. Prevent anaphylactic shock
3. Promote normal erythropoiesis
4. Prevent erythroblastosis fetalis

43. During a counseling discussion of nutrition, the nurse explains to a pregnant client that she will need additional calcium during pregnancy and that the best source is milk. The client states, "I never drink milk or eat milk products. They turn my stomach." The best reply by the nurse would be:
1. "How unfortunate; this may cause your teeth to loosen."
2. "Just make sure the rest of your diet is nutritionally sound."
3. "You will have to try and drink some milk so that the baby will have strong bones."
4. "There are many mineral and vitamin supplements the physician can order for you."

44. When discussing dietary needs during pregnancy, a client tells the nurse that milk constipates her at times. The nurse should explain that it is preferable to:
1. Substitute a variety of cheeses for the milk
2. Substitute skimmed or buttermilk for whole milk
3. Increase her prenatal capsules and omit the milk
4. Treat constipation in some way other than omitting milk

45. The nurse explains to a pregnant client who does not like milk that there are other foods that are good sources of calcium and advises the client to eat:
1. Corn
2. Liver
3. Broccoli
4. Lean meat

46. The nurse teaches a client that the increased need for vitamin A to meet rapid tissue growth during pregnancy may be met by using increased amounts of food such as:

1. Carrots
2. Nonfat milk
3. Citrus fruits
4. Extra egg whites

47. The nurse knows that a client in early pregnancy understands the need to increase her intake of complete proteins during her pregnancy when she reports she is eating more:
1. Nuts and seeds
2. Milk, eggs, and cheese
3. Beans, peas, and lentils
4. Whole grains and breads

48. A newly married client visits the clinic because she has not been feeling well. The nurse suspects that the client is probably pregnant when:
1. Her menses are already 7 days late
2. Her urine immunoassay test is positive
3. She relates that urinary frequency occurs every 2 to 3 hours
4. She complains of nausea and vomiting episodes every morning

49. The nurse understands that an ultrasound examination ordered for a pregnant client is used primarily to:
1. Estimate fetal age
2. Detect mental retardation
3. Rule out congenital defects
4. Approximate fetal linear growth

50. A client in the thirty-second week of pregnancy is scheduled for ultrasonography. When preparing the client for the procedure the nurse informs her that for this test it will be necessary to:
1. Have an enema the night before the examination
2. Monitor closely afterward for signs of precipitate labor
3. Fast for 12 hours to minimize the possibility of vomiting
4. Refrain from voiding for at least 3 hours before the test

51. The nurse understands that when a contraction stress test is interpreted as negative it means:

1. The fetus at this time is likely to tolerate the stress of labor but the test should be repeated weekly
2. The test should be repeated in 24 hours because the examination results indicate hyperstimulation
3. Immediate delivery should be considered because there is no fetal heart acceleration with fetal movement
4. A trial induction should be started because fetal heart rate acceleration with movement is indicative of a false result

52. Nursing care for a pregnant client who is to have a contraction stress test should include:
   1. Having the client empty her bladder
   2. Placing the client in a supine position
   3. Keeping the client on nothing by mouth
   4. Preparing the client for insertion of internal monitors

53. At 38 weeks an amniocentesis is done to determine fetal maturity. The proper L/S ratio for lung maturity is:
   1. 1:1
   2. 1:2
   3. 2:1
   4. 1.5:1

54. A primigravida, 36 weeks gestation, is admitted to the labor suite with ruptured membranes and a cervix that is 2 cm dilated and 75% effaced. The first question the nurse should ask is:
   1. "What is your expected date of delivery?"
   2. "Are you planning to breastfeed or to bottle-feed?"
   3. "What time was your last meal and what did you eat?"
   4. "How frequent are your contractions and how long do they last?"

55. The nurse uses phenaphthazine (nitrazine) paper to test the pH of the leaking vaginal fluid from a laboring client. If amniotic fluid is present, the nitrazine paper will become:
   1. Red
   2. Blue
   3. Purple
   4. Orange

56. For a client with a left breech presentation, the nurse should place the fetal heart transducer on the client's abdomen in the:
   1. Left lower quadrant
   2. Left upper quadrant
   3. Right upper quadrant
   4. Midline of the lower quadrant

57. When doing Leopold's maneuvers on a client who has just been admitted to the labor room suite, the nurse notes the presence of a firm round prominence over the pubic symphysis, a smooth convex structure down her right side, irregular lumps down her left side, and a soft roundness in the fundus. The nurse should conclude that the fetal position is:
   1. RSA
   2. LOA
   3. LOP
   4. ROA

58. When assessing a newly admitted laboring primigravada the nurse notes that the fetal heartbeat is loudest in the upper left quadrant. The nurse suspects that the position of the fetus is probably:
   1. Left sacral anterior
   2. Left occipital anterior
   3. Left mentum anterior
   4. Left occipital transverse

59. A laboring couple ask the nurse about the cause of low back pain during labor. The nurse replies, "This occurs most often when the position of the baby is:
   1. Breech."
   2. Transverse."
   3. Mentum anterior."
   4. Occiput posterior."

60. The membranes of a laboring client whose fetus is in a breech position rupture spontaneously. The nurse then notes fresh meconium in the vaginal introitus and realizes that this:
   1. Indicates that the cord will prolapse
   2. Is evidence of impending fetal distress
   3. Is a normal occurrence in breech presentations
   4. Requires immediate notification of the physician

61. The nurse encourages the husband of a client who is experiencing back pain during labor to comfort her by:
    1. Positioning her with her legs elevated
    2. Having her perform a panting breathing pattern
    3. Applying pressure to the sacrum during contractions
    4. Encouraging her to do Kegel exercises between contractions

62. In the 40th week of gestation, a client is admitted to the labor unit. On auscultation the fetal heart is heard in the lower right quadrant, and on palpation the occiput is identified as anterior. The nurse determines the fetal presentation to be:
    1. LOP
    2. LSA
    3. ROA
    4. RMA

63. The teaching plan for a father who is acting as a coach during labor would include the information that it would be best for him to:
    1. Leave his wife alone periodically so that she can rest between contractions
    2. Let his wife know the progress she is making and that she is doing a good job
    3. See that his wife remains supine so that the monitoring equipment is not disturbed
    4. Keep the conversation in the labor room to a minimum so that his wife can concentrate

64. For an actively laboring client whose cervix is 4 cm dilated and 100% effaced with the fetal head at 0 station the best nursing intervention should be to:
    1. Check the fetal heart rate every 5 minutes and record it on her chart
    2. Call the anesthesia department and alert them to an imminent delivery
    3. Ask the client how bad her pain is and whether she wants medication for it
    4. Continue to assist the client's husband to coach her in the use of breathing techniques

65. The nurse would be aware that the husband of a client in the early phase of labor had successfully learned his role and understood the teaching from childbirth classes when he is observed assisting his wife to:

    1. Pant-blow breathe
    2. Slow chest breathe
    3. Shallow chest breathe
    4. Accelerate-decelerate breathe

66. A husband, who is coaching his wife during labor, demonstrates an understanding of the transitional phase of labor when with each contraction he instructs his wife to:
    1. Take cleansing breaths and push
    2. Take quick shallow breaths and blow
    3. Use slow, rhythmic diaphragmatic breathing
    4. Switch from accelerated to decelerated breathing

67. A client has been in labor for the past 4 hours and is 5 cm dilated. In the past 30 minutes her contractions gradually became irregular and of fair quality. When caring for her the nurse should first check for:
    1. False labor
    2. A full bladder
    3. Uterine dysfunction
    4. A breech presentation

68. A client in active labor is admitted to the birthing room. A vaginal examination reveals a 6 to 7 cm dilation. Based on this finding the nurse should expect that this client would:
    1. Have a profuse bloody show
    2. Appear unable to control her shaking legs
    3. Be uncomfortable because of nausea and vomiting
    4. Have contractions every 5 to 7 minutes of 45-second duration

69. As the nurse inspects the perineum of a client who has been admitted in early labor, the client suddenly turns pale and says she feels as if she is going to faint even though she is lying flat on her back. The nurse should:
    1. Elevate her feet
    2. Elevate her head
    3. Turn her on her left side
    4. Start oxygen and IV fluids

70. A client is admitted in labor twelve hours after her membranes have ruptured. It is important for the nurse to assess the character of the client's amniotic fluid to prepare for potential:

1. Cord prolapse
2. Placenta previa
3. Maternal sepsis
4. Abruptio placentae

71. During labor a client begins to experience dizziness and tingling of her hands. The nurse instructs the client to:
    1. Use a fast deep-breathing pattern
    2. Pant during the next three contractions
    3. Hold her breath with the next contraction
    4. Breathe into her cupped hands or a paper bag

72. A client in active labor states, "I feel all wet. I think I urinated." The nurse should first:
    1. Give her the bedpan
    2. Change the bed linens
    3. Inspect the perineal area
    4. Auscultate the fetal heart rate

73. When monitoring of the fetal heart rate during the first stage of labor shows an irregular baseline with variability, a nursing priority is to:
    1. Administer oxygen
    2. Notify the physician
    3. Change the client's position
    4. Continue to monitor the client

74. During labor a client has a fetal monitor applied. The nurse should be concerned about a fetal heart rate that:
    1. Did not drop during contractions
    2. Varied from 130 to 140 beats per minute
    3. Dropped to 110 beats during a contraction
    4. Occasionally dropped to 90 beats unrelated to contractions

75. A client in early labor is receiving oxytocin. When observing a deceleration in the fetal heart rate, the nurse should first:
    1. Administer oxygen
    2. Place her on her left side
    3. Check the blood pressure
    4. Discontinue the oxytocin infusion

76. A client in late active labor is experiencing severe back pain. At this time, the best nursing intervention would be to:

1. Place the client in a supine position, using pillows for sacral support
2. Assist the client to walk about the room until her membranes rupture
3. Instruct the client to increase her effleurage and relaxation exercises
4. Apply external pressure manually in the area of the client's lower back

77. The position a client should be taught to avoid when she experiences back pain during labor is the:
    1. Sitting position
    2. Supine position
    3. Side-lying position
    4. Knee-chest position

78. A client's membranes rupture. The nurse, seeing a deceleration in the fetal heart rate, inspects the vaginal area and notes a prolapsed cord. The nurse should immediately:
    1. Administer oxygen by face mask at 7 L/minute
    2. Elevate the presenting part off the cord until delivery
    3. Notify the physician of the findings of the examination
    4. Instruct the client to assume a dorsal recumbent position

79. Priority nursing intervention for a laboring client with a sudden prolapse of the umbilical cord should focus on:
    1. Gently replacing the cord in the vaginal vault
    2. Checking the fetal heart rate every 15 minutes
    3. Covering the cord with a sterile moist dressing
    4. Starting oxygen at 2 L per minute via a face mask

80. After a client's membranes rupture spontaneously, the nurse observes the umbilical cord protruding from the vagina. The nursing action that should receive the highest priority in this situation is:
    1. Raising the foot of the bed
    2. Administering oxygen by mask
    3. Auscultating the fetal heart tones
    4. Preparing for a cesarean delivery

81. The nurse understands that a type of anesthetic block that will provide perineal anesthesia but allow the client to feel contractions and push during delivery is a:
    1. Saddle block
    2. Epidural block
    3. Pudendal block
    4. Paracervical block

82. A woman is receiving Pitocin IV to augment her labor. She suddenly begins to moan loudly and the nurse observes that the contractions are becoming more intense and prolonged with little or no rest periods in between. The nurse should:
    1. Continue fetal monitoring
    2. Discontinue the IV Pitocin
    3. Turn the client on her side
    4. Notify the physician immediately

83. When assessing a laboring client for signs that the transitional phase is beginning, the nurse would expect the client to have:
    1. Bulging of the perineum
    2. Pinkish vaginal discharge
    3. Crowning of the fetal head
    4. Rectal pressure during contractions

84. The nurse is aware that the management of a client in transition is primarily directed toward:
    1. Helping the client maintain control
    2. Having the client breathe simple patterns
    3. Decreasing the client's intravenous fluid intake
    4. Reducing the client's discomfort with medication

85. A laboring client who is 6 cm dilated is given an epidural. A common adaptation after receiving this regional anesthetic for which the nurse should monitor the client is:
    1. Urticaria
    2. Light-headedness
    3. Elevated temperature
    4. Sensation of chilliness

86. While having contractions every 2 to 3 minutes which last from 60 to 90 seconds, a client complains of having rectal pressure. The nurse should:
    1. Attach an external fetal heart monitor
    2. Inspect the client's perineum for bulging
    3. Determine when the client's labor began
    4. Ask the client if her membranes have ruptured

87. During the transition phase of labor, the nurse should be concerned primarily with:
    1. Monitoring intake and output
    2. Monitoring uterine contractions
    3. Assessing the client's vital signs
    4. Helping the client maintain control

88. When a client experiences the urge to push at 9 cm dilation, the breathing pattern that the nurse should instruct the client to use is the:
    1. Expulsion pattern
    2. Slow chest pattern
    3. Panting or blowing pattern
    4. Accelerated-decelerated pattern

89. When doing shallow breathing during the transitional phase of labor, a client experiences tingling and numbness of the fingertips. The nurse should instruct her to breathe into:
    1. A paper bag
    2. An oxygen mask
    3. The room's atmosphere
    4. A trichloroethylene (Trilene) mask

90. The nurse is aware that a client is beginning the second stage of labor when:
    1. The bloody show appears to lessen
    2. About a "dime's worth" of caput is showing
    3. A gush of watery fluid bursts from the vagina
    4. Beads of perspiration appear on the client's upper lip

91. The nursing action that has the highest priority for a client in the second stage of labor is to:
    1. Check the fetal position
    2. Help the client push effectively
    3. Administer medication for the pain
    4. Prepare the client to breastfeed on the delivery table

92. The nurse is aware that when local anesthesia is used for delivery:
    1. Labor is slowed after its administration
    2. There is a danger of maternal aspiration
    3. Maternal respirations may be depressed
    4. Reactions such as vertigo and tinnitus may occur

93. A client in active labor starts screaming, "The baby is coming!" The first nursing action should be to:
    1. Call the physician
    2. Check the perineum
    3. Tell her it is impossible
    4. Keep the client's knees together

94. A client arrives in the labor room suite with the caput emerging. The nurse recognizes that delivery is imminent and tells the client to:
    1. Push with all her power
    2. Use the pant-breathing pattern
    3. Assume the Trendelenburg position
    4. Hold her breath and turn to the left side

95. A client's membranes rupture during the transition phase of labor and the amniotic fluid appears pale green. Because of this finding, at delivery the nurse should be prepared to:
    1. Stimulate the baby to cry
    2. Administer oxygen by face mask
    3. Put a moist saline dressing on the cord stump
    4. Provide for suctioning of the oropharynx when the head emerges

96. Five minutes after delivery the nurse midwife assesses that the client's placenta is separating when:
    1. The fundus becomes completely relaxed
    2. There is a lengthening of the umbilical cord
    3. The client complains of unbearable abdominal pain
    4. Bright red blood continually seeps out of the vaginal opening

97. After repair of an episiotomy, the nurse notes that the client has a continuous trickle of blood from the vagina, but the fundus is firm and even with the umbilicus. The best nursing action is to:
    1. Have the client void
    2. Massage the uterus
    3. Notify the client's physician
    4. Monitor vital signs q30 minutes

98. After a cesarean delivery, a client is taken to the recovery room where the nurse performs fundal checks every 15 minutes. During one check the nurse notes that the fundus is soft and boggy. The priority nursing action at this time is to:
    1. Elevate the client's legs
    2. Massage the client's fundus
    3. Increase the Pitocin drip rate
    4. Examine the client's perineum for bleeding

99. An important nursing intervention during the fourth stage of labor is to:
    1. Vigorously massage the fundus
    2. Monitor the vital signs every hour
    3. Assist the client to the bathroom to void
    4. Turn the client on the side to check lochia

100. The nurse should assess a client in the fourth stage of labor for:
    1. Ability to relax
    2. Level of maternal love
    3. Distention of the bladder
    4. Knowledge of newborn behavior

101. After delivery the mother's vital signs are T 99.4°F, P 80 regular and strong, R 16 slow and even, and BP 148/92. The assessment the nurse should continue to monitor is the client's:
    1. Pulse
    2. Respiration
    3. Temperature
    4. Blood pressure

102. Thirty minutes after delivery a grand multipara is in the recovery room. Because of the client's obstetrical history, the nurse should monitor her for:
    1. Uterine atony
    2. Urinary distention
    3. Profuse diaphoresis
    4. Hypertensive episodes

103. In the second hour after delivery a client's uterus is found to be firm, above the level of the umbilicus, and to the right of midline. The appropriate intervention would be to:
1. Observe for signs of retained secundines
2. Tell the client that this is a sign of uterine stabilization
3. Assist the client to the bathroom to empty her bladder
4. Massage her uterus vigorously to prevent hemorrhage

104. Thirty minutes after delivery the nurse finds that a client's uterus is relaxed and the lochia is excessive. The first action by the nurse should be to:
1. Check the client's vital signs
2. Elevate the foot of the client's bed
3. Immediately notify the client's physician
4. Massage the client's uterus and expel any clots

105. The nurse is aware that a client could be at increased risk for postpartum hemorrhage if the client:
1. Breastfed in the delivery room
2. Received a pudendal block for delivery
3. Delivered a baby who weighed 9 lbs 8 ozs
4. Had a third stage of labor that lasted 10 minutes

106. After delivery, a client tells the nurse, "I'm so cold and I can't stop shaking." The nurse should tell the client:
1. "I am going to take your blood pressure and pulse."
2. "Let me check your fundus to see whether it is firm."
3. "Please turn on your side so I can check the amount of lochia."
4. "I will put some warm blankets on you; the chill will subside soon."

107. The best nursing intervention to minimize perineal edema following an episiotomy would be:
1. Hot sitz baths tid
2. Aspirin 10 grains po q4h
3. Ice packs to the perineum
4. Elevation of hips on a pillow

108. In the postpartum period the nurse anticipates that a client with a second degree laceration and repair is most likely to develop:
1. Posterior vaginal varicosities
2. Difficulty voiding spontaneously
3. Delayed onset of milk production
4. Maladaptive bonding and attachment

109. Following delivery a client is transferred to the postpartum unit. Of the newly delivered mothers on the unit, the one the nurse should observe most closely is:
1. A primipara who has delivered an 8 lb baby
2. A grand multipara who experienced a labor of only one hour
3. A primipara who received 100 mg of Demerol during her labor
4. A multipara in whom the placenta separated and delivered in 10 minutes

110. A primigravida has a right mediolateral episiotomy following a vaginal delivery of an 8 lb baby. While assisting the client with a sitz bath, the nurse recalls that a mediolateral episiotomy is associated with:
1. Less swelling
2. More comfort
3. Less bleeding
4. More infections

111. A client required an extensive episiotomy because her baby was large. A priority nursing intervention that will minimize edema and lessen discomfort at the episiotomy site would be:
1. Spraying the area with a local anesthetic
2. Applying some form of cold to the perineum
3. Giving the client an oral analgesic immediately
4. Positioning the client on her side, off the incisional area

112. The nurse teaches a recently delivered client how to care for her episiotomy at home. The nurse would know that the priority instruction was understood when the client states:
1. "I should discontinue the sitz baths once I am in my own home."
2. "I must not climb up or down stairs for at least 3 days after discharge."
3. "I must continue perineal care after I go to the bathroom until healing occurs."
4. "I should continue the sitz baths three times a day if it provides me with comfort."

113. Eight hours postpartum the nurse finds a client's fundus to be 3 cm above the umbilicus and displaced to the right. The statement by the client to the nurse that is most significant would be:
    1. "I've been so thirsty the past few hours."
    2. "I've changed my pads once since I got to my room."
    3. "I've had a lot of contractions, especially when nursing."
    4. "I've been up to the bathroom, but can't seem to urinate."

114. Twelve hours after a normal spontaneous delivery, a client's temperature is 100.4°F. This elevation is most likely an indication of:
    1. Mastitis
    2. Dehydration
    3. Puerperal infection
    4. Urinary tract infection

115. Twenty four hours after an uncomplicated labor and delivery, a client's CBC reveals a WBC count of 17,000/mm³. The nurse should interpret this WBC count as being indicative of:
    1. A normal decrease in white blood cells
    2. A normal response to the labor process
    3. An acute sexually transmitted viral disease
    4. A bacterial infection of the reproductive system

116. To help prevent postpartum infection the most important discharge instruction given by the nurse would be:
    1. "Don't take tub baths for at least six weeks after delivery."
    2. "Wash your hands before and after changing your sanitary napkins."
    3. "Tampons are better than napkins for inhibiting bacteria in the postpartum period."
    4. "Douche gently with Betadine solution twice a day for a week or more after delivery."

117. After delivery, a client tells the nurse she was very uncomfortable during her pregnancy because of varicose veins. In light of this information, the nurse's assessment should include:
    1. A daily clotting time
    2. Tests for platelet fragility
    3. Frequent Hgb and Hct values
    4. Testing for the presence of Homans' sign

118. The comment by a new mother of twins on the fourth postpartum day that indicates to the nurse the need for further assessment is:
    1. "I hope I'll be a good mother to these sweet babies."
    2. "I've been urinating large amounts ever since I delivered."
    3. "My breasts feel full, heavy, and tingly before I feed the babies."
    4. "My lochia is bright red with small brown clots the size of my thumb."

119. The type of lochia the nurse should expect to observe on the fifth postpartal day is:
    1. Scant rubra
    2. Moderate alba
    3. Moderate rubra
    4. Moderate serosa

120. A client vaginally delivers a 7 pound 2 ounce baby and has made the decision to breastfeed the infant. When instructing the client regarding breastfeeding, the nurse tells the client to expect that:
    1. Weight loss will occur rapidly
    2. Lochial flow will be increased
    3. Uterine involution will be delayed
    4. Use of heat will be contraindicated

121. When preparing a client to breastfeed, the nurse teaches the client that:
    1. High levels of progesterone stimulate the secretion of oxytocin
    2. High levels of estrogen stimulate secretion of lactogenic hormones
    3. Suckling stimulates the pituitary gland to release oxytocin which initiates lactation
    4. Milk secretion is under the control of hormones and starts immediately after delivery

122. A new mother asks the nurse how human milk compares with cow's milk. The information given to the client should include the following:
    1. Lactose content is significantly higher in cow's milk
    2. Protein content in human milk is higher than that in cow's milk
    3. Immunologic and antiallergic factors are now found in cow's milk
    4. Fat in human milk is easier to digest and absorb than that in cow's milk

123. A statement by a nursing mother that indicates that the nurse's teaching about stimulating the breastfeeding let-down reflex has been successful is, "I will:
    1. Drink at least two quarts of low-fat milk a day."
    2. Take a cool shower before each breastfeeding."
    3. Wear a snug-fitting breast binder 24 hours a day."
    4. Apply warm moist packs and massage my breasts before each feeding."

124. As a result of her newborn's vigorous sucking, a client's nipples become sore and tender. The best nursing action would be to:
    1. Apply continuous ice packs
    2. Give analgesic medication as ordered
    3. Expose the nipples to air several times a day
    4. Remove the baby from the breasts for a few days

125. A breastfeeding mother asks the nurse what she can do to ease the discomfort caused by a cracked nipple. The nurse should instruct the client to:
    1. Stop nursing for 2 days to allow the nipple to heal
    2. Manually express milk and feed it to the baby in a bottle
    3. Use a breast shield to keep the baby from direct contact with the nipple
    4. Nurse the baby on the unaffected breast first until the affected breast heals

126. A new mother wishes to breastfeed her infant and asks the nurse if she needs to alter her diet needs. The nurse can best respond:
    1. "Just eat as you have been doing during your pregnancy."
    2. "Just drink a lot of milk; you need the calcium to make your own milk."
    3. "Don't worry about it, your body will produce the amount of milk your baby needs."
    4. "You'll need greater amounts of the same foods you've been eating and more fluids."

127. A few weeks after discharge, a postpartal client develops mastitis and telephones for advice concerning breastfeeding. The nurse should tell the client to:

1. Start to wean the baby from the breast because it will reduce the pain
2. Get an antibiotic from the physician and start the baby on bottle feedings
3. Pump her breasts and wear a tight-fitting bra to suppress milk production
4. Breastfeed often because this will keep the breasts empty and reduce pain

128. The nurse discusses breast care with a mother who is bottlefeeding her infant. The nurse plans further teaching when the client states:
    1. "May I have my medication for the discomfort in my breasts?"
    2. "The discomfort I am feeling will go away in a couple of days."
    3. "How should I apply heat to my breast to help my milk dry up?"
    4. "I must call my husband and ask him to bring my new brassiere."

129. Before discharge the nurse should teach the non-nursing mother that if breast engorgement occurs she should:
    1. Wear a tightly-fitted brassiere
    2. Take 2 aspirins every 4 hours
    3. Cease drinking milk for 2 weeks
    4. Apply hot compresses to the breasts

130. A client who is not breastfeeding is taught how to care for her engorged breasts. The nurse realizes that the client does not understand the teaching when the client states:
    1. "I'm wearing a well-fitting, tight brassiere."
    2. "I am drinking 2 quarts of fluid every 24 hours."
    3. "I'm expressing milk from my breasts every 3-4 hours."
    4. "I do not let warm water run over my breasts when showering."

131. The nurse is aware that during the taking-in phase of the postpartum period the area of health teaching that the client will be most responsive to is:
    1. Perineal care
    2. Infant feeding
    3. Infant hygiene
    4. Family planning

132. A newly delivered adolescent mother confides to the nurse that she hopes her baby will be good and sleep through the night. The nurse should plan to teach the mother to:
1. Put a soft cuddly toy next to the baby at bedtime
2. Cuddle the baby and talk softly when crying occurs
3. Add cereal to the bedtime bottle to ensure deep sleep
4. Keep the baby awake for longer periods during the day

133. The nurse is planning for the discharge of a crack-addicted 17-year-old mother and her baby. To best meet the mother's and her baby's needs, the nurse should attempt to initiate a:
1. Legal aid referral
2. Foster care referral
3. Family court referral
4. Visiting nurse referral

134. The husband of a woman who had her fourth child three weeks ago states she has been irritable and crying since coming home from the hospital. The nurse tries to assist him in understanding the situation by stating that:
1. His wife probably has postpartum blues that will pass soon
2. Having four children is tiring and assistance may be needed
3. This behavior is common after delivery and he should not be too concerned
4. Often women express themselves by crying and he should allow her to continue

HIGH RISK PREGNANCY

135. A young couple on their first visit to the obstetrician ask the nurse if the wife should have an amniocentesis for genetic studies. The nurse responds that the indications for these studies include:
1. A recent history of drug use
2. Prior spontaneous abortions
3. First pregnancies in older women
4. A history of questionable genetic problems

136. A newly pregnant couple in their late thirties are having their first child and want to have an amniocentesis procedure. The nurse is aware that this procedure can be done:

1. In the last trimester only
2. Immediately after conception
3. As soon as the mother feels life
4. After the fourteenth week of pregnancy

137. The client who is scheduled for an amniocentesis states, "I'm glad this test will be able to tell if my baby is well." The nurse's best response would be:
1. "This is such a good test and the work in this field is amazing."
2. "A normal amniocentesis is a reliable indicator of a healthy baby."
3. "This test is useful in detecting potential defects due to chromosomal errors."
4. "Amniocentesis is a valuable tool for detecting congenital defects in the developing baby."

138. Before an amniocentesis the nurse should:
1. Obtain an informed consent from the client
2. Initiate the intravenous therapy as ordered by the physician
3. Inform the client that the procedure could precipitate an infection
4. Perform a vaginal examination on the client to assess cervical dilation

139. When obtaining informed consent from a client who is to have an amniocentesis, it is unnecessary for the nurse to give the client:
1. A copy of the Patient's Bill of Rights
2. An explanation of any usable alternative procedures
3. An offer to answer any questions about the procedure
4. A complete description of the possible dangers and discomforts

140. Before an amniocentesis a client is asked to drink 8 oz of fluid. This is done to:
1. Hydrate the mother and increase circulation
2. Improve ultrasonic visualization of the fetus
3. Hydrate the fetus and decrease its movement
4. Replace fluid that may be lost during the procedure

141. To detect possible complications immediately after an amniocentesis, the nurse caring for the client should first:
    1. Assess the fetal heart rate (FHR)
    2. Position the client on her left side
    3. Apply pressure for 5 minutes at the puncture site
    4. Check the client for vaginal bleeding or discharge

142. Following an amniocentesis, the nursing care should include:
    1. Giving perineal care
    2. Observing for signs of labor
    3. Encouraging fluids every hour
    4. Changing the abdominal dressing

143. A client at 16 weeks gestation is to have a sonogram followed by an amniocentesis. Nursing intervention would include directing this client to void:
    1. Just before each procedure is begun
    2. After the first sonogram tracing is obtained
    3. At least 1 hour before the procedures are scheduled to begin
    4. After the sonogram is completed and before the amniocentesis is begun

144. In addition to measuring fetal age, ultrasonography of a fetus can identify:
    1. Cleft palate
    2. Spina bifida
    3. Biliary atresia
    4. Mental retardation

145. In her 32nd week of pregnancy, a client's ultrasonography reveals a low lying placenta. The nurse is aware that when this client's pregnancy comes to term and labor begins, the client may first experience:
    1. Sharp abdominal pain
    2. Painless vaginal bleeding
    3. Increased lower back pain
    4. Early rupture of membranes

146. The nurse explains to a pregnant client undergoing a nonstress test that the test is a way of evaluating the condition of the fetus by comparing the fetal heart rate with:
    1. Fetal gestational age
    2. Fetal physical activity
    3. Maternal blood pressure
    4. Maternal uterine contractions

147. The nurse understands that a positive contraction stress test may be indicative of potential fetal distress, because the test demonstrates that during contractions the fetal heart rate shows:
    1. A normal baseline
    2. Late decelerations
    3. Early decelerations
    4. Variable decelerations

148. A client with a high risk pregnancy is to undergo a contraction stress test (CST). The nurse understands that this test would not be done if the client had:
    1. Blurred vision
    2. Vaginal bleeding
    3. Sickling of the red cells
    4. Increasing hypertension

149. Prior to the administration of RhIg, the nurse reviews the laboratory data of a pregnant client. RhIg is given to pregnant women who are:
    1. Rh positive and Coombs' positive
    2. Rh negative and Coombs' positive
    3. Rh positive and Coombs' negative
    4. Rh negative and Coombs' negative

150. During a prenatal visit, the nurse explains to a client who is Rh negative that RhoGAM will be administered:
    1. Weekly during the ninth month, because this is her third pregnancy
    2. Within 72 hours after delivery if her infant is found to be Rh positive
    3. During the second trimester, if an amniocentesis indicates a problem
    4. To her infant immediately after delivery if the Coombs' test is positive

151. Rho (D antigen) immune globulin (Rho-GAM) has been ordered for an Rh negative client who has just delivered. Before giving the medication, the nurse must verify that the infant is:

1. Rh positive, positive Coombs'
2. Rh positive, negative Coombs'
3. Rh negative, positive Coombs'
4. Rh negative, negative Coombs'

152. A client, who is pregnant for the first time and is carrying twins, is scheduled for a cesarean delivery. Preoperative teaching should include telling the client to expect to:
1. Be discharged between 7 days to 10 days post-partum
2. Need an enema to have an effective bowel movement
3. Be ambulating whenever desired the day after surgery
4. Take sponge baths until the incision is completely healed

153. On the first postpartum day a major concern of nursing intervention for a client who had a cesarean delivery would be:
1. Promoting dietary intake
2. Promoting bowel function
3. Relieving postoperative pain
4. Relieving gaseous distention

154. After the removal of a Foley catheter following a cesarean delivery, a client has difficulty voiding. The nurse can best evaluate if the client has emptied her bladder by:
1. Catheterizing the client for residual urine
2. Asking the client if she still feels the urge to void
3. Gently palpating the client's bladder for distention
4. Measuring the amount of urine the client has voided

155. When doing coughing and deep breathing exercises following a cesarean delivery, the client complains of sharp localized pain at the site of the wound. The nurse should:
1. Call the physician to secure an order for an abdominal binder
2. Place the client in a supine position and inspect the incisional site
3. Tell the client to splint the wound when she coughs and deep breathes
4. Assess the duration and intensity of pain and give analgesics as ordered

156. A pregnant client who has a history of heart problems asks how she can relieve her occasional heartburn. As part of the teaching plan the nurse should warn against taking antacids containing:
1. Sodium
2. Calcium
3. Aluminum
4. Magnesium

157. To facilitate delivery in a client with cardiac problems the nurse would expect that the physician will probably:
1. Use Pitocin induction
2. Use forceps to assist delivery
3. Schedule a cesarean delivery
4. Do nothing and let nature proceed

158. The nurse is aware that placenta previa occurs when:
1. There is premature separation of a normally implanted placenta
2. The placenta is not implanted securely in place on the uterine wall
3. There is premature aging of a placenta implanted in the uterine fundus
4. The placenta is implanted in the lower uterine segment covering part of the os

159. The nurse gently performs Leopold's maneuvers on a client with a suspected placenta previa and expects to find the:
1. Fetal head firmly engaged
2. Fetal small parts difficult to palpate
3. Uterus hard and tetanically contracted
4. Fetal presenting part high and floating

160. The nursing diagnosis that the nurse should consider in planning nursing care for a client with a placenta previa is:
1. Pain related to bleeding from placental tears
2. High risk for infection related to placental location
3. Impaired skin integrity related to placental damage
4. Anticipatory grieving related to possible genetic birth defects

161. The best way for the nurse to assess the blood loss of a client with placenta previa is to:
1. Count or weigh perineal pads
2. Measure the height of the fundus
3. Monitor pulse and blood pressure
4. Check hemoglobin and hematocrit

162. A client with heavy bleeding because of placenta previa is admitted. The nurse places the client in the knee-chest position to:
1. Prevent shock
2. Control bleeding
3. Keep pressure off the cervix
4. Move the placenta off of the cervix

163. A client with a suspected placenta previa is to have an ultrasonogram to determine the location of the placenta. In preparation for this procedure the nurse should:
1. Insert an indwelling urinary catheter
2. Cleanse her abdomen with a germicidal soap
3. Instruct her to drink two large glasses of water
4. Give a cleansing enema of 500 ml normal saline

164. The attending physician prepares to do a vaginal exam on a client with a confirmed diagnosis of placenta previa. In preparation for this examination the nurse plans to:
1. Have equipment ready for a fetal scalp pH after the examination
2. Prepare a supply of IV magnesium sulfate in case early labor begins
3. Attach the client to an internal monitor to closely watch the fetus' response
4. Prepare for a double set up that includes equipment for a cesarean delivery

165. If the physician plans to do a vaginal examination on a client with a placenta previa, the nurse should have available:
1. One unit of freeze-dried plasma
2. Vitamin K for intramuscular injection
3. Heparin sodium for intravenous injection
4. Two units of typed and cross-matched blood

166. A pregnant client is admitted with abdominal pain and severe vaginal bleeding. After assessment the nurse makes a nursing diagnosis of decreased cardiac output related to hemorrhage. The first nursing action should be to:
1. Administer oxygen
2. Elevate the head of the bed
3. Draw blood for Hgb and Hct
4. Give Demerol 50 mg IM for pain

167. The nurse is aware that the client most likely to be predisposed to placenta previa would be a:
1. 19 year old, gravida 1, para 0
2. 25 year old, gravida 2, para 1
3. 40 year old, gravida 2, para 1
4. 30 year old, gravida 6, para 5

168. The nurse instructs and encourages a client admitted with placenta previa about the importance of:
1. Breathing deeply to ensure that the fetus gets oxygen
2. Keeping all movement to a minimum to diminish bleeding
3. Remaining on her back to minimize pressure on the cervix
4. Lying on her side to avoid putting pressure on the vena cava

169. When caring for a laboring client with placenta previa, it would be most important for the nurse to:
1. Assess the fetal heart tones by fetoscope
2. Frequently assess the height of the fundus
3. Evaluate the external blood loss by pad count
4. Perform frequent vaginal and rectal examinations

170. To allay some of the concerns that a client with placenta previa has about herself and her baby, the nurse should tell her that:
1. Infant mortality from placenta previa is less than maternal mortality
2. With a very aggressive approach infant morbidity is almost nonexistent
3. With conservative therapy the dangers to mother and infant are greatly decreased
4. There is little danger to mother or child as long as the physician's orders are followed

171. Dietary counseling for a pregnant client with sickle cell anemia should include supplemental folic acid. The nurse recognizes that this is important because it:
1. Prevents sickle cell crises
2. Decreases the sickling of RBCs
3. Lessens the oxygen needs of cells
4. Compensates for a rapid turnover of RBCs

172. When a pregnant client with sickle cell anemia comes to the clinic each month, in addition to the routine observations, the nurse should also assess her for:
1. Signs of hypothyroidism
2. Hyperemesis gravidarum
3. Symptoms of pyelonephritis
4. Adult respiratory distress syndrome

173. Upon admission, a client, 42 weeks gestation, complaining of back pain and fluid leaking from the vagina is admitted and assessed. The findings are: contractions q 3 to 4 minutes, lasting 30 to 45 seconds; cervix 2 cm dilated and 70% effaced; presenting part floating; fetal heart rate; 140 bpm in the RLQ; streaks of blood from the vagina; and a positive nitrazine test. The nurse suspects that the finding that indicates that a problem with delivery may occur is the:
1. Nitrazine test is positive
2. Presenting part is floating
3. Streaks of blood from the vagina
4. Fetal heart tones of 140 beats/minute in the RLQ

174. When a breech presentation is suspected, the nurse should diligently observe the client for:
1. Symptoms of fetal distress, such as a prolapse of the cord
2. Signs of precipitate labor, such as rapid dilation of the cervix
3. Symptoms of primary uterine inertia, such as cessation of contractions
4. Signs that normal labor is progressing, such as increased contractions

175. A client has a history of multiple preterm births followed by neonatal deaths. During the prenatal period it is essential that the nurse teach this client that one of the most important danger signs to be aware of is:

1. Leg cramps
2. Pelvic pressure
3. Nausea and vomiting
4. Lack of fetal movement at 12 weeks

176. A client at 10 weeks gestation was admitted in preterm labor yesterday and is receiving terbutaline sulfate (Brethine) 5 mg q6h. The contractions continue but a vaginal examination reveals no cervical dilation. The nurse anticipates that the physician will:
1. Increase the terbutaline to q4h
2. Increase the terbutaline to 10 mg
3. Discontinue the terbutaline for the present
4. Maintain the terbutaline as ordered previously

177. While receiving tocolytic therapy for preterm labor, the client begins to experience muscle tremors, nervousness, and palpitations. The nurse should:
1. Get a medical order to discontinue the medication
2. Recognize that these are the usual symptoms of preterm labor
3. Review the client's laboratory results for electrolyte and glucose levels
4. Reassure the client that these are expected side effects of the medication

178. In her 30th week of gestation, a 16-year-old primigravida whose usual blood pressure is 120/70 has a blood pressure of 130/88. She is admitted to the labor room and says, "I don't know why the doctor is so worried about my blood pressure. According to a book I have it's normal." The nurse should respond:
1. "Your physician is just being very cautious."
2. "Your blood pressure is high for your age group."
3. "Your book is either for older women or outdated."
4. "Your blood pressure is slightly elevated by pregnancy guidelines."

179. A pregnant client who is experiencing contractions at 33 weeks gestation comes to the clinic. After a vaginal examination, the client is sent home and told to stay in bed. A teaching plan for this client should include the information that:
1. Blocks should be placed at the foot of the bed to raise it
2. She should lie on her side with her head raised on a small pillow
3. She should sit in an upright position with several pillows behind her back
4. For ten minutes every two hours she should assume the knee-chest position

180. The nurse explains to a client who is 33 weeks pregnant and is experiencing contractions that coitus:
1. Is permitted if penile penetration is not deep
2. Is safe as long as she is in the side-lying position
3. Need not be modified in any way by either partner
4. Should be restricted because it may stimulate labor

181. A client, 34 weeks gestation, is in labor and asks the nurse for some medication for the increasing discomfort. The nurse's response is best guided by the understanding that the use of analgesics during preterm labor is:
1. Reduced to a minimum
2. Not influenced by fetal age
3. Contraindicated at any time
4. Based on the client's comfort level

182. A women in labor at 34 weeks gestation receives two IM injections of betamethasone (Celestone). The nurse is aware that this medication is given to:
1. Stop the labor process
2. Help mature the fetus' lungs
3. Increase placental perfusion
4. Reduce the intensity of contractions

183. A client who is at 34 weeks gestation has been receiving terbutaline (Brethine) IV. Her contractions increase to every 10 minutes, and her cervix dilates to 4 cm. The Brethine is discontinued. Priority nursing care during this time should be directed toward:

1. Promotion of maternal-fetal well being during labor
2. Reduction of anxiety associated with preterm labor
3. Supportive communication with the client and her partner
4. Assisting the family to cope with the impending preterm birth

184. A client, 35 weeks gestation, is admitted with a small amount of bright red vaginal bleeding without contractions. After placing the client in bed, the nurse should:
1. Check fetal heart tones
2. Administer a Fleet's enema
3. Obtain an amniotomy setup
4. Perform a vaginal examination

185. Aware of a client's history of narcotic abuse, the nurse's initial plans for providing pain relief measures during labor should include:
1. Scheduling pain medication at regular intervals
2. Administering the medication just when the pain is severe
3. Avoiding the administration of medication unless it is requested
4. Recognizing that she will not need as much pain medication as others

186. The nurse should be aware that a newly delivered client with a history of drug abuse may be experiencing drug withdrawal if she develops:
1. Extreme hunger and thirst
2. Paranoia and evasiveness
3. Depression and tearfulness
4. Irritability and muscle tremors

187. A client is admitted with uterine tenderness and very minimal dark red vaginal bleeding. She is diagnosed as having abruptio placentae. Upon admission, the priority assessment would include vital signs, skin color, urine output, and:
1. Her past obstetrical history
2. Fundal height or abdominal girth
3. The time and amount of last meal
4. Family history of bleeding disorders

188. When performing a physical assessment of a pregnant woman, the nurse should recognize that 40% to 50% of all clients with abruptio placentae also have:
1. Hydramnios
2. Hypertension
3. Heart disease
4. Diabetes mellitus

189. A client with pregnancy-induced hypertension is being treated on an ambulatory basis and bed rest for three days is prescribed. The nurse encourages the client to stay in bed and assume the:
1. Supine position
2. Side-lying position
3. Semi-Fowler's position
4. Slight Trendelenburg position

190. A client in the 38th week of gestation develops a slight increase in blood pressure. The physician advises her to remain in bed at home in a side-lying position. The client asks why this is important. The nurse's response would be based on the knowledge that this position:
1. Decreases intraabdominal pressure
2. Lowers the blood pressure significantly
3. Prevents the development of generalized edema
4. Increases the circulation to the kidneys and uterus

191. A 16-year-old primigravida at 36 weeks gestation tells the nurse that her shoes and rings have been tight the past few mornings. Her blood pressure is found to be significantly elevated and there is 1+ proteinuria by dipstick. The client's blood pressure had been averaging 92/70 during her previous prenatal visits. By the accepted definition of hypertension in pregnancy, a significant rise in blood pressure would be manifested by a reading of:
1. 100/76
2. 118/82
3. 120/84
4. 122/86

192. A nonstress test is scheduled for a client with pregnancy-induced hypertension. During the nonstress test the nurse should be aware that if nonperiodic accelerations of the fetal heart rate occur with fetal movement it most likely indicates:
1. Fetal well-being
2. Head compression
3. Uteroplacental insufficiency
4. Umbilical cord compression

193. Although the exact cause of pregnancy-induced hypertension is unknown the nurse knows that it is often associated with:
1. A vitamin deficiency
2. A limited amount of calories
3. An inability to absorb minerals
4. An inadequate intake of protein

194. When providing health teaching for a client with pregnancy-induced hypertension, a therapeutic instruction that the nurse should give the client is:
1. Eat a sodium-free diet
2. Walk at least a mile a day
3. Limit fluid intake to 1000 ml a day
4. Rest frequently in the side-lying position

195. When doing a physical assessment on a client with worsening preeclampsia, the nurse should expect to find:
1. Vaginal spotting
2. Proteinuria of 3+
3. Difficulty in breathing
4. Blood pressure of 130/80

196. A nurse admits a client with severe pregnancy-induced hypertension (PIH). After obtaining the vital signs, the nurse should:
1. Check the client's reflexes
2. Call the physician immediately
3. Determine the client's blood type
4. Start an intravenous of normal saline

197. Before administering IV magnesium sulfate therapy to a client with pregnancy-induced hypertension, the nurse should assess the client's:
1. Urinary glucose, acetone, and specific gravity
2. Temperature, blood pressure, and respirations
3. Urinary output, respirations, and patellar reflexes
4. Level of consciousness, funduscopic appearance, and knee reflex

198. A client who is hospitalized with pregnancy-induced hypertension is encouraged to lie in the left lateral recumbent position because it maximizes:
1. Uterine and kidney perfusion and relieves compression of the major vessels
2. Intraabdominal pressure on the iliac veins and increases blood in the pelvic area
3. Aortic compression, decreases uterine arterial pressure, and increases uterine blood flow
4. Hemoconcentration, reduces blood volume and cardiac output, and increases placental perfusion

199. During her 6-month prenatal office visit a pregnant client states that she is getting fat all over and that she even needs bigger shoes because her old ones are too tight. The nurse should:
1. Reassure the client that weight gain is expected
2. Encourage the client to use a comfortable walking shoe
3. Teach the client about the groupings in the food pyramid
4. Obtain the client's weight, blood pressure, and fundal height

200. When assessing the effectiveness of a teaching plan about self-care and conservative management of mild pregnancy-induced hypertension (PIH), the nurse would know that the client understood the teaching when the client recognized the importance of:
1. Eating a low-protein diet
2. Joining a weight reduction program
3. Maintaining a normal sodium intake
4. Following the diuretic regimen as ordered

201. A client with worsening preeclampsia is hospitalized and placed in a private room. The nurse knows that this is important because a nonstimulating environment for a client with increased cerebral irritability:
1. Improves intracellular fluid reabsorption
2. Reduces the severity of frontal headaches
3. Reduces the probability of grand mal seizures
4. Prolongs the duration of hypotensive medications

202. A client with pregnancy-induced hypertension is suspected of having impending eclampsia. A characteristic symptom of eclampsia for which the nurse should assess is:
1. Anasarca
2. Convulsions
3. Excessive weight gain
4. Increased blood pressure

203. While a client is receiving magnesium sulfate for severe pregnancy-induced hypertension, a primary nursing intervention would be:
1. Limiting her fluid intake to 1000 ml/24 hours
2. Preparing for the possibility of a precipitate delivery
3. Restricting visitors and keeping the room darkened and quiet
4. Obtaining magnesium gluconate for use as an antagonist if necessary

204. A client is in the hospital undergoing therapy for severe pregnancy-induced hypertension. If eclampsia should occur, the nurse's first action should be to:
1. Assess fetal heart tones
2. Maintain an open airway
3. Protect the client from injury
4. Increase the infusion of magnesium sulfate immediately

205. A client with a history of phenylketonuria, who was maintained on a low-phenylalanine diet until 9 years of age, is now pregnant. The nurse teaches this client that:

1. Reinstitution of the low-phenylalanine diet will protect her baby from PKU
2. The baby will probably be mentally retarded because of her history of PKU
3. The fetus is at no risk prenatally but will require immediate care at birth to prevent PKU
4. Phenylalanine should be avoided even when not pregnant so that her body is able to support a pregnancy

206. Diet counseling for a breastfeeding client with a history of phenylketonuria should include providing a food list displaying the type of:
1. Lactose
2. Glucose
3. Fatty acids
4. Amino acids

207. The nurse knows that women with diabetes mellitus who become pregnant:
1. Have 30% or higher fetal mortality
2. Have decreased insulin requirements
3. Require intensive and thorough prenatal care
4. Should have their babies by cesarean delivery

208. The nurse explains to a newly pregnant client with diabetes mellitus that to minimize fetal neonatal complications the most important action for her to take is to:
1. Check her blood glucose level as ordered
2. Keep all the physician's appointments made for her
3. Adhere strictly to the prescribed diet to limit weight gain
4. Cooperate with the physician to maintain normal blood glucose

209. A client with insulin dependent diabetes mellitus is counseled during her second month of pregnancy. Teaching is based on the knowledge that this is a particularly crucial time because of the risk of:
1. Spontaneous abortion
2. Urinary tract infections (UTI)
3. Elevated serum glucose levels
4. Hypoglycemia (hyperinsulinism)

210. A primary long term goal for the pregnant client with diabetes mellitus is to:
1. Minimize dietary fluctuations
2. Keep blood sugar levels stable
3. Deliver an optimally healthy baby
4. Minimize the amount of insulin given

211. A client with diabetes mellitus has an amniocentesis in the thirty seventh week of gestation; the L/S ratio of the amniotic fluid indicates adequate lung maturity. Based on this information the nurse assesses that:
1. Labor will probably be induced very shortly
2. The baby will have to be delivered immediately
3. There will be no need for further fetal monitoring
4. The baby should be free from major respiratory problems

212. Aware of the signs of an impending postpartal hemorrhage, the nurse assesses a newly delivered client for:
1. A decrease in pulse rate
2. Continuous trickling of blood
3. Persistent muscular twitching
4. An increase in blood pressure

213. A client who has undergone a cesarean delivery because of the presence of active genital herpes is transferred to the postpartum unit 2 hours after delivery. The nurse on the unit should plan to institute:
1. Strict isolation
2. Enteric isolation
3. Contact isolation
4. Protective isolation

NORMAL NEWBORN

214. Gloves are being used when handling newborns whether they are HIV positive or not. However, the nurse understands that it is usually not necessary to wear gloves with unaffected infants when:
1. Giving a feeding
2. Changing the diaper
3. Suctioning the infant
4. Doing an admission bath

215. At 1 minute after birth the nurse notes that an infant is crying, has a heart rate of 140, has acrocyanosis, resists the suction catheter, and keeps the arms extended. The nurse should assign this infant an Apgar score of:
1. 4
2. 6
3. 8
4. 10

216. The obstetrician hands the neonate to the nurse after delivery. The nurse's first action should be to:
1. Dry and place the infant in a warm environment
2. Cut the umbilical cord and attach a Hesseltine clamp
3. Administer oxygen by face mask until cyanosis clears
4. Perform an abbreviated systematic physical assessment

217. During the physical assessment of a recently delivered newborn, the nurse palpates the infant's femoral pulses. This is done to detect the presence of:
1. Atrial septal defect
2. Coarctation of the aorta
3. Ventricular septal defect
4. Patent ductus arteriosus

218. An Apgar score recorded 5 minutes after birth helps to evaluate the:
1. Gestational age of the infant
2. Effectiveness of the labor and delivery
3. Adequacy of transition to extrauterine life
4. Possibility of respiratory distress syndrome

219. The nurse informs the parents of a newborn that the petechiae on their infant's face and neck is a result of:
1. A rash called erythema toxicum
2. Excessive superficial capillaries
3. Decreased vitamin K level in the newborn infant
4. Increased intravascular pressure during delivery

220. A newborn's total body response to noise or movement is often distressing to the parents. It is important for the nurse to teach the parents that this response is:

1. A reflexive response that indicates normal development
2. An involuntary response that will remain for the first year of life
3. An automatic response that may indicate that the baby is hungry
4. A voluntary response that indicates insecurity in a new environment

221. One minute after delivery, a newborn is crying vigorously and has an apical pulse of 110. The nurse notes acrocyanosis and flexion of the extremities. The baby's Apgar score is:
1. 7
2. 8
3. 9
4. 10

222. A baby weighing 5 lb 6 oz is born via a cesarean delivery and is admitted to the newborn nursery. The nurse expects the newborn's respiratory rate to range between:
1. 20 to 40 per minute
2. 30 to 60 per minute
3. 60 to 80 per minute
4. 70 to 90 per minute

223. On the afternoon following the birth of her daughter, a mother states to the nurse, "The nursery nurse told me that my baby has to have an injection of vitamin K. She's so small to be getting a shot. Why does she have to have it?" The nurse's most appropriate response would be:
1. "Your baby needs the injection to help her develop red blood cells."
2. "An injection of vitamin K will help to prevent your baby from becoming jaundiced."
3. "Newborns are deficient in vitamin K. This treatment protects your baby from bleeding."
4. "A newborn's blood clots faster than it should. This injection helps decrease the clotting time."

224. The nurse recognizes that in the healthy, full-term neonate heat production is accomplished by:
1. Oxidizing fatty acids
2. Shivering vigorously
3. Breaking down brown fat
4. Increasing muscular activity

225. On the third postpartum day, a mother asks why her newborn's skin has begun to appear yellow. The nurse should plan to teach her that the change in skin tone is a result of:
1. Breast milk ingestion
2. Inadequate fluid intake
3. Breakdown of red blood cells
4. An immature vascular system

226. To best assist new parents to understand the unique characteristics of a newborn, the nurse should discuss with them the:
1. Infant's response to routine feeding schedules
2. Testing of the normal newborn's auditory acuity
3. Newborn's behaviors and states of wakefulness
4. Importance of reading about parent-infant bonding

227. When inspecting her newborn after delivery, a mother asks the nurse if her newborn has flat feet. The nurse recalls that:
1. Flat feet are common in children and infants
2. This is difficult to assess because the feet are so small
3. Flat feet are associated with major deformities of the bones of the feet such as clubfoot
4. The arch of the newborn's foot is covered with a fat pad giving the appearance of being flat

228. The nurse recognizes that survival in the neonatal period is largely related to:
1. Gestational age and birth weight
2. Reproductive history of the mother
3. Timing and adequacy of prenatal care
4. Parental health habits and social class

229. A newborn is delivered spontaneously. Immediately after delivery the neonate is active, cries lustily, has a heart rate of 150 beats per minute, but the bottoms of the feet have a marked bluish tinge. The Apgar score for this infant at 1 minute would be:
1. 3
2. 5
3. 7
4. 9

230. The nurse, observing a sleeping newborn, notes periods of irregular breathing and occasional twitching movements of the arms and legs. The neonate's heart rate is 150 per minute; the respiratory rate is 50 per minute; and the glucose strip reading is 60 mg/100 ml. The nurse's most appropriate assessment would be:
1. The baby requires no intervention; all findings are normal
2. The twitching movements suggest the baby may be having seizures
3. The baby's blood sugar is low; twitching movements suggest hypoglycemia
4. The rapid respiratory rate and irregular breathing suggest respiratory distress

231. When assessing a newborn, the nurse notes several areas of raised white spots on the chin and nose. The nurse is aware that these are known as:
1. Milia
2. Lanugo
3. Vascular nevi
4. Erythema toxicum

232. After pushing for an hour, a client delivers a full-term male infant with an 8/9 Apgar score. The immediate nursing care of this newborn should include:
1. Assessing respirations, identifying the infant, and keeping him warm
2. Applying a prophylactic agent to the eyes, giving AquaMEPHYTON, and bathing him
3. Rushing him to the nursery while aspirating the oropharynx, and stimulating him often
4. Weighing him, placing him in a crib, and leaving him near until the physician is finished with the mother

233. After birth a neonate receives an intramuscular injection of vitamin K. The purpose of this medication is:
1. Stimulation of its production in the baby
2. Promotion or proliferation of intestinal flora
3. Maintenance of normal intestinal flora count
4. Prophylaxis until intestinal flora is established

234. A newborn infant has a PKU test after formula feedings have been initiated. This is done primarily to prevent:
1. Failure to thrive
2. Mental retardation
3. Growth retardation
4. Spread of the disease

235. A newborn male is circumcised. The nurse would recognize that the mother requires additional teaching regarding care of her son following the circumcision when she indicates that she plans to:
1. Change her son's diapers very frequently
2. Call the physician if there is excessive bleeding
3. Give the baby a tub bath the day after he is discharged
4. Place petrolatum gauze or A & D ointment on his penis with each diaper change

236. When changing her infant, a new mother notes a reddened area on the infant's buttock and reports it to the nurse. The nurse should:
1. Have the nursery staff change the infant's diaper
2. Use both lotion and powder to protect the involved area
3. Notify the pediatrician and request an order for a topical ointment
4. Encourage the new mother to cleanse and change the infant more often

237. A newborn develops jaundice 72 hours after birth. The nurse explains to the parents that the jaundice is probably due to:
1. An allergic response to the feedings
2. Normal physiological destruction of immature RBCs
3. An obstruction in the bile duct, which is common in newborns
4. Some Rh negative blood that is still present in the baby's bloodstream

238. The nurse is aware that the nursing action that would best promote parent-infant attachment behaviors would be:

1. Restricting visitation on the postpartum unit
2. Supporting rooming in with parental infant care
3. Encouraging the parents to choose breast-feeding
4. Keeping the new family together immediately postpartum

239. Following delivery a client wishes to begin nursing her infant. The nurse assists the client by:
1. Positioning the infant to grasp the nipple so as to express milk
2. Giving the infant a bottle first to evaluate the baby's ability to suck
3. Leaving them alone and allowing the infant to nurse as long as desired
4. Touching the infant's cheek adjacent to the nipple to elicit the rooting reflex

240. The best indication that correct attachment to the breast has occurred is when the:
1. Baby's tongue is securely on top of the nipple
2. Baby's mouth covers most of the areolar surface
3. Baby sucks each breast vigorously for 5 minutes before falling asleep
4. Baby makes frequent loud clucking sounds while nursing at each breast

241. The nurse assures the breastfeeding mother that she will know that her infant is getting an adequate supply of breast milk if the infant gains weight and:
1. Rarely sucks on a pacifier
2. Has several hard stools daily
3. Voids six or more times a day
4. Awakens to feed every 4 hours

242. A mother is breastfeeding her newborn. She asks when she can switch the baby to a cup. The nurse would recognize that the mother understands the teaching about feeding when she says she will start to introduce a cup when the baby is:

1. 4 months old
2. 6 months old
3. 12 months old
4. Eighteen months old

243. The mother who is bottle feeding her 1-month-old asks the nurse if any vitamin or mineral supplements are required. The nurse bases the reply on the knowledge that babies who are bottle fed with ready-to-use formula require:
1. Iron
2. Fluoride
3. Vitamin K
4. Vitamin B₁₂

HIGH RISK NEWBORN

244. An infant is born with an Apgar score of 3 at 1 minute. The nurse is aware that this score necessitates:
1. Oxygen by mask
2. Immediate resuscitation
3. Additional warming measures
4. Stimulation to the soles of the feet

245. A newborn of 30 weeks gestation has a heart rate of 86 beats per minute and slow irregular respirations. The infant grimaces in response to suctioning, is cyanotic, and has flaccid muscle tone. The nurse should assign the infant an Apgar score of:
1. 2
2. 3
3. 4
4. 5

246. After delivery, a neonate has an Apgar score of 4. Five minutes later the score is 6. The nurse should be aware that:
1. The infant is in immediate danger
2. The infant is probably hypoglycemic
3. There is an immediate need to resuscitate the infant
4. There is a chance the infant may be neurologically impaired

247. After delivery, a preterm neonate weighing 2300 g has Apgar scores of 3 and 8 at 1 and 5 minutes respectively. These scores indicate that:
1. Respiratory stimulation will be needed for the first 24 hours
2. The newborn was responding according to the preterm gestational age
3. Resuscitation was necessary and the measures used were appropriate to the need
4. Oxygen under pressure was not necessary because the 1 minute Apgar score was 3

248. The nurse would observe for symptoms of respiratory distress syndrome (RDS) in an infant whose mother:
1. Is a Class A diabetic
2. Had previously used heroin
3. Had been hypertensive during pregnancy
4. Was preeclamptic during labor and delivery

249. Since preterm infants are prone to respiratory distress, a nurse caring for an infant of 33 weeks gestation should observe the infant for:
1. Flaring nares
2. Acrocyanosis
3. Abdominal breathing
4. Respirations of 40 per minute

250. A client expresses a desire to breastfeed her preterm infant who is in the neonatal intensive care nursery. The nurse should:
1. Tell the client this is not possible because the infant is being fed by gavage
2. Discourage the client because of the time and effort it will take to pump her breasts
3. Instruct the client that breast milk is inadequate for a preterm infant because it does not contain all the necessary nutrients
4. Support the client's decision and explain that the infant will initially lose weight due to the energy expended when breastfeeding

251. A neonate, born at 33 weeks gestation, develops respiratory distress syndrome (RDS) at 6 hours of age. Assessment of the infant at this time would reveal:
    1. A high pitched cry
    2. A heart rate of 140
    3. Intercostal retractions
    4. Respirations of 20 per minute

252. Respiratory acidosis is confirmed in an infant with respiratory distress syndrome when the nurse notes that the laboratory report of blood gases reveals:
    1. A pH of 7.35
    2. An elevated P_{CO_2}
    3. A potassium level of 4.6 mEq/L
    4. An arterial O_2 level of 80 mmHg

253. Nursing care of an infant with respiratory distress syndrome (RDS) should be directed toward:
    1. Maintaining the infant in a warm environment
    2. Turning the infant frequently to prevent apnea
    3. Keeping the infant in oxygen concentrations of 40%
    4. Stimulating deep breathing by tapping the infant's toes

254. The nurse is aware that a finding consistent with the diagnosis of respiratory distress syndrome in an infant would be:
    1. Inspiratory stridor
    2. A pulse rate of 100
    3. Diminished breath sounds
    4. An arterial blood pH of 7.50

255. A preterm infant is receiving oxygen by an overhead hood. During the time the infant is under the hood it would be appropriate for the nurse to:
    1. Hydrate the infant q 15 min
    2. Put a hat on the infant's head
    3. Keep the O_2 concentration at 100%
    4. Remove the infant q 15 min for stimulation

256. Supplemental oxygen is ordered for a preterm infant with respiratory distress syndrome. To prevent retinopathy of prematurity (retrolental fibroplasia), the nurse plans to:

    1. Administer the oxygen by hood
    2. Apply eye patches to both eyes
    3. Warm and humidify all oxygen flow
    4. Analyze O_2 concentration frequently

257. A newborn with respiratory distress syndrome is placed on continuous positive-pressure ventilation therapy via an endotracheal tube. The nurse notes that the infant's right sided breath sounds are diminished, and the point of maximum impulse (PMI) of the heartbeat is in the left axillary line. Interpretation of this assessment data should lead the nurse to understand that:
    1. These are normal findings because infants with this disorder frequently have some degree of atelectasis
    2. The inspiratory pressure on the ventilator is probably too low and needs to be increased for adequate ventilation
    3. The infant may have a pneumothorax and the physician should be contacted immediately so treatment can be instituted
    4. The endotracheal tube has probably slipped into the left main stem bronchus and needs to be pulled back to ventilate both lungs

258. A nursing intervention for an infant with respiratory distress syndrome would be:
    1. Position carefully to promote respiratory efforts
    2. Set Isolette temperature at 85°F to prevent shivering
    3. Observe carefully for possible congenital birth defects
    4. Avoid handling to minimize overstimulation and conserve O_2

259. When estimating an infant's gestational age the nurse should take into consideration:
    1. Weight and length at birth
    2. Presence of a tonic neck reflex
    3. Size of breast tissue and genitalia
    4. Condition of skin on the extremities

260. When assessing a preterm infant, it is most important for the nurse to know the infant's gestational age and how it compares with the birth weight because:

1. This information will help identify potential newborn problems
2. This information must be documented on the admission record
3. The infant will lose 10% of birth weight the first few days of life
4. Evaluation and classification records are necessary for health insurance

261. After an emergency cesarean delivery a newborn, born at 35 weeks gestation, is admitted to the neonatal intensive care nursery. The neonate has a Silverman-Anderson Index of 3 which reflects a need for:
1. Continuous cardiac monitoring
2. Increased caloric intake and fluids
3. Assessment of neurologic reflexes
4. Respiratory support and observation

262. The nurse is aware that in an infant of 32 weeks gestation the:
1. Areola and nipple are barely visible
2. Palms have clearly defined creases
3. Ear pinna springs back when folded
4. Square window sign shows a 0-degree angle

263. When assessing a newly delivered neonate, the nurse notes the following findings: arms and legs slightly flexed; skin smooth and transparent; abundant lanugo on the back; slow recoil of pinna; and few sole creases. In light of these findings the care plan for this neonate should include nursing orders to monitor for:
1. Polycythemia
2. Hyperglycemia
3. Postmaturity syndrome
4. Respiratory distress syndrome

264. A newborn delivered at 39 weeks gestation weighing 2450 g (5.5 lb) would be classified as being:
1. Preterm and immature
2. Small for gestational age
3. Average for gestational age
4. Average for gestational age but preterm

265. A small for gestational age (SGA) newborn, who has just been admitted to the nursery, has a high-pitched cry, appears jittery, and has irregular respirations. The nurse is aware that these symptoms may be associated with:

1. Hypovolemia
2. Hypoglycemia
3. Hypercalcemia
4. Hypothyroidism

266. The nurse understands that oxygen concentrations for preterm infants must be carefully monitored to prevent the development of:
1. Cataracts
2. Strabismus
3. Ophthalmia neonatorum
4. Retinopathy of prematurity

267. A finding in the physical assessment of a neonate, that may indicate that the infant is preterm is:
1. Flexion of extremities
2. Many superficial veins
3. Absent femoral pulses
4. A positive Babinski reflex

268. The nurse suspects that a preterm infant may have necrotizing enterocolitis (NEC) when:
1. Circumoral pallor develops during gastric feeding
2. An increased number of explosive stools are noted
3. Several severe bouts of projectile vomiting are observed
4. Large amounts of residual formula are withdrawn before gavage

269. Nursing care for an infant with necrotizing enterocolitis includes:
1. Diluting the formula mixture as ordered
2. Measuring abdominal girth every 2 hours
3. Administering oxygen prior to gastric feeding
4. Giving $1/2$ strength formula by gavage feeding

270. Based on an assessment of 34 weeks gestation and a birth weight of 1000 g, the nurse would consider a neonate to be:
1. Term, small for gestational age (SGA)
2. Preterm, large for gestational age (LGA)
3. Term, average for gestational age (AGA)
4. Preterm, small for gestational age (SGA)

271. During the assessment of a preterm infant, the nurse determines that the infant is experiencing temperature instability. The nurse should:
    1. Rapidly rewarm the infant over the next hour until the temperature is stabilized
    2. Gradually rewarm the infant over the next several hours and monitor frequently
    3. Assess the infant for signs of hyperglycemia and begin temperature stabilization
    4. Assess and record the infant's skin temperature every hour until the temperature is stable

272. A mother delivers a male infant at 35 weeks gestation. When visiting her infant in the neonatal intensive care nursery (NICU) for the first time the mother asks, "When will I be able to breastfeed my son?" The nurse's most appropriate response would be:
    1. "Even though he is preterm, he is stable. You may try now if you would like."
    2. "Preterm infants should not breastfeed. It uses more calories than bottle feeding."
    3. "Pump your breasts now and then feed him the milk by bottle to conserve his energy."
    4. "He is preterm and sucks weakly so it will be several weeks before you may breastfeed."

273. As a client watches, the nurse does a nasogastric feeding on the client's preterm infant son who weighs 2350 g. The client asks, "Would it hurt for my baby to suck on a pacifier during the feeding?" The nurse's most appropriate response would be:
    1. "It might tire him out because he's still so small. We don't want him to use up all his energy."
    2. "If he sucks on a pacifier a lot now he may have problems learning how to suck from a bottle later."
    3. "There's no real benefit in using a pacifier and there is a relationship between the use of a pacifier and buck teeth."
    4. "Sucking on a pacifier during tube feedings may help him associate sucking with food so that he'll adjust better to bottle feedings."

274. The nurse caring for a 32 week appropriate for gestational age (AGA) neonate establishes the following list of potential interventions for the infant. The intervention that should receive the highest priority is:
    1. Promoting bonding
    2. Preventing infection
    3. Maintaining respirations
    4. Supporting body temperature

275. When an apnea monitor sounds an alarm 10 seconds after cessation of respirations, the nurse should respond first by:
    1. Assessing skin color and respirations
    2. Using tactile stimuli on chest or extremities
    3. Checking the device for signs of malfunction
    4. Resuscitating with face mask and Ambu bag

276. The nurse is aware that a preterm infant may have a potential nutritional problem because of:
    1. A poor sucking reflex
    2. A decreased metabolic rate
    3. Decreased caloric requirements
    4. Increased absorption of nutrients

277. To prevent the development of retinopathy of prematurity (retrolental fibroplasia) it would be most beneficial for the nurse to:
    1. Place a shield over the neonate's eyes
    2. Maintain low level of lighting around the neonate
    3. Assess the neonate every hour with a pulse oximeter
    4. Position the neonate in an elevated side-lying position

278. A preterm newborn is having some respiratory difficulty and is placed in an oxyhood. Nursing intervention for an infant in an oxyhood includes:
    1. Covering the infant's eyes
    2. Hydrating the infant frequently
    3. Placing a hat on the infant's head
    4. Turning the infant every two hours

279. The parents of a preterm infant are finally taking their child home. To evaluate the parent's competency level in the care of their infant it would be most effective to:
1. Ask the parents what they plan to do at home
2. Determine the rationale behind the parents' actions
3. Observe the parents in a return demonstration of care
4. Give the parents a simple test on infant care practices

280. After delivery, a large for gestational age (LGA) infant of a diabetic mother should be assessed for:
1. A blood glucose level below 45
2. An axillary temperature below 98° F
3. Elevated bilirubin levels in the first 24 hours
4. Cyanotic episodes accompanied by tremors

281. The nurse transporting a newly delivered infant with Apgar scores of 9/10 to the transition nursery reports that this delivery was difficult because the infant has wide shoulders. Based on this information, the nursery nurse's priority assessment would be to check for a normal:
1. Moro reflex
2. Plantar grasp
3. Babinski reflex
4. Stepping reflex

282. A newborn whose mother has Type I diabetes mellitus has been receiving a continuous infusion of fluids with glucose. When discontinuing the IV infusion, the nurse should:
1. Slowly decrease the rate
2. Observe for metabolic alkalosis
3. Withhold oral feedings for 4 to 6 hours
4. Check the urine for glucose every hour

283. A client developed a rubella infection during the fourth month of pregnancy. After delivery, the nursery nurse should:
1. Use enteric precautions
2. Institute blood precautions
3. Use universal precautions at all times
4. Place the baby in the isolation nursery

284. A newborn infant develops physiologic jaundice, and phototherapy is ordered to:
1. Activate the liver to dispose of the bilirubin
2. Break down the bilirubin into a conjugated form
3. Activate vitamin K to facilitate excretion of bilirubin
4. Dissolve the bilirubin and allow it to be excreted from the skin

285. When an infant is receiving phototherapy the nurse should plan to:
1. Use mineral oil on the skin to prevent excoriation
2. Cover the baby's head with a cap to minimize heat loss
3. Discontinue the therapy when feeding and hold the baby
4. Regulate radiant heat to keep the skin temperature at 99°F (37.3°C)

286. In doing a newborn assessment of a male infant after a cesarean delivery, the nurse notes that the infant's head circumference is $1\frac{1}{2}$ inches smaller than his chest. The nurse is aware that this finding:
1. Is indicative of anencephaly
2. Could indicate microcephaly
3. Commonly occurs in babies born by cesarean delivery
4. Is normal in male newborns regardless of mode of birth

287. The nurse is aware that an ABO incompatibility is most common when the mother is:
1. Type A
2. Type B
3. Type O
4. Type AB

288. The nurse understands that the effect PKU has on development will depend on:
1. Diagnosis within the first 3 days after birth
2. The level of phenylalanine in the blood at birth
3. Compliance with a corrective diet and how early it is instituted
4. The presence of phenylpyruvic acid in the urine at 1 week of age

289. The nurse is aware that the child with PKU has a characteristic urinary odor best described as:
1. Fishy
2. Ammoniacal
3. Mousy or musty
4. Aromatic or pungent

290. The nurse assesses a newborn and observes central cyanosis. Central cyanosis is indicative of congenital heart defects that affect cardiac circulation by:
1. Shunting blood right to left
2. Shunting blood left to right
3. Obstructing flow of blood from the left side of the heart
4. Preventing shunting of blood between left and right sides of the heart

291. The nurse understands that congestive heart failure is the usual sequela to congenital cardiac defects that result from left-to-right shunting of blood in the heart. With this knowledge, the nurse should be aware that a sign that would be most indicative of early onset of congestive heart failure in the infant would be:
1. Cyanosis of skin
2. Decreased heart rate
3. Increased respiratory rate
4. Liver 2 cm below costal margin

292. The newborn of a drug-addicted mother is suspected of having cytomegalovirus disease. The nurse recognizes that the infant's mother probably contracted the disease from:
1. Handling a cat litter box
2. Drinking contaminated water
3. Having sex with many partners
4. Eating improperly cooked meats

293. A mother's laboratory results indicate the presence of cocaine and alcohol. The characteristic in the baby that would indicate to the nurse that the baby has been affected by fetal alcohol syndrome would be:
1. Cleft lip
2. Polydactyly
3. Umbilical hernia
4. Small upturned nose

DRUG RELATED RESPONSES

294. The physician orders penicillin G benzathine suspension (Bicillin L-A) 2.45 million units for a client with a sexually transmitted disease. The drug is available in a multidose vial of 10 ml in which 1 ml = 300,000 units. The nurse should administer:
1. 8.8 ml
2. 8.2 ml
3. 0.8 ml
4. 0.008 ml

295. A client who is 33 weeks pregnant has contracted gonorrhea and is placed on probenecid (Benemid) and penicillin therapy. The nurse knows that the client understands the action of the drugs when she states that the probenecid will:
1. "Minimize any allergy to penicillin."
2. "Increase the penicillin in my blood."
3. "Reduce the side effects of the disease."
4. "Activate my immune defense mechanisms."

296. A pregnant client with an infection tells the nurse that she has taken tetracycline for infections on other occasions and would prefer to take it now. The nurse tells the client that tetracycline is avoided in the treatment of infection in pregnant women because it:
1. Adversely affects breastfeeding
2. Permanently stains the baby's teeth
3. Produces allergies to the drug in the baby
4. Increases the baby's tolerance to the drug

297. A client is placed on progesterone oral contraceptives (minipills) and is instructed by the nurse to take one pill daily:
1. Throughout the menstrual cycle
2. During the 5 days surrounding ovulation
3. During the first 5 days of the menstrual cycle
4. Throughout the first 21 days of the menstrual cycle

298. The nurse would know that a client taking oral contraceptives understood the teaching about the estrogen when the client indicates that the most common side effect of the estrogen would be:

1. Amenorrhea
2. Hypomenorrhea
3. Nausea and vomiting
4. Depression and lethargy

299. The nurse evaluates that a client understands the teaching about oral contraception when the client states that she will immediately cease taking the pill if she experiences:
1. Chest pain
2. Menorrhagia
3. Mittelschmerz
4. Increased leukorrhea

300. A pregnant client with iron-deficiency anemia is prescribed iron supplements daily. To increase iron absorption the nurse should suggest that the client eat foods high in:
1. Vitamin C
2. Fat content
3. Water content
4. Vitamin B complex

301. A 39-year-old who is Rh negative is seen by the physician during the first trimester of pregnancy. She has just been told that Rh sensitization is suspected. The nurse explains that Rho (D) immunoglobin (RhIg) will be given to reduce sensitization. The nurse's teaching is effective if the client understands that she will receive RhIg at:
1. 12 weeks' gestation
2. 28 weeks' gestation
3. 36 weeks' gestation
4. 40 weeks' gestation

302. The nurse should be aware that the only anticoagulant drug that a pregnant client with thrombophlebitis can safely receive is:
1. Dicumarol
2. Anisindione
3. Heparin sodium
4. Warfarin sodium

303. A pregnant client on anticoagulant therapy has blood drawn daily for activated partial thromboplastin time (APTT). One day her APTT is 98 seconds. The nurse notifies the physician because the anticoagulant should be:

1. Increased for better clotting results
2. Discontinued because the APTT is normal
3. Changed to one of the other effective anticoagulants
4. Omitted for today and the APTT should be rechecked tomorrow

304. To halt preterm labor a client is started on terbutaline (Brethine). The nurse is aware that a side effect of this drug is:
1. Bradycardia
2. Hypertension
3. Difficulty falling asleep
4. Hypertonic uterine contractions

305. When counseling a pregnant client with an iron deficiency the nurse teaches that iron use is more efficient if the prescribed iron supplement is taken:
1. At bedtime
2. At mealtime
3. With a milkshake
4. With orange juice

306. The physician orders meperidine hydrochloride (Demerol) and promethazine (Phenergan) prn for a client in active labor. The client asks why she is getting Phenergan. The nurse explains that this drug:
1. Initiates the analgesic effects of Demerol
2. Reverses the analgesic effects of Demerol
3. Decreases the analgesic effects of Demerol
4. Potentiates the analgesic effects of Demerol

307. A client has a paracervical block for delivery. Aware of the risk most often associated with administration of paracervical block, the nurse should observe for:
1. Fetal bradycardia
2. Maternal hypertension
3. Maternal respiratory paralysis
4. Aspiration of stomach contents

308. A client is to receive oxytocin (Pitocin) to augment labor. The physician's order states: add 10 units of Pitocin to 1000 ml of D5W and administer 0.01 units per minute. The IV set has a drop factor of 60 gtt/ml. To administer the correct amount of medication the nurse should set the flow rate at:
1. 20 gtt/min
2. 40 gtt/min
3. 60 gtt/min
4. 80 gtt/min

309. When a client is receiving Pitocin, the nurse, aware of the adverse effects of this oxytocic drug, should carefully observe the client for:
1. Intrauterine pressure of 60 mmHg
2. Contractions with a duration of 30 seconds
3. A fetal heart rate of 120 to 150 beats per minute
4. Contractions occurring more frequently than every 2 minutes

310. An adverse reaction from prolonged Pitocin administration for which a client in labor must be closely monitored is:
1. Hyperventilation
2. A change in affect
3. Water intoxication
4. An elevated temperature

311. A client, with severe preeclampsia, is receiving large doses of IV magnesium sulfate. To evaluate the effectiveness of this therapy, the nurse should assess for:
1. Increased urinary output
2. A decreased respiratory rate
3. Absent deep tendon reflexes
4. An increase in blood pressure

312. The nurse understands that when giving magnesium sulfate to clients with pregnancy-induced hypertension it can build to toxic levels. The nurse should withhold the drug and notify the physician if an assessment of the client revealed:
1. A BP of 140/100
2. Respirations of 12/min
3. A urinary output of 30 ml/hr
4. Deep tendon reflexes of plus 2

313. A client with severe preeclampsia who has a BP of 170/110, a pulse of 108, and respirations of 24 is placed on IV magnesium sulfate therapy. Eight hours later her BP is 150/110, the pulse is 98, and respirations are 14, and there is absence of the knee jerk reflex. The nurse should:
1. Eliminate the next dose of magnesium sulfate and notify the physician
2. Administer calcium gluconate as an antidote for the magnesium sulfate
3. Administer the next dose of magnesium sulfate because the blood pressure is still high
4. Wait 1 hour, monitor the vital signs and reflexes again, and then administer the next dose

314. A client with preeclampsia who is receiving magnesium sulfate (MgSO$_4$) is showing signs of magnesium sulfate toxicity. The nurse is aware these signs can be reversed by the administration of:
1. Edetate disodium (EDTA)
2. Calcium gluconate (Kalcinate)
3. Hydralazine hydrochloride (Apresoline)
4. Sodium polystyrene sulfonate (Kayexalate)

315. Before giving medications to a client who is 6 hours postpartum, the nurse assesses the client and notes the following findings: BP 178/110; TPR 98/60/18; fundus firm, one finger below umbilicus; episiotomy edematous, red, and approximated; and one Peri-pad saturated with lochia rubra in 6 hours. In light of these assessment findings the nurse should contact the physician before administering:
1. Cephradine (Velosef)
2. Hydrocortisone acetate (Epifoam)
3. Methylergonovine maleate (Methergine)
4. Casanthranol and docusate sodium (Peri-Colace)

316. Twelve hours postpartum, the nurse prepares to administer the client's medications and ascertains that the client is allergic to penicillin. Until contact with the client's physician is made, the nurse should withhold the prescribed:

1. Cephradine (Velosef)
2. Bromocriptine mesylate (Parlodel)
3. Methylergonovine maleate (Methergine)
4. Casanthranol and docusate sodium (Peri-Colace)

317. The nurse understands that a drug that is contraindicated for a woman who is breast-feeding would be:
1. Heparin
2. Propylthiouracil (PTU)
3. Gentamicin (Garamycin)
4. Diphenhydramine (Benadryl)

318. The nurse should withhold methylergonovine maleate (Methergine) from a postpartum client if the client is found to have a:
1. Positive Homans' sign
2. Negative Babinski reflex
3. Blood pressure of 160/90
4. Respiratory rate of 12 per minute

319. A client indicates correct understanding of postpartum discharge instructions when stating that she will take her iron supplements with:
1. Milk
2. Water
3. Each meal
4. Orange juice

320. A preterm infant is started on digoxin (Lanoxin) and furosemide (Lasix) for persistent patent ductus arteriosus. The nursing assessment that would provide the best indication that the Lasix is effective is that the:
1. Pedal edema is reduced
2. Fontanels appear depressed
3. Urine output exceeds fluid intake
4. Drug has not precipitated digitalis toxicity

EMOTIONAL NEEDS RELATED TO CHILDBEARING

321. A client comes to the infertility clinic for a work up and is told by the nurse to prepare for a Papanicolaou test. The client states, "I do not want this test. I want to speak to the doctor." The nurse should:

1. Recognize that the client is uncooperative
2. Inform the physician of the client's request
3. Encourage the client to comply with clinic procedures
4. Remind the client of the importance of cancer detection

322. A client in the infertility clinic is being treated for hypertension and obesity with a regimen of diet and exercise. During the past month she has lost 8 pounds and her blood pressure has gone down to 154/98. The client states that she is using self-control strategies to reduce her blood pressure and weight. The nurse should:
1. Acknowledge the client's achievement and encourage the continuation of the client's action program
2. Emphasize the importance of the client's exercising in addition to the reduction of sodium and calories
3. Encourage the client to take antihypertensive drugs until her blood pressure is reduced to normal limits
4. Point out to the client that her action program is inadequate, because her blood pressure remains abnormal

323. A client with preeclampsia is told that she must remain on bedrest at home. The client starts to cry and tells the nurse that she has two small children at home who need her. The nurse's best response would be:
1. "You'll need someone to care for the children."
2. "You are worried about how you will be able to manage."
3. "You can get a neighbor to help out, and your husband can do the housework in the evening."
4. "You'll be able to fix light meals, and the children can go to nursery school a few hours each day."

324. The best nursing intervention to achieve cooperation of an extremely anxious client during her first pelvic examination to confirm pregnancy would be to:
1. Assist the physician so that the examination can be finished quickly
2. Distract the client by asking her preference as to the sex of the child
3. Maintain eye contact, touch gently, and thoroughly explain the procedure
4. Encourage the client to close her eyes and hold her breath during the examination

325. A client whose first baby died from SIDS asks the nurse if the risk of having another infant die from SIDS is increased with subsequent pregnancies. The nurse should inform the client that a subsequent sibling of a SIDS infant is at:
1. No particular risk for the development of SIDS
2. Lower risk for SIDS than is the general population
3. Greater risk for SIDS than is the general population
4. The same risk for SIDS as is the general population

326. A pregnant client, whose first child has Down syndrome, is about to undergo an amniocentesis. The client tells the nurse that she does not know what she will do if this baby has the same diagnosis. The client asks the nurse, "Do you think abortion is the same as killing?" The nurse's best response would be:
1. "Some people think this is what an abortion is."
2. "No, I don't think so, but its your decision to make."
3. "I really can't answer that question. You seem ambivalent about abortion."
4. "I don't want to answer that question at this time. How do you feel about it?"

327. A client who has just delivered an infant with Down syndrome tells the nurse that she could not possibly take a retarded child home and asks if she should plan to place the child in an institution. An appropriate statement by the nurse at this time would be:

1. "I understand how you feel, and I will notify the nursery personnel of your decision."
2. "At this young age no one is able to predict your baby's ultimate level of functioning."
3. "Give yourself time to get acquainted and you will see that your baby isn't retarded yet."
4. "You should not make such a hasty decision, as your baby is like any other baby right now."

328. A client with severe pregnancy-induced hypertension (PIH), who has been admitted to the hospital, anxiously asks the nurse, "Will my baby be all right?" The nurse's most appropriate response would be:
1. "There is no way of telling at this time what the outcome will be."
2. "The baby will probably be all right; it's protected by the amniotic fluid."
3. "If you do what the doctor tells you to do, everything will progress normally."
4. "We will be constantly monitoring your baby's condition. Would you like to listen to the baby's heart beat?"

329. An infant born in a birthing center is experiencing respiratory distress and is being transferred to a regional neonatal intensive care unit. The nursing action that would best promote parent-infant attachment would be:
1. Encouraging the parents to call their infant by name
2. Allowing the parents to hold their infant before departure
3. Giving the parents a picture of their infant in the intensive care unit
4. Instructing the parents to phone the neonatal intensive care unit daily

330. The nurse should be aware of the stages of parental adjustment that follow delivery of an infant at risk who is in the neonatal intensive care unit. To better plan nursing care, nursing observations and assessments should be based on the recognition that the:

1. Mother should not see the infant until she has completed the necessary grief work
2. Parents should be encouraged to visit the newborn within the first 24 hours after birth
3. Mother should be reunited with her infant as soon as possible to enhance adjustment
4. Nurse should wait until the parents request to see the newborn before suggesting a visit

331. After being shown to the parents, a preterm male infant weighing 1500 g (3 lb 15 oz) is moved to the neonatal intensive care nursery. The nurse should plan to:
1. Ask the physician's permission to have the mother see her infant
2. Take the mother to the NICU to see the infant as soon as possible
3. Discourage the mother's involvement with the infant until the prognosis is favorable
4. Find out the condition of the infant and take the mother to see him if the infant is doing well

332. On her first visit to the neonatal intensive care unit to see her preterm newborn daughter, the mother stands 2 feet way and does not touch the infant. The mother's only comment to the nurse is, "She looks so fragile. Do you think she'll make it?" The most appropriate comment for the nurse to make would be:
1. "The staff is confident because all preterm babies look like this at first."
2. "The baby is small, but many infants born as small as she is have done just fine."
3. "I can understand that she looks fragile to you. What did the physician tell you about her condition?"
4. "She's not as fragile as she might appear. You need to get used to her and then it won't be so frightening."

333. When first seeing her preterm infant in the neonatal intensive care unit (NICU), the mother immediately starts to cry and refuses to touch the baby. The nurse understands that this behavior represents:

1. A normal detachment behavior
2. An incomplete bonding behavior
3. A normal reaction to the situation
4. A reaction to the NICU environment

334. While watching her preterm infant son in the neonatal intensive care unit, a mother exclaims, "My baby is so little. How will I ever care for him?" The nurse should explain to the mother that she:
1. Can watch his care to assist her in becoming familiar with the specific routines
2. Will be able to care for him in a special nursery for a few days prior to his discharge
3. Should find someone with training in preterm care to help her at home the first week
4. Will be encouraged to participate in his care as much as possible from the beginning

335. The nurse observes a newly delivered client's behavior but cannot decide whether the client is anxious about her baby or experiencing postpartum depression. The client's behaviors that would clarify this confusion for the nurse would be:
1. Decreased appetite, crying, and insomnia
2. Long periods of sleep, lethargy, and anorexia
3. Ambivalence, lethargy, and increased appetite
4. Increased appetite, insomnia, and ambivalence

336. A client, who has participated in caring for her infant in the neonatal intensive care unit for several days in preparation for the baby's discharge, comes to the unit on the last hospital day with alcohol on her breath and slurred speech. The nurse's most appropriate action would be to:
1. Talk with the mother about her condition and assess her willingness to participate in an alternate plan for discharge
2. Speak openly to the mother about her condition and have her see a social worker about discharge to a foster home
3. Continue with the discharge procedure alerting the home health nurse that immediate follow up is needed for the mother
4. Avoid confrontation by asking the mother to wait in the hospital lobby and calling the physician to cancel the discharge order

337. Before an amniocentesis both parents express nervousness about the fetus' safety during the test. The nursing intervention that would best promote the parents' ability to cope is:
1. Initiating a parent-physician conference
2. Reassuring them that the procedure is safe
3. Informing them about the procedure step by step
4. Arranging for the father to be present during the test

338. During preterm labor, a client tells the nurse that she and her husband are very concerned because the baby is coming a whole month early. The nurse's best response would be:
1. "I don't blame you for worrying; there is some danger."
2. "Your physician is very good; try not to worry about it now."
3. "I can understand why you and your husband are so worried."
4. "Don't worry; the care of preterm babies has greatly improved."

339. A neonate born at 32 weeks gestation and weighing 3 pounds is admitted to the neonatal intensive care nursery. The nurse plans to take the neonate's mother to visit the infant in the intensive care unit:
1. As soon as the mother feels up to it
2. When the infant's condition has stabilized
3. When the infant is out of immediate danger
4. After the physician writes an order permitting it

340. The mother of an infant in the neonatal intensive care nursery expresses concern about her infant. To best facilitate mother-infant bonding the nurse should:
1. Assure the mother that her baby will be fine
2. Have the mother stroke the baby whenever possible
3. Avoid discussing negative aspects of the baby's condition
4. Encourage the mother to let the nursing staff care for the baby

341. A common concern of the mother after an unexpected cesarean delivery that the nurse should anticipate is the:

1. Postoperative pain and scarring
2. Prolonged period of hospitalization
3. Inability to assume her mothering role
4. Sense of failure in the birthing process

342. After an unexpected emergency cesarean delivery, the client tells the nurse that she is a "natural childbirth flunkie." The postpartal phase of adjustment that this statement most closely typifies is:
1. Taking in
2. Letting go
3. Taking hold
4. Working through

343. A client who has just had her second child wishes to breastfeed. When the nurse brings the baby to be breastfed, the mother asks if she may drink a small glass of wine to help her relax. The nurse's best response would be:
1. "I'm sure that drinking one glass of wine would not cause any harm."
2. "Yes it's relaxing, but I do think you should find another, better way to relax."
3. "You seem a little tense. Tell me about your past breastfeeding experiences."
4. "I'm sure a glass of wine would be okay, but you had better check with your doctor."

344. On the first postpartum day, a client who is rooming in asks the nurse to return her baby to the nursery and bring the baby to her only at feeding time. The best response by the nurse would be:
1. "I think you are having difficulties caring for the baby."
2. "All right, I will inform the other nurses of your decision."
3. "It seems like you have changed your mind about rooming in."
4. "Oh, you must be tired. I'll bring the baby back at feeding time."

345. The nurse is aware that babies born to very young mothers are at risk for neglect or abuse because adolescents characteristically:
1. Do not plan for their pregnancies
2. Cannot anticipate the baby's needs
3. Are involved in seeking their own identity
4. Resent having to give constant care to the baby

346. The parents of a male newborn ask the nurse whether they should have their son circumcised. The nurse's most appropriate response would be:
1. "It would probably be a good idea because circumcision is known to prevent penile cancer."
2. "That's something you both will have to decide after you discuss it thoroughly with your doctor."
3. "I'm sure you have discussed this with your doctor, but let's discuss the benefits and risks of circumcision"
4. "The Academy of Pediatrics recommends that circumcision not be done routinely because of the risks associated with the procedure."

347. A mother of an infant begins to cry as she readies her infant for discharge from a neonatal intensive care unit. She says to the nurse, "I know I should not be crying but I have to work. I know my baby will suffer in a day-care center without me." The best response by the nurse would be:
1. "Children fare better when taken to a sitter's home for care."
2. "Motor development is advanced in children attending day-care centers."
3. "Only a few children suffer mentally from being placed in a high-quality day-care center."
4. "No ill effects have been noted when children are placed in high-quality day-care centers."

REPRODUCTIVE CHOICES

348. A client, 16 weeks gestation, is being treated for Trichomonas vaginitis. The statement that best indicates to the nurse that the client has learned measures to prevent recurrence is, "I will:
1. Void immediately after intercourse."
2. Persuade my sexual partner to be treated."
3. Insert a vaginal suppository after intercourse."
4. Douche immediately after having sexual intercourse."

349. A client, admitted for surgery for an ectopic pregnancy, asks the nurse why she has shoulder pain. The nurse would base a response on the fact that the pain is caused by:
1. Anxiety about the diagnosis
2. Cardiac changes from hypovolemia
3. Blood accumulation under the diaphragm
4. Rebound tenderness from the ruptured tube

350. The most appropriate nursing diagnosis for a client with a ruptured ectopic pregnancy would be:
1. Fluid volume excess
2. High risk for infection
3. Decreased cardiac output
4. Altered health maintenance

351. A 17-year-old client tells the nurse that her sister had a tubal pregnancy about 3 months ago and had to have her tube removed. The nurse knows that this young woman needs further explanation when she states:
1. "This kind of thing can happen to my sister again."
2. "I guess I'll have to wait awhile to become an aunt."
3. "This kind of thing can happen after a pelvic infection."
4. "My sister is lucky because she'll never have a period again."

352. After 5 years of unprotected intercourse, a childless couple comes to the infertility clinic. The husband tells the nurse that his parents have promised to make a down payment on a house for them if his wife gets pregnant this year. The nurse's best response to this comment would be:
1. "How do the two of you feel about having a baby?"
2. "You're lucky; I wish someone would give me a down payment for a house."
3. "Five years without a pregnancy is a long time. Do you think there is something wrong with both of you?"
4. "You know, you don't have to worry about satisfying your parents. Having a child should be a decision you make."

353. A 37-year-old female comes to the gynecology clinic with a history of being unable to conceive after 4 years of unprotected intercourse. The client complains of recurring headaches with pain radiating down the neck. The physical examination reveals a blood pressure of 170/100. The client is advised to limit salt intake and take her basal temperature for 3 months. The health professionals are:
    1. Not helping the client
    2. Avoiding the major problem
    3. Overlooking the hypertension
    4. Encouraging self-responsibility

354. A client comes to the infertility clinic for a carbon dioxide insufflation test to determine if her Fallopian tubes are patent. As part of the teaching before the test the nurse tells the client:
    1. "You will receive a local anesthetic to lessen the pain of the test."
    2. "You will have to rest in bed for 8 hours after the test is completed."
    3. "You may have some persistent shoulder pain for 24 hours after the test."
    4. "You may become nauseated during the test but the nausea will subside."

355. Because an infertility workup involves both partners, a male client is to have a semen analysis. As part of his instructions the nurse should tell him to:
    1. Use a condom to collect the semen specimen
    2. Make sure that the specimen is collected as soon as he awakens
    3. Ejaculate 2 to 3 days before collection to ensure a pure specimen
    4. Refrigerate the specimen until it can be delivered to the laboratory

356. On a return visit to the infertility clinic a client whose temperature charts demonstrate an ovulatory pattern and a normal menstrual cycle despite an inability to become pregnant requests fertility drugs. The nurse should recognize that the client:
    1. Has a right to receive this drug
    2. Will require an endometrial biopsy
    3. Has to be scheduled for a culdoscopy
    4. Needs to bring her husband's semen in to be examined

357. A client who is to have a uterine aspiration abortion at 10 weeks gestation should be told that:
    1. A general anesthetic will be used to insert the laminaria tent
    2. The uterine lining will be scraped after removal of the laminaria
    3. The laminaria tent will have to be retained in the cervical canal for 4 to 24 hours
    4. An increased amount of bleeding will be present for 3 to 5 hours after the abortion

358. After a first-trimester aspiration abortion, the nurse knows that the instructions are understood when the client states:
    1. "I will be able to resume intercourse in 4 to 5 days."
    2. "After 24 hours I can substitute tampons for sanitary pads."
    3. "I can expect my menstrual period to resume in 2 to 3 weeks."
    4. "I will call the physician if I must change my sanitary pad more than once in 4 hours."

WOMEN'S HEALTH

359. When reviewing the role of hormones in the reproductive process, the nurse recalls that the corpus luteum secretes:
    1. Cortisol
    2. Prolactin
    3. Oxytocin
    4. Progesterone

360. When discussing immunity with a prenatal client during her first visit to the prenatal clinic, the nurse recalls that active immunity occurs when:
    1. Protein antigens are formed in the blood to fight invading antibodies
    2. Protein substances are formed by the body to destroy or neutralize antigens
    3. Blood antigens are aided by phagocytes in defending the body against pathogens
    4. Sensitized lymphocytes from an immune donor act as antibodies against invading pathogens

361. A 13-year-old client whose menses began 2 years ago complains of having some mild upper abdominal pain between each period. The nurse explains that this:

1. Requires immediate medical attention
2. Usually occurs when menses first begin
3. Will disappear when ovulation is well established
4. Is a common occurrence known as mittelschmerz

362. A young client tells the nurse that her mother complains about having dysmenorrhea and asks the nurse what this means. The nurse can best describe dysmenorrhea as:
1. Cessation of menstruation
2. Abnormal vaginal bleeding
3. Uterine pain with menstruation
4. Spotting between menstrual periods

363. A 35-year-old woman is admitted to the hospital complaining of polyuria and pain and burning when urinating. Her medical diagnosis is a urinary tract infection. When assisting this client it is important to:
1. Have her void every two hours
2. Select the appropriate type bedpan for voiding
3. Pour warm water over her vulva when she voids
4. Teach her to wash her hands before and after voiding

364. A client is to receive a tuberculin test as part of her prenatal workup. Before administering the test, the most important information for the the nurse to collect is whether or not the client has:
1. Previously had a tuberculin test
2. Ever had a positive tuberculin test
3. A history of tuberculosis in the family
4. Had any serious respiratory diseases

365. A pregnant client asks the nurse for information about toxoplasmosis during pregnancy. The nurse teaches the client that:
1. Pork and beef should be properly cooked before eating
2. Toxoplasmosis is a disease that is prevalent just in foreign countries
3. Eating salads with mayonnaise should be avoided during the summer
4. Raw shellfish are intermediary hosts and should be avoided during pregnancy

366. A client, age 16, has a steady boyfriend and is having sexual relations with him. She is seeking advice as to how she can protect herself from contracting AIDS. The nurse advises her to:
1. Have her partner withdraw before ejaculating
2. Make certain their relationship is monogamous
3. Have her partner use a condom during sexual activity
4. Seek counseling about various contraceptive methods

367. When assessing a female client who is suspected of having early syphilis, the nurse should expect the client to exhibit the early symptom of:
1. Flat wart-like plaques around the vagina and anus
2. An indurated painless nodule on the vulva that begins to drain
3. Glistening patches in the mouth covered with a yellow exudate
4. A maculopapular rash on the palms of the hands and soles of the feet

368. A client who has been diagnosed as having syphilis tells the nurse that it must have been contracted from a toilet seat. The nurse knows that this cannot be true because the causative agent of syphilis is:
1. Immobilized by body contact
2. Chelated by wood and plastic
3. Destroyed by warmth and moisture
4. Inactivated when exposed to dryness

369. The major body system affected in tertiary syphilis is the:
1. Reproductive
2. Integumentary
3. Cardiovascular
4. Lower respiratory

370. To perform breast self-examination correctly, a premenopausal female should be examining her breasts:
1. When she ovulates
2. The first of every month
3. The day her menses begins
4. Three days after her menses ends

371. When performing breast self-examination a client should be:
    1. Squeezing the nipples to check for discharge
    2. Using the right hand to examine the right breast
    3. Placing a pillow under the shoulder opposite the side being examined
    4. Pressing the palm of the hand against the breast to compress it to the chest wall

372. A 26-year-old female, whose sister recently had a mastectomy, calls the local women's health center for an appointment for a mammography. To prepare for the test, the nurse should teach the client that:
    1. The room will be darkened throughout the procedure
    2. Each breast will be firmly compressed between 2 plates
    3. Food and fluid must be avoided for 6 hours before the test
    4. She does not need a mammography until she is 50 years old

373. A client is scheduled for a modified radical mastectomy for an adenocarcinoma of the right breast. It would be inappropriate for the nurse developing the client's preoperative teaching plan to include:

    1. Allowing the client time to ventilate her feelings
    2. Urging the client to have immediate reconstructive surgery
    3. Explaining the dressings and drains that the client will have after surgery
    4. Teaching the client the postoperative pulmonary routines that will be followed

374. After a mastectomy or hysterectomy many clients feel incomplete as women. The statement that should alert the nurse to this feeling in a client following a total hysterectomy would be:
    1. "I can't wait to see all my friends again."
    2. "I feel washed out; there isn't much left."
    3. "I can't wait to get home to see my grandchild."
    4. "My husband plans for me to recuperate at our daughter's home."

375. The nurse's history and physical assessment reveal that a client has previously received estrogen replacement therapy as a treatment for osteoporosis. The nurse should recognize that the client has an increased risk of developing:
    1. Endometrial cancer
    2. Accelerated bone loss
    3. Vaginal tissue atrophy
    4. A myocardial infarction

Answers and Rationales for Childbearing and Women's Health Nursing Questions

REPRODUCTIVE CHOICES

1. 1 Unless the condom is held, it can be displaced, allowing the sperm to enter the vagina. (2) (CW; IM; ED; RC)

2 Spermicidal cream is needed because the diaphragm may be displaced in some positions.

3 This is not true; sperm can be deposited at the beginning of intercourse without the man's knowledge.

4 When the woman has a rise in her basal temperature, she is most fertile and should avoid intercourse.

2. 3 Oral contraceptives may cause hypertension and place the client at risk for the development of a CVA. (2) (CW; AS; TC; RC)

1 Oral contraceptives are contraindicated in women older than age 40 because of an increased risk of myocardial infarction.

2 Clients should be strongly cautioned about smoking even 15 cigarettes a day.

4 There is no relationship between oral contraceptives and multiple births.

3. 4 Headaches, either sudden or persistent, may indicate hypertension or a cardiovascular event; visual disorders, such as partial or complete loss of vision or double vision, may indicate neuroocular lesions which are associated with the use of oral contraceptives. (2) (CW; IM; TC; RC)

1 These are expected side effects and the client may need an adjustment in the dose or have to change to another product; these are not among the reportable symptoms.

2 While there is controversy over the contribution of oral contraceptives to the development of breast cancer, the presence of breast pain, which may occur, is not a sign of this disorder and is not reportable; weight gain, not loss, occurs because of edema.

3 Hypotension and amenorrhea do not occur; hypertension may occur with oral contraceptives and subsides when they are discontinued.

4. 3 This is the preferred method for clients with diabetes because it has no physiologic side effects. (1) (CW; IM; ED; RC)

1 This requires a great deal of self-control and a strong desire to avoid pregnancy, and it is not as effective as a diaphragm.

2 Because of the possibility of perforation, this method increases the risk of infection for diabetic women.

4 Oral contraceptives have a diabetogenic effect; they alter carbohydrate metabolism, and insulin dosage must be adjusted.

5. 4 The diaphragm holds the spermicide against the cervix for the length of time it takes to kill the sperm; the diaphragm may be placed ahead of time but additional spermicide should be added before repeated intercourse. (2) (CW; IM; ED; RC)

1 The diaphragm must always be used with a spermicide to be effective.

2 The diaphragm may be inserted with the dome facing either up or down and still be effective.

3 Puckering, especially near the rim, could indicate thin spots which could rupture during intercourse; the diaphragm should not be used if puckering is noted.

6. 3 In a normal, regular cycle, ovulation occurs 2 weeks (14 days) before the onset of the next menses. (1) (CW; IM; ED; RC)

1 This would occur in a woman who menstruates every 28 days.

2 This is too early in the cycle; ovulation generally occurs 14 days before the onset of the next menses.

4 This is just the first week of the cycle; ovulation usually occurs 14 days before the onset of the next menses.

7.   2   The fertile period is determined by subtracting 18 days from the length of the shortest cycle to determine the first unsafe day and subtracting 11 days from the length of the longest cycle to determine the last unsafe day. (2) (CW; EV; ED; RC)

   1   This is how the last day, not the first day, of the unsafe period is determined.

   3   This is only true if the shortest cycle is 28 days; the date is dependent upon a calculation based on the length of the woman's shortest and longest cycles.

   4   This is incorrect; the longest and shortest cycles are used, not the average length of a cycle.

8.   1   The IUD may cause irritability of the myometrium, inducing uterine contractions and expulsion of the device; the presence of the IUD thread should be verified both before menstruation and coitus. (2) (CW; IM; ED; RC)

   2   It is not common to have discomfort during coitus with an IUD in place; it is one of the warning signs that should be reported.

   3   This is a rare, rather than a common, occurrence.

   4   The incidence of vaginal infections is not increased with the use of an IUD; also, the risk of pelvic inflammatory disease is not increased if there is only one sexual partner.

9.   4   This is the most common side effect of the implantation of non-biodegradable Silastic capsules containing Progestin. (2) (CW; IM; ED; RC)

   1   Although this is a side effect, it is less common than irregular menstrual bleeding.

   2   This may occur with some types of contraceptives that contain estrogen, not progestin.

   3   This is a side effect of estrogen excess; this product contains progestin, not estrogen.

10.   4   This is true; some women find it emotionally unnerving to handle their genitals and discharges. (2) (CW; AN; PS; EC)

   1   The data do not support this conclusion.

   2   Same as answer 1.

   3   Same as answer 1.

HEALTHY CHILDBEARING

11.   1   Add 7 days to the beginning of the last menstrual period and subtract 3 months. (2) (CW; AN; PA; HC)

   2   This is an incorrect calculation; this is too late.

   3   This is an incorrect calculation; this is too early.

   4   Same as answer 3.

12.   2   Development proceeds in a cephalic to caudal progression. (1) (CW; AN; PA; HC)

   1   Both sides of the brain develop at the same time; which side of the brain becomes dominant develops later.

   3   Development proceeds in a cephalic to caudal progression, not caudal to cephalic.

   4   Both sides of the brain develop and begin functioning at the same time.

13.   3   Auscultation of the fetal heart is a positive sign of pregnancy. (1) (CW; AS; PA; HC)

   1   The feeling of movement is a presumptive sign of pregnancy.

   2   The bluish color of the cervix caused by pelvic congestion and edema is a probable sign of pregnancy.

   4   The presence of chorionic gonadotropin in the urine is a probable sign of pregnancy.

14.   4   Increased levels of HCG may cause nausea and vomiting, but the exact reason for this is unknown. (1) (CW; AN; PA; HC)

   1   Some women do not experience nausea and vomiting.

   2   Lightening occurs at the end of the third trimester; nausea and vomiting usually cease at the end of the first trimester.

   3   Nausea and vomiting are unrelated to whether or not the pregnancy is planned or desired.

15.   3   There is reduced GI motility during pregnancy because of the high level of placental progesterone and displacement of the stomach superiorly and the intestines laterally and posteriorly. (3) (CW; AN; PA; HC)

   1   The glomerular filtration rate increases during pregnancy.

   2   This is unrelated to the absorption of drugs.

   4   HCl secretion decreases during pregnancy.

16. 1 This amount is recommended by the Food and Nutrition Board of the National Academy of Sciences. (1) (CW; IM; ED; HC)
2 This is more than the recommended requirement; an increase of 15 g is recommended.
3 Same as answer 2.
4 Same as answer 2.

17. 3 Often there is a decrease in sexual desire in the first trimester, probably related to nausea and vomiting; if couples are informed about this, they are less likely to become distressed. (2) (CW; IM; ED; HC)
1 Calling the situation a problem may cause further anxiety in the client.
2 The client is asking the nurse for information; the client may be unable to answer this question.
4 This does not tell the client why this feeling is occurring; this provides false reassurance.

18. 4 Fasting results in hypoglycemia, which can cause nausea; in addition, the developing fetus should not be deprived of nutrients for any length of time. (2) (CW; PL; ED; HC)
1 Fluids need not be increased but should be consumed between meals.
2 Calcium intake will not change the nausea.
3 This intake would not be sufficient to meet the normal nutritional needs of the mother and fetus.

19. 4 The recommended weight gain is 25 to 30 pounds for a woman who was of average weight for her height before pregnancy. (1) (CW; AN; PA; HC)
1 This is below the recommended weight gain for a woman who was of average weight for her height before pregnancy.
2 Same as answer 1.
3 Same as answer 1.

20. 4 The fetal heartbeat can be heard with an electronic doppler between 10 and 12 weeks gestation; a fetoscope cannot pick up the fetal heartbeat before the seventeenth week. (1) (CW; IM; ED; HC)

1 This is too early for the heartbeat to be heard with a fetoscope.
2 Same as answer 1.
3 This is late; the fetal heart can be first heard with an electronic doppler between 10 to 12 weeks.

21. 4 Because the cervical os is closed, tub bathing cannot cause an ascending infection and may be continued until the onset of labor. (2) (CW; IM; ED; HC)
1 This is untrue; infection may occur only if the cervical os is open and the bathtub is dirty.
2 Tub bathing is permitted throughout pregnancy, usually until the onset of labor when the cervical os begins to open.
3 Same as answer 2.

22. 3 During pregnancy the need for water is increased; it is related to the increased metabolic rate and expanded blood volume; there is no indication of urinary infection. (1) (CW; PL; TC; HC)
1 Fluids must be increased, not decreased.
2 This is unnecessary; there is no indication of urinary infection.
4 The bladder needs to be emptied frequently to prevent urinary stasis and potential ascending infection into the kidneys.

23. 2 The issue of pregnancy is resolved by this time; more awareness of the fetus as a person and the body changes of pregnancy lead to a desire to learn about fetal growth, body changes, and nutrition. (2) (CW; IM; ED; HC)
1 This information would be appropriate for the last trimester.
3 This information would be appropriate for the first trimester.
4 Same as answer 1.

24. 1 Twins should be suspected with a more rapid increase in fundal height than normal; the nurse should assess for two distinct heartbeats. (3) (CW; AS; PA; HP)

2 Fundal height, not the size of the baby, should lead the nurse to suspect a multiple pregnancy.

3 This cannot be determined until an ultrasound is done.

4 Weight gain will not influence the height of the fundus; a multiple pregnancy is more likely the factor.

25. 3 The funic souffle is blood rushing through the fetal umbilical cord and is therefore the same rate as the fetal heart rate. (3) (CW; AN; PA; HC)

1 Twins would have different heart rates.

2 The maternal heart rate should be much slower than the fetal heart rate.

4 The uterine souffle is blood moving through the maternal side of the placenta and is the same as the mother's heart rate; the maternal heart rate should be less than 100.

26. 4 This provides the opportunity for an evaluation of the client's food intake. (2) (CW; AS; TC; HC)

1 This may prevent further exploration of the diet because the client may answer yes or no.

2 Same as answer 1.

3 This assumes the client is not eating properly.

27. 3 Pelvic rocking exercises in which the lower back can be pressed onto the floor by contracting the abdominal muscles reduce back pain. (3) (CW; EV; PA; HC)

1 Leg lifts help to strengthen the abdominal muscles and promote circulation in the lower extremities.

2 Tailor sitting stretches the muscles of the inner thighs and tones the muscles of the outer thighs.

4 Kegel exercises are used to tone pelvic floor muscles.

28. 3 This is the time when the fetus is laying down fat deposits and gaining the most weight. (2) (CW; IM; ED; HC)

1 There is weight gain throughout pregnancy, but it is most marked in the third trimester.

2 There is little weight gain during this period of organ development.

4 Same as answer 1.

29. 3 Nägele's rule takes the first day of the last menstrual period, subtracts 3 months, and then adds 7 days. (1) (CW; AN; PA; HC)

1 This would be one month too early.

2 This would be one week too early.

4 This would be too late.

30. 4 This is the content of childbirth classes to adequately prepare parents for childbirth. (2) (CW; IM; ED; HC)

1 This is only part of the class content.

2 This is not an absolute; most childbirth methods inform parents that drugs are available if necessary.

3 Same as answer 1.

31. 2 There is much to be learned and practiced so that the client can vary the techniques through the stages of labor. (3) (CW; IM; ED; HC)

1 The Read method can be quickly taught to an "unprepared" woman in labor.

3 This is untrue, because small amounts of medication can be used if required.

4 The Read method focuses on naturalness and denial of pain.

32. 4 Effleurage is gentle massage of the abdomen. (1) (CW; EV; ED; HC)

1 This is the pelvic rock; it is used during pregnancy to relieve backache.

2 This is a technique of breathing.

3 Same as answer 2.

33. 4 Kegel exercises develop and strengthen the pubococcygeal muscle; they are done through repeated contractions of the perineum. (3) (CW; EV; ED; HC)

1 Tailor sitting aids in relaxing the muscles of the pelvic floor.

2 This is effective in relieving backaches.

3 Same as answer 2.

34. 3 Conception occurs when one sperm penetrates one ovum and creates a viable zygote. (1) (CW; AN; ED; RC)

1 A high sperm count is optimum, but only one sperm is needed to penetrate the ovum.

2 Conception takes place in a fallopian tube, not the uterus.

4 The sperm penetrates the ovum in a fallopian tube and then the impregnated ovum travels down the tube to the uterus.

35. 2 The amniotic fluid is a protective environment; the fetus depends on the placenta, along with the umbilical blood vessels, for obtaining nutrients and oxygen. (2) (CW; EV; ED; HC)

1 This is a true statement and would not require further teaching.

3 Same as answer 1.

4 Same as answer 1.

36. 1 Fatigue will influence the successful use of other coping strategies such as distraction; this may lead to the client's requiring pain medication. (2) (CW; IM; ED; HC)

2 Progesterone is decreased at this time.

3 Energy will enhance the quality of contractions.

4 The client does not push during the first stage of labor; pushing is done during the second stage.

37. 4 Kegel exercises tone the pelvic floor muscles and prepare the area for the second stage of labor. (3) (CW; IM; ED; HC)

1 This alleviates backache and strengthens the abdominal muscles.

2 This helps the abdominal musculature.

3 Same as answer 1.

38. 2 There are various foods that can be substituted for meat or animal-related products in planning nutritious meals for the pregnant women who is a vegetarian. (1) (CW; PL; TC; HC)

1 This would be difficult for a client who is a vegetarian.

3 The client may know good nutrition; this client needs help to adapt the vegetarian diet to meet pregnancy needs.

4 Same as answer 1.

39. 4 Beans are economical and a high source of iron. (2) (CW; IM; ED; HC)

1 This is an iron rich food but expensive and often unpalatable to many people.

2 This is a moderate source of iron but the leaner cuts of meat are expensive and not as good a source of iron as the 3 bean salad.

3 This is expensive and a lower source of iron than a 3 bean casserole.

40. 3 The recommended daily food plan during pregnancy includes 6 to 7 ounces of protein daily; protein is necessary for growth and development of the fetus. (2) (CW; EV; ED; HC)

1 This is unnecessary; 3 to 4 servings of milk products such as whole milk, ice cream, and yogurt are permitted; in addition, 8 glasses of fluid should be taken daily.

2 This is contraindicated; some salt is needed to maintain the increased blood volume associated with pregnancy.

4 This increase would probably exceed the 2200 to 2500 calories daily recommended during pregnancy.

41. 3 Liver as well as kidney, green leafy vegetables, and asparagus are rich sources of folic acid, a member of the B vitamin group. (1) (CW; IM; ED; HC)

1 Celery has a negligible amount of folic acid.

2 Bananas are high in potassium, not folic acid.

4 Turkey has 7.5 mg of folic acid per 3.5 ounces compared to beef liver which has 290 mg of folic acid per 3.5 ounces.

42. 3 During pregnancy, a blood volume increase of 30% to 60% and an elevated basal metabolic rate produce an increased need for red blood cells. (2) (CW; AN; PA; HC)

1 There are no data to support the presence of pernicious anemia.

2 This is not the action of folic acid.

4 This is related to the Rh factor and is not prevented by folic acid.

43. 4 Calcium supplements are available for people who do not consume milk or milk products. (1) (CW; PL; TC; HC)
1 Good dental care and proper mouth hygiene will be more beneficial for maintaining healthy teeth.
2 Calcium is essential to the pregnant woman's diet for the development of the fetal skeleton; it must be supplemented if the client dislikes milk and milk products.
3 If milk makes the client ill, this would be poor advice and compliance would be suspect.

44. 4 Unless a lactose intolerance is present, the client should drink milk; eating dried fruits, high fiber foods, and increasing fluids and activity will aid in lessening constipation. (2) (CW; IM; ED; HC)
1 These can cause constipation.
2 These are not as beneficial as whole milk and will cause constipation as well.
3 Megadoses of vitamins can be harmful; prenatal vitamins are not a substitute for milk.

45. 3 Broccoli is a good source of calcium because it contains approximately 150 mg of calcium per 6 oz cup, compared with a 6 oz cup of milk, which contains 216 mg. (2) (CW; PL; ED; HC)
1 Corn contains about 5 mg calcium per 6 oz cup.
2 Liver contains about 18 mg calcium per 6 oz serving.
4 Lean meat contains about 20 mg calcium per 6 oz serving.

46. 1 Carrots provide the precursor pigment, carotene, which the body converts to vitamin A. (1) (CW; AN; PA; HC)
2 This contains only about one half the needed vitamin A precursor.
3 These contain a very small amount of vitamin A precursor.
4 These do not contain any vitamin A precursor.

47. 2 These animal proteins are complete proteins containing all eight essential amino acids; plant proteins are incomplete. (2) (CW; EV; ED; HC)

1 These are not as good a source of protein as milk, eggs, and cheese.
3 Same as answer 1.
4 These are incomplete proteins; also, comparatively small amounts of protein are contained in these foods.

48. 2 A positive sign of pregnancy is a urine immunoassay pregnancy test because it is 95% accurate in detecting pregnancy; the basis for this test is the presence of the beta subunit of HCG in the urine. (2) (CW; AS; PA; HC)
1 This is a presumptive sign of pregnancy; there are many other causes of amenorrhea.
3 This is a presumptive sign of pregnancy; there are other causes of frequency, such as urinary tract infection.
4 This is a presumptive sign of pregnancy; although nausea can occur during the first trimester because of the secretion of HCG, there are many causes of nausea other than pregnancy.

49. 1 Measurement of the fetal structures provides information that is useful in approximating fetal age. (1) (CW; AS; PA; HC)
2 This test can detect only physical defects.
3 Ultrasound can detect some, but not all, birth defects.
4 Ultrasound is done primarily to estimate fetal age, not to approximate linear growth.

50. 4 A full bladder is required for effective visualization of the uterus. (1) (CW; IM; ED; HC)
1 This is unnecessary; the procedure does not involve the colon.
2 This is a noninvasive procedure that does not irritate the uterus nor initiate labor.
3 This is a noninvasive procedure that does not affect the alimentary tract; fasting is contraindicated during pregnancy.

51. 1 A negative test implies that placental support is adequate and the fetus is likely to tolerate the stress of labor should it ensue within the week. (2) (CW; AN; PA; HC)
2 Interpretable data did not show signs of hyperstimulation if a negative result was reported.

3   A positive test indicates that the fetus is at increased risk; the fetus has persistent and consistent late decelerations with contractions.

4   Fetal heart rate accelerations with movement do not require doing a trial induction.

52.   1   The detection of the fetal heartbeat may be impeded by a full bladder. (1) (CW; IM; TC; HC)

2   The client should be in the semi-Fowler's position to avoid supine hypotension.

3   The client should eat so that the fetus does not become hyperactive.

4   Only external monitoring is done.

53.   3   The lecithin concentration rises abruptly at 35 weeks, reaching a level that is twice the amount of sphingomyelin, which decreases concurrently. (1) (CW; AS; PA; HC)

1   At about 30 to 32 weeks gestation the amounts of lecithin and sphingomyelin are equal; this result indicates lung immaturity.

2   The ratio is 2:1 when lung maturity is adequate; it is only early in pregnancy that the sphingomyelin concentration is higher than the lecithin concentration.

4   It is not until the L/S ratio is 2:1 that fetal lung maturity is attained.

54.   4   The priority is to evaluate the progress of labor so that the nurse can plan care. (2) (CW; AS; PA; HC)

1   This question should be asked but is not the first priority.

2   Same as answer 1.

3   Same as answer 1.

55.   2   Amniotic fluid is alkaline and turns nitrazine paper blue; acidic fluid turns nitrazine paper yellow. (1) (CW; AN; TC; HC)

1   Amniotic fluid does not turn nitrazine paper this color.

3   Same as answer 1.

4   Same as answer 1.

56.   2   The left breech position indicates that the sacrum is presenting on the left side and the head is in the fundus; fetal heart sounds are best heard in the left upper quadrant. (2) (CW; AS; TC; HC)

1   Fetal heart sounds would be in the left upper, not the lower, quadrant.

3   Fetal heart sounds would be in the left, not right, upper quadrant.

4   Same as answer 1.

57.   4   This is an ROA presentation because the prominence over the symphysis suggests a vertex and the fetal occiput and back are in the right anterior quadrant. (3) (CW; AN; TC; HC)

1   This is ruled out; this fetus is in a vertex, not a breech, presentation.

2   This is ruled out by the presence of irregular lumps on the left side, suggesting that the fetal back is in the mother's right quadrant.

3   The occiput is not located in the left posterior quadrant; the occiput and back are on the mother's right side.

58.   1   If the heart is heard in the upper left quadrant, the baby must be lying in a breech position with the head upright and the heart uppermost. (2) (CW; AS; PA; HC)

2   Fetal heart tones are heard best in the lower quadrants of the abdomen in cephalic presentations.

3   Same as answer 2.

4   Same as answer 2.

59.   4   A persistent occiput-posterior position causes intense back pain because of fetal compression of the sacral nerves. (1) (CW; IM; ED; HC)

1   This would not cause back pain.

2   Same as answer 1.

3   Same as answer 1.

60.   3   This occurs because pressure on the fetal abdomen from the contractions forces meconium from the bowel. (2) (CW; AN; PA; HC)

1   Cord prolapse is not an absolute, but it may occur if the presenting part does not fill the pelvic cavity.

2   This is unusual unless there are some accompanying signs of fetal distress, such as prolapsed cord or decelerations.

4   This is unnecessary; this is a normal occurrence caused by pressure on the fetal abdomen during contractions when the fetus is in the breech position.

61. 3   Counterpressure alleviates some of the discomfort from the pressure of the fetal head on the sacrum. (1) (CW; IM; ED; HC)

1   Elevating the legs will increase tension and discomfort.

2   Panting may lead to hyperventilation, which will cause maternal respiratory alkalosis and fetal acidosis.

4   Kegel exercises tone the pelvic musculature, not the back.

62. 3   This describes the right occiput anterior presentation; the fetal heart is on the right and the head is anterior. (1) (CW; AS; PA; HC)

1   In the left occiput posterior presentation, the back is on the left and the occiput is posterior.

2   In the left sacrum anterior presentation, the breech is the presenting part, not the head.

4   In the right mentum anterior presentation, the chin is the presenting part, not the occiput.

63. 2   Identifying progress and providing encouragement motivates the client and promotes positive feelings about the self. (1) (CW; PL; PS; HC)

1   A client in active labor should not be left alone.

3   Lying flat on her back may induce supine hypotension; side-lying should be encouraged to promote venous return.

4   During this early stage of labor, diversion is therapeutic because the client is not totally involved with herself.

64. 4   The client is in the early part of the first stage of labor, and it is important to help the partner with the role of coach. (2) (CW; IM; ED; HC)

1   It is not necessary to measure the fetal heart rate this often until the second stage of labor; the client may be on an external monitor, which constantly records FHR.

2   Delivery is not imminent at this time.

3   Suggesting that the pain is bad may increase anxiety and produce greater discomfort.

65. 2   This is used during the early phase of labor when mild contractions dilate the cervix to 3 cm. (2) (CW; EV; ED; HC)

1   This is used during the transition phase of labor.

3   This is used in combination with other breathing patterns; it is a part of the accelerated-decelerated pattern.

4   This is used during the active phase of the first stage of labor.

66. 2   This is done to prevent pushing, because full dilation has not yet occurred. (1) (CW; EV; TC; HC)

1   This is not done until full dilation; it may tire the mother and cause cervical edema.

3   This is done in the early part (preliminary phase) of the first stage of labor.

4   This is done in the middle part (accelerated phase) of the first stage of labor.

67. 2   A full bladder will push the presenting part against the uterus; this can result in irregular, poor-quality contractions. (2) (CW; AS; PA; HC)

1   The client has been dilating and is therefore in true, not false, labor.

3   Before this conclusion is considered, the client's bladder should be emptied to relieve the pressure of the bladder on the uterus; the client can then be observed to see if regular contractions resume.

4   This would have been established in the admission examination.

68. 4   This is a description of the contractions during the active portion of the first stage of labor. (2) (CW; AS; PA; HC)

1   This adaptation occurs in the transitional phase of the first stage of labor.

2   Same as answer 1.

3   Same as answer 1.

69. 3   The client is experiencing supine hypotension, which is caused by the gravid uterus compressing the large vessels; side-lying will relieve the pressure, increase venous return, improve cardiac output, and raise blood pressure. (1) (CW; IM; PA; HC)

1 This will not relieve uterine compression of large vessels; the client should be placed on her side.
2 Same as answer 1.
4 Same as answer 1.

70. 3 After 12 hours, amniotic fluid must be assessed for odor and appearance indicating infection for either mother or infant. (3) (CW; AS; PA; HC)
1 A prolapsed cord usually occurs shortly after the membranes rupture; it is very unlikely that it will occur 12 hours after the membranes rupture.
2 This is an abnormally implanted placenta; it is totally unrelated to ruptured membranes.
4 This is premature separation of a normally implanted placenta; it is totally unrelated to ruptured membranes.

71. 4 The client is hyperventilating; these actions promote rebreathing of carbon dioxide, relieving respiratory alkalosis. (1) (CW; IM; ED; HC)
1 This may cause the client to hyperventilate further.
2 Same as answer 1.
3 This will not improve the client's respiratory alkalosis, the problem that is causing the client to hyperventilate.

72. 3 Examining for a prolapsed cord is the first priority after the membranes rupture. (2) (CW; AS; TC; HC)
1 The client probably does not have to void; the priority action is checking for a prolapsed cord.
2 This can be done after checking for a prolapsed cord and assessing the fetal heart rate.
4 The fetal heart rate should be assessed after it has been determined that the cord has not prolapsed.

73. 4 This is a normal occurrence caused by the action of the sympathetic and parasympathetic nervous systems. (3) (CW; IM; TC; HC)
1 There is no need for this intervention because this is a normal response.

2 This is not an abnormal finding.
3 Unless the fetal heart decelerates, indicating hypoxia, there is no need to change the client's position.

74. 4 This fetal heart pattern is known as type III dip or deceleration; it indicates cord compression that may lead to fetal hypoxia. (3) (CW; AN; PA; HC)
1 The fetal heart rate does not always drop with a contraction in all labors.
2 Beat-to-beat variability indicates a fetus with no nervous system depression and warrants no concern.
3 This is a type I dip that results from fetal scalp compression during a contraction and is considered normal.

75. 2 The most common cause of deceleration is compression of the great vessels; placing the client on her side relieves compression, enhances venous return, increases cardiac output, and improves placental perfusion. (1) (CW; IM; TC; HC)
1 This can be done after the client is placed on her side; it is important to relieve compression on the great vessels first.
3 This will not improve the fetal heart rate; it is more important to place the mother in the left lateral position.
4 If deceleration does not improve after the client is placed on her side, then the infusion should be stopped.

76. 4 External pressure is useful for reducing intense sensations caused by a posterior presentation. (1) (CW; IM; TC; HC)
1 The supine position increases the weight of the uterus and baby on the muscles of the back; it can also cause supine hypotension.
2 Walking aids in increasing labor contractions but does not decrease the pain of back labor.
3 Effleurage or breathing techniques may not be enough to reduce the pain associated with back labor.

77. 2 Low back pain is aggravated when the client is in the supine position because of increased pressure from the fetus as the head rotates. (1) (CW; IM; ED; HC)
1 This position relieves back pain.
3 Same as answer 1.
4 The knee-chest position is not used in labor except in an emergency situation such as cord prolapse.

78. 2 If cord compression is allowed to occur, fetal hypoxia results in central nervous system damage or death; therefore manual elevation of the presenting part is indicated. (2) (CW; IM; TC; HC)
1 This can be done after elevating the presenting part off the cord; this is necessary because with each contraction the umbilical cord becomes compressed between the maternal pelvis and the presenting part.
3 This is unsafe and too time consuming; immediate intervention is necessary to prevent fetal hypoxia.
4 This would be unsafe; compression of the cord would continue in this position; the knee-chest or Trendelenburg positions could be used to allow gravity to reduce pressure on the cord.

79. 3 This prevents the cord from drying and the umbilical vessel, which supplies oxygen to the fetus, from collapsing. (2) (CW; IM; TC; HC)
1 This action may lead to further reduction of the fetal oxygen supply because the cord may be compressed.
2 This is insufficient monitoring; electronic monitors will be applied; the priority is to keep the cord from drying.
4 Moistening the cord and preserving the oxygen supply to the infant are more critical.

80. 1 This eases the pressure of the presenting part on the umbilical cord and receives the highest priority. (2) (CW; IM; TC; HC)
2 Oxygen can be given, but this is not the priority.
3 Time should not be wasted trying to locate the fetal heart when the fetus is at risk for hypoxia because of cord compression.
4 A cesarean delivery may be necessary; however, the priority is to ease the pressure on the cord to prevent fetal hypoxia.

81. 3 This block relieves vaginal and perineal pain but does not impair the ability to push. (3) (CW; AN; PA; HC)
1 This block relieves pain from the umbilicus to the lower perineum; the client will not feel the urge to push.
2 This relieves pain from the umbilicus to the midthigh; the client will not feel the urge to push.
4 This relieves uterine pain, not vaginal or perineal pain; the client will not feel contractions.

82. 2 The uterus is being overstimulated and becoming tetanic; this must be interrupted because it may cause fetal hypoxia. (2) (CW; IM; TC; HC)
1 This is unsafe; continuing fetal monitoring without first discontinuing the Pitocin keeps the fetus at risk for developing hypoxia.
3 Turning the client on her side will increase placental perfusion but will not decrease the intensity and length of contractions; discontinuing the Pitocin is the priority.
4 This should be done after the Pitocin is discontinued.

83. 4 Pressure on the rectum during contractions would indicate that a laboring client is beginning transition. (3) (CW; AS; PA; HC)
1 This occurs when transition is complete; that is, when the client is fully dilated.
2 This occurs when labor begins, not in the beginning of the transitional phase.
3 Same as answer 1.

84. 1 This is the most difficult part of labor, and the client needs encouragement and support to cope. (2) (CW; AN; TC; HC)
2 Breathing patterns should be complex and should require a high level of concentration to distract the client.
3 Fluids should be increased because of the increase in metabolism.
4 Medication at this time will depress the infant's respirations and is contraindicated.

85. 2 This common response to local anesthesia occurs for a short period because of a fall in the blood pressure. (2) (CW; EV; TC; HC)

　1 This is associated with an allergic response, which is not a common adaptation to a local anesthetic.

　3 This could be a response to a developing infection or dehydration but rarely to local anesthesia.

　4 Same as answer 1.

86. 2 All signs indicate imminent delivery; the perineum should be inspected for the appearance of caput. (2) (CW; AS; PA; HC)

　1 This is essential but not the initial action.

　3 This is important to know, but inspection is the most important action.

　4 Same as answer 1.

87. 4 The client becomes very introverted, starts to lose control, and needs assistance and support to help her through this most difficult phase of labor. (1) (CW; PL; TC; HC)

　1 This is done throughout labor.

　2 Same as answer 1.

　3 Same as answer 1.

88. 3 Clients should use a panting or blowing pattern to overcome the premature urge to push. (2) (CW; IM; ED; HC)

　1 Expulsion breathing should not be used at this time because the cervix is not fully dilated and cervical edema and lacerations can occur.

　2 Slow chest breathing is used during the early phase of the first stage of labor.

　4 Accelerated-decelerated breathing is used during the first stage of labor.

89. 1 A paper bag helps the client to rebreathe CO_2, which helps correct the respiratory alkalosis. (2) (CW; IM; ED; HC)

　2 The client's O_2 level is already elevated; the client needs to elevate the CO_2 level.

　3 CO_2 is too dilute in room atmosphere.

　4 Anesthesia will further deplete CO_2 and is therefore contraindicated.

90. 4 Transition is the most difficult part of labor, which has just been completed and the client has been working very hard; beads of perspiration are prominent on the upper lip. (1) (CW; AS; PA; HC)

　1 The bloody show increases during the transitional phase; this occurs from the increased pressure by the presenting part.

　2 This would be seen at the end, not the beginning, of the transitional phase.

　3 This signifies that the client has ruptured the membranes.

91. 2 Effective pushing will hasten the passage of the baby through the birth canal. (1) (CW; EV; PA; HC)

　1 The fetal position should have been established before the second stage.

　3 Delivery is imminent, and medication given at this time will depress the infant's respirations at birth.

　4 The mother will breastfeed in the fourth stage of labor.

92. 3 Mild toxic reactions occur because of vasodilation from direct action of these medications on maternal blood vessels; vertigo, dizziness, and hypotension may occur. (3) (CW; EV; TC; HC)

　1 Labor is not affected because there is no systemic effect.

　2 Local anesthesia will not lower the level of consciousness, thus the loss of the swallowing reflex is avoided.

　4 Local anesthesia does not affect the respiratory center in the central nervous system.

93. 2 The first action by the nurse should be to confirm if delivery is imminent by seeing if caput is emerging. (1) (CW; IM; TC; HC)

　1 The client should not be left alone, if indeed, delivery is imminent.

　3 This response demeans the client; she may be correct.

　4 If delivery is imminent this could cause injury to the baby.

94. 2 Panting will slow the process so the nurse can support the head as it is delivered. (1) (CW; IM; PA; HC)
1 Pushing will speed up the delivery and could injure the mother and the baby.
3 This will have no effect on the progress of the delivery.
4 Usually holding the breath causes involuntary pushing and it also depletes the mother and baby of oxygen; there are no signs of impaired placental perfusion so a left side-lying position is not necessary.

95. 4 Pale green amniotic fluid denotes potential meconium aspiration syndrome; appropriate action is to suction immediately at delivery to avoid possible complications from meconium aspiration. (1) (CW; PL; PA; HC)
1 The newborn should not be stimulated to cry until the airway is patent.
2 This should be done after oropharyngeal suctioning.
3 There is no indication that an umbilical transfusion will be necessary.

96. 2 As the placenta separates and drops down, the cord appears to lengthen. (2) (CW; AS; PA; HC)
1 The fundus contracts and becomes rounded and firmer.
3 The client may feel a contraction, but it is not nearly as uncomfortable as the painful contractions at the end of the first stage of labor.
4 Continual seepage occurs when there is hemorrhaging; a large sudden gush of blood heralds placental separation.

97. 3 A continuous trickle is indicative of hemorrhage; immediate medical intervention is required. (2) (CW; IM; TC; HC)
1 There are no data to indicate a full bladder; the fundus is firm and not dextroverted.
2 Data indicate that the fundus is firm and at the appropriate level.
4 This should be done more frequently; however, vital signs do not always change markedly until a large amount of blood is lost.

98. 2 Gentle massage stimulates muscle fibers and results in firming the tone of the fundus; it also helps expel any clots that may be interfering with the firming of the fundus. (1) (CW; IM; PA; HC)
1 Elevating the client's legs would increase return of blood from the extremities but it would not firm the tone of the client's fundus.
3 This would be done only if massaging the uterus were ineffective; a physician's order is required.
4 This would not be the first action at this time; gentle massage to firm the fundus is the priority.

99. 4 Lochia can accumulate under the buttocks; cannot be accurately observed when client is supine. (2) (CW; IM; TC; HC)
1 Overstimulation can cause uterine atony.
2 Vital signs should be taken q 15 minutes during fourth stage of labor which continues for 1 hour after delivery.
3 Too soon for ambulation.

100. 3 A distended bladder impedes uterine contractions, predisposing the client to hemorrhage. (1) (CW; AS; PA; HC)
1 Relaxation is a priority before delivery; in the fourth stage the client is often euphoric.
2 Love grows with care and responsibility.
4 The mother is egocentric at this point and is not yet totally involved with the infant.

101. 4 This blood pressure is elevated and exceeds the 140/90 designated by the National Institutes of Health as Stage I hypertension; intervention may be necessary. (1) (CW; AS; TC; HC)
1 This is within normal limits.
2 Same as answer 1.
3 This is a slight elevation which is consistent with the physiology of labor.

102. 1 Grand multiparas have decreased uterine muscle tone as a result of the repeated distension of pregnancy; consequently, the uterine muscles have difficulty in contracting after delivery. (1) (CW; PL; TC; HC)

2 This can occur in all clients after delivery; it is not specific to grand multiparas.

3 This occurs in all postpartal clients; it is the body's attempt to dispose of excess fluid now that the placenta and baby are no longer present.

4 This may be indicative of preeclampsia, which is more common in primiparas and teenage clients.

103. 3 A full bladder frequently elevates the uterus and displaces it to the right; even though the uterus feels firm, it may relax enough to foster bleeding; therefore, the bladder needs to be emptied to increase uterine tone. (1) (CW; IM; TC; HC)

1 If part of the placenta, umbilical cord, or fetal membranes are not fully expelled during the third stage of labor, their retention limits uterine contraction and involution; a boggy uterus and bleeding would be evident.

2 This is not a sign of uterine stabilization; the uterus cannot remain contracted over a full bladder.

4 Vigorous massage tires the uterus and even with massage the uterus cannot contract over a full bladder.

104. 4 Massaging the uterus will induce contraction and cause expulsion of clots; frequent massage should be continued to keep the uterus firm and inhibit bleeding. (2) (CW; IM; TC; HC)

1 Pulse and blood pressure do not change significantly unless large amounts of blood are lost.

2 This would be done if the client were in shock; the priority intervention now is to massage the uterus and prevent hemorrhage.

3 This is unnecessary; the client's fundus is boggy and needs to be massaged to help it contract.

105. 3 Chances of postpartal hemorrhage are 5 times greater with large infants because uterine contractions may be impaired after delivery. (2) (CW; AN; PA; HC)

1 On the contrary, early breastfeeding will stimulate uterine contractions and lessen the chance of hemorrhage.

2 This does not contribute to postpartum hemorrhage because anesthesia for a pudendal block does not affect uterine contractions.

4 This is a short third stage; a prolonged third stage of labor, 30 minutes or more, may lead to postpartum hemorrhage.

106. 4 A postpartum chill is a normal occurrence of unknown cause. (1) (CW; EV; PA; HC)

1 This measure is part of the routine postpartum assessment but does not need to be done in relation to the chill.

2 Same as answer 1.

3 Same as answer 1.

107. 3 Initially, cold therapy reduces edema and discomfort. (2) (CW; PL; TC; HC)

1 Heat therapy usually begins after 8 to 12 hours of cold therapy; warm, not hot, water would be used.

2 ASA is contraindicated in the puerperium; there is too great a risk for hemorrhage.

4 This provides little or minimal perineal relief.

108. 2 Voiding will be difficult because of periurethral edema and discomfort. (2) (CW; EV; PA; HC)

1 This rarely occurs with primigravidas, even when a lot of pushing occurs.

3 A second degree laceration is unrelated to lactation.

4 A second degree tear is unrelated to maladaptive bonding and attachment.

109. 2 Increased parity contributes to an increased incidence of uterine atony because the uterine muscle may not contract effectively, thus leading to postpartal hemorrhage; a one hour labor in a grand multipara is not uncommon. (3) (CW; AS; TC; HC)
1 A primipara should maintain a well contracted uterus because with only one pregnancy the uterus usually maintains its tone.
3 100 mg of Demerol is not considered excessive for a primipara and would not contribute to uterine atony.
4 The delivery of the placenta 10 minutes after delivery of the fetus is normal and would not affect tone of the uterus; while multiparity contributes to uterine atony, the woman who is a grand multipara is at a higher risk for hemorrhage.

110. 4 There is a greater chance for infection to occur because with this type of episiotomy there is more tissue damage and healing is slower. (2) (CW; AN; TC; HC)
1 There is more tissue damage so there would be more edema.
2 The mediolateral episiotomy cuts large muscles used in ambulation so there is more discomfort with movement.
3 More blood vessels are injured so there is more bleeding and bruising.

111. 2 Cold causes vasoconstriction and reduces edema by lessening the accumulation of blood and lymph at the episiotomy site; cold also deadens nerve endings and lessens the pain. (2) (CW; IM; TC; HC)
1 This is not used after an episiotomy.
3 This may diminish the pain but will not lessen the edema.
4 This position will not lessen pain or reduce edema.

112. 3 Prevention of infection is the priority. (2) (CW; EV; ED; HC)
1 Not necessary to stop sitz baths as long as they provide comfort.
2 Stair climbing may cause some discomfort but is not detrimental to healing.
4 Provides comfort but is not the priority.

113. 4 The client's statement, in conjunction with the other findings, suggests urinary retention. (1) (CW; AS; PA; HC)
1 This is unrelated to the other findings; thirst is related to dehydration, whereas the other signs are related to urinary retention.
2 This is an expected postpartal response.
3 This is expected; oxytocin secretion, which is stimulated by infant suckling, causes the uterus to contract.

114. 2 A client's temperature may be elevated to 100.4°F during the first 24 hours postpartum as a result of dehydration from labor. (2) (CW; AN; PA; HC)
1 Mastitis usually develops after breastfeeding has been established and mature milk is present.
3 This usually begins with a fever of 100.4°F or above on 2 successive days, excluding the first 24 hours postpartum.
4 Urinary tract infections usually become evident later in the postpartum period.

115. 2 During the postpartum period a leukocytosis (WBC count of 15,000 to 20,000/mm^3) is normal and related to the physical exertion experienced during labor and delivery, not infection. (2) (CW; EV; PA; HC)
1 This is not a drop in the WBC count because the normal postpartal white blood cell count is between 15,000 and 20,000/mm^3.
3 The leukocytosis is normal and related to physical exertion of labor and delivery, not infection.
4 Same as answer 3.

116. 2 Infection is most commonly transmitted through contaminated hands. (2) (CW; IM; ED; HC)
1 Tub baths are permitted.
3 This is contraindicated in the postpartum period until the cervix is completely closed.
4 Douching is contraindicated until the cervix is closed, usually six weeks after delivery.

117. 4 Varicose veins predispose the client to thrombophlebitis; Homans' sign, calf pain with dorsiflexion of the foot, is an indication that this may be occurring. (1) (CW; AS; TC; HC)
1 The clotting mechanism is not affected; clot formation results because of venous pooling and decreased venous return caused by the impaired vasculature.
2 These tests, while concerned with clotting factors, are not related to the development of thrombophlebitis.
3 These would be affected by the amount of bleeding incurred during delivery and usually are not severe enough to impair circulatory competency.

118. 4 This indicates subinvolution and needs further assessment. (1) (CW; EV; TC; HC)
1 This is a normal postpartal concern, especially with twins.
2 This is normal postpartal diuresis.
3 This is the normal milk let-down reflex.

119. 4 On the 3rd to 4th day the uterine discharge becomes pink to brown; it lasts to the 10th day approximately. (1) (CW; AS; PA; HC)
1 It is unusual to have scant lochia rubra.
2 After about 10 days the uterine discharge becomes yellow to white; it may continue until 2 to 6 weeks after the birth of the baby.
3 Lochia rubra lasts from the 1st to the 3rd or 4th day; it is usually heavy but may be moderate after a few days.

120. 2 Breastfeeding stimulates oxytocin release and uterine contractions resulting in increased lochial flow. (2) (CW; IM; ED; HC)
1 Weight loss may occur more slowly in the breastfeeding mother because of increased nutritional and caloric needs.
3 The increased levels of oxytocin and subsequent uterine contractions will enhance involution.
4 Heat is not contraindicated and the client may take warm showers; heat is also used if the mother experiences problems such as engorgement or sore nipples.

121. 3 If suckling or nipple stimulation is discontinued, acini cells degenerate, regressive changes occur, and lactation ends. (2) (CW; IM; ED; HC)
1 Other than suckling, the stimulant for oxytocin secretion is unknown.
2 High levels of estrogen inhibit anterior pituitary gland secretion of lactogenic hormones.
4 Milk secretion starts on the third or fourth day after delivery.

122. 4 This is due to the arrangement of fatty acids on the glycerol molecule and is related to the natural lipase activity that is present in human milk that has not been heat treated. (2) (CW; AN; ED; HC)
1 The converse is true; lactose content is higher in human milk.
2 It is lower, but protein in human milk is easier for the infant to digest.
3 This is untrue; these factors are found only in human milk.

123. 4 This dilates milk ducts, promotes emptying of the breasts, and stimulates further lactation. (1) (CW; EV; ED; HC)
1 A large consumption of milk products is not required to stimulate the production of milk.
2 This will contract the milk ducts and interfere with the milk let-down reflex.
3 Breast binders may inhibit lactation; they fool the body into thinking that milk secretion is no longer needed.

124. 3 Exposure to air dries the nipples by evaporation; exposure also tends to harden the nipples, making them less tender. (2) (CW; IM; TC; HC)
1 Continuous ice packs are used to relieve the discomfort caused by engorged breasts, not sore nipples.
2 This may relieve discomfort but will do nothing to toughen the nipples.
4 If kept from the breast for a prolonged period, the baby may become accustomed to the bottle and not wish to nurse again; in addition, absence of suckling will inhibit lacation.

125. 4 The most vigorous sucking will occur during the first few minutes of nursing when the infant would be on the unaffected breast; later sucking is less traumatic. (3) (CW; IM; PA; HC)
1 Stopping nursing for 2 days is unnecessary and would interfere with lactation.
2 Manual expression may not completely empty the breast, interfering with lactation.
3 A breast shield confuses an infant because it is necessary to use a different sucking pattern to obtain milk.

126. 4 Compared with the prenatal diet, the diet for lactation requires an increased intake of all food groups, vitamins, and minerals, plus increased fluid to replace that lost with milk secretion; calories should be increased by 500 daily and protein by 10 to 15 g daily. (2) (CW; IM; ED; HC)
1 Breastfeeding mothers need to consume an additional 500 calories and 10 to 15 g of protein per day to maintain adequate milk production.
2 The client needs a well-balanced diet, not just milk, and she must consume an additional 500 calories a day.
3 This denies the client's concern; optimal nutrition is necessary to produce an adequate milk supply.

127. 4 This keeps the breast as empty as possible, limiting pressure within the ducts, thereby reducing pain. (1) (CW; IM; ED; HC)
1 Weaning will cause stasis of milk ducts and increase the fullness of the breasts at this time, thereby increasing pain.
2 The causative organism is probably already in the baby's nose and mouth; weaning is not always necessary with mastitis.
3 This is false; a tight fitting bra will increase pain and suppress milk production; this will impede breastfeeding.

128. 3 Heat increases milk flow, and because the client is not breastfeeding, this is an undesired outcome; application of cold is recommended to restrict milk flow. (1) (CW; EV; ED; HC)
1 This is a correct statement; analgesics will help lessen the discomfort of engorgement; no further teaching is needed.

2 This is a correct statement; engorgement lasts 48 to 72 hours; no further teaching is needed.
4 This is a correct statement; a tight, supportive bra will suppress milk production; no further teaching is needed.

129. 1 This is like binding the breasts; it reduces pain and prevents further engorgement. (1) (CW; IM; ED; HC)
2 Medication would reduce pain but would not prevent further engorgement.
3 Milk and fluids should not be restricted after delivery.
4 Cold compresses would prevent further engorgement in the nonnursing mother; this is not an independent function of the nurse; it would require a physician's order.

130. 3 This is an incorrect statement; if the client expresses milk from her breasts, she is stimulating milk production and this will not relieve engorgement; therefore additional teaching will be necessary. (2) (CW; EV; ED; HC)
1 This is a correct statement; this measure is used to give the body the message that milk production is not needed.
2 This is a correct statement; non-breastfeeding mothers do not need extra fluids.
4 This is a correct statement; warm water will promote vasodilation, lead to emptying of breasts, and support further milk production.

131. 1 During the taking-in phase, a woman is primarily concerned with being cared for and being cared about. (2) (CW; PL; PS; EC)
2 Infant feeding is best taught during the taking-hold phase of postpartum adjustment.
3 Same as answer 2.
4 This is not a primary concern during the immediate postpartum period.

132. 2 The mother needs to learn the realities of infant behavior and how to cope with them; holding and talking to the baby are consoling measures. (2) (CW; PL; ED; HC)
1 At this age a toy would not be meaningful and would be an inadequate substitute for parental attention.

3 The infant is too young to be given cereal at this time.

4 It is unhealthful to disrupt the baby's sleep pattern.

133. 4 The nurse, by going into the home, would be able to monitor both the mother's and baby's health, as well as the mother's parenting skills and evidence of drug rehabilitation. (3) (CW; PL; TC; EC)

1 This is unnecessary; the court system is already involved because of the baby's positive toxicology screen.

2 Foster care is not automatic if the mother has been determined to be able to care for the baby.

3 Same as answer 1.

134. 2 This statement acknowledges the situation and suggests a possible solution to the problem. (3) (CW; IM; PS; HC)

1 If it were true that the mother had postpartum depression, it would be inappropriate for the nurse to dismiss it so lightly.

3 This is not true and the response does not address the problem that is evident in the situation.

4 This is stereotyping and would not be therapeutic.

HIGH RISK PREGNANCY

135. 4 An amniocentesis is commonly used to diagnose genetic problems, as well as to diagnose fetal maturity and fetal hemolytic disease. (1) (CW; IM; ED; HP)

1 This is not a reason for doing this invasive procedure.

2 Same as answer 1.

3 An amniocentesis is no longer done routinely if the mother is an older primipara; a sonogram is usually done.

136. 4 In the fourteenth week, amniotic fluid is present and small amounts can be withdrawn for testing. (1) (CW; IM; ED; HP)

1 This is untrue; an amniocentesis can be performed any time after the fourteenth week.

2 There is no amniotic fluid present at the time of conception.

3 It is more appropriate to do an amniocentesis before quickening is established.

137. 3 Amniocentesis has proven useful in detecting potential defects resulting from chromosomal errors such as Down syndrome, Tay-Sachs disease, hemophilia, and thalassemia. (2) (CW; IM; ED; HP)

1 This is false reassurance and it may stop further communication by the mother.

2 Not all fetal defects can be detected prior to birth; an amniocentesis can identify some.

4 An amniocentesis does not detect all congenital defects.

138. 1 An invasive procedure such as amniocentesis requires consent. (1) (CW; IM; ED; HP)

2 Intravenous therapy is unnecessary.

3 The infection rate is 1%; this is not an appropriate nursing intervention.

4 No vaginal examination is done before amniocentesis.

139. 1 A copy of the Patient's Bill of Rights is not necessary to give informed consent for treatment. (2) (CW; IM; ED; HP)

2 Alternative treatment regimens should be discussed so that the client is able to make an informed choice about which course of treatment to pursue.

3 All questions should be answered honestly and in terms that the client can understand.

4 This information is required to give informed consent.

140. 2 A full bladder facilitates accuracy during ultrasonic visualization of the fetus and placenta prior to the amniocentesis. (2) (CW; AN; TC; HP)

1 Eight ounces of fluid will do little to hydrate a person or improve circulation.

3 Giving 8 ounces of fluid will not hydrate the fetus or decrease its movement.

4 This is unnecessary; a small amount of fluid is withdrawn from the amniotic sac; excessive fluid is not lost.

141. 1 This is done to determine if any injury has occurred to the fetus or placenta during the procedure. (1) (CW; EV; TC; HP)

2 This position enhances placental perfusion, but it serves no purpose in detecting complications.

3 This is unnecessary; the puncture site seals by itself immediately after removal of the needle.

4 There is no entry into the vaginal canal with this procedure; bleeding or discharge is not expected.

142. 2 It is possible that stimulation of the uterus due to the amniocentesis may cause uterine contractions. (1) (CW; AS; TC; HP)

1 This is not necessary because an amniocentesis is not done via the vagina.

3 This is irrelevant because amniotic fluid is in no way influenced by the intake of fluid.

4 This should not be necessary because the pinprick opening seals up immediately.

143. 4 A full bladder is required for effective visualization of the uterine contents during the sonogram; the bladder should be emptied before an amniocentesis to prevent accidental puncture of the bladder during the procedure. (2) (CW; PL; TC; HP)

1 A full bladder is required for effective ultrasonography.

2 The client voids only after all abdominal tracings are obtained.

3 The bladder may fill within 1 hour; a full bladder is undesirable before an amniocentesis.

144. 2 Ultrasound can detect anomalies that can be visualized on the body surface. (1) (CW; AS; PA; HP)

1 This is an internal problem that cannot be identified by ultrasound.

3 Same as answer 1.

4 Same as answer 1.

145. 2 As the process of effacement occurs in the latter part of pregnancy, placental separation from the uterus may occur, causing painless bleeding. (2) (CW; AN; PA; HP)

1 This occurs in separation of a normally implanted placenta (abruptio placentae).

3 This is generally not associated with placenta previa at its onset; it may occur later.

4 This is not usually the first thing to occur; it may occur after the placenta separates.

146. 2 Under normal conditions the heart rate increases with physical activity; the test looks for accelerations of 10 to 15 beats with fetal movements. (2) (CW; AS; PA; HP)

1 This is not a part of the evaluation of the fetus in the nonstress test.

3 Same as answer 1.

4 This is used in the contraction stress test (CST).

147. 2 The fetus with a borderline cardiac reserve will show hypoxia by a decreased heart rate when there is minimal stress, making the test positive. (2) (CW; AS; PA; HP)

1 The normal baseline measurement would be taken before the test or early in the test to provide a basis of comparison.

3 These decelerations are a response to head compression.

4 There are non-uniform drops in FHR before, during, or after a contraction; they are related to partial, brief cord compression that can be eliminated by changing the mother's position.

148. 2 Bleeding could indicate placenta previa or abruptio placentae, which would be aggravated by the contractions from the use of Pitocin. (1) (CW; AS; TC; HP)

1 A contraction stress test is indicated; blurred vision may indicate PIH; cardiac problems may diminish O_2 perfusion to the placenta and compromise the infant during labor.

3 A contraction stress test is indicated; sickling may reduce O_2 perfusion to the placenta and compromise the infant during labor.

4 A contraction stress test is indicated; arteriolar spasms may diminish O_2 perfusion to the placenta and compromise the infant during labor.

149. 4 RhIg is given to prevent active formation of antibodies when a negative individual is at risk for sensitization; if given to an Rh positive person an injection of RhIg would cause hemolysis of RBCs. (3) (CW; AN; TC; HP)

1 RhIg is never given to an individual with Rh antibodies.

2 A positive Coombs' test indicates that the woman has Rh antibodies; RhIg is never given to an individual with Rh antibodies.

3 Administration of RhIg to an Rh positive woman causes hemolysis of RBCs.

150. 2 RhoGAM will be given only if the infant is Rh positive and the Coombs' test is negative. (3) (CW; PL; ED; HP)

1 This is not done; however, a minimal dose of RhoGAM may be given in the twenty-eighth week of gestation to decrease antibody response in the presence of transplacental bleeding.

3 RhoGAM might be given after the twenty-eighth week if the amniocentesis procedure resulted in the escape of some fetal blood into the maternal circulation.

4 RhoGAM is given only to Rh negative mothers to prevent antibody formation and protect future pregnancies; it is never given to the baby.

151. 2 All Rh negative mothers with Rh positive infants are candidates for RhoGAM; a negative Coombs' indicates an absence of Rh antibodies. (3) (CW; AS; TC; HP)

1 The positive Coombs' indicates the presence of circulating antibodies; therefore RhoGAM is of no use.

3 When mother and baby both have Rh negative blood, RhoGAM is not required.

4 Same as answer 3.

152. 3 Early postoperative ambulation helps prevent many postpartal complications such as thrombophlebitis and constipation. (2) (CW; PL; ED; HP)

1 Clients are generally discharged by the fifth postpartal day.

2 A bowel movement can occur spontaneously if early ambulation and adequate fluids are encouraged.

4 Clients are permitted to shower after 48 hours.

153. 3 Just as after any surgery, pain is a major postoperative problem during the first 24 hours after cesarean delivery. (3) (CW; AN; PA; HP)

1 Oral intake is usually limited for the first 24 to 48 hours postoperatively.

2 Bowels ordinarily do not move for 48 to 72 hours postoperatively.

4 Gaseous distention is more likely to occur on day three.

154. 3 Palpation will indicate if bladder distention is present; the increased intraabdominal space available after delivery can result in bladder distention without discomfort. (2) (CW; EV; TC; HP)

1 A physician's order is needed for catheterization.

2 Trauma to the area makes surrounding organs atonic; the client may have a full bladder and not feel the urge to void.

4 Measurement alone is not sufficient for 24 to 48 hours postpartum.

155. 2 These are symptoms of separation of the incision; further evaluation should be made because dehiscence is always a possibility. (3) (CW; EV; TC; HP)

1 This would not be done without further evaluation of the source of the pain experienced by the client.

3 A sharp, severe pain may result from a variety of causes, and a continuation of the activity even with splinting is unsafe.

4 This is only part of the assessment; an analgesic would alleviate the pain but do nothing about the underlying problem.

156. 1   Excess fluid retention is an undesirable effect of sodium intake. (2) (CW; PL; ED; HP)

2   There is no concern about fluid retention when taking antacids that do not contain sodium.

3   Same as answer 2.

4   Same as answer 2.

157. 2   This will decrease the workload of the heart during expulsion and permit a vaginal delivery. (3) (CW; PL; TC; HP)

1   This can increase the cardiac workload.

3   Many clients with cardiac problems can deliver vaginally when precautionary measures are instituted; it is preferable to avoid the secondary stresses that surgery may impose.

4   During the second stage cardiac output can be increased and this might cause cardiac arrest; the client needs assistance to decrease the cardiac workload.

158. 4   This is the accepted definition of partial placenta previa. (2) (CW; AN; PA; HP)

1   This occurs in abruptio placentae.

2   Same as answer 1.

3   This will not lead to placenta previa but will place the fetus in jeopardy.

159. 4   With a low implanted placenta (placenta previa) the presenting part may have difficulty entering the pelvis. (3) (CW; AS; PA; HP)

1   Engagement is difficult with a low-lying placenta.

2   Placenta previa does not make it difficult to palpate small fetal parts.

3   This occurs with abruptio placentae.

160. 2   Blood loss and anemia cause a lowered resistance to infection; the placental site is in the lower uterine segment and is more exposed to the entry of organisms through the vagina in both the antepartal and postpartal periods. (2) (CW; AN; TC; HP)

1   Placenta previa is characterized by painless bleeding.

3   There is a separation from the uterine wall as the uterus expands; there is no tearing of the placenta.

4   Placenta previa is not caused by a genetic factor and would not cause genetic birth defects in the fetus.

161. 1   By counting or weighing pads, an accurate measurement of the amount of blood loss may be obtained. (1) (CW; AS; TC; HP)

2   The fundus may be higher than normal because the low-lying placenta prevents the descent of the fetus into the pelvis, but the height cannot be used to measure blood loss.

3   The vital signs will reflect the effects of the blood loss rather than the amount.

4   Laboratory results demonstrate the effects of the blood loss rather than the amount.

162. 1   This position shunts blood to the upper body and vital organs. (3) (CW; AN; TC; HP)

2   The bleeding will continue regardless of this position.

3   Pressure on the cervix is thought to have no bearing on bleeding episodes.

4   The placenta is implanted and positioning will not move it off the cervix.

163. 3   A full bladder helps to stabilize the uterus during the ultrasonogram; this allows for better visualization of the fetus; two full glasses of water, drunk about 1 hour before the test, will fill the bladder. (2) (CW; IM; TC; HP)

1   Emptying the bladder is inadvisable because a full bladder supports the uterus and improves visualization of the uterus.

2   Because the procedure is noninvasive, it is unnecessary to cleanse the skin.

4   An enema is contraindicated when bleeding occurs.

164. 4   Vaginal examination may cause separation of the entire placenta with resulting hemorrhage; an immediate cesarean delivery is done to prevent fetal demise. (2) (CW; PL; TC; HP)

1 This would do nothing to save the infant if total placental separation occurs.

2 Delaying labor would not be helpful; immediate cesarean delivery is necessary in this emergency.

3 Same as answer 1.

165. 4 A vaginal examination may result in a sudden, severe hemorrhage because of the location of the placenta near the cervical os; whole blood should be ready for administration to prevent shock. (2) (CW; PL; TC; HP)

1 This is an incorrect response; fresh plasma may be used to restore coagulation factors when DIC occurs after severe blood loss.

2 Adults manufacture their own vitamin K, and an injection would not help to prevent bleeding from the placenta.

3 Giving heparin sodium is contraindicated in the presence of hemorrhage.

166. 1 The symptoms indicate loss of blood; to compensate for the decreased cardiac output, oxygen is needed to maintain the well being of both the mother and fetus. (1) (CW; IM; PA; HP)

2 This would decrease blood flow to the vital centers in the brain.

3 This would not be the first action; in view of the blood loss, providing oxygen is the priority.

4 This could mask abdominal pain and sedate an already compromised fetus.

167. 4 Multiple past pregnancies tend to make the endometrial lining more vulnerable to abnormal implantation. (1) (CW; AN; PA; HP)

1 Primigravidas are the least prone; the endometrium is receptive to normal implantation.

2 Two pregnancies have not compromised the endometrium too much; abnormal implantation is less likely to occur.

3 Age is not known to be a significant factor; also, two pregnancies have not compromised the endometrium too much.

168. 4 The side-lying position decreases pressure on the vena cava from the gravid uterus, assuring more adequate oxygenation of the fetus. (1) (CW; IM; TC; HP)

1 Without proper positioning, breathing techniques will be less effective.

2 This is not likely to have a significant effect if the client is in active labor.

3 Lying on the back will increase pressure on the vena cava, further compromising the fetus.

169. 3 This will indicate whether bleeding may be progressing toward maternal and fetal distress. (2) (CW; AS; TC; HP)

1 A fetal monitor would be indicated, because it more accurately records fetal well-being.

2 This is done in the postpartum period, not while the client is in labor.

4 This is contraindicated; these examinations may stimulate greater bleeding if the placenta is accidentally dislodged.

170. 3 Conservative therapeutic approaches have decreased risks to both mother and infant. (2) (CW; IM; PS; HP)

1 This is not true; the infant is compromised more than the mother is.

2 This is not true; conservative approaches are more effective.

4 Although the prognosis has improved, there is still danger for both mother and infant.

171. 4 Folic acid is needed to produce heme for hemoglobin. (3) (CW; AN; PA; HP)

1 Folic acid may reduce the risk of a sequestration crisis but it will not prevent it.

2 There is no relationship between folic acid and the reduction of sickling.

3 There is no change in needs; sickling decreases the oxygen-carrying capacity of hemoglobin.

172. 3 When a woman with sickle cell anemia becomes pregnant, she should be assessed carefully for pyelonephritis, leg ulcers, and cardiopathy; pregnancy usually causes worsening of most aspects of sickle cell anemia. (2) (CW; AS; TC; HP)
   1 Hypothyroidism affects 1 in 1500 women during pregnancy; women with sickle cell anemia are not at any higher risk for hypothyroidism than the general population.
   2 Women with sickle cell anemia are not at an increased risk for this problem during pregnancy.
   4 Same as answer 2.

173. 2 A floating fetal head in a primigravida of 42 weeks gestation, who is in early labor, is suggestive of disproportion because engagement usually occurs 2 weeks before term in primigravidas. (3) (CW; AN; TC; HP)
   1 This test confirms the presence of ruptured membranes, which should not cause any problems with delivery.
   3 This occurs during early labor when the presenting part bears down on the capillary structure of the cervix.
   4 This falls within the normal range of 120 to 160 beats per minute.

174. 1 The feet or buttocks are not effective in blocking the cervical opening, and the cord may slip through and be compressed. (2) (CW; AS; TC; HP)
   2 Rapid dilation and precipitate labor can occur with infants in cephalic positions as well.
   3 Uterine inertia may result from fatigue or cephalopelvic disproportion and is not directly related to fetal position.
   4 This is a normal occurrence.

175. 2 Pelvic pressure or a feeling that the baby is pushing down is one of the earliest symptoms of preterm labor and should be taught to the client so that she can present herself early for care. (3) (CW; IM; ED; HP)
   1 This is not a danger sign of preterm labor.
   3 These are not danger signs of preterm labor.
   4 Fetal movement is not normally felt until approximately 16 weeks.

176. 1 Increasing the frequency may decrease or stop the contractions and prevent dilation. (3) (CW; PL; TC; HP)
   2 This could cause toxic side effects.
   3 This would be unsafe because labor would continue.
   4 This will do nothing if labor is beginning.

177. 4 Betamimetics have the unpleasant side effects of nervousness, tremors, and palpitations; clients should be informed that these side effects are expected. (3) (CW; EV; PA; DR)
   1 The medication, if contractions are lessened, is performing as expected and does not need to be discontinued.
   2 These are not the usual symptoms of preterm labor.
   3 There is no correlation between electrolyte levels and these symptoms.

178. 4 This provides accurate information; an increase of 30 mmHg in the systolic reading or an increase of 15 mmHg in the diastolic reading indicates hypertension during pregnancy. (2) (CW; IM; ED; HP)
   1 This is false reassurance.
   2 This could be frightening and elevate the blood pressure even more.
   3 This response is demeaning.

179. 2 Bed rest keeps the pressure of the fetal head off the cervix; the side-lying position keeps the gravid uterus from impeding major vessels, thus enhancing uterine perfusion. (2) (CW; PL; TC; HP)
   1 These are used only when the cord is prolapsed or the client is in shock.
   3 Sitting up in bed increases pressure on the cervix; this may lead to further dilation.
   4 This may aid in relieving pressure of the fetus on the cervix, but it will not enhance uterine perfusion.

180. 4 Prostaglandins in semen may stimulate labor, and penile contact with the cervix may increase myometrial contractability. (1) (CW; IM; ED; HP)
   1 Sexual intercourse may cause labor to progress; delivery is not desired in the thirty-third week of pregnancy.
   2 Same as answer 1.
   3 Same as answer 1.

181. 1 Preterm infants are at risk for respiratory distress and would be compromised by excessive use of narcotic analgesics; other supportive measures should be used initially to relieve discomfort. (2) (CW; AN; TC; HP)

    2 This is untrue; preterm infants are at risk for respiratory distress, and respiratory depression from analgesia may further compromise their immature lungs.

    3 This is untrue; however, use is limited as much as possible.

    4 Although this is taken into consideration, fetal safety is primary, and analgesia is reduced to a minimum.

182. 2 Betamethasone helps increase the lecithin/sphingomyelin (L/S) ratio, which is an indicator of fetal lung maturity. (2) (CW; AN; PA; HP)

    1 Betamethasone does not affect the labor process.

    3 Betamethasone does not increase placental perfusion.

    4 Betamethasone does not affect the intensity of contractions.

183. 1 Labor is continuing and the promotion of the well-being of the client and fetus is the most important priority for nursing care during this period. (2) (CW; PL; PA; HP)

    2 This response addresses only one aspect of this client's needs; this problem must be dealt with in the context of her other needs.

    3 Same as answer 2.

    4 Same as answer 2.

184. 1 In light of the vaginal bleeding, the priority nursing action is ascertaining if a viable fetus is present. (2) (CW; AS; TC; HP)

    2 This is absolutely contraindicated; bright red bleeding is suggestive of placenta previa.

    3 Same as answer 2.

    4 Same as answer 2.

185. 1 This client will have lower tolerance for pain and greater need for pain relief. (2) (CW; PL; TC; HP)

    2 Larger doses may be needed if this is done.

    3 Delays increase anxiety and discomfort, and larger doses are needed.

    4 Individuals who abuse drugs need more medication than do others because of tolerance.

186. 4 The earliest sign of drug withdrawal is CNS overstimulation. (2) (CW; AS; PA; HP)

    1 These have no relation to drug abuse; most postpartum women are hungry and thirsty.

    2 These have no relation to drug abuse.

    3 Same as answer 2.

187. 2 It is vital that a baseline measurement be obtained because increasing size is a sign of concealed hemorrhage; in abruptio placentae there is bleeding behind the placenta. (3) (CW; AS; PA; HP).

    1 This would be an appropriate assessment but it is not a priority at this time.

    3 Same as answer 1.

    4 Same as answer 1.

188. 2 Abruptio placentae occurs in about 1% of all pregnancies; the problem is much more common in women with hypertension; the causative factors are not clear. (1) (CW; AN; PA; HP)

    1 Hydramnios occurs about 10 times more frequently in pregnancies when the clients have diabetes mellitus.

    3 Spontaneous abortion, preterm labor and birth, and intrauterine fetal growth retardation (IUGR) are more common in pregnant clients with heart disease.

    4 There is no higher incidence of abruptio placentae in the client with diabetes mellitus; about 25% to 30% of the clients with diabetes mellitus develop pregnancy-induced hypertension (PIH) or preeclampsia.

189. 2 The side-lying position improves venous return to the heart and increases stroke volume and cardiac output. (1) (CW; PL; TC; HP)

    1 This position impairs venous return and may cause supine hypotension syndrome.

    3 This position does not promote optimal venous return to the heart.

    4 This will cause dyspnea because of increased pressure on the diaphragm from the abdominal organs and fetus.

190. 4   This position moves the gravid uterus off the great vessels of the lower abdomen which increases venous return, improves cardiac output, and promotes kidney and placental perfusion. (2) (CW; AN; PA; HP)

1   The side-lying position does not influence intraabdominal pressure.

2   This is not accomplished by positioning; this is accomplished with magnesium sulfate therapy when symptoms of pregnancy-induced hypertension worsen.

3   The side-lying position does not reduce edema.

191. 4   The accepted definition of hypertension during pregnancy is an elevation of 30 mmHg systolic and/or 15 mmHg diastolic over previous normal levels; this reading is above that level and could be indicative of developing preeclampsia in a young primigravida. (2) (CW; AS; TC; HP)

1   These increases are within the acceptable elevations in blood pressure during pregnancy.

2   Same as answer 1.

3   Same as answer 1.

192. 1   Nonperiodic accelerations on movement and a baseline variability of 5 to 15 beats indicate fetal well-being. (3) (CW; AS; PA; HP)

2   Early decelerations are associated with fetal head compression.

3   Late decelerations are associated with uteroplacental insufficiency.

4   Variable decelerations are associated with cord compression.

193. 4   There is strong evidence that low protein intake is associated with pregnancy-induced hypertension. (1) (CW; AN; PA; HP)

1   This may cause other problems, but it is not generally associated with pregnancy-induced hypertension.

2   This is too vague; it addresses calories but not the type of calories.

3   Same as answer 1.

194. 4   Rest is advised to reduce arteriolar spasm, and side-lying promotes more efficient venous return to heart; this improves cardiac output and placental perfusion. (1) (CW; PL; ED; HP)

1   Sodium is necessary to maintain circulatory volume and is not removed from the diet.

2   This may increase general arteriolar spasm; also, venous return is inhibited in the upright position.

3   Because of the increased circulatory volume with pregnancy, the client needs 2000 ml of fluids per day.

195. 2   Blood pressure rises, edema increases, and degenerative changes of the kidney cause increasing proteinuria (3+) as preeclampsia worsens. (2) (CW; AS; PA; HP)

1   This may be indicative of placenta previa but is not a common adaptation to worsening of pregnancy-induced hypertension.

3   This is indicative of a cardiac or respiratory problem; it is not found with worsening hypertension.

4   This is within normal limits; there is insufficient information to identify if it is elevated in this client.

196. 1   The client is exhibiting symptoms of preeclampsia; the presence of hyperreflexia will help confirm this diagnosis and direct the physician to appropriate interventions while alerting the nurse to the possibility of seizures. (3) (CW; AS; TC; HP)

2   The physician will need to be called, but a complete assessment should be done first to provide the physician with the most information.

3   The client's blood type is not necessary at this time; assessment of the neurological status is the priority.

4   An IV may need to be started but should not precede a proper assessment; normal saline would not be preferred.

197. 3   An adequate urinary output, an indicator of adequate renal function, is necessary to prevent toxicity because $MgSO_4$ is excreted by the kidneys; signs of $MgSO_4$ toxicity are reduced respirations and absent patellar reflexes; therefore baseline assessments should be done. (2) (CW; PL; TC; HP)

1   These are urine tests; they are not significant to $MgSO_4$ toxicity.

2   Deviations in temperature do not indicate $MgSO_4$ toxicity.

4   These are assessments that may indicate worsening preeclampsia, not $MgSO_4$ toxicity.

198. 1 The gravid uterus no longer compresses major vessels; cardiac output is maintained; glomerular filtration and uterine perfusion rates increase. (2) (CW; IM; TC; HP)

2 Maximizing intraabdominal pressure on the iliac veins will decrease blood flow to the pelvic area.

3 Maximizing aortal compression will decrease uterine blood flow.

4 Hemoconcentration occurs in the standing and sitting positions and decreases uterine perfusion.

199. 4 From these assessments the nurse can determine unusual weight gain and an increase in blood pressure; both of these are early symptoms of pregnancy-induced hypertension. (3) (CW; IM; TC; HP)

1 The data indicate fluid retention.

2 This would be therapeutic for a backache; this answer ignores the possible edema and increased weight gain.

3 The weight gain may not be caused by inappropriate dietary intake but rather by fluid retention.

200. 3 Sodium is not restricted because restriction decreases blood volume, which in turn reduces placental perfusion. (3) (CW; EV; ED; HP)

1 Women at risk for this condition are advised to eat a high-protein diet.

2 Losing weight is contraindicated during pregnancy and does not reduce the incidence of pregnancy-induced hypertension.

4 Diuretic therapy is dangerous because it decreases blood volume, which in turn reduces placental perfusion.

201. 3 Even minimal sensory stimuli can trigger exaggerated cerebral responses such as convulsions; therefore a nonstimulating environment is therapeutic. (2) (CW; AN; TC; HP)

1 This is an undesired action; intracellular volume should be increased during pregnancy.

2 Non-stimulating environments do not reduce headaches resulting from hypertension.

4 A non-stimulating environment has no relation to the length of time antihypertensive drugs are effective.

202. 2 This is the unique characteristic symptom of eclampsia that occurs because of CNS irritation. (2) (CW; AS; PA; HP)

1 This is a symptom of preeclampsia.

3 Same as answer 1.

4 Same as answer 1.

203. 3 A quiet room helps to reduce stimuli, which is essential for limiting or preventing seizures. (2) (CW; PL; PA; HP)

1 The urinary output for someone receiving magnesium sulfate should be at least 100 ml in 4 hours; thus, fluid would not be restricted.

2 Precipitous delivery is not an usual side effect of magnesium therapy.

4 Calcium gluconate, not magnesium gluconate, is the antagonist for magnesium sulfate and should be on hand if symptoms of toxicity appear.

204. 3 When a client is eclamptic she will be experiencing seizures; protecting the client from injury is always the first priority with any seizure. (3) (CW; IM; TC; HP)

1 With a rigid abdomen and seizure activity occurring, accurate assessment is improbable.

2 This is done immediately following the seizure; injury can occur if force is applied to maintain the airway during the seizure.

4 IV effects are immediate, and increasing the dose may cause immediate toxicity.

205. 1 The fetus is at risk for retardation prenatally from a buildup of metabolites in the PKU-affected mother if a prescribed diet is not followed by the mother. (3) (CW; IM; ED; HP)

2 This will not occur if the proper diet is maintained by the mother.

3 The fetus is at risk for mental retardation if the maternal diet contains phenylalanine; also, the infant can inherit phenylketonuria via an autosomal-recessive gene.

4 The client should remain on a phenylalanine restricted diet during, not necessarily before, pregnancy to prevent negative effects on the fetus.

206. 4   PKU is an inborn error of metabolism involving an inability to properly metabolize phenylalanine, an essential amino acid. (2) (CW; AN; TC; HP)

1   This is metabolized normally in those with PKU.

2   Same as answer 1.

3   Same as answer 1.

207. 3   There is a constant need for evaluation of diabetic status, fetal maturity, and placental functioning. (2) (CW; AN; TC; HP)

1   Fetal mortality in pregnancies in which diabetes is present is 10% to 15% higher than for pregnancies in which diabetes is not present.

2   Insulin requirements vary and are usually increased during the second and third trimesters of pregnancy.

4   Many clients with diabetes deliver vaginally with no problems.

208. 4   The blood glucose level is important because hypoglycemia in early pregnancy can lead to congenital abnormalities; hyperglycemia in late pregnancy may lead to fetal hyperinsulinism and subsequent neonatal hypoglycemia. (2) (CW; PL; ED; HP)

1   This is too limited a response; assessment without intervention is useless.

2   Appointments should be made by the client; an authoritative approach takes control away from the client and may increase anxiety.

3   Dietary regulation is usually minimal, with a restriction on excessive carbohydrate ingestion; a limited diet to control weight gain could jeopardize both the fetus and the mother's nutritional status.

209. 4   During the first trimester, hypoglycemia is a factor in managing the pregnant woman who is diabetic; this is because the fetus needs the glucose for its growth and also because of the nausea and vomiting that often occur during this time. (3) (CW; PL; ED; HP)

1   Abortion is not necessarily more common at this time; it is, in fact, most common during the earlier weeks of gestation.

2   Diabetes does not increase the risk of UTI; however, these occur most frequently about the fifth month as more mechanical pressure is placed on the ureters.

3   During the first trimester the serum glucose levels may be low, not elevated, because of nausea and vomiting and the use of glucose by the fetus for growth.

210. 3   In any prenatal situation the goal is an optimally healthy mother and baby, no matter what other factors are involved. (3) (CW; PL; TC; HP)

1   This is important, but delivery of an optimally healthy baby is the priority.

2   This is an ongoing goal, not a long-term goal.

4   This is false; insulin is given as necessary to maintain acceptable glucose levels.

211. 4   An L/S ratio indicates adequacy of pulmonary function, and the baby should be free from major respiratory problems. (1) (CW; AN; ED; HP)

1   There is no correlation between L/S ratio and the need for induced labor.

2   There is no indication of fetal distress; immediate delivery is unnecessary.

3   The L/S ratio only determines fetal lung maturity; further fetal monitoring will be necessary in the future as with any pregnancy.

212. 2   Blood pressure and pulse may not change significantly until large amounts of blood have been lost; the trickling of blood indicates continuous bleeding. (2) (CW; AS; TC; HP)

1   The pulse becomes very rapid, but not until a significant amount of blood is lost.

3   This is not a sign of impending hemorrhage.

4   Blood pressure is normotensive; it usually does not change significantly until a large amount of blood is lost.

213. 3   Wound and skin precautions include wearing gown and gloves; these protect the nurse from the virus. (1) (CW; PL; TC; HP)

1   A mask is not needed because the virus is not airborne.

2　This is used for fecal contamination.

4　This is done for the client's protection, not the nurse's; when caring for a client with herpes the nurse needs to be protected.

NORMAL NEWBORN

214. 1　When an infant is HIV negative and does not have a history of vomiting, the nurse does not have to wear gloves when administering a feeding; however, if the nurse has a cut on a hand or if the mother or infant is HIV positive, the nurse should wear gloves. (1) (CW; IM; TC; NN)

2　Wearing clean gloves for diaper changes in all newborns is a standard protocol.

3　Sterile gloves should be worn when performing suctioning of an infant.

4　Clean gloves should be worn for all admission baths because the nurse will be exposed to blood and amniotic fluid.

215. 3　A perfect score is 10; one point is deducted for lessened muscle tone, the baby's arms do not flex, and one point for acrocyanosis, which is manifested by bluish hands and feet. (2) (CW; AS; PA; NN)

1　The infant must have a higher score based on the data.

2　Same as answer 1.

4　This infant would not have a perfect score of 10; the muscle tone is somewhat lessened, and there is acrocyanosis.

216. 1　Preventing heat loss conserves the infant's oxygen and glycogen reserves, and this is a first priority. (2) (CW; IM; TC; NN)

2　This can be done after provision has been made to prevent heat loss.

3　Warming the infant will reduce cyanosis if no respiratory obstruction is present.

4　This is important but not a priority; assessment should be delayed until the infant is warm.

217. 2　Coarctation of the aorta results in diminished or absent femoral pulses. (3) (CW; AS; PA; NN)

1　This has no impact on the volume of peripheral circulation (minimal shunting occurs in the newborn period).

3　This has minimal impact on the volume of peripheral circulation (left-to-right shunt).

4　Same as answer 3.

218. 3　The score at 5 minutes evaluates the adequacy of the cardiac and respiratory systems' responses to the environment. (1) (CW; AS; ED; NN)

1　The Dubowitz score relates to gestational age.

2　The score represents the neonate's response to the environment and has no relationship to the actual process of labor and delivery.

4　Respiratory distress syndrome in full term infants is a condition that usually does not appear until 24 to 48 hours after birth.

219. 4　Increased pressure during the birth process causes increased intravascular pressure, which may result in capillary rupture. (2) (CW; AN; PA; NN)

1　This is caused by the collection of eosinophils.

2　These are intact capillaries; they may be distinguished from petechiae if they disappear when the area is blanched.

3　Bloody stools or oozing from the umbilicus is the most frequent sign of vitamin K deficiency.

220. 1　This is a normal Moro response, which indicates an intact nervous system. (2) (CW; IM; ED; NN)

2　This total body reaction is the Moro response, which is normally not present after the third month of life; if it persists, there may be a neurologic disturbance.

3　The Moro response has no relationship to hunger.

4　The Moro response is an involuntary reflex to environmental stimuli.

221. 3 Apical pulse of 110 = 2; acrocyanois = 1; active motion and flexion = 2; vigorous cry = 2; effective respiratory effort with crying = 2; total Apgar score = 9. (2) (CW; AS; PA; NN)
1 This is too low; the infant loses only 1 point for not being all pink.
2 Same as answer 1.
4 This is inaccurate; the infant loses 1 point because of a lack of all-pink color.

222. 2 After the respirations are established, the rate ranges from 30 to 60 breaths per minute with short periods of apnea. (1) (CW; AS; PA; NN)
1 Twenty breaths per minute is too slow.
3 Over 60 breaths per minute is too rapid.
4 Same as answer 3.

223. 3 The absence of normal intestinal flora in the newborn results in low levels of vitamin K causing a transient blood coagulation deficiency; an injection of vitamin K is given prophylactically to all infants on the day of birth. (1) (CW; IM; ED; NN)
1 Vitamin K has no effect on erythropoiesis.
2 Vitamin K is important in the synthesis of clotting factor in the liver, but will not prevent jaundice.
4 Newborns have a blood coagulation deficiency; the blood clots more slowly, not more quickly.

224. 3 This metabolic process releases energy and increases heat production in the newborn. (3) (CW; AN; PA; NN)
1 Fatty acids are by-products of the breakdown of brown fat.
2 Shivering is the mechanism of heat production for the adult, not for the newborn.
4 This will not be successful unless plentiful brown fat is present.

225. 3 Physiologic jaundice is caused by elevated bilirubin levels resulting from breakdown of excessive fetal red blood cells; this occurs on the second or third day of life. (1) (CW; PL; ED; NN)
1 Breast milk jaundice usually does not occur until the fifth or sixth postpartal day.

2 This would be evidenced by a decreased urinary output and depressed fontanels.
4 Mottling in the newborn is related to an immature vascular system.

226. 3 This information assists parents to understand the unique features of their newborn and promotes interaction and care during periods of wakefulness. (3) (CW; PL; ED; NN)
1 Most infants are on a demand feeding schedule, not a routine schedule; demand feeding provides for individuality.
2 This is too limited; the parents need a broader discussion of infant behaviors.
4 Printed instructions are inadequate if unaccompanied by a discussion.

227. 4 The fat pad is present in newborns and infants; the arch develops when the child begins to walk. (2) (CW; AN; PA; NN)
1 Flat feet are no more common in children than in adults.
2 The size of the feet is not relevant; arch development is related to walking.
3 Flat feet are not associated with a deformity such as clubfoot.

228. 1 Adaptation to the extrauterine environment is largely dependent on the functional capacity of vital organ systems, which is established during intrauterine development; this is measurable in terms of gestational age and weight. (2) (CW; AN; PA; NN)
2 Although this factor may influence health, it is not critical to neonatal survival.
3 Although these factors may influence health, they are not critical to neonatal survival.
4 Same as answer 3.

229. 4 Using the Apgar score, a value of 1 will be assigned to the color category; the other four categories have values of 2, making the Apgar score 9, demonstrating a healthy baby. (2) (CW; AS; PA; NN)
1 This infant would be cyanotic and apneic and would have very diminished muscle tone and reflex responsiveness.

2 Diminished muscle tone and reflexes are characteristic of these infants; they would not be active or crying lustily.

3 This would apply to a healthy infant whose bluish color would be more generalized and who lost 1 point in one of the other categories.

230. 1 During periods of active or irregular sleep it is normal for newborns to have some twitching movements and irregular respirations; the vital signs and blood glucose levels are normal. (1) (CW; AN; PA; NN)

2 Twitching is a common finding in normal neonates; it often occurs with crying or stimulation.

3 Hypoglycemia in normal newborns would be characterized by a blood glucose level below 30 mg/dl.

4 The normal respiratory rate is 30 to 60; irregular breathing is normal.

231. 1 These are raised sebaceous cysts commonly found on the chin and nose of a newborn; they disappear spontaneously in a few days or weeks. (1) (CW; AS; PA; NN)

2 This is the fine downy hair covering the back and arms of the newborn.

3 These are elevated lesions of immature capillaries and endothelial cells that regress over a period of years; these are commonly called birthmarks.

4 This is an innocuous pink papular neonatal rash; it appears within 24 to 48 hours after birth and resolves spontaneously within a few days.

232. 1 Establishing a patent airway and diminishing cold stress are the priorities; identification is necessary before the infant leaves the delivery area. (1) (CW; PL; PA; NN)

2 Application of eye prophylaxis and administration of vitamin K are often delayed to allow the parents to bond with the infant; a bath at this time would increase the risk of cold stress.

3 These measures would be appropriate in a compromised infant; an 8/9 Apgar is indicative of a healthy uncompromised newborn.

4 The newborn needs constant monitoring and should be placed in a warmer rather than a crib; the infant can be weighed later.

233. 4 There is an absence of normal intestinal flora which results in low levels of vitamin K; vitamin K is necessary for the formation of prothrombin and is administered to prevent hemorrhagic disorders. (1) (CW; AN; PA; NN)

1 Exogenous vitamin K compensates for the vitamin K deficiency that exists until newborns are able to produce their own.

2 Exogenous vitamin K does not produce or maintain normal intestinal flora; vitamin K is produced in the gastrointestinal tract soon after microorganisms are introduced with feedings; within 8 days after birth normal newborns can produce their own vitamin K.

3 Same as answer 2.

234. 2 Screening for the disease results in early diagnosis and treatment, which can prevent mental retardation. (1) (CW; PL; TC; HN)

1 These children have no problem with physical growth; their problem is mental retardation.

3 This is not the problem; the major manifestations are mental or neurologic in origin.

4 The disease is genetic and cannot be acquired other than by inheritance; testing is done for early identification and treatment.

235. 3 Circumcision is a surgical procedure, and infection can occur; the area should not be exposed to organisms in tub water. (1) (CW; EV; ED; NN)

1 The diaper should be changed frequently to prevent irritation from the urine.

2 There should be only minimal bleeding; excessive bleeding requires immediate attention.

4 Petrolatum gauze or A&D ointment prevents the diaper from adhering to the operative site.

236. 4 Proper cleansing and frequent changing will limit the presence of irritating substances. (1) (CW; IM; ED; NN)
  1 Having the nurses change the diaper may lower the mother's self-esteem.
  2 Powder and lotion will cake and retain moisture in the area.
  3 This is a nursing, not a medical, problem.

237. 2 Once the infant breathes the oxygen in the air, the need for an increased amount of immature erythrocytes decreases. (2) (CW; AN; PA; NN)
  1 Jaundice is not an allergic response.
  3 This is not a common occurrence in newborns; also, symptoms would occur more quickly.
  4 The infant and mother have independent blood supplies, and Rh negative blood does not enter the baby's bloodstream.

238. 4 Research strongly supports the theory that there is a sensitive period during the first few hours of life that is extremely important in the promotion of parent-infant attachment. (2) (CW; PL; PS; NN)
  1 Contact with the entire family is important during the taking-in phase of postpartum adjustment.
  2 Encouraging rooming-in is also helpful because it increases the amount of contact between the parents and the newborn; however, this contact is after the first few critical hours.
  3 Contact with the baby can be achieved with breastfeeding or bottle feeding; it is the contact, not the method, that promotes bonding.

239. 4 Stimulating the rooting reflex is effective in making the infant grasp the nipple. (1) (CW; IM; PA; NN)
  1 For milk to be expressed the infant must grasp the entire areola, which contains the secretory ducts.
  2 Bottle feeding may interfere with the infant's learning to accept the breast.
  3 The mother should be supervised for correct positioning of the infant's mouth on the nipple to avoid nipple soreness.

240. 2 This is the proper attachment and helps compress the milk glands. (1) (CW; EV; PA; NN)
  1 The nipple must be on top of the tongue.
  3 This is not a good indication; the infant may be sucking on the nipple only.
  4 This indicates improper attachment.

241. 3 The presence of at least 6 to 8 wet diapers each day indicates sufficient breast milk intake. (2) (CW; EV; ED; NN)
  1 This is a poor indicator; not all babies need extra sucking stimulation.
  2 This could indicate an inadequate amount of fluid ingestion.
  4 This is not a reliable indicator; sleep patterns may vary.

242. 2 At about 6 months of age infants are able to swallow independently of sucking and a cup can be introduced. (3) (CW; PL; ED; NN)
  1 This would be inappropriate because the infant does not have the ability to swallow independently of sucking at this time.
  3 Between 9 and 12 months of age infants can swallow 4 to 5 times consecutively and hold and carry a cup to the mouth; introduction of a cup at 6 months of age makes the weaning easier at 9 to 12 months of age.
  4 This is too late; by this time the child has teeth and sucking on a bottle promotes the development of caries as well as a preference for milk over solid foods.

243. 2 Unless fluoridated water is used by the manufacturer, fluoride supplementation of 0.25 mg daily is required. (3) (CW; AN; PA; NN)
  1 Commercial formulas are iron fortified.
  3 The supply of vitamin K is adequate after the first week of life.
  4 This is unnecessary; vitamin B_{12} may be needed if the mother is a vegetarian and is breastfeeding.

HIGH RISK NEWBORN

244. 2 An Apgar score of 3 indicates a severely depressed infant with apnea, lowered heart rate, and absent reflexes. (2) (CW; AS; PA; HN)

1 The priority is intubation to obtain a patent airway; the infant is usually apneic and not able to breathe independently.

3 Although this is important, establishing a patent airway and initiating respirations are of greater importance.

4 This would be ineffective; this infant requires resuscitative measures.

245. 2 Heart rate below 100 beats per minute = 1; slow and irregular respirations = 1; grimaces in response to suctioning = 1; flaccid muscle tone = 0; and cyanosis = 0; the Apgar score would total 3. (3) (CW; AN; PA; HN)

1 This score is too low; the infant should receive 1 point for heartbeat, 1 point for respirations, and 1 point for grimacing; thus the assigned score is 3.

3 This is too high; the infant should receive 1 point for heartbeat, 1 point for respirations, and 1 point for grimacing; thus the assigned score is 3.

4 Same as answer 3.

246. 4 When the 5-minute Apgar score is 7 or less, there is a 66% chance that the infant will be neurologically impaired. (3) (CW; AN; PA; HN)

1 This may or may not be true; assessment of other factors is necessary.

2 The Apgar score does not evaluate serum glucose levels.

3 An Apgar score between 0 and 3 necessitates immediate resuscitative measures.

247. 3 The 1-minute Apgar score indicates the need to take resuscitative action, and the 5-minute Apgar score indicates whether the action was successful. (2) (CW; AN; TC; HN)

1 The scores do not indicate a need for this.

2 Apgar measurements are for infants of all gestational ages; these scores indicate difficulty regardless of gestational age.

4 Moist oxygen over the face through a funnel to the nose and mouth or stimulation of crying to increase respirations may be sufficient with Apgar scores as low as 5; oxygen under pressure is used when the Apgar score is below 4 at 1 minute.

248. 1 Infants of Class A diabetic mothers may be delivered before 38 weeks; therefore, these infants would be predisposed to the development of respiratory distress syndrome (RDS, hyaline membrane disease) which occurs in preterm infants. (3) (CW; PL; PA; HN)

2 The use of heroin by the mother does not predispose the infant to RDS.

3 The baby of a mother with hypertension may be small for gestational age but not necessarily preterm and at risk for RDS.

4 Preeclampsia does not necessarily predispose the infant to the development of RDS.

249. 1 Flaring nares are a compensatory mechanism that attempts to lessen resistance of narrow nasal passages and increase oxygen intake. (1) (CW; AS; PA; HN)

2 Acrocyanosis is not related to respiratory distress but is caused by vasomotor instability; this is a normal occurrence in the newborn.

3 This is a normal finding in the newborn.

4 Same as answer 3.

250. 4 Weight loss results from the extra sucking effort required to obtain milk flow from the breast. (2) (CW; IM; PS; HN)

1 If the infant is being fed by gavage, the mother's breasts can be pumped and the breast milk can be used for gavage feedings.

2 Time consumption and effort are insufficient reasons to discourage breastfeeding.

3 Breast milk provides adequate nutrition, protects the infant from necrotizing enterocolitis, and provides antibodies.

251. 3 This is a classic sign of respiratory distress in the newborn. (1) (CW; AS; PA; NN)

1 This is associated with neurologic impairment, not respiratory distress.

2 This is within normal limits.

4 The respiratory rate increases, not decreases.

252. 2   In respiratory acidosis, the pH falls and the CO_2 level rises. (2) (CW; AN; PA; HN)
1   This is a normal pH.
3   This is very high but is unrelated to acidosis.
4   The arterial oxygen level may or may not change with acidosis.

253. 1   This is done because any attempt by the infant to maintain temperature further compromises physical status by increasing metabolic activity and O_2 demands. (2) (CW; PL; PA; HN)
2   Increased activity will increase oxygen demands.
3   This is not accurate; the O_2 percentage will vary with PO_2 values of the infant.
4   Same as answer 2.

254. 3   This is a finding consistent with respiratory distress syndrome because of atelectasis and underinflation of alveoli resulting from decreased surfactant in immature lungs. (3) (CW; AS; PA; HN)
1   Expiratory stridor is present in RDS.
2   The rate is much higher in RDS.
4   A lowered pH is more consistent with RDS.

255. 2 O_2 has a cooling effect, and the baby should be kept warm so that metabolic activity and O_2 demands are not increased. (1) (CW; IM; PA; HN)
1   This could produce fluid overload which would lead to increased cardiac output, an undesired outcome especially for an infant with respiratory distress.
3   O_2 concentration is determined by blood gas levels and is changed accordingly.
4   This would tire the baby and increase the need for O_2.

256. 4   Prolonged use of oxygen concentrations above those required to maintain adequate oxygenation has been found to contribute to the occurrence of retinopathy of prematurity (retrolental fibroplasia). (1) (CW; PL; TC; HN)
1   Retinopathy of prematurity cannot be prevented by using any preferred route of O_2 administration.

2   Retinopathy of prematurity is caused by high blood concentrations of O_2, not by eye exposure to oxygen.
3   Warming and humidifying O_2 will not affect the level in the environment.

257. 3   These are key signs of a pneumothorax, which can occur when an infant is receiving oxygen by positive pressure. (2) (CW; AN; PA; HN)
1   The findings are not normal and need immediate attention.
2   The findings do not indicate this occurrence.
4   Same as answer 2.

258. 1   Positioning with the head slightly hyperextended and changing the position q 1 to 2 hours helps to drain secretions and can increase O_2 available for use by promoting respiratory efforts in a premature infant with immature lung tissue. (2) (CW; AN; TC; HN)
2   This is too low; preterm infants do not shiver.
3   Congenital birth defects are observed for in all infants, not just those with RDS.
4   Extensive handling is not desired, but infants do need to be touched.

259. 3   The breast buds and genitalia develop at a specified rate and are good indicators of gestational age. (3) (CW; AS; PA; HN)
1   Weight and length may be influenced both by genetic factors and by prenatal stresses and are not accurate indicators of gestational age.
2   This provides information about the infant's neuromuscular status and is not a specific indicator of gestational age.
4   This is not a good indication of gestational age.

260. 1   A preterm, small for gestational age infant is at risk for problems not seen in the term or average for gestational age infant because of immaturity; this information will help the nurse to anticipate potential problems and aim interventions at prevention. (1) (CW; AN; TC; HN)

2 The information is documented on the infant's chart, but this is not the overriding reason for obtaining this data.

3 The infant will lose weight, but the comparison of weight and gestational age is important for the planning of appropriate nursing measures.

4 Same as answer 2.

261. 4 The Silverman-Anderson Index reflects respiratory status. (3) (CW; EV; PA; HN)

1 The Silverman-Anderson Index does not reflect cardiac function.

2 The Silverman-Anderson Index does not reflect caloric needs.

3 The Silverman-Anderson Index does not reflect neurologic status.

262. 1 Breast tissue is not palpable in an infant of less than 33 weeks gestation. (1) (CW; AS; PA; HN)

2 Creases in the palms and on the soles of the feet are not clearly defined until after the thirty-seventh week of gestation.

3 Ear pinnae spring back in an infant of 36 weeks gestation.

4 A zero-degree square window sign is present in an infant of 40 to 42 weeks gestation.

263. 4 The assessment findings are indicative of a preterm infant; therefore the nurse should closely monitor the infant for signs of respiratory distress syndrome; this occurs frequently in preterm infants because their lungs are immature. (2) (CW; AS; PA; HN)

1 Preterm AGA infants do not develop polycythemia; preterm LGA infants may develop polycythemia, but there are no data to indicate the infant is LGA.

2 Preterm AGA infants may become hypoglycemic.

3 The neonate is preterm, not postterm.

264. 2 The infant would be classified as small for gestational age (SGA) because the weight is below the 10th percentile on the growth curve for a term infant. (1) (CW; AN; PA; HN)

1 An infant is considered to be preterm if born before the end of the thirty-seventh week of gestation; the term small for gestational age rather than immature is used.

3 This is untrue; the infant's weight is below the 10th percentile for a term infant; the infant is SGA.

4 Same as answer 3.

265. 2 SGA infants may exhibit hypoglycemia, especially during the first 2 days of life, because of depleted glycogen stores and inhibited gluconeogenesis. (2) (CW; AN; PA; HN)

1 Decreased BP, pallor with cyanosis, tachycardia, retractions, lethargy, and weak cry are present in hypovolemia.

3 Hypercalcemia is uncommon in newborns.

4 These signs are unrelated to hypothyroidism; symptoms of hypothyroidism are difficult to identify in the newborn.

266. 4 Retinopathy of prematurity (ROP), which used to be called retrolental fibroplasia, is caused by high concentrations of oxygen that may occasionally have to be used with the preterm infant; oxygen must be administered cautiously and the infant's blood oxygen level monitored carefully. (3) (CW; EV; TC; HN)

1 Cataracts are not caused by high oxygen concentrations.

2 Strabismus, which is crossed eyes, is not caused by high oxygen concentrations.

3 This refers to an inflammation of the eyes caused by gonorrheal or Chlamydial infection contracted as the infant passes through the birth canal.

267. 2 Many superficial veins are common in the preterm infant because of the lack of subcutaneous fat deposits. (1) (CW; AS; PA; HN)

1 Flexion of extremities is the posturing of normal term infants; preterm infants usually posture with extremities extended and flaccid.

3 Absent femoral pulses are indicative of coarctation of the aorta, a congenital heart defect.

4 A positive Babinski reflex is a normal newborn reflex.

268. 4 Primary manifestations of NEC are feeding intolerance, increased gastric residual of undigested formula, and bile-stained emesis. (3) (CW; AS; PA; HN)
1 This may occur with a cardiac anomaly, not NEC.
2 This occurs with diarrhea; stools in those with NEC are generally reduced in number and contain glucose and blood.
3 This occurs with pyloric stenosis.

269. 2 Prolonged gastric emptying occurs when the baby has NEC; an increase in abdominal girth of greater than 1 cm in 4 hours is significant and needs immediate intervention. (2) (CW; PL; TC; HN)
1 Formula is stopped and the baby is placed on parenteral fluids.
3 This will have no therapeutic value for a child with NEC.
4 Same as answer 1.

270. 4 An infant of less than 37 weeks gestation is considered preterm; a weight of 1000 grams is under the 10th percentile for the gestational age. (2) (CW; AS; PA; HN)
1 A term infant is gestationally 37 weeks or greater.
2 The infant is preterm, but the weight is under the 10th percentile for the gestational age.
3 Same as answer 1.

271. 2 Gradually rewarming an infant experiencing cold stress is essential to avoid compromising the infant's cardiopulmonary status. (3) (CW; IM; PA; HN)
1 Rapid rewarming of an infant may result in apnea and neonatal stress.
3 An infant experiencing cold stress will become hypoglycemic; the infant uses up glycogen and glucose to maintain the core temperature.
4 Skin temperatures should be taken at least every 15 minutes until stable.

272. 1 A preterm infant may have a weak suck but usually can be breastfed; the mother may at least attempt it, if the infant is stable. (2) (CW; IM; ED; HN)

2 It does not necessarily use more calories to breastfeed; also, there are immunologic benefits to the preterm infant who receives antibodies through breast milk.
3 Pumping the breasts may be necessary, but bottle feeding is not needed because this only deters the mother and infant; at 34 weeks if the infant is stable and the mother so desires, breastfeeding should be attempted.
4 The suck may or may not be weak, but a supervised attempt to breastfeed may help the mother get to know the infant and feel competent in providing care.

273. 4 Research has demonstrated that preterm infants who are allowed to suck on a pacifier during tube feedings take bottle feedings more readily and are discharged sooner. (2) (CW; IM; TC; HN)
1 There is no evidence that non-nutritive sucking is harmful for a preterm infant this size.
2 On the contrary, sucking on a pacifier promotes adaptation to later bottle feedings.
3 Research has identified a benefit of non-nutritive sucking; buck teeth are associated with thumb sucking.

274. 3 If the airway is not patent and gas exchange is inadequate, life cannot be sustained, thus this must be the top priority. (3) (CW; PL; TC; HN)
1 Although bonding is important to the parent-child relationship, without oxygen, life could not be sustained.
2 Although preventing infection is important because the baby lacks immunity from the mother, without oxygen, life could not be sustained.
4 Although body temperature is important because the baby is lacking brown fat and other defense mechanisms needed to maintain temperature, without oxygen, life could not be sustained.

275. 2 The nurse applies tactile stimulation after validating that respirations are absent; this action may be sufficient to reestablish respirations in the high-risk neonate with frequent episodes of apnea. (2) (CW; IM; TC; HN)

1 Assessment will not interrupt the period of apnea; respirations must be immediately reestablished.

3 The monitor should be assessed for proper functioning before use.

4 These measures are too invasive and aggressive for initial intervention; gentle stimulation should be attempted first.

276. 1 The reflexes and muscles of sucking and swallowing are immature; this makes oral feeding ineffectual and exhausting. (3) (CW; AN; PA; HN)

2 The metabolic rate is increased because of fatigue and growth needs.

3 Caloric requirements are increased because of extra growth needs.

4 Absorption of nutrients is decreased because of immaturity of the intestines.

277. 3 Retinopathy of prematurity (ROP) is a complex disease of the premature infant; hypoxemia and hyperoxemia are two of the numerous causes implicated and both can be monitored for with pulse oximetry. (3) (CW; EV; TC; HN)

1 This will not prevent the development of ROP.

2 Light levels are not considered to be a factor in the cause of ROP.

4 Same as answer 1.

278. 3 Oxygen is cooling and the preterm infant already has a predisposition to cold stress; the head accounts for a large proportion of the neonate's body surface and should be covered to retain warmth. (1) (CW; IM; TC; HN)

1 This is unnecessary; this is done when the infant is receiving phototherapy.

2 Too much fluid will cause a full stomach which can put pressure against the diaphragm resulting in respiratory embarrassment.

4 There are no prescribed intervals for turning; this in fact may further compromise an already stressed neonate.

279. 3 Observing the care that the parents actually give the infant provides direct validation of their skill and comfort levels. (1) (CW; EV; ED; HN)

1 This action is helpful in anticipatory guidance but is only a small part of competency evaluation.

2 Although this is helpful in identifying empirical knowledge, it does not test their skill or comfort level.

4 Same as answer 2.

280. 1 At birth, circulating maternal glucose is removed; however, the infant still has a high level of insulin and may develop a rebound hypoglycemia. (2) (CW; AS; TC; HN)

2 The temperature-regulating ability of a neonate born to a mother with diabetes mellitus is similar to that of a normal neonate unless the infant is preterm.

3 Pathologic jaundice is associated with hemolytic diseases such as Rh and ABO incompatibility, and sepsis, not diabetes mellitus.

4 Cyanotic episodes, with or without tremors, may be indicative of cardiac problems, not diabetes mellitus.

281. 1 A difficult delivery because of broad fetal shoulders may result in a fractured clavicle, which can be assessed by the findings of a knot or lump, limited arm movement, and a unilateral Moro response. (2) (CW; AS; PA; HN)

2 This is unrelated to a difficult delivery of a baby with broad shoulders.

3 This reflex involves the feet; it is in no way related to a difficult delivery because of broad shoulders.

4 Same as answer 3.

282. 1 Decreasing IV glucose slowly is necessary to prevent a hypoglycemic response. (3) (CW; IM; PA; HN)

2 Metabolic alkalosis will not occur with discontinuation of the glucose; it occurs with excessive amounts of bicarbonate.

3 Withholding oral feedings while withdrawing IV glucose may result in hypoglycemia.

4 Glycosuria is unlikely to occur when decreasing the IV glucose because blood glucose levels will decrease.

283. 4   Because the virus is found in the respiratory tract and the urine, isolation is necessary; rubella is spread by droplets from the respiratory tract. (2) (CW; PL; TC; HN)

1   Enteric precautions are indicated when pathogens are transmitted in the feces; however, since the rubella virus may be found in the urine, gloves should be used when changing diapers.

2   This is not necessary; it would be necessary to prevent transmission of diseases, such as malaria and serum hepatitis, that have blood borne pathogens.

3   Universal precautions alone would be unsafe; additional precautions must be taken to protect the nurse from droplet infection.

284. 2   Phototherapy changes unconjugated bilirubin in skin to conjugated bilirubin bound to protein, permitting excretion. (1) (CW; EV; TC; HN)

1   Phototherapy does not affect liver function; the liver does not dispose of bilirubin.

3   Vitamin K has no effect on bilirubin excretion; it is necessary for prothrombin formation.

4   The bilirubin is not excreted via the skin but in the urine and feces.

285. 3   This is necessary to provide for some normal psychosocial contact. (2) (CW; PL; PS; HN)

1   This may block light rays from acting on bilirubin deposits; frequent cleansing after voiding and defecation will prevent skin excoriation.

2   All parts of the body may contain bilirubin deposits and should be exposed to the light.

4   Radiant heaters are not used; only fluorescent bulbs are used.

286. 2   The head circumference is usually 1 inch larger than the chest; a head circumference $1\frac{1}{2}$ inches smaller than the chest could indicate microcephaly. (3) (CW; AS; PA; HN)

1   In anencephaly, the disparity between the head and chest circumference would be much larger than $1\frac{1}{2}$ inches.

3   No molding takes place in cesarean delivery; therefore the head should be about 1 inch larger than the chest at birth.

4   According to growth charts, the range of head circumference for boys is just slightly ($\frac{1}{2}$ inch) larger than the chest.

287. 3   Mothers with Type O blood have anti-A and anti-B antibodies that are transferred across the placenta; this is the most common incompatibility because the mother is Type O in 20% of all pregnancies. (2) (CW; IM; PA; HN)

1   This is usually not a problem.

2   Same as answer 1.

4   Same as answer 1.

287. 3   Adherence to the diet is necessary for optimal physical growth with no adverse effects on mental development; a diet that is instituted late will not reverse brain damage. (1) (CW; AN; PA; HN)

1   Detection cannot occur until the infant has taken milk or formula that contains phenylalanines for 24 hours and metabolites accumulate in the blood; behaviors indicating mental retardation and CNS involvement usually are evident by about 6 months of age in the untreated infant.

2   There is no phenylalanine at birth; it first becomes measurable after the infant ingests milk or formula.

4   This is untrue; it is related to compliance with the prescribed diet once the diagnosis is made.

289. 3   The term phenylketonuria is derived from phenylpyruvic acid, which gives urine a mousy, musty odor. (2) (CW; AS; PA; HN)

1   This odor is not present with phenylketonuria.

2   Same as answer 1.

4   Same as answer 1.

290. 1   Right-to-left shunts result in inadequate perfusion of blood; not enough blood flows to the lungs for oxygenation. (3) (CW; AN; PA; HN)

2   Left-to-right shunts result in too much blood flowing to the lungs; blood is adequately perfused.

3 Left-sided obstruction to the flow of blood results in decreased peripheral pulses, not cyanosis.

4 Normally there should be no shunting of blood between the right and left sides of the heart after the ductus arteriosus closes.

291. 3 Because the lungs are stressed by increased fluid, increased respirations are the first and best indicators of early congestive heart failure. (3) (CW; AS; PA; HN)

1 Cyanosis is not an early sign because there is adequate perfusion of blood.

2 The heart rate would not decrease; it would increase in an attempt to compensate.

4 This is a normal finding in the newborn.

292. 3 The cytomegalovirus has been recovered from semen, vaginal secretions, urine, feces, and blood; it is commonly found in clients with AIDS. (3) (CW; AN; PA; HN)

1 This is associated with toxoplasmosis.

2 This is associated with hepatitis A.

4 Same as answer 1.

293. 4 The abnormal facies associated with fetal alcohol syndrome includes a small, up-turned nose, which is distinctive in these infants. (3) (CW; AS; PA; HN)

1 A cleft lip may occur without a precursor or with the trisomies.

2 Multiple fingers are associated with the trisomies.

3 An umbilical hernia can develop in early infancy and is not related to fetal alcohol syndrome.

DRUG RELATED RESPONSES

294. 2 Use ratio and proportion:
2,450,000 u / 300,000 u = x ml / 1 ml
300,000 x = 2,450,000
x = 8.2 ml.
(2) (CW; AN; TC; DR)

1 This would deliver more than the ordered amount.

3 This would deliver less than the ordered amount.

4 Same as answer 3.

295. 2 Probenecid reduces renal tubular excretion of penicillin. (2) (CW; EV; ED; DR)

1 This is unrelated to the concomitant administration of penicillin and probenecid.

3 Same as answer 1.

4 Same as answer 1.

296. 2 Tetracycline has an affinity for calcium; if used during tooth bud development, it may cause discoloration of teeth. (2) (CW; IM; ED; DR)

1 This is untrue; it is associated only with the discoloration of teeth.

3 Same as answer 1.

4 Same as answer 1.

297. 1 Maintenance of serum progesterone levels keeps cervical mucus thick and hostile to sperm at all times. (1) (CW; IM; ED; DR)

2 Progesterone-only pills do not interfere with ovulation.

3 Fertility drugs are often taken during the first part of the cycle to encourage ovulation, not contraception.

4 Combined estrogen and progesterone oral contraceptives are taken during the second, third, and fourth weeks of the cycle.

298. 3 Nausea and vomiting are related to excessive amounts of estrogen; these symptoms can usually be controlled by reducing the dose. (1) (CW; EV; TC; DR)

1 Amenorrhea is associated with pregnancy; breakthrough bleeding is more common than amenorrhea with estrogen.

2 Hypomenorrhea is caused by estrogen deficiency.

4 Depression and lethargy can be related to both excessive estrogen and progesterone but are not common side effects.

299. 1 Oral contraceptives should be discontinued with any symptom that could be related to emboli. (1) (CW; EV; TC; DR)

2 Menorrhagia is a side effect related to excessive amounts of estrogen; immediate discontinuance of contraceptives is unnecessary.

3 Mittelschmerz is pain midway in the menstrual cycle, usually at ovulation.

4 This may be a sign of infection, not a side effect of oral contraceptives.

300. 1 Vitamin C aids in absorption of iron because of its ability to reduce acidity. (2) (CW; PL; ED; DR)
    2 This is unrelated to the absorption of iron.
    3 Same as answer 2.
    4 Same as answer 2.

301. 2 RhIg administration during the 28th week of gestation reduces an active antibody response in an Rh negative individual exposed to the positive blood; this drug is used during pregnancy. (3) (CW; EV; ED; DR)
    1 It would be difficult to determine whether Rh sensitization had occurred this early in pregnancy.
    3 RhIg is given earlier in the pregnancy; it is a preventive measure, not a treatment for a woman already sensitized.
    4 RhIg will not be effective if given this late in the pregnancy because sensitization has already occurred.

302. 3 Heparin can be used during pregnancy because it does not cross the placental barrier and will not cause hemorrhage in the fetus. (3) (CW; IM; TC; DR)
    1 This drug can cross the placental barrier and cause hemorrhage in the fetus.
    2 Same as answer 1.
    4 Same as answer 1.

303. 4 Heparin should not be given because 98 seconds is almost three times the normal time it takes a fibrin clot to form (25 to 36 seconds) and prolonged bleeding may result; the therapeutic range with heparin is $1\frac{1}{2}$ to 2 times the normal range. (3) (CW; EV; TC; DR)
    1 Heparin must not be increased; the client already has received too much.
    2 The APTT is not normal but prolonged; it is almost three times the normal rate.
    3 The medication does not need to be changed; it needs to be stopped.

304. 2 This is a frequently occurring side effect of this drug. (2) (CW; EV; TC; DR)
    1 Tachycardia, not bradycardia, frequently occurs.
    3 This is not an expected side effect.
    4 These do not occur with terbutaline.

305. 4 Ascorbic acid enhances the absorption of iron. (2) (CW; IM; ED; DR)
    1 Iron should be taken in the morning before meals to allow for maximum absorption.
    2 Same as answer 1.
    3 Although milk will decrease stomach irritation, it will not enhance iron absorption.

306. 4 Phenergan potentiates the analgesic effect of Demerol; it also acts as an antiemetic if Demerol causes nausea and vomiting. (1) (CW; IM; ED; DR)
    1 This is untrue; Phenergan potentiates the analgesic effects of Demerol.
    2 Same as answer 1.
    3 Same as answer 1.

307. 1 This is caused by the local anesthetic passing rapidly through the placenta to the fetus and having a quinidine-like effect on the myocardium. (3) (CW; EV; PA; DR)
    2 The opposite is true; hypotension may occur.
    3 This can occur with epidural or spinal anesthesia when the anesthetic is injected too high.
    4 This can occur with general anesthesia.

308. 3 This is the correct flow rate; 10 units of the drug added to 1000 ml of IV results in a solution where 1 ml = 0.01 mg of the drug; therefore, 1 ml must be administered per minute; multiply the amount to be infused (1 ml) by the drop factor (60) and divide the result by the amount of time in minutes (1). (3) (CW; AN; TC; DR)
    1 This is too slow; it should be 60 gtt/min.
    2 Same as answer 1.
    4 This is too fast, it should be 60 gtt/min.

309. 4 Frequent contractions with short relaxation periods may lead to fetal hypoxia. (2) (CW; AN; PA; DR)
    1 This intensity is within the normal limits of 50 to 75 mmHg.
    2 An adverse response to Pitocin is a contraction lasting more than 90 seconds; contractions lasting 30 seconds usually occur in early labor.
    3 This is within the normal fetal heart rate range of 120 to 160 during labor.

310. 3 Oxytocin (Pitocin) has an antidiuretic effect, acting to reabsorb water from the glomerular filtrate. (3) (CW; EV; PA; DR)

1 Hyperventilation is caused by inappropriate breathing patterns, not by prolonged use of Pitocin.

2 Affect is not altered by the use of Pitocin.

4 Fever occurs with infection or dehydration, not with prolonged use of Pitocin.

311. 1 Effective magnesium sulfate therapy reduces edema, thus leading to increased urinary output. (3) (CW; EV; TC; DR)

2 This is a sign of toxicity.

3 Same as answer 2.

4 The goal of this therapy is to reduce the blood pressure.

312. 2 A side effect of this drug is respiratory depression; therefore, a reduction of respirations to this level indicates toxicity and the drug should be withheld. (3) (CW; EV; TC; DR)

1 The blood pressure is already known to be high and the drug must be given to prevent a seizure from occurring.

3 This drug has a sodium retention effect so urinary output is important but 30 ml per hour is within the acceptable range of 100 ml per 4 hours.

4 This is considered a therapeutic effect of this drug.

313. 1 Near-toxic levels of magnesium sulfate are indicated by the disappearance of the knee-jerk reflex and by depressed respirations below 12 per minute. (3) (CW; EV; TC; DR)

2 This is given as an antidote only when ordered by the physician.

3 This is unsafe; this would cause an overdose and exacerbate the toxic signs.

4 Waiting could put the client in jeopardy of respiratory arrest; toxic symptoms require medical intervention.

314. 2 Hypermagnesemia causes extreme muscle depression; calcium gluconate, the MgSO$_4$ antidote, promotes muscle function. (2) (CW; AN; TC; DR)

1 This is used in chelation therapy for lead poisoning.

3 This is an antihypertensive.

4 This is used for hyperkalemia.

315. 3 Methergine, an oxytocic, is used to promote uterine contractions; its vasoconstrictive action can also lead to hypertension, and it should not be used when hypertension is already present. (2) (CW; EV; TC; DR)

1 This medication generally is not given to a postpartum client unless an infection is present; there are no data to support the presence of an infection.

2 There is no contraindication to using this medication to relieve the discomfort of an episiotomy.

4 There is no contraindication for use of this drug; there are no data to support the fact that the client is constipated.

316. 1 Clients with allergies to penicillin must be evaluated carefully because they may have an allergic response to Velosef as well. (3) (CW; AS; TC; DR)

2 This is unrelated to penicillin hypersensitivity.

3 Same as answer 2.

4 Same as answer 2.

317. 2 The concentration of propylthiouracil excreted in breast milk is 3 to 12 times higher than its level in maternal serum; this may cause agranulocytosis or goiter in the infant. (3) (CW; IM; EV; DR)

1 Heparin is not excreted in breast milk.

3 The amount of breast milk excretion of gentamicin is unknown, but it can be given to infants directly without adverse effects.

4 Diphenhydramine is excreted in breast milk, but it does not adversely affect the infant when therapeutic doses are given to the mother.

318. 3 Methergine can cause hypertension and should not be given to a client with an elevated blood pressure. (2) (CW; EV; PA; DR)
1 This indicates thrombophlebitis and is not related to Methergine.
2 This is a normal adult finding.
4 Methergine does not affect respirations.

319. 4 Iron is best utilized when given in an acid medium. (2) (CW; EV; ED; DR)
1 This would decrease the acidity of the stomach; an alkaline medium does not promote absorption of iron.
2 Same as answer 1.
3 Same as answer 1.

320. 3 This is the expected outcome; if output exceeds intake, it indicates that the infant is diuresing from the Lasix. (1) (CW; EV; PA; DR)
1 Although important to assess, this is subjective; intake and output would be an objective assessment.
2 This is not the desired outcome; this would indicate dehydration, which could occur with excessive administration of Lasix.
4 Although Lasix can cause hypokalemia, which can precipitate digitalis toxicity, this is not the desired effect of Lasix administration.

EMOTIONAL NEEDS RELATED TO CHILDBEARING

321. 2 The client has the right not to accept the Papanicolaou test; the nurse must recognize the client's need to talk with the physician first. (2) (CW; IM; PS; EC)
1 This is a subjective conclusion; the client has the right to refuse the test.
3 This is inappropriate; this action is not client centered.
4 The client's need must be recognized first.

322. 1 This recognizes achievement and reinforces the client's positive behavior. (2) (CW; IM; PS; EC)
2 This implies that the client is not doing enough; the focus should be on the positive, and the gains should be reinforced.

3 This is inappropriate; the client has been successful in reducing her blood pressure and weight with nonpharmacologic strategies.
4 This focuses on the negative rather than the positive; small gains should be reinforced.

323. 1 The therapeutic regimen includes bed rest; peace of mind can best be achieved if the children are adequately cared for. (3) (CW; IM; PS; EC)
2 This explores feelings without including a therapeutic regimen.
3 This is giving solutions rather than exploring the situation with the client.
4 Complete bed rest has been prescribed.

324. 3 Doing this will help the client relax and will lessen discomfort. (2) (CW; IM; PS; EC)
1 The client may become more anxious if the procedure is hurried.
2 This may distract the client but will not produce relaxation.
4 This may make the client more anxious; holding the breath causes tightening of the perineum.

325. 3 One of the characteristics of SIDS is that subsequent siblings of a SIDS infant have a five times greater risk for SIDS than do infants in the general population. (2) (CW; IM; ED; EC)
1 This is untrue; they have a greater risk for SIDS.
2 The opposite is true.
4 Same as answer 1.

326. 3 This response is nonjudgmental; it permits the client to recognize her own feelings. (2) (CW; IM; PS; EC)
1 This is judgmental; it leaves no room for the client's feelings.
2 This is judgmental; it gives the nurse's opinion on a moral question for the client.
4 This response leaves the burden of the decision to the client without offering assistance.

327. 2 This is an accurate and nonjudgmental response. (2) (CW; IM; PS; EC)

1 This response recognizes the client's feelings but cuts off communication because it ends the discussion.

3 This is a judgmental response that questions the mother's decision making and deals only with the present.

4 Same as answer 3.

328. 4 This reassures the client that her baby is alright at the moment and that the nurses are aware of and monitoring the baby's status. (1) (CW; IM; PS; EC)

1 This response does not provide the mother with any reassurance of the baby's status or that anything is being done to monitor the baby.

2 This provides false reassurance; amniotic fluid will not protect the fetus if the mother has a seizure.

3 This provides false reassurance; following instructions does not guarantee a healthy baby.

329. 2 Because seeing and touching the newborn infant is a species-specific behavior for human attachment, allowing them to hold the infant will promote bonding. (2) (CW; IM; PS; EC)

1 Although this is a viable action, holding and touching will promote bonding more effectively.

3 After touching and holding, this action can also contribute to bonding.

4 Actual holding and touching promotes bonding more than does just hearing about the baby.

330. 3 The mother should be reunited with the baby at the first opportunity and when the mother is prepared and feeling well enough to do so. (2) (CW; PL; PS; EC)

1 Grief work will go on for an extended period of time and has no relationship to when the baby is seen.

2 There is no magic about the first 24 hours; some mothers are too ill or both parents may be too frightened to see the baby that soon.

4 Some parents may be too frightened to think to ask to see the baby; the nurse can prepare the parents and then suggest a visit.

331. 2 The development of bonding between mother and infant is an important psychologic goal and should be facilitated. (2) (CW; PL; PS; EC)

1 This is a nursing action and does not require a physician's order.

3 It is important for mothers to develop a relationship with ill newborns even if the prognosis is poor.

4 Same as answer 3.

332. 3 This statement conveys acceptance by the nurse and encourages the mother to verbalize additional concerns; it also explores the mother's understanding of the physician's explanation. (2) (CW; IM; PS; EC)

1 This reply belittles the mother's concern and cuts off further communication.

2 Although this response does acknowledge part of the mother's concerns, it denies her the opportunity of further exploration of her fears that her infant may not respond to therapy.

4 Same as answer 1.

333. 3 To cry in this situation is a normal response; it is also normal to be frightened about touching a small preterm infant but the nurse should provide support and encourage the mother to do so. (2) (CW; AN; PS; EC)

1 Bonding does not have a detachment behavior phase; the behavior indicates apprehension in a difficult situation.

2 This is not incomplete bonding, but fear in a difficult situation.

4 The reaction to the baby is more complex than merely fear of the NICU.

334. 4 By participating in the infant's care, the client will gain confidence in her own ability to meet the infant's needs. (2) (CW; IM; PS; EC)

1 Watching the provision of care by others would only increase the client's sense of inadequacy.

2 If she is not permitted to care for the infant sooner, the client will have to develop these skills under stress.

3 There is no need for a specialist to care for the infant after discharge.

335. 1 If the client demonstrates anorexia, crying, and insomnia, the nurse should recognize these as symptoms of depression, not anxiety. (2) (CW; AS; PS; EC)

2 Lethargy and anorexia are manifestations of depression, but they are usually accompanied by insomnia rather than prolonged sleep.

3 Ambivalence and lethargy can be associated with depression, but they are usually accompanied by anorexia, not increased appetite.

4 Insomnia and ambivalence may be seen with depression, but they are accompanied by anorexia, not increased appetite.

336. 1 Confrontation about the active substance abuse and the mother's diminished ability to safely care for the infant at this time is necessary to help the mother get help and to also protect the baby. (2) (CW; IM; PS; EC)

2 Decisions should not be made without input from the mother.

3 This would be unsafe; the mother may not be capable of caring for the infant.

4 Same as answer 2.

337. 3 Giving the parents true information about what to expect during the procedure will help to allay their fears and encourage their cooperation. (2) (CW; IM; PS; EC)

1 The nurse should be able to provide information and interpretation of procedures for clients; delay in answering their questions may increase clients' concerns.

2 Reassurance is nontherapeutic; an amniocentesis is a low-risk procedure, but some complications may occur.

4 If the father is uninformed, viewing the procedure may increase his anxiety even though his presence may be comforting to the mother.

338. 3 This response encourages the client to verbalize concerns; verbalization is an outlet for discharging tension. (1) (CW; IM; PS; EC)

1 This response reinforces the client's fears.

2 This response denies the client's feelings and gives false reassurance.

4 Same as answer 2.

339. 1 The mother should see her infant as soon as possible so that she can acknowledge the reality of the delivery and begin bonding. (2) (CW; PL; PS; EC)

2 A delay retards maternal-infant bonding.

3 Same as answer 2.

4 This is an independent nursing action.

340. 2 Touching and holding the infant is the most effective way of promoting mother-infant bonding. (1) (CW; IM; PS; EC)

1 This provides false reassurance; the nurse does not know if this is true.

3 This is an unreal approach; it does not prepare the mother to deal with her ill child.

4 This would prevent the mother from touching and holding the baby; the mother must do this to foster bonding.

341. 4 Unplanned cesarean delivery can result in guilt, disappointment, anger, and a sense of failure as a woman. (1) (CW; AN; PS; EC)

1 This is not usually a common concern.

2 The hospital stay is not exceptionally prolonged; the client usually is discharged within 2 to 5 days.

3 Mothers who deliver by cesarean delivery can assume the mothering role.

342. 1 By discussing the experience, the client is bringing it into reality; this is characteristic of the taking-in phase. (3) (CW; AN; PS; EC)

2 The client is not ready to assume the tasks of the letting-go phase until completing the tasks of the taking-in and taking-hold phases.

3 The taking-hold phase is marked by an increased desire to resume independence; this statement reveals the client is still in the taking-in phase.

4 The working-through phase is not a separate phase of adjustment to parenthood; this is not relevant.

343. 3 This recognizes the client's feelings, encourages ventilation, and does not encourage the use of alcohol for relaxation. (1) (CW; IM; PS; EC)

1 This gives false reassurance; the use of alcohol should not be encouraged for relaxation.

2 This does not recognize the client's underlying feelings and could put the client on the defensive.
4 The nurse cannot ensure the physician's response; the use of alcohol should not be encouraged for relaxation.

344. 3 This opens communication and allows the client to verbalize thoughts and feelings. (2) (CW; IM; PS; EC)
1 This is judgmental; there are not enough data to make this assumption.
2 This ignores the client's needs and cuts off communication.
4 This does not give the client the opportunity to verbalize feelings and needs.

345. 3 Adolescent parents are still involved in the developmental stage of resolving their own self-identity; they have not sequentially matured to intimacy and generativity. (1) (CW; AN; ED; EC)
1 Although this may be true, it is not the reason the baby is at risk for neglect or abuse.
2 Same as answer 1.
4 Same as answer 1.

346. 3 This statement allows parents an opportunity to obtain additional information and review their options to make an informed decision. (3) (CW; IM; ED; EC)
1 Recent studies do not support any connection between circumcision and penile cancer.
2 This information may have already been discussed with the physician; it may be more helpful for the nurse to review the information at this time.
4 This is a partially true statement; however, the Academy primarily emphasizes that there are no medical indications for this procedure.

347. 4 This has been validated by the literature; also, children thrive as long as their caregivers provide an opportunity for stable relationships to occur. (1) (CW; IM; PS; EC)
1 This is not validated by current literature.
2 Same as answer 1.
3 Same as answer 1.

REPRODUCTIVE CHOICES

348. 2 The male should be treated to prevent the infection from passing back and forth between him and his sexual partner. (1) (CW; EV; ED; RP)
1 The organism is most likely present in the partner's urogenital tract; voiding will not prevent recurrence.
3 This is an ineffective remedy and will not prevent recurrence.
4 A douche is not recommended during pregnancy.

349. 3 Any blood from the rupture will accumulate; pressure from this accumulation pushing on the diaphragm causes pain. (3) (CW; AN; PA; RP)
1 Anxiety can cause many things, but shoulder pain is an atypical symptom.
2 The cardiac changes caused by hypovolemia do not cause shoulder pain.
4 This does not cause shoulder pain, but could cause rebound abdominal pain.

350. 3 This is an appropriate nursing diagnosis; the bleeding is causing a decreased circulating blood volume and therefore a decreased cardiac output. (3) (CW; AN; PA; RP)
1 This would not be an appropriate nursing diagnosis for this client; there would be a fluid volume deficit, not excess.
2 Infection could occur later but is not a problem at this time.
4 This client is not incapable of making decisions for herself.

351. 4 Removing the tube does not bring a halt to menses; endometrial proliferation and shedding will occur as long as the ovaries and uterus are present. (1) (CW; EV; ED; RP)
1 This is a correct statement; there is evidence that clients who have one tubal pregnancy are highly susceptible to having another.
2 This is a correct statement; pregnancy should be delayed 6 to 12 months after a tubal pregnancy.
3 This is a correct statement; pelvic infections can lead to constriction of tubes, and a fertilized ovum may become trapped.

352. 1 This response encourages the clients to verbalize their feelings. (1) (CW; IM; PS; RP)

2 The clients are not interested in the nurse's wishes; the focus should be on them.

3 This is a very insensitive and incorrect statement; there may be nothing wrong with either client.

4 The clients are not seeking advice about dealing with their parents.

353. 2 Only superficial attention has been directed to hypertension; ongoing health supervision is needed. (1) (CW; AN; TC; RP)

1 Teaching and encouraging the client to engage in self-care is helping the client.

3 This is untrue; however, limiting sodium intake is too superficial.

4 Involving the client is important, but professional supervision is required.

354. 3 This is referred pain from the passage of carbon dioxide through the tubes; this is usually indicative of tubal patency. (2) (CW; IM; ED; RP)

1 No anesthesic is given; the client's awareness of pain is necessary to evaluate whether carbon dioxide is able to pass through the tubes.

2 The client can resume normal activities as soon as the test is over.

4 The client does not usually experience nausea and/or vomiting.

355. 4 This is necessary to keep the sperm viable; if the specimen becomes warm, the sperm will die. (1) (CW; IM; ED; RP)

1 Rubber solvents and preservatives may affect the semen specimen.

2 The specimen can be collected at any time.

3 This may lessen the amount of ejaculate needed for the specimen.

356. 4 Because the client is ovulating, the infertility may be due to a seminal factor; the partner's semen should be examined before more extensive studies or treatments are begun with the woman. (2) (CW; AN; PA; RP)

1 All other potential problems should be ruled out first; the client does not have a right to receive the drug unless it is appropriate for the problem.

2 Other potential problems should be ruled out first.

3 Same as answer 2.

357. 3 As the laminaria tent is left in place for this length of time it increases in size from absorption of moisture and dilates the cervix two to three times its original diameter before the suction procedure is done. (2) (CW; IM; ED; RP)

1 A local anesthetic agent is usually injected into the cervix (paracervical block) and may cause mild cramping or light spotting.

2 Suction is used after removal of the laminaria; a D&C procedure would be used subsequently only if placental tissue were retained.

4 Cervical bleeding is reduced by the use of laminaria and is usually equivalent to a heavy menstrual period; the client is usually observed for 1 to 3 hours following the procedure.

358. 4 This indicates that the bleeding is excessive and the physician should be notified. (1) (CW; EV; ED; RP)

1 Although instructions vary among health care providers, sexual intercourse usually may be resumed in 1 to 3 weeks.

2 Although instructions vary among health care providers, tampons usually are denied for 3 days to 3 weeks.

3 The menstrual period will usually resume in from 4 to 6 weeks.

WOMEN'S HEALTH

359. 4 This is known as the hormone of pregnancy; together with estrogen it helps prepare the endometrium for the fertilized ovum, helps maintain pregnancy, and prepares the mammary glands for milk secretion. (1) (CW; AN; PA; WH)

1 This is secreted by the adrenal cortex, and it affects carbohydrate metabolism.

2 This is secreted by the anterior lobe of the pituitary gland; it starts and maintains milk secretion by the mammary glands.

3 This is secreted by the posterior pituitary gland; it stimulates labor contractions and contractile tissue around the nipple during nursing.

360. 2   Active immunity occurs when the individual's cells produce antibodies in response to an agent or its products; these antibodies will destroy the agent (antigen) should it enter the body again. (3) (CW; AN; PA; WH)

   1   Antigens do not fight antibodies; they trigger an antibody formation that in turn attacks the antigen.
   3   Antigens are foreign substances that enter the body and trigger antibody formation.
   4   Sensitized lymphocytes do not act as antibodies.

361. 4   Mittelschmerz is pain that sometimes occurs at ovulation when the ova erupts from the follicle. (1) (CW; AN; ED; WH)

   1   The pain is mild, cyclic, and characteristic of mittelschmerz; it requires no medical intervention.
   2   When menses first begin the client is usually anovulatory and would not experience the pain known as mittelschmerz.
   3   The pain will probably occur most frequently when ovulation is well established.

362. 3   This is the only correct definition of dysmenorrhea. (1) (CW; AS; ED; WH)

   1   This occurs with menopause and during pregnancy, not dysmenorrhea.
   2   This is any bleeding that occurs at any time other than during the menstrual period; there may or may not be any pain.
   4   This is known as menometrorrhagia.

363. 4   This medical aseptic technique should limit the spread of microorganisms and help prevent future urinary tract infections if incorporated into her health practices. (1) (CW; IM; TC; WH)

   1   This is unnecessary; also, the client is probably experiencing frequency.
   2   The client does not have to use a bedpan; if intake and output are being measured, the use of a container to collect the urine is sufficient.
   3   This is unnecessary while urinating; it may be employed as a part of perineal care after urinating.

364. 2   A tuberculin test should not be administered to a client with a previous positive tuberculin test because severe reactions can occur at the test site in individuals previously sensitized. (2) (CW; EV; TC; WH)

   1   It is more important to know whether the test was positive than if it was done.
   3   Although this may provide exposure to tuberculosis it does not necessarily mean the client will have a positive tuberculin test.
   4   Unless it was tuberculosis, this would not affect giving the tuberculin test.

365. 1   This avoids the possibility of ingesting infected cysts. (3) (CW; IM; ED; WH)

   2   This disease, though more prevalent in foreign countries, is seen in the United States.
   3   This is not related to toxoplasmosis.
   4   Same as answer 3.

366. 3   A condom covers the penis and contains the semen when it is ejaculated; semen contains a high percentage of HIV in infected individuals. (1) (CW; IM; ED; WH)

   1   This is poor advice; pre-ejaculatory fluid carries the HIV in an infected individual.
   2   This is unsafe; although a monogamous relationship is less risky than having multiple sexual partners, if the one partner is HIV positive, the other person is at high risk for acquiring the HIV.
   4   This is not what the client is asking; most contraceptives do not provide any protection from the HIV.

367. 2   This is a description of a chancre which is the initial sign of syphilis. (3) (CW; AS; PA; WH)

   1   These are condylomata lata which are typical of the secondary stage.
   3   This is typical of the secondary stage of systemic involvement which occurs from 2 to 4 years after the disappearance of the chancre.
   4   This is typical of the secondary stage.

368. 4 Dryness inactivates the *Treponema pallidum* making it incapable of causing disease. (1) (CW; AN; PA; WH)

1 The organism is transferred by sexual contact; warm, moist body contact supports growth of the organism.

2 This is not true; nothing chelates the organism.

3 These support the growth of the organism.

369. 3 Syphilis is primarily a vascular disease; aortitis, valvular insufficiency, and aortic aneurysms are the most prevalent problems in tertiary syphilis. (2) (CW; AN; PA; WH)

1 Although lesions occur on the genitalia during primary and secondary syphilis, the reproductive system is not the major body system affected in tertiary syphilis.

2 A gumma skin lesion is the least commonly occurring lesion associated with tertiary syphilis; skin lesions such as macular and papular eruptions most commonly occur in secondary syphilis.

4 Although lesions can occur about the mouth (chancre in primary syphilis and mucous patches in secondary syphilis), the structures of the lower respiratory tract are not the major structures involved in tertiary syphilis.

370. 4 The least amount of breast engorgement occurs at this time, limiting lumps that may occur because of fluid accumulation. (1) (CW; AS; PA; WH)

1 Breast engorgement begins before ovulation and does not subside until several days after menses ends; engorgement interferes with accurate palpation.

2 Inaccurate assessment could result because examination would occur at different times of the menstrual cycle; accurate comparisons could not be made from month to month; this is appropriate for postmenopausal women.

3 Same as answer 1.

371. 1 Serous or bloody discharge from the nipple is abnormal. (2) (CW; AS; PA; WH)

2 The right hand should examine the left breast because this allows the flattened fingers to palpate the entire breast including the tail (upper, outer quadrant toward the axilla) and axillary area.

3 A small pillow or rolled towel should be placed under the scapula of the side being examined.

4 The flat part of the fingers, not the palm or finger tips, should be used for palpation.

372. 2 Compression of the breast flattens mammary tissue and maximizes the penetration of the breast by x-rays; this is especially important for the dense breast tissue of adolescents, young nulliparous women, and women with large breasts. (1) (CW; IM; ED; WH)

1 This is usually done with sonography.

3 This is not necessary.

4 The American Cancer Society recommends that women at high risk for breast cancer (the client's sister had breast cancer) should have routine mammographies regardless of age or relationship to menopause.

373. 2 Pressure to follow a course of therapy is never appropriate, especially at such a stressful time. (1) (CW; PL; ED; WH)

1 This would be therapeutic.

3 Knowledge of procedures decreases anxiety and would be therapeutic.

4 This would help decrease postoperative complications and would be therapeutic.

374. 2 The client's statement infers an emptiness with an associated loss. (1) (CW; EV; PS; WH)

1 Resumption of social activities indicates an acceptance of her condition and a willingness to move on with life.

3 This is a typical response of a grandmother anxious to resume her life.

4 The client is sharing planning and concern by her husband, not expressing a sense of loss.

375. 1 Statistics indicate a relationship between estrogen therapy and an increased incidence of endometrial cancer, although mortality is not increased. (3) (CW; AN; PA; WH)
2 Estrogen retards bone loss.
3 Estrogen maintains vaginal tissue turgor and lubrication.
4 Estrogen appears to play a protective role against myocardial infarction.

Praevia → low linning
over os
Painless brightred

Abrupt → seperated
Pain
bleeding

Childbearing and Women's Health Nursing Quiz

1. A client, 38 weeks gestation, who is having periods of bright red, painless bleeding is in the high risk unit because of a placenta previa. The nurse is aware that the client's labor has started when assessment demonstrates:
   1. Decreased fetal heart rate
   2. Increased vaginal bleeding
   3. Decreased vaginal spotting
   4. Rhythmic uterine contractions

2. A grand multigravida, recognizing that her labor is progressing very rapidly, calls her neighbor, a nurse, to help. The nurse assesses the client's perineum and notes that it is bulging. The nurse's priority action would be to:
   1. Place a clean drape under the perineal area
   2. Encourage her to pant during the contraction
   3. Accurately time the length of each contraction
   4. Contact the physician by phone for instructions

3. A pregnant client develops vaginitis for which the physician prescribes daily douches. The nurse provides the client with instructions for douching. The most important aspect of these instructions would be that the client should:
   1. Use a sterilized bulb syringe
   2. Insert the douche tip 5 to 6 inches
   3. Recline with head and shoulders elevated slightly
   4. Hold the labia together while instilling the douche solution

4. The physician tells the parents of a newborn that their child may have Down syndrome and additional diagnostic studies will need to be done. In the plan of care the nurse should prepare the infant for:
   1. Karyotyping
   2. A buccal smear
   3. An amniocentesis
   4. An enzyme assay

5. After doing a nursing assessment on a newly delivered male child, the nurse suspects that this neonate is postmature. It is most likely that this classification is based on the assessment finding of:
   1. Abundant lanugo and vernix caseosa
   2. Skin thick with desquamation over most of body
   3. Sole creases over anterior two thirds of each foot
   4. Testicles undescended with few rugae over scrotum

6. The nurse is aware that a common adaptation during pregnancy is:
   1. Increased ovarian activity
   2. Increased pulmonary capacity
   3. Decreased glomerulofiltration rate
   4. Decreased gastrointestinal motility

7. A client attending the prenatal clinic for the first time tells the nurse that her last menstrual cycle began on January 11. The client also states that she had 1 day of light spotting on February 7. The client's expected day of delivery is calculated to be:
   1. October 14
   2. October 18
   3. November 14
   4. November 18

8. A client with pregnancy-induced hypertension is placed on intravenous magnesium sulfate therapy. The nurse caring for this client should immediately notify the physician if the client's:
   1. Respirations are 18 per minute
   2. Patellar reflexes can be elicited
   3. Blood pressure begins to decrease
   4. Output is less than 100 ml in 4 hours

9. After taking clomiphene citrate (Clomid) for 3 months to treat anovulatory cycles, a client complains of difficulty with penetration during intercourse because of vaginal dryness. An appropriate response by the nurse would be:
   1. "Good, this means you are probably beginning to ovulate."
   2. "I know you are concerned about it, but this is only temporary."
   3. "Stop the Clomid immediately; the physician will have to prescribe another drug."
   4. "This is a common side effect; use a water soluble lubricant to ease penetration."

10. As part of the physical examination of a newborn, the nurse palpates the baby's abdomen. The organ that the nurse would normally expect to palpate is the:
    1. Liver
    2. Stomach
    3. Pancreas
    4. Gall bladder

11. When assessing a client with an abruptio placentae, the nurse would expect to observe:
    1. A flaccid uterus
    2. Painless bleeding
    3. Bright red bleeding
    4. A board-like abdomen

12. The nurse is aware that diabetes can affect pregnancy by:
    1. Promoting abnormal placental implantation
    2. Predisposing the client to hypertensive states
    3. Decreasing the amount of amniotic fluid present at term
    4. Increasing the appetite and causing excessive weight gain

13. Upon discovering the presence of a prolapsed cord, the nurse anticipates that the client's delivery will be:
    1. Induced with oxytocin
    2. Via a cesarean delivery
    3. A low forceps vaginal delivery
    4. Postponed as long as possible

14. In the eighth month of pregnancy, a client tells the nurse that she is experiencing dyspareunia. The nurse should plan to teach the client to:
    1. Avoid intercourse
    2. Try alternative positions
    3. Douche to lubricate the vaginal mucosa
    4. Consult a therapist for sexual counseling

15. A client is in the recovery room following a cesarean delivery. She is receiving IV fluids and has a Foley catheter. The client's fluid intake should be increased when the nurse notes:
    1. Urinary suppression
    2. A blood pressure of 100/60
    3. Tinges of blood in the urine
    4. A urine specific gravity of 1.030

16. A newborn is suspected of having toxoplasmosis. Toxoplasmosis, one of the TORCH diseases, may have been transmitted to the infant through:
    1. The placenta in utero
    2. Breastfeeding after delivery
    3. Contact with the maternal genitals
    4. A blood transfusion given to the mother

17. A client admitted with a threatened abortion anxiously asks the nurse, "Could this have happened because I had the flu?" The nurse's best response would be:
    1. "You feel that you did something to cause the bleeding? Tell me more about what you think."
    2. "We know that maternal infections sometimes result in miscarriages. Perhaps the flu did cause it."
    3. "The doctor will be here soon and at that time will tell you what is causing the bleeding. Wait until then."
    4. "I'm sure that there is absolutely nothing you could have done to cause this. You need not worry about that."

18. A primigravida, complaining of vaginal spotting and a sharp, shooting pain in the lower abdomen, is diagnosed as having a ruptured tubal pregnancy. When questioning the client about the initial appearance of symptoms, the nurse would expect the client to indicate that her symptoms started:

1. About the sixth week of pregnancy
2. At the beginning of the last trimester
3. Midway through the second trimester
4. Immediately after implantation occurred

19. After a spontaneous vaginal delivery the obstetrician hands the neonate to the nurse. The nurse's first action should be to
1. Stimulate the baby to cry
2. Administer oxygen by mask
3. Dry and place the infant in a warm environment
4. Perform a physical assessment and instill eye drops

20. The nurse tells a primigravida who is attending the prenatal clinic for the first time that the most common emotional reaction to pregnancy in the first trimester is:
1. Rejection
2. Narcissism
3. Depression
4. Ambivalence

21. Before a client signs the informed consent for a modified radical mastectomy, the nurse should be certain that the client knows the surgery includes the removal of:
1. Pectoral muscles
2. Skin overlying the breast tissue
3. Axillary lymph nodes on the affected side
4. The involved half of the breast and nodes

22. An 18-year-old primigravida in the 36th week of gestation is admitted with a diagnosis of pregnancy-induced hypertension. The nurse admitting this client is aware that nursing care measures will be directed chiefly toward reducing:
1. Anxiety
2. Bleeding
3. Vasospasms
4. Blood pressure

23. A client, wishing to postpone having children until she and her husband were financially sound, has been on oral contraceptive pills for several years. The nurse is aware that an assessment finding that would indicate a potential risk with continuing use of birth control pills is:

1. Dysmenorrhea
2. A B/P of 140/90
3. Mid-cycle bleeding
4. The lack of ovulation

24. A female client finds a lump in her breast and is hospitalized for a biopsy and possible mastectomy. As the nurse is preparing her for surgery, the client says, "I'm really scared. My mother and sister went through this. It was awful." The nurse's most appropriate response would be:
1. "You know most breast lumps are benign."
2. "Breast cancer has an excellent cure rate."
3. "You are worried about the results tomorrow?"
4. "What happened with your mother and sister?"

25. Immediately after a client has completed the second stage of labor the nurse administers 10 units of oxytocin (Pitocin) as ordered by the physician. The desired response from this medication will:
1. Lessen the discomfort of the episiotomy
2. Relax the uterus so that it can be emptied
3. Aid in the separation of the placenta from the uterine wall
4. Stimulate the client's breasts so that breast-feeding can be started

26. The nurse uses the Leopold maneuvers when a client is admitted in labor to palpate the abdomen and assess the:
1. Station of the fetus
2. Rate of uterine involution
3. Position of the fetus in utero
4. Strength and duration of contractions

27. A client is in active labor. Her contractions are now 2 to 3 minutes apart and last approximately 45 seconds. The fetal heart rate between contractions is about 100 beats per minute. The nurse should:
1. Obtain the mother's vital signs
2. Notify the physician immediately
3. Record this normal fetal response
4. Continue to monitor the fetal heart rate

28. A 15-year-old who is in true labor asks that her mother remain at her bedside but refuses her mother's assistance with comfort measures, stating, "I can do this myself." The client's conflicting behavior is representative of the adolescent's attempt to achieve the developmental task of:
    1. Identity
    2. Integrity
    3. Industry
    4. Intimacy

29. A 30-year-old client with a 35 day menstrual cycle is attempting to become pregnant. The client and her husband are counseled by the nurse about the optimal timing of intercourse during the cycle. The nurse would know that the counseling was effective when the couple state that they should have intercourse on the:
    1. Twelfth day of the cycle
    2. Fourteenth day of the cycle
    3. Twenty-first day of the cycle
    4. Twenty-fifth day of the cycle

30. During a contraction stress test the nurse should place the client in a:
    1. Sims' position to promote examination
    2. Lithotomy position to facilitate visualization
    3. Semi-Fowler's position to avoid hypotension
    4. Trendelenburg position to prevent cervical pressure

31. During an emergency delivery, as the fetal head begins to crown, the nurse should:
    1. Press firmly on the fundus
    2. Apply gentle perineal pressure
    3. Suggest that she push down vigorously
    4. Encourage the client to take prolonged deep breaths

32. When assessing an infant born at 42 weeks gestation, the nurse is most likely to find:
    1. Large amounts of lanugo over the shoulders
    2. Ample fatty tissue distributed over the entire body
    3. That the infant seems to want to sleep for long periods
    4. That the infant is constantly putting the fists in the mouth

33. After a cesarean delivery, a client is transferred to the recovery room. A nursing diagnosis of altered tissue perfusion is made related to the:
    1. Inability of the client to turn from side to side
    2. Unfavorable position of the fetus during labor
    3. Use of regional anesthesia during the delivery
    4. Increased risk for hemorrhage after a cesarean delivery

34. A client seeking family planning information asks the nurse during which phase of the menstrual cycle should an IUD be inserted. The nurse responds that the insertion is usually done on the:
    1. First to fourth day
    2. Fifth to eleventh day
    3. Fourteenth to sixteenth day
    4. Twenty-fifth to twenty-eighth day

35. Because preterm infants are at risk for respiratory distress syndrome, immediate nursing intervention is required when the infant develops:
    1. An expiratory grunt
    2. Substernal retractions
    3. Tachycardia of 160 per minute
    4. A respiratory rate of 50 per minute

36. At 30 weeks gestation a client with Class 1 cardiac disease expresses concern about her delivery and asks the nurse what to expect. The nurse should be aware that the physician will probably:
    1. Induce her labor with Pitocin
    2. Prematurely rupture her membranes
    3. Perform an elective cesarean delivery
    4. Use prophylactic forceps after a pudendal block

37. While a client is receiving intravenous magnesium sulfate therapy, the nurse should have at the bedside:
    1. Adrenalin
    2. Neo-Cortef
    3. Calcium chloride
    4. Calcium gluconate

38. When assessing a newborn in the nursery immediately after arrival from the delivery room, the nurse notes that the baby's skin is mottled. The nurse should first:
1. Administer oxygen
2. Notify the physician
3. Encourage an oral feeding
4. Check the baby's temperature

39. The nurse assesses the hips of a newborn for dislocation and is aware that dislocation would be indicated by:
1. Legs of equal length
2. Limitation in flexion of the hips
3. Limitation in abduction of either hip
4. Ability to abduct each hip 90 degrees

40. A client, gravida III, is admitted to the labor room. The nurse knows that gravida III means that the client:
1. Had one premature baby
2. Is pregnant for the third time
3. Has had an induced abortion
4. Has three living children at home

41. In the 37th week of gestation, a client with diabetes mellitus undergoes an amniocentesis. The nurse is aware that this is being done primarily to determine the:
1. Exact gestational age
2. Lung maturity of the fetus
3. Presence of genetic disorders
4. Glucose level of the amniotic fluid

42. About 6 hours after delivery the nurse notes that a client's fundus is two fingerbreadths above the umbilicus and is deviated to the right of the midline. The nurse suspects that the client has:
1. Begun involution
2. Bladder distention
3. Second-degree uterine atony
4. Retained placental fragments

43. A couple, expecting their first child, have a history of congenital defects in the family. They have been advised to have an alpha fetoprotein test of amniotic fluid to detect the presence of neural tube defects. They ask when the test will have to be performed. The nurse tells them that the test will be scheduled sometime during the:
1. Eighth to tenth week
2. Fourteenth to sixteenth week
3. Twentieth to twenty-fourth week
4. Thirty-second to thirty-sixth week

44. The day after a client's cesarean delivery, the Foley catheter is removed. The nurse can best evaluate that the client's urinary function has returned to normal when:
1. The client's daily urinary output is at least 1500 ml
2. The client's urinalysis indicates no bacteria present
3. The client has a residual urine of 90 ml after voiding
4. The client voids at least 300 ml 4 hours after catheter removal

45. A client who has just begun breastfeeding her infant complains that her nipples feel very sore. The mother should be encouraged to:
1. Apply continuous ice packs to her nipples to reduce the pain
2. Take the analgesic medication prescribed to limit the discomfort
3. Remove the baby from the breast for a few days to rest the nipples
4. Assume a different position when breastfeeding to adjust the infant's sucking

Childbearing and Women's Health Nursing Quiz Rationales

1. 4 Rhythmic uterine contractions are positive signs of beginning labor. (2) (CW; AS; PA; HP)
  1 This is not a sign of labor but a sign of fetal distress that demands medical attention.
  2 This has no relation to the onset of labor; it is more likely a sign of further placental separation.
  3 This is not a sign of labor; it may indicate that placental separation has stopped.

2. 1 Delivery is imminent; contamination will be minimized by catching the infant on a clean surface. (2) (CW; AN; TC; HC)
  2 Panting will hold back the infant and exhaust the mother.
  3 This is not the priority; delivery is imminent.
  4 It is too late; the nurse is capable of assisting the mother and should remain with her.

3. 4 Because the vagina has no sphincter, holding the labia permits the solution to enter, fill, and irrigate the vaginal vault. (2) (CW; IM; ED; WH)
  1 A bulb syringe should never be used because it may cause an air embolism.
  2 The douche tip should never be inserted more than 3 inches during pregnancy.
  3 This is a possible position to empty the vaginal vault after the fluid has been instilled; the client should be in the lithotomy position while the fluid is being instilled.

4. 1 This is a pictorial analysis of chromosomes usually done on peripheral blood, which will show chromosomal abnormalities such as the translocation found in Down syndrome. (2) (CW; PL; PA; HN)
  2 Karyotyping, not a buccal smear, is done to identify chromosomal aberrations.
  3 This is a test that is done before delivery.
  4 This test does not assess chromosomal aberrations.

5. 2 The desquamation occurs from prolonged exposure to amniotic fluid, causing cracking, peeling, and drying of skin in the postterm baby. (2) (CW; AS; PA; HN)
  1 This indicates a preterm infant.
  3 Creases would cover the entire sole of each foot.
  4 Same as answer 1.

6. 4 The influence of progesterone and the pressure of the gravid uterus slow GI motility. (1) (CW; AN; PA; HC)
  1 There is a decrease in ovarian activity.
  2 The pulmonary capacity stays relatively stable as the thoracic cage widens to accommodate lung volume.
  3 There is an increase in the glomerulofiltration rate because of the increased fluid volume.

7. 2 Using Nägele's rule to calculate, the estimated date of delivery (EDD) is the date of the last menstrual period (LMP) plus 7 days minus 3 months; spotting is fairly common at the time of the expected menstrual period. (1) (CW; AN; PA; HC)
  1 This is an incorrect calculation; this is too early.
  3 This is an incorrect calculation; this is too late.
  4 Same as answer 3.

8. 4 An output of of 25 ml/hr would not permit proper excretion of the magnesium sulfate; excess magnesium levels can cause respiratory and cardiac depression. (2) (CW; EV; TC; DR)
  1 Respirations at this rate are normal; a rate of at least 16 breaths per minute should be present before each dose of magnesium sulfate.
  2 Loss of patellar reflex is indicative of magnesium sulfate toxicity and the next dose should not be given.
  3 This is the expected response to magnesium sulfate.

9. 4 This shows understanding and offers reassurance that this is a normal side effect; this response also offers a possible solution. (1) (CW; EV; ED; RP)

1 This side effect has nothing to do with ovulation.

2 This side effect continues as long as the drug is continued.

3 This indicates a problem where one probably does not exist.

10. 1 The liver is usually palpable in the newborn at 2 cm below the costal margin. (1) (CW; AS; PA; NN)

2 The stomach is never palpable, and the borders are not detectable.

3 The pancreas is never palpable because it is located in the posterior portion of the abdominal cavity.

4 The gall bladder is not palpable because it is a posterior structure.

11. 4 Extravasation of blood at the separation site into the myometrium causes a tetanic, board-like uterus. (2) (CW; AS; PA; HP)

1 The uterus is rigid because of filling with blood and clots.

2 This is associated with placenta previa; pain and possible minimal external bleeding can occur in abruptio placentae.

3 This occurs with placenta previa; there is little external bleeding with abruptio placentae; if any does occur, it is dark red.

12. 2 The likelihood of pregnancy-induced hypertension increases fourfold in clients with diabetes mellitus, probably because of a preexisting vascular condition. (1) (CW; AN; PA; HP)

1 Abnormal implantation may occur because of scarring or uterine abnormalities, not because of diabetes.

3 Clients with diabetes have increased, rather than decreased, amniotic fluid.

4 Most pregnant women have increased appetites; excessive weight gain may be caused by a macrosomic infant and hydramnios.

13. 2 Immediate cesarean delivery is necessary to prevent fetal hypoxia and death from pressure on the cord. (1) (CW; PL; TC; HP)

1 This is unsafe; contractions would increase pressure on the cord, causing fetal hypoxia.

3 This is unsafe; this would increase pressure on the cord.

4 This is unsafe; the fetus is in distress, and immediate delivery is necessary.

14. 2 Pain caused by deep penetration by the male partner is common in late pregnancy and can be reduced by using alternative positions such as rear entry. (1) (CW; PL; ED; HC)

1 This should not be suggested until other alternatives have been tried.

3 Douching is not recommended and does not lubricate the vagina; a water-soluble lubricant is more effective.

4 This is unnecessary because this is common during the third trimester.

15. 4 This value indicates a highly concentrated urine and requires additional hydration of the client. (1) (CW; IM; PA; HP)

1 Increasing the IV rate in the presence of urinary suppression would be unsafe because it could cause hypervolemia.

2 This reading is meaningless unless a comparison with other readings indicates a decrease and the possibility of shock.

3 Tinges of blood in the urine may indicate bladder injury and are not related to the client's fluid status.

16. 1 This is the most frequent route of transmission. (2) (CW; AN; PA; HN)

2 There is no evidence of toxoplasmosis being transmitted via this route.

3 The genital tract is not locally affected.

4 Same as answer 2.

17. 1 This response encourages the client to discuss her fears and anxieties. (1) (CW; IM; PS; EC)

2 This gives inaccurate information; this conclusion has not been documented, and this response adds to the guilt felt by the client.

3 This response does not focus on the client's feelings; it cuts off communication between the nurse and the client.

4 This is false reassurance; it denies the client's feelings and cuts off communication.

18. 1 At this time the tube is unable to expand to the size of the growing pregnancy. (1) (CW; AS; PA; RP)

2 Tubal pregnancies cannot advance to this stage because of the tube's inability to expand with the growing pregnancy.

3 Same as answer 2.

4 The size of the fertilized egg at this time is miniscule and will cause no problem.

19. 3 The first action should be to dry and place the infant under a warmer to prevent chilling, thereby decreasing the possibility of development of metabolic acidosis. (2) (CW; IM; PA; NN)

1 This would not be done until after the baby is warmed.

2 This is useless without an adequate airway.

4 This is not the priority at this time; conserving body heat takes precedence.

20. 4 This is most common as the disbelief of actually being pregnant is experienced. (2) (CW; IM; PS; EC)

1 Rejection is more commonly seen in the third trimester.

2 Narcissism is more commonly seen in second and third trimesters.

3 Depression is more commonly seen in the third trimester and postpartum.

21. 3 Axillary lymph nodes are an early site of metastasis and thus are removed. (1) (CW; EV; ED; WH)

1 Pectoral muscles are not removed in a modified radical mastectomy.

2 This is not removed in this type surgery; leaving the skin intact improves healing.

4 The entire breast is removed in this type surgery.

22. 4 Treatment is directed primarily toward reducing the blood pressure to prevent seizures. (1) (CW; PL; TC; HP)

1 Anxiety may be present but the elevated blood pressure is the priority problem.

2 Bleeding is not generally a problem with pregnancy-induced hypertension unless abruptio placentae occurs.

3 Unless the client is in a very salt-poor state that contributes to hypovolemia, the compensatory state of vasospasm will not occur.

23. 2 The estrogen and progesterone in birth control pills increase the amount of renin, which in turn increases production of angiotensin, a potent pressor substance. (1) (CW; EV; TC; RC)

1 This is untrue.

3 This is not usually serious; it often indicates a low hormone level; it is corrected by changes in the type of medication prescribed.

4 Anovulation is the desired effect of oral contraceptives.

24. 3 Reflecting these feelings gives the client the opportunity to express fears and provides a chance to explore the family history. (2) (CW; IM; PS; WH)

1 Although true, this provides false reassurance.

2 This supports the client's fears of cancer and blocks communication.

4 This statement is probing and does not address the client's fears.

25. 3 Pitocin will cause the uterus to contract, which will assist in separating the placenta from the uterine wall. (2) (CW; EV; TC; DR)

1 Pitocin has no analgesic effect.

2 Relaxation of the uterus is undesirable and would not result in separation of the placenta.

4 Prolactin, not pitocin, stimulates milk production.

26. 3 The nurse palpates the abdomen to locate the head, back, and small parts of the fetus; the location of these parts reveals the position of the fetus. (1) (CW; AS; PA; HC)
   1 The station can be ascertained only on vaginal examination, which is not part of the Leopold maneuvers.
   2 Uterine involution is measured during the postpartum period.
   4 This can be done by lightly placing the hand on the fundus during a contraction; no other maneuver is necessary.

27. 2 Bradycardia (baseline FHR below 120 beats per minute) may indicate fetal distress and may require medical intervention. (2) (CW; IM; TC; HC)
   1 There is no indication of maternal distress; the fetus may be in distress.
   3 The normal fetal heart rate is 120 to 160 beats per minute.
   4 This is dangerous; the fetus may be in distress, and time should not be spent on monitoring.

28. 1 According to Erikson, identity vs role confusion is the developmental conflict of the adolescent. (1) (CW; AN; ED; EC)
   2 Ego integrity vs despair is the developmental conflict of the older adult.
   3 Industry vs inferiority is the developmental conflict of the school-age child.
   4 Intimacy vs isolation is the developmental conflict of the young adult.

29. 3 Ovulation usually occurs 14 days before menses; in a 35-day cycle, ovulation may occur as late as the twenty-first day. (2) (CW; EV; ED; RC)
   1 This is the proliferative phase of the cycle; ovulation has not yet occurred.
   2 If the woman has a 28-day cycle, ovulation could be expected at this time.
   4 The ovum has already passed out of the fallopian tube and can no longer be fertilized.

30. 3 A semi-Fowler's position will avoid hypotension and is recommended for safety and comfort. (1) (CW; PL; TC; HP)
   1 The Sims' position would make monitoring very difficult.

2 Usually no vaginal examination is necessary, and the lithotomy position is very uncomfortable for long periods.
4 This position is used for shock or a prolapsed cord, not for a CST.

31. 2 This prevents too rapid expulsion of the head, which can lead to increased intracranial pressure in the infant and a perineal laceration in the mother. (3) (CW; IM; TC; HC)
   1 This is unnecessary; precipitate delivery is caused by forceful uterine contractions that expel uterine contents.
   3 Vigorous pushing will cause too rapid expulsion, leading to increased intracranial pressure in the infant and laceration in the mother.
   4 At this time the urge to push is uncontrollable and she will be unable to take prolonged deep breaths.

32. 4 These babies have been nutritionally deprived by placental insufficiency and put their fists in their mouths to try to satisfy their hunger. (1) (CW; AS; PA; HN)
   1 This is not present in the postmature infant but in the preterm infant.
   2 Postmature infants lose weight because of insufficient nutrition from the aging placenta.
   3 The postmature infant is alert and awake immediately after birth and tends to stay awake for long periods.

33. 4 Abdominal surgery, especially pelvic surgery, predisposes the client to the risk of hemorrhage. (2) (CW; AN; TC; HP)
   1 An impaired gas exchange would be the appropriate diagnosis for a client who is immobilized.
   2 The position of the fetus is unrelated to tissue perfusion.
   3 Regional anesthesia is related to impaired physical mobility and sensory-perceptual alterations, not altered tissue perfusion.

34. 1 Intrauterine devices should be inserted during menses because the cervical os is slightly dilated and the chance of pregnancy is slim. (3) (CW; IM; ED; RC)

2 An IUD should not be inserted at this time; this is the proliferative phase of the menstrual cycle.

3 An IUD should not be inserted at this time because pregnancy may have occurred.

4 Same as answer 3.

35. 2 Retractions are a prominent feature of respiratory problems in preterm infants because of their compliant chest walls. (2) (CW; AS; PA; HN)

1 This is more indicative of low body temperature, not respiratory distress.

3 This rate is still within the normal range of 120 to 160 per minute.

4 A rapid respiratory rate of 40 to 60 is normal in neonates.

36. 4 Forceps reduce the mother's need to push, thereby conserving energy; regional anesthesia does not compromise cardiovascular function. (2) (CW; PL; TC; HP)

1 Induced labor is often more stressful and painful than natural labor.

2 Same as answer 1.

3 Major abdominal surgery is performed on clients with cardiac problems only when absolutely necessary because surgery adds additional stress to a compromised heart.

37. 4 Calcium gluconate is the antidote for magnesium sulfate toxicity. (1) (CW; PL; TC; DR)

1 Adrenalin is a vasoconstrictor and is not used as an antidote for magnesium sulfate toxicity.

2 Neo-Cortef is a steroid and is not used to counteract magnesium sulfate toxicity.

3 Calcium gluconate, not calcium chloride, is the antidote.

38. 4 Mottling of the skin results from hypothermia in the newborn. (1) (CW; IM; PA; NN)

1 This is not necessary; this is a normal phenomenon that usually indicates falling temperature; the baby requires warming.

2 This is not necessary; the baby requires warming.

3 Feeding will not increase temperature.

39. 3 Dislocation of the hip limits abduction to less than 90 degrees. (2) (CW; AS; PA; HN)

1 It is normal for the legs to be of equal length.

2 Flexion of the hips is not affected by dislocation.

4 This is a normal finding in the newborn; maternal hormones cause loosening of ligaments, which allows abduction to 90 degrees.

40. 2 Gravid means pregnant, so gravida III indicates a third pregnancy. (1) (CW; AN; PA; HC)

1 Para and gravida do not refer to the gestational age of babies at birth.

3 Gravida does not identify either induced or spontaneously aborted pregnancies.

4 Neither para nor gravida indicates whether there are living children.

41. 2 An amniocentesis at this stage of gestation is performed to determine L/S ratios, which indicate fetal lung maturity. (1) (CW; AS; PA; HP)

1 This is determined by the less invasive procedure of ultrasonography.

3 Amniocentesis would be done between the sixteenth and twentieth weeks to determine genetic disorders.

4 This is irrelevant; this is not the primary purpose for examining amniotic fluid at this time.

42. 2 Bladder distention causes uterine displacement, which interferes with uterine contractions and may lead to postpartum hemorrhage. (1) (CW; AS; PA; HC)

1 During normal involution the uterus is not deviated to the right.

3 There is no such thing as second-degree uterine atony.

4 Retained placental fragments often cause bright red bleeding and a boggy uterus; there are no data to support this.

43. 2 In pregnancies in which the fetus has a neural tube defect, alpha fetoprotein leaks into the amniotic fluid, causing abnormally high levels; at 14 to 16 weeks there is a sufficient amount of amniotic fluid present to obtain a sample and to perform the test. (3) (CW; AS; PA; HC)
   1 This is too early to safely obtain amniotic fluid.
   3 This is not the optimal time for diagnostic testing for birth defects; the optimal time for an amniocentesis is when the uterus enters the abdominal cavity, there is sufficient amniotic fluid available, and the fetus is still small.
   4 Same as answer 3.

44. 4 This would indicate that the kidneys are secreting adequate urine and the urinary sphincter tone has not been affected by the catheter. (2) (CW; EV; TC; HP)
   1 Although the total amount of urine indicates adequacy of kidney function, it does not reflect sphincter control or the possibility of retention.

2 The absence of bacteria indicates the absence of infection but does not portend the return of urinary function.
3 This indicates retention with overflow; the client urinates small amounts but does not completely empty the bladder.

45. 4 Altering the breastfeeding position may ensure that the entire nipple and as much of the areola as possible is in the infant's mouth; when the infant is latched on the nipple correctly and a finger is used to release suction at the end of a feeding, trauma to the nipple is reduced. (2) (CW; PL; PA; HC)
   1 This is contraindicated because it suppresses lactation; also, ice applications of any kind should never be continuous because it can result in tissue damage.
   2 This is unnecessary; soreness is common; it usually occurs only at the beginning of a feeding and is temporary until the nipples become accustomed to the infant's sucking.
   3 This is usually unnecessary; removing the infant from the breast will result in engorgement which will increase the discomfort.

CHAPTER 4

Pediatric Nursing Review Questions

GROWTH AND DEVELOPMENT

1. To bring about effective communication with any child, the nurse must first take into consideration the child's:
   1. State of health
   2. Developmental level
   3. Ability at self-expression
   4. Fear of authoritarian figures

2. The nurse understands that the first activity of daily living that should be taught to a developmentally disabled child is:
   1. Toileting
   2. Dressing
   3. Self feeding
   4. Combing hair

3. An appropriate toy for a 3-month-old infant would be a:
   1. Push-pull toy
   2. Metallic mirror
   3. Stuffed animal
   4. Large plastic ball

4. The nurse is aware that the play of a 5-month-old infant is most likely to consist of:
   1. Picking up a rattle or toy and putting it into the mouth
   2. Exploratory searching when a cuddly toy is hidden from view
   3. Simultaneously kicking the legs and batting the hands in the air
   4. Waving and clenching fists and dropping toys placed in the hands

5. The nurse counsels a mother of an 8-month-old child to make sure the floors are free of small objects when her child is crawling on the floor. The major rationale for this instruction is that:
   1. An 8-month-old infant can easily pick up small objects
   2. Sharp objects can injure the fragile skin of an 8-month-old
   3. It is a health hazard for babies to pick things up off the floor
   4. The infant could hide small objects making them difficult to locate

6. The nurse notes that a 22-month-old uses two- or three-word phrases (telegraphic speech), has a vocabulary of about 200 words, and frequently uses the word "me." The nurse would interpret the child's language development as being:
   1. A severe lag
   2. Slow for the child's age
   3. Normal for the child's age
   4. Advanced for the child's age

7. Based on an understanding of normal preschool behavior, during hospitalization the nurse is aware that a 4-year-old will probably:
   1. Refuse to cooperate with nurses during the parents' absence
   2. Demonstrate despair if parents do not visit at least once a week
   3. Cry when the parents leave and return but not during their absence
   4. Be unable to relate to peers in the playroom if there are parents present

8. A 2½-year-old male child who has fallen from a tree tells his parents, "Bad, bad tree." The nurse recognizes that the child is within the cognitive developmental norm of Piaget's:
   1. Concrete operations
   2. Concept of reversibility
   3. Preconceptual operations
   4. Sensorimotor development

9. The nurse is aware that the most reliable indicator of pain in a 4-year-old child is:
   1. Crying and sobbing
   2. Changes in behavior
   3. Decreased heart rate
   4. Verbal reports of pain

10. To properly visualize the auditory canal of a 4-year-old during an otoscopic examination, the nurse should pull the pinna of the ear:
    1. Up and back
    2. Up and forward
    3. Down and back
    4. Down and forward

11. The nurse is aware that the toy that would be most appropriate for a 4-year-old would be a:
    1. Fuzzy stuffed animal
    2. Six piece jigsaw puzzle
    3. Lunch box filled with plastic figures
    4. Blunt scissor and pictures to cut out

12. The nurse is aware that corrective surgery for a newborn's hypospadias will be done:
    1. Shortly after birth
    2. Within a few months after birth
    3. At approximately 5½ years of age
    4. When the child is between 3 and 4 years old

13. An 8-year-old child, admitted for intrathecal methotrexate chemotherapy, is prescribed allopurinol (Zyloprim) and asks the nurse why this medication has to be taken. The nurse's best response would be:
    1. "Because this pill helps the other medicines get rid of the things that are making you sick."
    2. "To protect your body from developing other problems after your treatment has been stopped."
    3. "To stop your sick white cells from going to other parts of your body where they can cause problems."
    4. "Because your doctor ordered it. Your doctor would not order anything for you unless it was very important."

14. The primary nurse, assigned to a 5½-month-old girl being admitted to the hospital, understands that the infant's emotional development should make the infant:
    1. Cry when the nurse approaches her for the first time
    2. Welcome the attention that the primary nurse gives her
    3. Smile socially in recognition of the primary nurse's face
    4. Cling furiously to her mother when the nurse tries to take her away

15. After teaching a mother about the appropriate play for an 8-month-old infant, the nurse is aware that the mother needs additional teaching when the mother states that she will buy a:
    1. Stuffed animal
    2. Play telephone
    3. Hanging mobile
    4. Book with textures

16. A 2½-year-old girl, whose older sibling has recently died, has started hitting her mother and refusing to go to bed at night. The nurse in the pediatric well-child clinic tells the mother that the toddler is probably:
    1. Fearful of dying in her sleep
    2. Trying to get more of her mother's attention
    3. Just going through the "terrible twos" developmental stage
    4. Reacting appropriately to anxiety generated by the family upheaval

17. When talking with a 4-year-old the nurse observes that the child is shy and stutters. The nurse is aware that stuttering in a 4-year-old child is considered:
    1. A sign of a delay in neural development
    2. A normal characteristic for a preschooler
    3. The result of a serious emotional problem
    4. An indication of a serious permanent impairment

18. The most appropriate toys for a 6-month-old infant would be:
    1. Push-pull toys
    2. Wooden blocks
    3. Soft stuffed animals
    4. Shape-matching toys

19. A mother indicates to the nurse in the pediatric clinic that she is concerned that her 20-month-old baby's bedtime thumb-sucking will cause the teeth to protrude. The nurse's most appropriate response would be:
    1. "You should seek counseling, the thumb-sucking may indicate an emotional problem."
    2. "You should switch the baby to a pacifier in the next two months to avoid protrusion of the teeth."
    3. "You need to restrain the baby from sucking the thumb because it prematurely loosens the first teeth."
    4. "You need not be concerned about the teeth protruding unless it persists after permanent teeth appear."

20. The nurse knows that an appropriate toy for a 6-year-old in a spica cast would be a:
    1. Ball and jacks
    2. Game of checkers
    3. Set of building blocks
    4. Coloring book and crayons

21. A developmental assessment of a 9-month-old would be expected to reveal:

    1. A two-to-three word vocabulary
    2. An ability to feed self with a spoon
    3. The ability to sit steadily without support
    4. Closure of both anterior and posterior fontanels

22. The nurse would assess a 4-year-old child's pain by:
    1. Asking the child to point to where the hurt is
    2. Auscultating the abdomen for bowel sounds
    3. Asking the parents about the child's bowel movements
    4. Observing the position and behavior while the child is moving

23. The nurse is aware that a 6-month-old infant on a regular diet could be fed:
    1. Applesauce, carrots, chicken, and formula
    2. Pears, green beans, turkey, and whole milk
    3. Bananas, sweet potatoes, ham, and formula
    4. Peaches, corn, cottage cheese, and whole milk

24. When assessing a 4-year-old the nurse would expect the child to:
    1. Ask the definitions of new words
    2. Have a vocabulary of 1500 words
    3. Name two or three different colors
    4. Use just three- or four-word sentences

25. When teaching parents to instill ear drops in an 18-month-old child, the nurse shows them how to:
    1. Cleanse the ear canal by pulling the pinna up and down
    2. Apply medicated ear wicks tightly before instilling the ear drops
    3. Straighten the auditory canal by pulling the earlobe up and back
    4. Straighten the auditory canal by pulling the pinna down and back

26. The nurse is reinforcing previous learning about cystic fibrosis and its treatment with a 9-year-old with the disease. The most suitable information for this child's stage of development would be:
    1. "The postural drainage will help you feel better."
    2. "The dietitian says this meal schedule is best for you."
    3. "Your medication is scheduled at this time because your doctor has prescribed it this way."
    4. "Your mucus is thick because cystic fibrosis interferes with how your mucous glands work."

27. While caring for a 6-month-old infant, it is likely that the nurse will observe the presence of the reflex called:
    1. Startle
    2. Babinski
    3. Extrusion
    4. Tonic neck

28. Developmentally, 2-year-old children are at risk for lead poisoning primarily because:
    1. Lead is easily available to them
    2. Their vascular system is very fragile
    3. They have a high level of oral activity
    4. Motor vehicle use and pollution have increased

29. Specific preoperative teaching before an orchiopexy in a 4-year-old child should include a:
    1. Doll with an intravenous tube in the arm
    2. Demonstration of the use of the abdominal binder
    3. Picture of a boy with a bandage on his lower abdomen
    4. Doll with a rubber band stretched from perineum to thigh

30. The nurse knows that a child is performing normal developmental tasks for a 5-year-old when the child:
    1. Is ritualistic when playing
    2. Makes up rules for a new game
    3. Asks for a pacifier when uncomfortable
    4. Plays near others quietly, but not with them

31. The nurse recognizes that behaviors typical of an 8-month-old include:
    1. Drinking from a cup, using the words "Mama" and "Dada," and standing alone
    2. Smiling spontaneously, clasping hands, and keeping the head steady when sitting
    3. Being shy with strangers, playing peek-a-boo, and standing by holding onto furniture
    4. Removing some clothing, building a tower of two cubes, and stooping to pick up toys

32. Preparation for surgery on a 4-year-old must include consideration of the child's age-related fear of:
    1. Strangers
    2. Intrusive procedures
    3. Disruption of routines
    4. Separation from parents

33. The nurse is aware that the most therapeutic play for a 4-year-old child on bedrest would be:
    1. Finger painting on blank sheets of paper
    2. Using crayons to color in a coloring book
    3. Engaging in a checker game with the father
    4. Playing dominos with an 8-year-old roommate

34. When listing all the problems of a teenaged client who has sickle cell anemia, the nurse recognizes that priority must be given to the client's:
    1. Restriction of movement during periods of arthralgia
    2. Altered body image resulting from skeletal deformities
    3. Separation from family during periods of hospitalization
    4. Interruption of learning as a result of multiple hospitalizations

35. A one-year-old visits the hospital playroom. The toy selected and used that would indicate an appropriate growth and developmental level would be a:
    1. Picture book
    2. Rocking horse
    3. Stuffed animal
    4. Plastic toy that squeaks

36. When planning self-care that would foster independence, the nurse would expect a 4-year-old child to be able to:
    1. Button a shirt
    2. Tie shoe laces
    3. Part and comb hair
    4. Cut the meat at dinner

37. The nurse should understand that to a preschooler, death is thought of as:
    1. An end to life
    2. A reversible separation
    3. Something that happens to old people
    4. A persona who takes one away from one's family

38. When caring for a 15-year-old client receiving chemotherapy for leukemia, the nurse should keep in mind that an adolescent of this age will:
    1. Feel dependent and enjoy the "sick role"
    2. Be most bothered by having to limit activities
    3. Feel different because of an altered body image
    4. Be preoccupied by concerns about missed schoolwork

39. When evaluating growth and development of a 6-month-old infant, the nurse would expect the infant to be able to:
    1. Sit alone, display pincer grasp, wave bye-bye
    2. Crawl, transfer toy from one hand to the other, display fear of strangers
    3. Pull self to a standing position, release a toy by choice, play peek-a-boo
    4. Turn completely over, sit momentarily without support, reach to be picked up

40. The parents of an 18-month-old child are anxious to know why their child has experienced several episodes of suppurative otitis. The nurse should explain the:
    1. Immunologic difference between the young child and the adult
    2. Structural difference between the eustachian tube of younger and older children
    3. Difference between the size of the middle ear cavity in infants and older children
    4. Functional difference between an infant's eustachian tube and that of an older child

41. Following surgery, a 5-year-old is experiencing intense pain and an analgesic is prescribed. When administering the prescribed analgesic the nurse should consider that:
    1. Even though children do not like medicines, analgesics will make them more comfortable
    2. Pain is not as strongly felt by children as by adults, so analgesics are not needed frequently
    3. Children should rarely receive analgesics because this may result in addiction or respiratory depression
    4. Children do not need analgesics because they are easily distracted and quickly return to playing or sleeping

42. An 11-year-old is diagnosed with acute lymphocytic leukemia (ALL) and the physician discusses the diagnosis and treatment with the family. The assessment data that indicate age-appropriate behavior for an 11-year-old regarding a diagnosis implying death and dying is the child:
    1. Is rude, impolite, and insolent
    2. Says that an uncle died and went to heaven
    3. Is afraid to go to sleep for fear of not awakening
    4. Tells the nurse that death is punishment for not being good

43. An assessment of a 6-month-old infant's growth and developmental level should reveal that the infant can:
    1. Say, "Mama"
    2. Crawl forward
    3. Turn pages in a book
    4. Hold a bottle without help

44. At the well-baby clinic, the nurse discusses the food and feeding needs of a toddler with the mother of a two-year-old. Considering a toddler's food and feeding needs the nurse should teach the mother that:
   1. Growth rate is increased at the age of 2 years, so the child needs more protein per unit of body size
   2. A child's energy requirements during the toddler stage are so high more calories are needed to meet them
   3. A child's normal struggle for independence at this age often involves refusal of food, but children will eat the amount they need
   4. Because the child often refuses food, the mother should prepare only the food the child likes and avoid snacks between meals

45. The nurse is aware that 5-year-olds engage in play that is known as:
   1. Parallel
   2. Ritualistic
   3. Aggressive
   4. Cooperative

46. The social development of a 9-month-old is best promoted by having the infant:
   1. Manipulate soft clay
   2. Pound on a peg board
   3. Play peek-a-boo and bye-bye
   4. Play with a large ball with a bell

47. The nurse is aware that 18-month-old children with normal hearing have usually acquired a vocabulary sufficient to enable them to communicate by:
   1. Pointing and grunting
   2. Using at least six words
   3. Making babbling sounds
   4. Using complete sentences

48. A fifteen-year-old girl is grounded for 2 weeks by her parents for smoking in school. The adolescent tells the school nurse, "It's not fair that I get punished when my friends get away with doing the same thing." The nurse's most appropriate response would be:
   1. "The others will pay someday for lying to school authorities."
   2. "I intend to report your friends to the principal so they can also be punished."
   3. "It is difficult enough to get teenagers to tell the truth. When parents don't act it reinforces deceptive behavior."
   4. "When errors in judgment are made, people must be prepared to take the consequences of their actions."

49. The nurse is aware that the kind of play two-year-old children engage in is called:
   1. Group play
   2. Parallel play
   3. Dramatic play
   4. Cooperative play

50. The play activity that would be appropriate for a 6-year-old whose energy level has improved following an acute episode of Hirschsprung's disease would be:
   1. Using a set of building blocks
   2. Finger painting on a large paper surface
   3. Taking apart and putting together a truck
   4. Drawing or writing with a pencil or marker

51. The mother of a 15-year-old female who is being treated for allergies privately tells the nurse that she thinks her daughter is becoming a hypochondriac. The nurse can be most therapeutic by:
   1. Discussing the underlying causes of hypochondriasis
   2. Discussing the developmental behavior of adolescents
   3. Explaining the potentially serious complications of allergies
   4. Explaining that the mother may be transferring her own fears to her daughter

52. A 15-year-old insulin dependent diabetic has a history of noncompliance with therapy. The nurse is aware that the noncompliance is developmentally related to:
   1. The need for attention
   2. A denial of the diabetes
   3. The struggle for identity
   4. A regression associated with illness

EMOTIONAL NEEDS RELATED TO HEALTH PROBLEMS

53. Three days after being admitted with meningococcal meningitis, a twelve-year-old client is afebrile and asymptomatic but appears very sad and cries frequently. To assist the child to verbalize thoughts and feelings, the nurse should:
1. Encourage the parents to speak with their child
2. Ask the child directly what seems to be the trouble
3. Show the child some photos of hospitalized children and have the child tell stories about them
4. Have the child watch videotapes about sick children and answer any questions that the child may have

54. To be most therapeutic when giving a 3-year-old toddler an intramuscular injection, the nurse should approach the child and say:
1. "Act like a big child and we can be done real quick."
2. "You are afraid of having a shot because of the pain."
3. "I know this might hurt, but it's important that you hold still."
4. "I brought another nurse along to help me give you your medicine."

55. A 9-year-old male child, who has been newly diagnosed with diabetic mellitus, is being discharged. The nurse suspects that there may be a problem with family dynamics when the child's mother states:
1. "We want to encourage our son to do as much as he can for himself."
2. "We know our child is special and we'll have to go easy on the discipline for him."
3. "We know our child and the rest of the family are in for a lot of ups and downs over the years."
4. "We really hope our son can still be in the Boy Scouts and participate with his Little League baseball team."

56. A 16-month-old male infant has been in the hospital for 3 weeks and has become increasingly withdrawn and mute. It would be most appropriate for the nurse to:

1. Move him in with other children
2. Provide him with distracting toys
3. Encourage the parents to stay with him as much as possible
4. Assign different nurses to be with him to provide sensory stimuli

57. A 5-year-old, newly arrived from Latin America, attends a nursery school where everyone speaks English. The child's mother tells the nurse in the well-child clinic that her child is no longer outgoing and is very passive in the classroom. The nurse suspects that the child:
1. May be experiencing discrimination
2. Lacks adequate motivation for school
3. Is not mature enough for kindergarten
4. Is undergoing a state of cultural shock

58. As the nurse plans to teach a 9-year-old male with a learning disability about his diabetes, the parents intervene and state, "That won't be necessary. With our son's disability we recognize that he is unable to care for himself." The best response by the nurse would be:
1. "Then I will just teach you what he needs to have done."
2. "This material is not difficult; even a slow child can learn it."
3. "Your son cannot always depend on you for his health needs."
4. "Your son seems bright enough to me. I think he can learn this."

59. The nursing plan for an 8-year-old boy with celiac disease should include helping the child to:
1. Express his feelings, while focusing on ways in which he can still be normal like his friends
2. Select meals from those high-residue, high-carbohydrate foods that are gluten-free and permitted
3. Understand the relationship of diet to disease so that he will be more willing to adhere to his diet and refrain from eating snack foods
4. Learn which snack foods can be substituted for the hot dogs and hamburgers that have wheat fillers, because occasional noncompliance is permitted

60. In the management of a child newly diagnosed with chronic celiac disease the primary nursing goal is to:
    1. Prevent celiac crisis and resulting complications
    2. Prevent complications from respiratory involvement
    3. Teach the parents to control the diet to promote normal growth
    4. Help the parents and child adjust to the life-long dietary restrictions

61. Before a four-year-old child with a new colostomy is discharged, the nurse prepares a teaching plan for the parents which includes telling them that:
    1. An enterostomal therapist is available to assist with home care
    2. They should try correcting the child's poor eating habits at mealtime
    3. Fluids should be limited between meals, although permitted at meals
    4. The child should not take part in physical education when attending school

62. The parents of a sick child constantly blame each other for their child's illness. The response by the parents that would indicate that the nurse's attempts to point out reality had been successful would be:
    1. The father bringing the child many expensive gifts
    2. The parents promising the child a trip to Disney World
    3. The parents making an appointment with a family counselor
    4. The mother assuming the blame for not paying attention to the child's complaints

63. A child who has barely survived a near drowning episode is in critical condition in an intensive care unit. At one point the child opens the eyes and smiles prompting the mother to say to the nurse, "Look, I think my child will get better now." The nurse's best response would be:
    1. "Yes, you are right; this is a very good sign."
    2. "See if you can get your child to hold your hand too."
    3. "God must have certainly been watching over your child."
    4. "We are doing everything we can to help your child to recover."

64. Following treatment for Lyme disease, a child expresses fear of going camping again because of the ticks. The nurse's best response would be:
    1. "Tell me more about your fears about camping."
    2. "You are afraid to go camping just because of a tick?"
    3. "Frequent checks for ticks are a defense against infection."
    4. "Oh, camping is fun. Just think of what you will be missing."

65. An infant is scheduled for emergency surgery. The nurse notes that the baby's mother is 13 years old and the father is 16 years old. The baby's father and the paternal grandmother who cares for the baby, are at the bedside. The nurse should obtain the informed consent from the:
    1. Paternal grandmother
    2. Hospital administrator
    3. Sixteen-year-old father
    4. Thirteen-year-old mother

66. When caring for children in a family that is economically deprived, the nurse should understand that the characteristic most common to those living in poverty is:
    1. Long-term feelings of powerlessness
    2. A willingness to postpone gratification
    3. Open and direct expressions of anger
    4. Compliance with health recommendations

67. When working with a family as the unit of service, the public health nurse should consider that:
    1. Separating health problems from other aspects of this family's life is essential to help them
    2. Certain members of the family may be capable of providing more support than the nurse can
    3. Assessing each member of this family is not necessary to plan the care for the family as a whole
    4. Values, beliefs, and attitudes held by the family have limited influence on how they will perceive assistance

68. When planning teaching for the parents of a child with tetralogy of Fallot, who are both employed full time, the nurse should:

1. Schedule a whole evening for teaching
2. Insist both parents attend the teaching sessions
3. Provide written and oral information in short sessions
4. Point things out to them when they are visiting their child

69. A 16-year-old, her 1-month-old baby, and the baby's grandmother come to the emergency room saying that the infant accidentally fell down the stairs. Legally, consent for the baby's medical care:
    1. Should be obtained from the grandmother who must sign the consent
    2. Must be decided by Family Court because the baby's mother is a minor
    3. Is not necessary because this is an emergency and no consent is needed
    4. Is the responsibility of the baby's mother, and she should sign the consent

70. The nursing diagnosis that would apply to families of all children with cerebral palsy is "High risk for alteration in parenting related to":
    1. Lack of social support
    2. An unrealistic expectation of self
    3. Having a mentally retarded child
    4. Loss of the expected normal child

71. A 6-year-old boy is receiving chemotherapy for a neuroblastoma, Stage 4. He had his first chemotherapy session last week and has arrived with his mother for this week's session. The nurse should approach the child and his mother by asking:
    1. "Did your son vomit after the last dose?"
    2. "How did you feel after your last medicine?"
    3. "Aren't you happy that two sessions will be finished?"
    4. "How are you feeling this week? Ready for another dose?"

72. A 16-year-old with full thickness burns of the entire right arm states, "I'll never be able to use my arm again. I'll be scarred forever." The nurse's best initial response would be:

1. "The staff will take steps to minimize scarring."
2. "Think about how lucky you are. You are alive."
3. "I know you're worried but it is still too early to tell."
4. "Try not to worry; concentrate on doing your range-of-motion exercises."

73. A child who had been severely beaten was found wandering in the streets and was admitted to the hospital. The nursing diagnosis that will most profoundly influence the planning of care for this child would be:
    1. Altered parenting
    2. Impaired skin integrity
    3. Post-trauma response
    4. Sensory/perceptual alteration: visual

74. An abused child, after being hospitalized for severe injuries, is being placed in temporary foster care. The foster family is coming into the hospital to meet the child. The nurse should plan to facilitate this meeting by:
    1. Decorating the child's room with "welcome" signs
    2. Providing a private room for the foster family and the child
    3. Encouraging the child to draw a picture for the new mother
    4. Answering all the child's questions about the foster family ahead of time

75. When the adolescent mother of an infant admitted with multiple trauma sees her infant in the intensive care unit for the first time she cries out, "I didn't mean to hurt her." The nurse should:
    1. Encourage the young mother's family to come and comfort her
    2. Notify the Child Abuse Hotline of this probable instance of abuse
    3. Respond by saying, "You caused your baby's injury and feel guilty."
    4. Put an arm around the young mother and say, "This must be difficult for you."

76. The nurse is aware that abusing parents:
    1. Are mature independent individuals
    2. Have few available personal resources
    3. Are aware of the abilities of young children
    4. Often have been raised with little discipline

77. When assessing the family dynamics of a suspected abusing family, the nurse would be surprised to observe that the:
    1. Parents provide little emotional support to the child
    2. Parents offer consistent, detailed stories about the injuries
    3. Child cringes and appears unduly afraid when approached
    4. Child has many unexplained old injuries, scars, and bruises

78. A mother of three children who was abandoned by her husband shortly after the birth of her youngest daughter brings the child, now 9 months old, into the hospital with a diagnosis of failure to thrive. As the mother leaves, the nurse is not surprised to see the daughter react by:
    1. Clinging to the mother and expressing fear of the nurse
    2. Crying at first but then letting the nurse hold and comfort her
    3. Sustaining eye contact with the mother and refusing the nurse's arms
    4. Readily allowing the nurse to take her but remaining stiff while being held

FLUIDS AND ELECTROLYTES

79. In children with renal disease the best indicator of fluid balance is the daily measurement of:
    1. Body weight
    2. Urinary output
    3. Abdominal girth
    4. Urine osmolality

80. A 4-year-old child with nephrotic syndrome has been restricted to 600 ml of fluid for 24 hours. The nursing intervention that would be most appropriate in assisting the child to cope with such a limitation is:

1. Dividing fluid intake equally among each shift (200 ml/each shift)
2. Allowing the child to drink fluids as desired until the 600 ml limit is reached
3. Withholding fluids from 7 PM to 7 AM and giving the entire 600 ml from 7 AM to 7 PM
4. Providing the child with a minimum of 1 ounce of fluid in small 1 ounce cups each waking hour

81. Children with acute glomerulonephritis are placed on diets low in:
    1. Fat
    2. KCl
    3. Protein
    4. Glucose

82. A $5\frac{1}{2}$-month-old infant is admitted with a fever and a history of vomiting for 48 hours. In view of this infant's responses, the assessment by the nurse that would initially influence the child's care is:
    1. Inspecting the baby's skin for poor turgor
    2. Determining the baby's vital signs and weight
    3. Checking the baby's neurologic status and urinary output
    4. Asking the mother whether the baby is breastfed or bottle-fed

83. To best ascertain the magnitude of fluid loss in an infant with gastroenteritis and diarrhea, the nurse should:
    1. Evaluate the infant's skin turgor carefully
    2. Note the elevation of the infant's hematocrit
    3. Assess the moistness of the infant's mucous membranes
    4. Compare the infant's pre-illness weight with current weight

84. An initial nursing assessment of an infant with severe dehydration will most likely reveal:
    1. Stools that are frothy
    2. A weak, decreased pulse
    3. Bulging of the occipital fontanel
    4. An elevated urine specific gravity

85. A 3-month-old infant with gastroenteritis and dehydration is admitted and placed on enteric precautions. Nursing assessment of this child will probably reveal:

1. A bulging fontanel
2. Resilient skin turgor
3. Marked restlessness
4. Decreased urinary output

86. When assessing a 4-month-old infant with gastroenteritis and dehydration, the nurse would expect to find a:
    1. Specific gravity of 1.014
    2. Urinary output of 50 ml/hr
    3. Depressed anterior fontanel
    4. History of allergies to various foods

87. A 5-month-old with a history of frequent bouts of diarrhea is to be discharged. A priority concern that the nurse should include in the teaching plan for the mother is the:
    1. Effects of antibiotics on viral gastroenteritis
    2. Potential hazards of fluid loss in young children
    3. Importance of a well-balanced diet for the infant
    4. Need for cleanliness of foods and feeding utensils

88. The nurse is aware that normal arterial blood gas values in the child would be most accurately reflected by readings of:
    1. pH 7.40, P_{O_2} 85 mmHg, P_{CO_2} 40 mmHg, base excess 0
    2. pH 7.50, P_{O_2} 85 mmHg, P_{CO_2} 35 mmHg, base excess 0
    3. pH 7.25, P_{O_2} 60 mmHg, P_{CO_2} 50 mmHg, base excess −4
    4. pH 7.45, P_{O_2} 70 mmHg, P_{CO_2} 25 mmHg, base excess +4

89. The nurse should recognize that the sequence of events that occurs in the respiratory response to acidosis is:
    1. Hypoventilation; increased CO_2 elimination; decreased blood H ions; increased pH
    2. Hypoventilation; decreased blood H ions; increased CO_2 elimination; decreased pH
    3. Hyperventilation; increased CO_2 elimination; decreased blood H ions; increased pH
    4. Hyperventilation; decreased CO_2 elimination; decreased blood H ions; decreased pH

90. A critically ill child develops Cheyne-Stokes respirations and the nurse suspects an increasing acid-base imbalance related to:

1. Respiratory alkalosis from overbreathing and excess carbon dioxide output
2. Respiratory acidosis from impeded breathing and the retention of carbon dioxide
3. Metabolic alkalosis from an increase in base bicarbonate due to the primary health problem
4. Metabolic acidosis from the concentration of cations in body fluids which displace bicarbonate

91. The physiologic compensatory mechanism that is activated to counteract the effects of acid-base imbalance in a child with severe dehydration is:
    1. Profuse diaphoresis
    2. Renal retention of H^+
    3. Elevated temperature
    4. Increased respirations

92. The blood gas report that would most likely reflect the acid-base balance found in a child admitted with severe dehydration is:
    1. A pH of 7.50 and a P_{CO_2} of 34
    2. A pH of 7.20 and a P_{CO_2} of 20
    3. A pH of 7.23 and a P_{CO_2} of 70
    4. A pH of 7.56 and a P_{CO_2} of 20

93. Following surgery for the repair of a meningomyelocele, an infant develops diarrhea and metabolic acidosis with a decreased urinary output. Because of the infant's status, the nurse anticipates that the physician will order:
    1. Plasmanate
    2. Isotonic saline
    3. Sodium lactate
    4. Potassium chloride

94. A specimen for arterial blood gases is obtained from a 3-month-old who has a 3 day history of diarrhea. The results are: pH 7.30; P_{CO_2} 35 mmHg; HCO_3 17mEq/L. The nurse recognizes that this infant is in:
    1. Metabolic acidosis
    2. Metabolic alkalosis
    3. Respiratory acidosis
    4. Respiratory alkalosis

95. A 9-year-old with insulin dependent diabetes mellitus is admitted to the hospital with deep, rapid respirations; flushed, dry cheeks; abdominal pain with nausea; and increased thirst. Laboratory tests would be expected to show:
1. A blood pH of 7.25 with a blood glucose of 60 mg/dl
2. A blood pH of 7.50 with a blood glucose of 60 mg/dl
3. A blood pH of 7.50 with a blood glucose of 460 mg/dl
4. A blood pH of 7.25 with a blood glucose of 460 mg/dl

96. When a three-month-old infant is receiving IV fluids via a scalp vein, the nurse should:
1. Check the baby's pupils for reaction every hour
2. Observe behind the baby's ear and occiput for infiltration
3. Restrain the baby's arms and legs when nobody is present
4. Explain to the parents why they can't hold the baby during IV therapy

97. The nurse notes that an infant with failure to thrive, who has been on tube feedings for three days, has very dry skin and mucous membranes. The nurse verifies that all feedings have been retained but the urinary output is consistently 250 ml and the infant has lost weight. The nurse should:
1. Increase the intravenous flow of half-normal saline and call the physician
2. Realize this is probably normal for babies and infants with failure to thrive
3. Recognize undernutrition and call the physician to increase the caloric intake
4. Recognize underhydration and call the physician to increase the infant's fluid intake

98. The best method for assessing an infant's response to rehydration therapy is for the nurse to:
1. Measure the infant's abdominal girth
2. Assess the color of the infant's stools
3. Weigh the infant at the same time daily
4. Monitor the infant's skin turgor frequently

99. After abdominal surgery, a priority nursing intervention for a young infant with an IV is:
1. Administering oral fluids
2. Limiting handling by the parents
3. Weighing the diapers after voiding
4. Placing elbow restraints on both arms

100. An IV of D5W is infusing when a child returns to the pediatric unit from the recovery room. The postoperative orders do not indicate the desired rate of infusion. The most appropriate action for the nurse to take is to:
1. Adjust the flow to the rate the child was receiving prior to surgery
2. Reduce the flow rate to keep the vein open and call the physician
3. Regulate the flow rate to 25 ml an hour until the physician makes rounds
4. Maintain the present flow rate and call the recovery room to verify the correct rate

101. An 8-month-old child who weighs 18 lbs 12 oz is receiving 8 oz of full strength formula every 4 hours. Based on the recommended caloric intake for an 8-month-old infant (108 kcal/kg) this child's caloric intake:
1. Is difficult to evaluate without further information
2. Meets the recommended requirements for growth
3. Exceeds the recommended requirements for growth
4. Is less than the recommended requirements for growth

102. The physician orders multielectrolyte solution (MES) 150 ml per kg of body weight per 24 hours for a child weighing 13 pounds. The nurse is aware that the intake of MES for this child should be:
1. 500 ml/24hr
2. 750 ml/24hr
3. 885 ml/24hr
4. 965 ml/24hr

103. The physician has ordered 500 ml of a balanced electrolyte solution to run over 18 hours for a 5-year-old. The IV set delivers 60 gtt/ml. To administer the 500 ml over 18 hours the nurse should set the IV drip rate at:

1. 0.5 gtt/min
2. 3.0 gtt/min
3. 28.0 gtt/min
4. 36.0 gtt/min

104. The physician orders 700 ml of IV fluid over 24 hours. The IV tubing has a drop factor of 60 gtt/ml. The nurse should set the flow to provide:
    1. 15 gtt/min
    2. 20 gtt/min
    3. 29 gtt/min
    4. 34 gtt/min

105. A child is to receive 500 ml of D5NS and 250 ml of RL over 24 hours. The tubing delivers 60 gtt/ml. The nurse should set the flow to provide:
    1. 11 gtt/min
    2. 21 gtt/min
    3. 31 gtt/min
    4. 41 gtt/min

BLOOD AND IMMUNITY

106. The nurse is aware that children with AIDS are even more prone to infection than adults with AIDS because:
    1. Even the immune system of a healthy child is incapable of producing antibodies
    2. The AIDS virus attacks children's immune systems through different mechanisms
    3. Children with AIDS are exposed to many more pathogens than are adults with AIDS
    4. Children have fewer circulating antibodies due to a lack of previous exposure to pathogens

107. The nurse is aware that immunization of infants does not begin until 2 months of age because:
    1. The neonatal spleen is unable to produce efficient antibodies
    2. Infants under 2 months are rarely exposed to infectious diseases
    3. The immunization would attack the immature infant's body and produce the disease
    4. Maternal antibodies interfere with the development of active antibodies by the infant

108. Before giving a 2-month-old child the first DTP immunization, the nurse discusses with the mother the possible reactions that may occur because these reactions are:
    1. Often serious and may require hospitalization
    2. Quite common and may be either local or systemic
    3. Often responsible for permanent neurological damage
    4. Sometimes responsible for deep ulceration at the site of injection

109. An infant receives the first DTP immunization at 2 months. The nurse instructs the parent to:
    1. Apply heat to injection site for the first day; afterwards apply ice if the arm is sore
    2. Apply ice to injection site if soreness present; call the physician if a fever develops
    3. Give Tylenol for fever; call the physician if marked drowsiness or convulsions occur
    4. Give the baby aspirin for pain; if swelling at injection site develops, call the physician

110. If a 5½-month-old infant's immunizatons are on schedule, the nurse can assume that the baby has already received:
    1. Measles, mumps, and rubella vaccines
    2. A booster dose of trivalent oral polio virus vaccine
    3. Two doses of diphtheria, tetanus, and pertussis vaccine
    4. The first booster dose of diphtheria, tetanus, and pertussis vaccine

111. If a 9-month-old's immunization schedule is up to date, the next immunization that the infant should receive at 12 to 15 months of age is:
    1. Tetanus toxoid
    2. Trivalent oral polio vaccine
    3. Measles, mumps, rubella vaccine
    4. Diphtheria, tetanus, pertussis vaccine

112. A newborn's immunization schedule is started. When discussing the immunization schedule for the first 6 months with the parents the nurse should inform them that children are not usually immunized against:
    1. Polio
    2. Tetanus
    3. Diphtheria
    4. Hepatitis B

113. A child with leukemia is to continue taking prednisone at home after discharge. The nurse discovers that the child's sibling is home with the chickenpox. The nurse plans the discharge teaching based on the knowledge that:
    1. Chickenpox can be fatal to clients with leukemia
    2. The child must be immunized before going home
    3. Clients receiving prednisone are immune to chickenpox
    4. If direct contact between the two children is avoided the client can go home

114. The nurse should suggest to the mother of an 18-month-old infant with anemia that the child be fed:
    1. Pieces of pumpkin pie
    2. Slices of a whole apple
    3. A cup of seedless grapes
    4. Bread pudding with raisins

115. A mother tells the nurse that her 8-month-old will eat only mashed potatoes and drink only milk and she is concerned about the baby's diet even though the baby is receiving infant vitamins daily. The nurse recognizes that the child's diet could lead to:
    1. A potassium deficit
    2. A vitamin deficiency
    3. An amino acid deficiency
    4. An iron deficiency anemia

116. The nurse, preparing a 12-year-old child for a bone marrow aspiration, would know that the child does not understand the teaching about the procedure when the child states:

1. "I can get out of bed after the doctor is finished."
2. "I will have a tight dressing to put pressure on the area."
3. "The doctor is going to inject a needle into the center of one of my hip bones."
4. "The only pain I should feel is when the doctor puts in the shot so it won't hurt."

117. The mother of a child, who has been recently diagnosed as having hemophilia, is pregnant with her second child and asks the nurse what the chances are that this baby will also have hemophilia. The nurse's best response would be:
    1. "There is no chance the baby will be affected."
    2. "There is a 25% chance the baby will be affected."
    3. "There is a 75% chance the baby will be affected."
    4. "There is a 50% chance the baby will be affected."

118. The most common area for bleeding to develop in a child with hemophilia is the:
    1. Brain
    2. Joints
    3. Abdomen
    4. Pericardium

119. In addition to the relief of pain, the nurse should direct the care for a client with sickle cell crisis toward:
    1. Antibiotics and narcotic regulation
    2. Oxygenation and adequate hydration
    3. Hydration and psychologic counseling
    4. Oxygenation and Factor VIII replacement

120. A 10-year-old is admitted in thrombocytic sickle cell crisis. When assigning a room, it is most appropriate for the nurse to place the child with a roommate who has:
    1. Pneumonia
    2. Thalassemia
    3. Osteomyelitis
    4. Acute pharyngitis

121. The nurse recognizes that the teaching about sickle cell anemia was understood when a 16-year-old with the disease states, "I know that symptoms will appear when I have:
    1. A low iron intake."
    2. A breakdown of RBCs."
    3. An increased WBC production."
    4. A fluid and electrolyte imbalance."

122. A nursing intervention for a child with sickle cell anemia would be:
    1. Teaching the child how to prevent sickling
    2. Explaining how excess oxygen sickles the RBCs
    3. Preparing the child for occasional blood transfusions
    4. Teaching the child about the prophylactic medications

123. When obtaining a health history from the parents of a toddler who is admitted with acute lymphocytic leukemia (ALL), the nurse would expect them to report that the first sign they observed was:
    1. A loss of appetite
    2. Sores in the mouth
    3. A paleness of the skin
    4. Purplish spots on the skin

124. When giving nursing care to a child with leukemia, the nurse notes blood on the pillow case and several bloody tissues. The nurse should check the child's laboratory report for the:
    1. Platelet count
    2. Uric acid level
    3. Prothrombin time
    4. Red blood cell count

125. When discharging a 5-year-old girl who is to continue chemotherapy at home, the nurse would know that the parents understood the discharge instructions when they say, "We should:

1. Isolate her from other children her age."
2. Allow her to eat her food at her own pace."
3. Have her rinse her mouth with mouthwash."
4. Provide her with structured activities each day."

126. A child with leukemia is to be sent home on a protocol that includes several antineoplastics after an intrathecal administration of methotrexate. Before discharge the nurse instructs the child's parents to:
    1. Limit contact with peers because they tend to have communicable diseases
    2. Return weekly for bone marrow aspiration to determine effectiveness of therapy
    3. Schedule routine laboratory appointments for evaluation of response to medication
    4. Withhold medications when nausea occurs to prevent additional episodes of vomiting

127. Caring for an infant who is HIV positive can best be accomplished in:
    1. The pediatric unit
    2. A critical care unit
    3. The home environment
    4. An extended care facility

128. When a child is admitted with a diagnosis of AIDS, to protect the staff the nurse should immediately institute:
    1. Strict isolation
    2. Protective isolation
    3. Enteric precautions
    4. Body secretion precautions

129. The nursing diagnosis with the highest priority for a child with AIDS would be:
    1. High risk for injury
    2. High risk for infection
    3. Alteration in growth and development
    4. Alteration in nutrition: less than body requirements

INTEGUMENTARY

130. A 3-month-old with severe dehydration has an excoriated diaper area. The infant's mother is quite upset when she finds the nurse has left her infant without a diaper. The nurse should explain that:
    1. Air-drying of the skin prevents the diaper from sticking to it
    2. Increasing the exposed areas helps to reduce the infant's fever
    3. Cleansing of the skin followed by air-drying reduces excoriation
    4. This action allows the nurse to observe more quickly when the infant stools

131. During a health history on the 4-month-old child of a migrant worker, the nurse learns that the child recently had a fever, runny nose, cough, and white spots in the mouth for 3 days. The child then developed a rash that started on the face and spread to the whole body. The nurse should suspect that the child had:
    1. Rubella
    2. Rubeola
    3. Varicella
    4. Scarlet fever

132. The nurse is aware that eczema in infants is a nonspecific ailment that is:
    1. Easily treated
    2. Highly contagious
    3. Predominantly found in infants
    4. Associated with chronic respiratory infections

133. The most important nursing care for infants with eczema is:
    1. Promotion of physical growth
    2. Provision of sufficient hydration
    3. Identification of causative factors
    4. Prevention of secondary infections

134. Allergic reactions in eczematous infants and young children are most often caused by:
    1. Fruit, eggs, and wheat
    2. Milk, eggs, and peanuts
    3. Woolens, meat, and milk
    4. Woolens, house dust, and dog hairs

135. The nurse evaluates that the mother of a 6-month-old with eczema needs more teaching regarding her baby's care when the mother states:
    1. "I will be careful not to cut the baby's nails short."
    2. "I have given all of the baby's woolen blankets to my nephew."
    3. "I will make sure not to give the baby any whole milk products."
    4. "I am going to buy my baby a whole new wardrobe of cotton clothing."

136. The symptoms that would most probably lead the nurse to suspect that a 3-year-old child has rubella are:
    1. Conjunctivitis and sensitivity to light
    2. Severe headache and nuchal rigidity
    3. Koplik's spots on the soft palate and buccal mucosa
    4. Enlargement of the posterior cervical and postauricular nodes

137. A child with rubella should be isolated from an unimmunized:
    1. 20-year-old brother living at home
    2. 3-year-old girl friend who lives next door
    3. 12-year-old sister who had rubeola as a child
    4. 18-year-old female cousin who has recently married

138. When extensive eschar formation is present on the arms of a child hospitalized with severe burns, the priority nursing action would be to:
    1. Remove blisters
    2. Check radial pulses
    3. Perform range of motion
    4. Enforce respiratory isolation

139. A 12-year-old has incurred partial thickness burns of the entire right arm, upper left arm, and anterior chest trying to start a campfire. According to the "rule of nines," the nurse estimates burn injury for this child would be:
    1. 15-24 percent
    2. 25-34 percent
    3. 35-44 percent
    4. 45-54 percent

140. When doing a dressing change the nurse understands that a basic principle of surgical asepsis is:
1. The entire sterile field is considered sterile
2. Sterile items held below the waist are considered sterile
3. Sterile objects in contact with clean objects are considered clean
4. Wounds with exudates are contaminated and dry wounds are sterile

141. When teaching a mother about communicable diseases, the nurse informs her that chickenpox is:
1. Still communicable until all the vesicles have dried
2. Still communicable even when just dry scabs remain
3. No longer communicable after a high fever has subsided
4. Not communicable as long as the vesicles are intact and surrounded by a red areola

142. Understanding that there is a need to protect susceptible persons from exposure to chickenpox during the acute phase, the nurse should question the mother of a child with chickenpox about relatives or friends who are receiving:
1. Long-term anticonvulsant therapy
2. Prolonged topical antibiotic therapy
3. High doses of systemic steroid therapy
4. Therapeutic doses of vitamins and minerals

143. To hasten the drying of the lesions and relieve the itch in a child with chickenpox, the nurse suggests that the mother should try:
1. Using wet to dry saline dressings over the oozing vesicles
2. Rubbing bacitracin (Bacitin) ointment into the open lesions
3. Having the child wear mittens and cutting the fingernails short
4. Patting the lesions gently with a paste of baking soda and warm water

144. As a mother leaves the hospital with her infant, the nurse notes that the mother covers the infant with a blanket. The nurse understands that the mother is preventing heat loss by the principle of:
1. Radiation
2. Conduction
3. Active transport
4. Fluid vaporization

145. The nurse teaches a teenager about the need for special mouth care because of the potential for lesions from the chemotherapy being administered. The nurse evaluates that the instructions were understood when the teenager says, "I should:
1. Brush my teeth with a toothbrush."
2. Rinse my mouth with hydrogen peroxide."
3. Rinse my mouth with undiluted mouthwash."
4. Brush my teeth with a foam-tipped applicator."

146. The nurse recognizes that when fever is suspected in preschool children with leukemia who are receiving chemotherapy that:
1. Rectal temperatures are too upsetting for this age group
2. Oral temperatures alone are inaccurate in children with leukemia
3. Ear temperatures alone are not accurate when fever is suspected
4. Rectal temperatures are avoided to reduce the risk of rectal trauma

147. The nurse is aware that rubeola is commonly known as:
1. Measles
2. Chickenpox
3. Whooping cough
4. German measles

148. The nurse is aware that rubeola often causes children to have:
1. A macular rash
2. A paroxysmal cough
3. Enlarged parotid glands
4. Generalized vesicular lesions

149. The nurse is aware that the most common secondary infection to head lice (pediculosis capitis) is:
1. Eczema
2. Cellulitis
3. Impetigo
4. Tinea capitis

150. A child, recently returned from a camping trip, complains of a rash, chills, fever, and a headache, and is brought to the clinic by the parents. The nurse in the clinic recognizes that this child's history and physical assessment should include:
1. A history of allergies and duration of symptoms
2. A developmental screening and history of exposure to chickenpox
3. Sports played on the trip and when the child has to return to school
4. The date the child received a flu vaccination and a history of any sunburn

151. When a 12-year-old boy, who received several tick bites on a camping trip, becomes ill, he is told that he may have Lyme disease. He asks the nurse, "What is Lyme disease?" The nurse's best response would be:
1. "It's a spirochetal infection that penicillin will treat."
2. "You sound upset, but we have medicine that will make you better."
3. "You are concerned. Why don't you ask me what you want to know."
4. "The insect bites gave you an infection but there is medication that will stop it."

152. A client asks the nurse what is the best way to remove a tick from the skin. The nurse should reply:
1. "Touch the tick with a lighted cigarette."
2. "Remove the tick carefully with tweezers."
3. "Pour ammonia over the tick and it will shrivel up."
4. "Spray the tick with insect repellent and it will fall off."

SKELETAL

153. When doing an assessment of a child who has just had a cast applied to the right arm, the nurse finds that the fingers of the child's hand are cool. The nurse should first:
1. Elevate the right arm to reduce the swelling
2. Clip the edge of the cast to reduce pressure
3. Compare the temperature of the right and left hands
4. Call the physician to report the circulatory impairment

154. The nurse, when teaching parents how to care for their child's plaster cast, tells them that to keep the cast clean they should:
1. Cover the cast with a piece of plastic
2. Remove surface dirt with a damp cloth
3. Rub the dirty area with a diluted bleach solution
4. Scrub the cast with a soft brush and mild abrasive

155. After giving a bed bath to a 2½-year-old child in Bryant's traction for a fractured femur, the nurse should be sure that the child's hip angle is maintained at:
1. 45 degrees
2. 60 degrees
3. 90 degrees
4. 180 degrees

156. Nursing care specific for a child in Bryant's traction should include:
1. Checking site of pins for bleeding or infection
2. Applying topical or antibiotic ointment as ordered
3. Removing the bandages daily to lubricate the skin
4. Assessing that the elastic bandages are not too loose or too tight

157. A child sustains a fractured femur in a bicycle accident. However, the admission x-ray films reveal evidence of fractures of other long bones in various stages of healing. The nurse determines that this child should be assessed for:
1. Child abuse
2. Vitamin D deficiency
3. Osteogenesis imperfecta
4. Inadequate calcium intake

158. A newborn with talipes equinovarus has a unilateral boot cast applied to the involved foot. When moving the infant with a newly applied plaster cast, the nurse should:
1. Touch the cast with just the fingertips
2. Turn the infant without touching the cast
3. Handle the cast with the palms of the hands
4. Move the infant's body and let the cast slide on the bed

159. Teaching for parents whose baby is undergoing frequent casting to correct a foot deformity should include information on plaster cast care such as:
1. Covering damp cast edges with adhesive petals
2. Applying lotion to the skin at cast edges to keep it soft
3. Checking the skin at the edges of the cast daily for redness
4. Immersing the cast briefly during the tub bath and wiping it lightly

160. During a newborn assessment a positive Ortolani sign would be indicated by:
1. A unilateral droop of the hip
2. A broadening of the perineum
3. An apparent shortening of one leg
4. An audible click on hip manipulation

161. When assessing a child suspected of having congenital hip dysplasia, the nurse would expect that an assessment of the child's orthopedic status would reveal:
1. An apparent shortening of one leg
2. A limited ability to adduct the affected leg   *Abduct*
3. A narrowing of the perineum with an anal stricture
4. An inability to palpate movement of the femoral head

162. The statement by the mother of a 6-week-old female infant that would lead the nurse to assess the child for the presence of an abnormality is:
1. "She wants to sleep curled up on her stomach all the time."
2. "Her feet look very flat when I put both of her booties on her."
3. "I seem to have a hard time getting her diaper between her legs."
4. "I can't get her to straighten out her legs when I try to stand her up."

163. Six weeks after birth, an infant is diagnosed as having congenital hip dysplasia. The infant is admitted to the hospital for immediate corrective measures because:

1. Infants are easier to manage in spica casts than toddlers
2. Mobility will be delayed if correction is postponed until later
3. The infant's hip joint is still cartilaginous and molding of the acetabulum is possible
4. Bryant's traction cannot be used effectively after a child reaches the age of 2 years

164. Before discharging a newborn infant with congenital hip dysplasia, the nurse teaches the parents that hip dislocation can be minimized if the infant is:
1. Carried straddling the hip
2. Tightly swaddled in blankets
3. Periodically strapped to a cradleboard
4. Placed in an infant seat on a set schedule

165. When planning home care for a 6-month-old infant who has just been placed in a hip spica cast, the nurse should emphasize to the parents that:
1. No special precautions will be necessary when diapering
2. The entire cast should be wrapped in plastic wrap to prevent soiling
3. Baby oil and powder should be used liberally around the diaper area
4. The edges of the cast in the perineal area should be covered with plastic wrap

166. When providing care for a child immediately after returning from surgery for the application of a spica cast, the nurse should plan to:
1. Dry the cast with a hair dryer
2. Turn the child by using the crossbar
3. Touch the cast using only the palms of the hands
4. Logroll the child every six hours until the cast is dry

167. The priority of care in the immediate postoperative period for a youngster with a newly applied spica cast would be:
1. Giving the child oral fluids
2. Checking the child's peripheral circulation
3. Encouraging the child to take deep breaths
4. Teaching the child to use the overhead trapeze

168. Three days following the application of a spica cast, a child has a temperature of 101.4°F. Suspecting an infection the nurse should first assess the child for:
    1. Rapid irregular respirations
    2. A foul smell coming from the cast
    3. Any complaints of tingling in the toes
    4. The presence of itching around the top of the cast

169. After giving a teenager discharge instructions regarding cast care, the nurse evaluates that the instructions were understood when the teenager says, "If I am itchy around the cast I will:
    1. Gently scratch the itchy area."
    2. Pat the area with an alcohol swab."
    3. Ask the physician for an antihistamine."
    4. Sprinkle a layer of powder around the itchy spots."

170. The nurse understands that the correct way to turn a 10-year-old in a spica cast is to:
    1. Log-roll the body as one unit
    2. Use the cross bar between the legs
    3. Have the child assist by using the overhead trapeze
    4. Teach the child to sit up and help when changing position

NEUROMUSCULAR

171. The parents of an infant with cerebral palsy should be taught to:
    1. Focus on cognitive rather than motor skills
    2. Preserve muscle tone to prevent contractures
    3. Maintain prolonged immobility of limbs with splints
    4. Encourage strenuous exercise to build muscle tone

172. A 3-year-old male has recently been diagnosed with X-linked Duchenne's muscular dystrophy. Neither parent has muscular dystrophy. The statement by the parents that indicates an understanding of the disease's transmission is:

1. "Our daughters could be carriers."
2. "Our sons or daughters could have the disease."
3. "We each contributed a gene that caused our son to have the disease."
4. "By Mendelian law, our son's having muscular dystrophy limits its occurrence in other children."

173. The nurse is aware that discharge planning related to care of a child with Duchenne's muscular dystrophy should include teaching the parents about:
    1. Range of motion exercises
    2. Maintaining a high caloric diet
    3. Instituting seizure precautions
    4. Restricting the use of larger muscles

174. The nurse understands that when a child with Duchenne's muscular dystrophy reaches adolescence, additional problems will probably develop with the:
    1. GI system
    2. Neurological system
    3. Musculoskeletal system
    4. Cardiopulmonary system

175. The nurse understands that the genetic etiology of Down's syndrome is an:
    1. Extra chromosome
    2. Intrauterine infection
    3. X-linked chromosome
    4. Autosomal recessive gene

176. The nurse should recognize that the most common serious anomaly associated with Down's syndrome is:
    1. Renal disease
    2. Hepatic defects
    3. Congenital heart disease
    4. Endocrine gland malfunction

177. The nurse suspects that the concept that a developmentally disabled child could probably learn the fastest is:
    1. Love vs hate
    2. Life vs death
    3. Large vs small
    4. Right vs wrong

178. When parents ask the nurse what to do about their preschooler's stuttering, the nurse should suggest that they:
1. Identify situations that increase stuttering and avoid or ignore the hesitancy
2. Avoid looking at the child when the child has difficulty forming or expressing words
3. Help the child by supplying the correct word when the child is experiencing a block
4. Stop the conversation and tell the child to speak slowly and think before starting again

179. Shortly following birth, a newborn is diagnosed as having Erb's palsy. The nurse is aware that this problem is caused by:
1. A disease acquired in utero
2. An X-linked inheritance pattern
3. A tumor arising from muscle tissue
4. An injury to the brachial plexus during birth

180. The nurse recognizes that a couple who have a newborn with Erb's palsy have an accurate understanding of their infant's prognosis when they state:
1. "This is a progressive disease with no cure."
2. "A year of physical therapy will be necessary."
3. "Correction can be achieved only through surgery."
4. "Complete recovery should occur in about 3 months."

181. The nurse is aware that a high level of lead in the blood of children with lead poisoning (plumbism) can lead to:
1. Liver damage
2. Marked anemia
3. Increased urination
4. Severe malnutrition

182. The nursing diagnosis that is most appropriate for children with lead poisoning is:
1. Chronic pain
2. Altered nutrition
3. Unilateral neglect
4. High risk for injury

183. After a craniotomy for the removal of a hematoma sustained in a fall, a child is returned to the recovery room. The nurse places the child in a semi-Fowler's position to:
1. Increase cranial drainage and prevent accumulation of fluid
2. Reduce subdural pressure and promote reaction from anesthesia
3. Decrease pressure on the diaphragm and increase thoracic expansion
4. Decrease the cardiac work load and facilitate oxygenation after surgery

184. The day after brain surgery, a nine-year-old child with diabetes mellitus develops a temperature of 103°F. The nurse understands that:
1. A slight fever is to be expected following any surgery
2. Anyone with diabetes will develop an infection following surgery
3. Edema following the surgery often causes pressure on the hypothalamus
4. An excess of viscid secretions has caused inadequate respiratory ventilation

185. The nurse is aware that infants with a myelomeningocele, not just a meningocele, usually have:
1. Hydrocephalus
2. Lower extremity paralysis
3. A sac over the lumbar area
4. Infections of the spinal fluid

186. The abnormal finding that a nurse would expect to observe during an assessment of a one-month-old infant admitted with hydrocephalus would be that:
1. The infant's anterior fontanel is tense on palpation
2. The infant demonstrates poor eye muscle coordination
3. The infant is unable to support the head and shoulders while prone
4. The infant's head circumference is larger than the chest circumference

187. An infant with a myelomeningocele is scheduled for surgery to close the defect. The nursing action which would best facilitate parent-child relationships in the preoperative period is:
1. Allowing the parents to cuddle the child in their arms
2. Demonstrating feeding techniques in the prone position
3. Encouraging the parents to stroke and comfort the child
4. Referring the parents to the Spina Bifida Association of America

188. A 1-month-old infant with hydrocephalus is scheduled for surgery for the insertion of a ventriculoperitoneal (VP) shunt. A short-term preoperative goal for the infant would be to:
1. Keep the infant as comfortable as possible to limit crying
2. Use a thick head bandage to protect the infant's head from injury
3. Establish and maintain a strict fixed feeding schedule to ensure hydration
4. Provide a wide variety of play objects to maintain age-appropriate stimulation

189. Preoperatively, the parents of a child undergoing an insertion of a ventriculoperitoneal (VP) shunt for hydrocephalus are taught about postoperative positioning. The nurse can evaluate their understanding of the teaching when they state, "We will avoid putting pressure on the valve site by positioning our baby:
1. In the position that provides the most comfort."
2. On the back with a small support beneath the neck."
3. On the abdomen with a small support against the left side of the head."
4. Flat and side lying with a small support against the right side of the head and back."

190. Following the repair of a myelomeningocele in a newborn the nurse should:
1. Keep the child in the supine position
2. Apply sterile moist dressings to the incision
3. Observe for signs of leakage of cerebrospinal fluid
4. Teach the parents intermittent clean catheterization

191. On the day after surgery for insertion of a ventriculoperitoneal shunt for hydrocephalus, an infant's temperature rises to 103°F. The nurse should first notify the physician and then:
1. Sponge the infant with tepid alcohol
2. Recheck the temperature in 2 hours
3. Remove any excess clothing from the infant
4. Record the temperature on the infant's chart

192. Following the insertion of an atrioventricular shunt, the nurse evaluates the function of the shunt by:
1. Noting the frequency of voiding
2. Assessing for periorbital edema
3. Palpating the child's anterior fontanel
4. Observing for symmetrical Moro reflexes

193. A 2½-year-old undergoes a shunt revision. Before discharge, the nurse, recognizing abnormal behavior for this age group, tells the parents to call the physician if the child:
1. Tries to copy all of the father's mannerisms
2. Talks incessantly regardless of the presence of others
3. Becomes fussy when frustrated and displays a shortened attention span
4. Frequently starts arguments with playmates by claiming all toys are "mine"

194. Upon return from surgery for placement of a ventricular peritoneal shunt for hydrocephaly, the nurse should place the child in:
1. A flat position on the unoperated side
2. The Sims' position on the operated side
3. A low-Fowler's position on the operated side
4. The semi-Fowler's position on the unoperated side

195. In addition to systemic chemotherapy, the nurse is aware that cranial radiation is done on children with leukemia to:
1. Improve the quality of the child's life
2. Reduce the risk of systemic infection
3. Avoid metastasis to the lymphatic system
4. Prevent central nervous system involvement

196. While in the playroom a 7-year-old child has a myoclonic seizure of the right arm and leg that almost immediately progresses to a tonic-clonic seizure with clenched jaws. The nurse's best initial action would be to:
1. Take the other children to their rooms
2. Put a plastic airway into the child's mouth
3. Place a large pillow under the child's head
4. Move the toys and furniture away from the child

197. During a tonic-clonic seizure a child becomes cyanotic. The nurse should:
1. Insert an oral airway
2. Administer oxygen by mask
3. Continue to observe the seizure
4. Notify the physician immediately

198. A 4½-year-old admitted with a diagnosis of cerebellar astrocytoma has surgery and a large tumor is excised. When preparing for the child's admission to the intensive care unit it would be inappropriate for the nurse to:
1. Place a hypothermic blanket on the bed
2. Raise the foot of the bed on shock blocks
3. Secure an IV pump to closely monitor fluids
4. Obtain a cardiorespiratory monitor and sphygmomanometer

199. The nurse knows that among infants and children otitis media is considered the most common:
1. Viral infection
2. Fungal infection
3. Bacterial infection
4. Rickettsial infection

200. When explaining a myringotomy procedure, the nurse should emphasize that the incision:
1. Provides immediate relief of pressure in the middle ear
2. Takes several days to heal and frequently leaves a scar
3. Widens the perforation in the eardrum to allow for drainage
4. Often results in permanent perforation of the tympanic membrane

201. The most important nursing responsibility during a myringotomy procedure on an 18-month-old child is to:

1. Collect the aspirated drainage in a culture tube
2. Maintain the continuous flow of local anesthetic
3. Have the mother stay and hold the child in her arms
4. Keep the child restrained and completely immobilized

202. To help the parents promote the effectiveness of their child's myringotomy procedure, the nurse suggests that they should:
1. Maintain the child in the supine position
2. Position the child with the affected ear down
3. Keep the child with the affected ear uppermost
4. Observe the child for bleeding from the operative site

203. Upon discharge after a myringotomy, a potential complication the nurse teaches the child's parents to report is:
1. Bleeding and diminished pain
2. Mild or moderate hearing loss
3. Lack of drainage and increased pain
4. Low-grade temperature and headache

204. The purpose of isolation for a child with an infectious disease is to:
1. Separate the infected child from noninfected persons
2. Interrupt the infectious process as quickly as possible
3. Protect the child with a decreased resistance to infection
4. Prevent nosocomial infection during the hospitalized period

205. A child with measles develops encephalitis and is admitted to the hospital. The physician orders strict isolation. After teaching the parents about the proper isolation precautions, the nurse would know that they understood the directions when they:
1. Put on gowns when they entered the room
2. Washed their hands and stood at the foot of the bed
3. Put on gowns, gloves, and masks before entering the room
4. Requested sterile gowns and gloves before entering the room

206. A child is admitted with a diagnosis of meningococcal meningitis. The nurse is aware that isolation:
    1. Of any kind is not required
    2. Will be required for seven days
    3. Must be maintained during the incubation period
    4. Is required for 24 to 72 hours after onset of antibiotic therapy

207. When obtaining the nursing history from the mother of a child with Reye's syndrome, the nurse would probably learn that the child recently recovered from:
    1. Rubella
    2. Chickenpox
    3. Rheumatic fever
    4. Bacterial meningitis

208. The early symptoms that usually bring the child with Reye's syndrome to the hospital are:
    1. Diarrhea and a rash
    2. Jaundice and oliguria
    3. Low-grade fever and petechiae
    4. Intractable vomiting and confusion

209. The nurse should expect that a child with Reye's syndrome will be:
    1. Placed on strict isolation
    2. Taken to surgery immediately
    3. Admitted to the intensive care unit
    4. Treated on an ambulatory basis initially

210. When caring for a child with Reye's syndrome the nurse must be alert for such manifestations as:
    1. Bladder distention and overflow
    2. A macular rash on face and trunk
    3. Marked periorbital edema from renal shutdown
    4. Bleeding and ecchymosis from liver involvement

211. In the well-child clinic a nurse teaches a group of parents guidelines that will possibly avoid Reye's syndrome in their young children. The nurse tells the parents:

1. "If your children's temperature reaches 101°F, begin sponge bathing with alcohol."
2. "Ask your doctor about inoculating your children with a specific immunization serum."
3. "Restrict your children's carbohydrate intake when they have the symptoms of a cold."
4. "Use an antipyretic other than aspirin when your children have a respiratory infection."

ENDOCRINE

212. The regulation of diabetes mellitus in a newly diagnosed juvenile is best accomplished by:
    1. Insulin, dietary control, and exercise
    2. Dietary control, exercise, and urine testing
    3. Dietary control, exercise, and blood glucose monitoring
    4. Oral hypoglycemic agents, dietary control, and exercise

213. After assessing what a newly diagnosed juvenile knows about diabetes, the nurse should:
    1. Develop a rapport with the client
    2. Set goals with the client and the client's family
    3. Teach the client how to do blood glucose testing
    4. Teach the client how to administer the insulin injections required daily

214. Since prevention of infection is of utmost importance in children with diabetes mellitus, the nurse should emphasize to the child and parents the importance of:
    1. Inspecting both feet frequently and carefully
    2. Soaking the feet at least once daily for 30 minutes in hot water
    3. Drying the feet thoroughly after a bath by rubbing vigorously with a towel
    4. Treating minor cuts on the feet immediately with a strong antiseptic such as iodine

215. The statement that reflects why the nurse teaches the mother of a young child with diabetes how to test the child's urine at home even though blood glucose testing is being done 4 times a day is:
1. The urine should be tested for acetone during illness and when the blood glucose is above 250
2. Blood glucose testing before meals and at bedtime may be stopped once the child is stabilized on insulin
3. Urine testing remains the most accurate way to check for high glucose if double voided specimens are used
4. It is now thought that voided urine specimens reflect short-term glucose levels more accurately than blood glucose, especially in children

216. When reviewing the plan of care for a child with diabetes mellitus, the nurse is aware that the most accurate method to evaluate the effectiveness of diet and insulin therapy over time is the laboratory test that measures:
1. Urine ketones
2. Serum protein levels
3. Serum glucose levels
4. Glycosylated hemoglobin

217. If surgery is to be performed on a child with diabetes mellitus the nurse should be cognizant that:
1. Urine test results provide the best gauge of diabetic control after the surgery
2. The greatest danger during the surgical procedure is from diabetic ketoacidosis
3. The stress of surgery causes a rise in blood glucose levels during the postoperative period
4. If insulin was not required before surgery it generally will not be required in the postoperative period

218. An 8-year-old child is receiving 45 units of Humulin N (NPH) insulin at 7 AM and 7 PM. The most appropriate information for the nurse to give the parents concerning a bedtime snack would be:

1. Provide a snack at bedtime to prevent hypoglycemia during the night
2. Give the child a snack at bedtime if any signs of hyperglycemia are displayed
3. Keep the snack in the refrigerator in case the child becomes hungry during the night
4. Bedtime snacks are not recommended for diabetic children treated with long acting insulin

219. A young girl with diabetes has just joined the school's soccer team and her mother is unsure of whether or not to tell the coach of her child's condition. The mother asks the nurse in the pediatric clinic for guidance. The nurse's response to the mother's concern should be based on the fact that:
1. The coach might discuss the child's condition with other faculty members
2. Hyperglycemia can be treated by the school nurse if symptoms are recognized early
3. The child would be dropped from the team if school authorities learn she has a chronic disease
4. Episodes of hypoglycemia are associated with children with diabetes who participate in sports activities

220. A 9-year-old child with diabetes mellitus is hospitalized for dosage regulation of insulin. The child appears to be very manipulative and has been observed sneaking food and trying to talk the mother into providing sweets. Based on this behavior, when the child complains of hypoglycemia, the most appropriate nursing action would be to:
1. Test the urine for glucose
2. Obtain a blood glucose level
3. Administer orange juice with sugar
4. Ask the child the last time food was eaten

221. A child with diabetes mellitus who is also learning disabled has trouble correctly measuring the required insulin dose. The child frequently draws up 42 units of insulin instead of the prescribed 24 units. The most appropriate intervention to ensure dosage safety would be to:
    1. Teach the child to use a magnifying glass to read the numbers on the syringe
    2. Exchange the insulin syringe the child has been using for a tuberculin syringe
    3. Provide the child with pre-set syringe guides that were developed for the blind
    4. Allow the child to have the number written down on paper when filling the syringe

222. A child with diabetes mellitus is receiving 15 units of Humulin R insulin and 30 units of Humulin N insulin at 7 AM each morning. The nurse should expect that a hypoglycemic reaction from the Humulin N insulin is most likely to occur:
    1. During the night
    2. Within 30 minutes
    3. In the late morning
    4. In the late afternoon

223. A nurse suspects that a child with diabetes mellitus might be hypoglycemic when the child manifests:
    1. Redness of the face and deep, rapid breathing
    2. A change in behavior, hunger, and diaphoresis
    3. Increased thirst, sleepiness, and some vomiting
    4. A decreased level of consciousness and dry mouth

224. When teaching about insulin self-administration to a 10-year-old child newly diagnosed with diabetes mellitus, the nurse should teach the child to:
    1. Always wash the hands prior to preparing the insulin injection
    2. Shake the bottle of insulin thoroughly before drawing the dose
    3. Briskly rub the injection site for a minute after giving the injection
    4. Give the insulin injections primarily in the opposite arm or either leg

225. The nurse plans to teach a child with diabetes mellitus, who is receiving both Humulin N and Humulin R insulin daily, how to self-administer the insulin before discharge. When learning to give the injections the child should:
    1. Alternate the sites until the best one to use is found
    2. Learn to use the needle and syringe by practicing on an orange first
    3. Administer the injections immediately after being taught the technique
    4. Draw up the Humulin N insulin first and then draw up the Humulin R insulin

226. A 13-year-old insulin-dependent diabetic with a history of poor adherence to therapy is admitted with a blood sugar of 700 mg/dl. A continuous insulin infusion is begun. When developing a plan of care for this adolescent the nurse should be alert for possible:
    1. Hypovolemia
    2. Hypokalemia
    3. Hypernatremia
    4. Hypercalcemia

227. A 16-year-old insulin-dependent diabetic adolescent is brought to the emergency room unconscious. The adolescent's blood glucose is 742 mg/dl. During the initial assessment the nurse would expect to note:
    1. Pyrexia
    2. Hyperpnea
    3. Bradycardia
    4. Hypertension

228. A primary long-term goal for a 16-year-old admitted for the control of insulin-dependent diabetes mellitus is to:
    1. Keep free of glucosuria
    2. Adhere to a routine exercise program
    3. Develop a life-style that will be nonstressful
    4. Maintain normoglycemia with few episodes of hypoglycemia or hyperglycemia

RESPIRATORY

229. An adolescent has an order for placement of a pulse oximeter. To ensure accuracy of the pulse oximeter reading the nurse should:

1. Place the probe on a finger or earlobe
2. Calibrate the oximeter at least every 8 hours
3. Place the probe on the abdomen or upper thigh
4. After application wait 30 minutes before obtaining a reading

230. The nurse understands that in the child, as in the adult, respiratory patterns are controlled by the:
1. Medulla
2. Cerebellum
3. Hypothalamus
4. Cerebral cortex

231. When examinining the throat of a 5-year-old, the nurse should position a tongue blade to the side of the child's tongue primarily to avoid:
1. Eliciting the gag reflex
2. Obstructing the airway
3. Hurting any of the teeth
4. Interfering with the visual examination

232. Immediately after being placed flat a child experiences shortness of breath and must sit up to breathe. The nurse knows that the term that best describes this phenomenon is:
1. Apnea
2. Dyspnea
3. Orthopnea
4. Hyperpnea

233. The nurse is aware that in administering routine oxygen therapy to a child the oxygen:
1. Should be labeled as flammable
2. Is warmed before administration
3. Must be humidified before administration
4. May be administered without a prescription

234. A 15-year-old high school student with hay fever has been taking a prescribed long-acting antihistamine/decongestant q8h for the past 3 days. The adolescent tells the nurse, "This medication is making me sleepy. Can you change it to something else?" The nurse's best response would be:

1. "Take only half a tablet before school."
2. "I think you should omit the early morning dose."
3. "The drowsiness will usually diminish after a few days."
4. "I'll ask the physician to change you to a medication containing ephedrine."

235. A 14-year-old develops sinusitis and is placed on a broad spectrum oral antibiotic to be taken 4 times a day. To maintain the blood level, the nurse should recommend that the medication be taken at:
1. 8 AM, 12 PM, 4 PM, and 8 PM
2. 8 AM, 4 PM, 12 AM, and 4 AM
3. 6 AM, 12 PM, 6 PM, and 12 AM
4. 10 AM, 2 PM, 10 PM, and 2 AM

236. A 10-year-old child is receiving 30% O_2 via mask. Pulse oximetry is ordered by the physician. The nurse should obtain the reading by placing the oximetry probe on the child's:
1. Great toe
2. Index finger
3. Radial pulse point
4. Popliteal pulse point

237. When making an assessment of a 6-month-old infant with bronchiolitis, the nurse would expect:
1. A decreased heart rate
2. Increased breath sounds
3. A prolonged expiratory phase
4. Intercostal and subcostal retractions

238. Based on the problems associated with bronchiolitis, the treatment of choice for a child with this illness should consist of:
1. Croupette and adequate hydration
2. Postural drainage and corticosteroids
3. Adequate hydration and bronchodilators
4. Croupette and broad spectrum antibiotics

239. The nurse organizes care for an infant with bronchiolitis to allow for uninterrupted periods of rest. This plan is:
    1. Inappropriate because constant care is necessary in the acute stage
    2. Appropriate because the cool mist helps to maintain hydration status
    3. Appropriate because this action promotes decreased oxygen demands
    4. Inappropriate because frequent assessment by auscultation is required

240. An important nursing measure for a 6-month-old infant with bronchiolitis is:
    1. Promoting stimulating activities that meet the infant's developmental needs
    2. Making frequent observations of the infant's skin color, anterior fontanel, and vital signs
    3. Discouraging visits from the parents during the acute phase to conserve the infant's energy
    4. Keeping the infant on strict isolation and using a gown, cap, mask, and gloves when giving care

241. A 3-year-old is admitted to the pediatric unit with a diagnosis of acute asthma. The child is short of breath, the respirations are 56, the pulse is 102, and there is a nonproductive cough. The nurse would expect the child's blood gas values to indicate a:
    1. pH of 7.32
    2. PO_2 of 95 mmHg
    3. HCO_3 of 26 mEq/L
    4. PCO_2 of 40 mmHg

242. An 8-year-old has a tonsillectomy. During the immediate postoperative period it is most important for the nurse to ensure that the child maintains:
    1. Hydration by providing cool liquids frequently
    2. Aeration by assisting with coughing and deep breathing
    3. Airway patency by placing the child in a side-lying position
    4. Consciousness by encouraging the mother to interact with the child

243. In the immediate postoperative period following a tonsillectomy, the mother of a 9-year-old should be encouraged to give her child:
    1. Ice cream
    2. Cold soda
    3. Tepid milk
    4. Orange juice

244. A young male client with cystic fibrosis (CF) becomes romantically involved with a young female with the same disease. He asks the nurse about the chances of having an affected child like himself. The most appropriate response by the nurse would be:
    1. "Use condoms for protection from pregnancy."
    2. "Young women with cystic fibrosis are not fertile."
    3. "All of your children would be carriers of cystic fibrosis."
    4. "You are probably not able to father children because of your cystic fibrosis."

245. The nurse understands that a male teenager, who has a sibling with cystic fibrosis (CF), understands genetic counseling when he states, "To determine if I am a carrier, I will have to undergo:
    1. A chest x-ray."
    2. Enzyme assays."
    3. DNA probe testing."
    4. Sweat chloride tests."

246. The nurse should be aware that the physiologic adaptations to cystic fibrosis are related to the:
    1. Sweat glands
    2. Endocrine glands
    3. Cilia of respiratory tract
    4. Mucus-secreting glands

247. The nurse understands that the pathophysiology primarily responsible for respiratory manifestations of cystic fibrosis is that:
    1. There is acute inflammation of the lung parenchyma
    2. Increased irritability of the airways causes obstruction
    3. Endocrine glands secrete abnormal levels of hormones
    4. Abnormally thick mucus leads to obstruction of the airways

248. A twenty-year-old female is known to be heterozygous for the cystic fibrosis (CF) gene. Her husband's genotype is unknown at present and the couple are expecting their first child. The chance that their baby will have cystic fibrosis is:
    1. 25% or less
    2. 50% or more
    3. Extremely rare
    4. Unknown at this time

249. A male adolescent with cystic fibrosis, whose parents are both carriers of the disease, asks the nurse, "When I have children could they have cystic fibrosis like me?" The nurse should base a response on the knowledge that:
    1. Men with cystic fibrosis generally have a 50% chance of having children with the disease
    2. Only women pass this disease to their children because it is carried on the sex chromosome
    3. This client has a greater chance of passing the disease to his children because his parents were only carriers
    4. Men with cystic fibrosis are frequently unable to father a baby, although sexual functioning is not affected

250. When assessing a newborn who has been diagnosed as having a diaphragmatic hernia, the nurse would expect to note the presence of:
    1. Blood in the stool
    2. A barrel-shaped chest
    3. Breath sounds over the abdomen
    4. An increased abdominal circumference

251. A nursing diagnosis of "impaired gas exchange" is made for an infant with a diaphragmatic hernia. The etiology of this diagnosis is the:
    1. Diaphragmatic hernia
    2. Decrease in oxygen intake
    3. Presence of excessive secretions
    4. Increase in the basal metabolic rate

252. In addition to raising the head of the bed of an infant who has had a surgical repair of a diaphragmatic hernia, the nurse should place the infant in the:

    1. Contour position in an infant seat
    2. Supine position with the knees flexed
    3. Prone position with the head to the side
    4. Side-lying position on the operative side

253. After the repair of a diaphragmatic hernia, the nurse would assess that the infant's respiratory condition is improving when:
    1. The infant stops crying
    2. The blood pH decreases to 7.31
    3. Breath sounds are heard bilaterally
    4. One oz of formula is ingested and retained

254. A child who was found face down in a water-filled ditch is brought to the emergency room. The child, who has a pulse of 50 beats per minute but no spontaneous respirations, is intubated and bagged with 100% oxygen. The most important nursing measure at this time is to:
    1. Start an intravenous line to provide fluid and electrolytes
    2. Assist the physician in delivering intracardiac medications
    3. Suction the endotracheal tube, mouth, and nasal passages
    4. Call the pediatric ICU to inform them of the child's admission

255. A child survives a near drowning episode in a cold pond, but still has many problems to overcome. The nurse is aware that the ultimate prognosis will depend mainly on the extent of damage resulting from the:
    1. Hypoxia
    2. Hyperthermia
    3. Emotional trauma
    4. Aspiration pneumonia

256. A young baby has an open repair of a fractured sternum and has a chest tube. The nurse explains to the baby's mother that the chest tube:
    1. Will be removed once the baby is feeding well and is afebrile
    2. Does not cause discomfort and is put in place for emergency use
    3. Is left in to drain the air from the chest cavity that entered during surgery
    4. Drains the extra air in the baby's chest that accumulated following the punctured lung

CARDIOVASCULAR

257. An infant born at 39 weeks gestation is sent to the intensive care nursery. The nurse suspects a possible cardiac anomaly when the admission assessment reveals:
1. Projectile vomiting
2. An irregular respiratory rhythm
3. Hyperreflexia of the extremities
4. Unequal peripheral blood pressures

258. A newborn with a cardiac defect is fed in the semi-Fowler's position. After the nurse feeds and burps the infant, and changes the infant's position, the infant has a bowel movement and almost immediately becomes cyanotic, diaphoretic, and limp. These symptoms are most likely caused by the:
1. Burping
2. Formula
3. Position change
4. Bowel movement

259. When examining the laboratory report of a child with the diagnosis of rheumatic fever, the nurse would expect the findings to demonstrate:
1. A negative C-reactive protein
2. A positive antistreptolysin titer
3. An elevated reticulocyte count
4. A decreased erythrocyte sedimentation rate

260. A cardiac catheterization is scheduled for a 5-year-old with a ventricular septal defect to:
1. Identify the degree of cardiomegaly present
2. Demonstrate the exact location of the defect
3. Confirm the presence of a pansystolic murmur
4. Establish the presence of ventricular hypertrophy

261. A child returns to the unit following a cardiac catheterization. The statement on the child's progress made during the change-of-shift report 2 hours after the catheterization that should be questioned by the oncoming nurse would be that the child:

1. Is on bedrest with bathroom privileges
2. Has a pressure dressing over the entry site
3. Has voided only 100 ml since the procedure
4. Has to have the blood pressure checked every 2 hours

262. Discharge instructions for a child following a cardiac catheterization should include:
1. Giving a sponge bath for the first 3 days at home
2. Using ice compresses to relieve swelling at the entry site
3. Limiting fluid intake for the next 3 days to prevent nausea
4. Returning to the clinic in 5 days for removal of the pressure dressing

263. The physician orders a complete blood work-up for a 5-month-old infant with tetralogy of Fallot. Due to the infant's heart disease the nurse would expect the report to show:
1. Polycythemia
2. Agranulocytosis
3. Thrombocytopenia
4. Decreased hematocrit

264. When caring for a 4-month-old infant with tetrology of Fallot and congestive heart failure, the nurse should:
1. Force nutritional fluids
2. Provide small frequent feedings
3. Measure the head circumference daily
4. Position the infant flat on the abdomen

265. The nurse is aware that the aim of palliative surgery for children with tetralogy of Fallot is to directly increase the blood flow to the:
1. Brain
2. Lungs
3. Myocardium
4. Right ventricle

266. A newborn is diagnosed with coarctation of the aorta. The baby is discharged with a prescription for digoxin (Lanoxin) 0.01 mg po q12h. The bottle of digoxin is labeled 0.01 mg in $1/2$ teaspoon. The nurse should teach the mother to administer the medication by using:

1. A plastic baby spoon
2. A nipple to deliver the medication
3. The calibrated dropper in the bottle
4. The small-size baby bottle with 1 oz of water

267. The nurse is aware that in infants with congestive heart failure (CHF):
1. The illness is an acquired congenital anomaly
2. The treatment differs vastly from adult treatment
3. Treatment is experimental because infants rarely develop congestive heart failure
4. Digoxin (Lanoxin) and furosemide (Lasix) are the most commonly used medications

268. A 4-month-old, who has a congenital heart defect, develops congestive heart failure and is exhibiting marked dyspnea at rest. This finding is attributed to:
1. Anemia
2. Hypovolemia
3. Pulmonary edema
4. Metabolic acidosis

269. The mother of a 5-month-old infant with congestive heart failure questions the necessity of weighing the infant every morning. The nurse's response should be based on the fact that this daily information is important in determining:
1. Renal failure
2. Fluid retention
3. Nutritional status
4. Medication dosage

270. When attempting to identify the presence of tetralogy of Fallot in an infant the nurse should understand that:
1. In the absence of cyanosis, poor sucking is insignificant
2. Many infants retain mucus that may interfere with feeding
3. Feeding problems are fairly common in infants during the first year
4. Poor sucking and swallowing may be early indications of heart defects

271. The nurse is aware that a common adaptation of children with tetralogy of Fallot is:

1. Clubbing of fingers
2. Slow, irregular respirations
3. Subcutaneous hemorrhages
4. Decreased red blood cell count

272. An infant with tetralogy of Fallot becomes cyanotic and dyspneic after a crying episode. To relieve the cyanosis and dyspnea, the nurse should place the infant in the:
1. Orthopneic position
2. Knee-chest position
3. Lateral Sims' position
4. Semi-Fowler's position

273. A 3½-year-old child returns to the room after a cardiac catheterization. Post-procedure nursing care for the child should include:
1. Encouraging early ambulation
2. Monitoring the insertion site for bleeding
3. Restricting fluids until blood pressure is stabilized
4. Comparing blood pressure in affected and unaffected extremities

274. A 5-year-old returns from the surgical recovery room following cardiac surgery. The child has a left chest tube attached to water-seal drainage, an IV of D5 ½ NS at 40 ml/hr, and a nasogastric tube to gravity. The child is attached to a cardiac monitor and has a left chest dressing. Upon admission to the unit, the nurse should first:
1. Take the vital signs
2. Check the identification bracelet
3. Measure the chest and gastric drainage
4. Check the suction pressure of the water seal drainage

REPRODUCTIVE AND GENITOURINARY

275. The nurse understands that surgery is needed in a 4-year-old child with undescended testes because:
1. Future malignancy may be prevented
2. Maturation of the testes starts around age 7
3. The puboscrotal ring is more elastic at this age
4. Early surgery produces less psychologic damage

276. The nurse is aware that uncorrected bilateral cryptorchidism can cause:
1. Sterility
2. Hydrocele
3. Varicocele
4. Epididymitis

277. The nurse explains to parents whose infant son has a hypospadias that this defect occurred in the:
1. First trimester
2. Third trimester
3. Second trimester
4. Implantation phase

278. The nursing care plan for a newborn with hypospadias should include:
1. Keeping the penis wrapped with petrolatum gauze
2. Preparing the infant for the insertion of a cystostomy tube
3. Explaining to the parents why a circumcision will not be done
4. Carefully explaining the genetic basis for the defect to the parents

279. After a child has a surgical correction for hypospadias, it is important for the nurse to:
1. Ensure that the child's privacy is maintained
2. Maintain the surgically implanted tension device
3. Keep the child properly immobilized with restraints
4. Gradually increase the time the catheter is clamped

280. A nursing diagnosis that should have priority for an infant born with exstrophy of the bladder is:
1. Urinary retention
2. Fluid volume deficit
3. High risk for infection
4. High risk for sexual dysfunction

281. An infant has exstrophy of the bladder. To protect the actual exposed bladder area, the nurse should expect the physician to order:
1. Antibacterial ointments
2. Pediatric urine collectors
3. Warm moist compresses
4. Sterile nonadherent dressings

282. After surgical repair of a urinary tract malformation, a child is to be discharged with an indwelling catheter. The parents should be taught that if no urine appears in the urinary drainage bag for a period of an hour or longer they should first:
1. Call the physician
2. Give the child extra fluids to drink
3. Check for blockage of the drainage tubing
4. Place firm pressure on the abdominal wall just above the bladder

283. The mother of a 6-year-old brings the child to the pediatric clinic and complains the child has malaise, weakness, lethargy, anorexia, headaches, and smoky urine. When taking the nursing history, the nurse asks the mother if the child has had a:
1. Pain in the shoulders and knees
2. Recent weight loss of at least 2 pounds
3. Streptococcal infection within the last two weeks
4. Rash on the palms and feet within the last 3 weeks

284. The nurse is aware that in order to confirm a diagnosis of acute glomerulonephritis in a 6-year-old the tests that the physician will order will include:
1. A routine urinalysis, a chest x-ray film, blood glucose levels, and an IVP
2. An electrocardiogram, a heterophile antibody test, a routine urinalysis, and a chest x-ray film
3. A routine urinalysis, a complete blood chemistry, a nasopharyngeal culture, and an ASO titer
4. An upper GI series, a 24-hour urine specimen, a complete blood chemistry, and a nasopharyngeal culture

285. A child is admitted to the pediatric unit with a diagnosis of acute glomerulonephritis. The nursing action that has priority is:
1. Assessing for dysuria
2. Observing for jaundice
3. Monitoring blood pressure
4. Testing vomitus for occult blood

286. A mother whose child has glomerulonephritis is fearful that her other child may get the disease. To allay the fears of the mother the nurse should tell her that:
1. "The cause of acute glomerulonephritis is unknown, so it is difficult to know how to prevent it."
2. "Acute glomerulonephritis is inherited by an autosomal recessive trait but usually occurs only in males."
3. "Acute glomerulonephritis is caused by clot formation in the small renal tubules secondary to systemic infection."
4. "Acute glomerulonephritis is caused by an antigen-antibody response secondary to group A beta hemolytic streptococcus."

287. When assessing a child with glomerulonephritis the nurse should expect to find:
1. A decrease in joint mobility
2. An increase in urine volume
3. The presence of periorbital edema
4. The occurrence of an intermittant fever

288. The nurse encourages a child with glomerulonephritis to choose combinations of foods that include:
1. Corn on the cob, baked chicken breast, rice, applesauce, milk
2. Hot dog on a bun, potato chips, dill pickle slices, brownie, milk
3. Baked potato, ground beef, canned carrots, banana, buttermilk
4. Canned green beans, baked ham, bread and butter, peach, milk

289. When testing the urine and assessing the condition of a child with acute glomerulonephritis, the nurse would not be surprised to note a:
1. Normal blood pressure, anorexia, 1+ proteinuria, and 3+ glycosuria
2. Decreased blood pressure, anorexia, hematuria, and 1+ proteinuria
3. Decreased blood pressure, periorbital edema, 1+ proteinuria, and a specific gravity of 1.001
4. Moderately elevated blood pressure, periorbital edema, 4+ proteinuria, and a specific gravity of 1.030

290. When caring for a child with acute glomerulonephritis the nurse plans to:
1. Maintain bedrest, use isolation techniques, encourage fluids, and provide meticulous skin care
2. Maintain bedrest, provide a low-sodium diet, monitor blood pressure every hour, and monitor IV therapy
3. Prevent chilling, monitor vital signs every 2 hours, provide a no-sodium diet, and get the child up in a chair
4. Promote rest, monitor intake and output, weigh the child daily, and provide a regular diet with no added salt

291. Before discharging a child who has been treated for acute glomerulonephritis, the nurse should plan to provide the parents with:
1. Suggestions about activities that will keep the child active for long periods of time
2. The nurse's phone number so that the parents can call if they have any questions
3. Instructions as to when the child should return for a work-up for a kidney transplant
4. A sample of a sodium-restricted diet because the child will continue on this diet at home

292. Close monitoring of the urine of a child with nephrotic syndrome who has been admitted with massive edema and decreased urinary output would be expected to reveal:
1. High protein levels
2. Crystalline particles
3. Normal specific gravity
4. Numerous red blood cells

293. When admitting a four-year-old child with nephrotic syndrome, the nurse should assess for:
1. Severe lethargy
2. Chronic hypertension
3. Dark, frothy urine output
4. Flushed, ruddy complexion

294. The nurse assigns a four-year-old boy, admitted with nephrotic syndrome, to a room with a:
1. 2-year-old boy with croup
2. 3-year-old boy with impetigo
3. 4-year-old girl with conjunctivitis
4. 5-year-old girl with a fractured femur

295. When planning nursing care for a child with nephrotic syndrome, the nurse includes:
    1. Provision of meticulous skin care
    2. A diet low in carbohydrates and protein
    3. Restriction of fluids to 500 ml each shift
    4. A laboratory test for type and crossmatch

296. The adaptation that indicates that a child may have nephrotic syndrome rather than glomerulonephritis is the presence of:
    1. Edema
    2. Lethargy
    3. Protein in the urine
    4. A slightly decreased blood pressure

297. The nurse realizes that the parents of a child with nephrotic syndrome need further discharge instructions when they state, "We will:
    1. Ignore any weight gain since it's normal."
    2. Look at our child's eyelids every morning."
    3. Need to test our child's urine for specific gravity."
    4. Give our child the prednisone with meals or milk."

298. The nurse teaches the parents of a 5-year-old boy with nephrotic syndrome about urine testing at home. The statement by them that alerts the nurse to the fact that the teaching has been effective is:
    1. "Our child is old enough to do his own urine testing."
    2. "We should notify the doctor if there is protein in the urine."
    3. "We will discard the first urine before we test it for acetone."
    4. "We realize the urine will show a false positive if it is cloudy."

299. A child in renal failure, who has had the creation of an arteriovenous fistula access, begins hemodialysis 3 times a week. The nurse would know the child's mother needs further teaching when the mother states, "I will:
    1. Call the doctor if my child develops vomiting or diarrhea."
    2. Check the pulse at the wrist of the arm with the fistula daily."
    3. Take a blood pressure in the arm with the fistula once a day."
    4. Ensure that my child drinks the appropriate amount of fluid in warm weather."

300. A 4-year-old child has a nephrectomy because of a Wilms' tumor. Following a nephrectomy it is essential that the parents:
    1. Maintain fluid restrictions
    2. Prevent urinary tract infections
    3. Restrict the child's intake of sodium
    4. Prepare the child for a kidney transplant

301. When a child with a history of hypospadias with chordee becomes an adult, he will be at increased risk for:
    1. Renal failure
    2. Testicular torsion
    3. Testicular cancer
    4. Sexual inadequacy

302. The statement by a teenage female with cystic fibrosis that best reflects her understanding of healthy sexuality would be:
    1. "I can never become pregnant."
    2. "Having sex is not possible for me."
    3. "A diaphragm is my best protection."
    4. "I will not have sex without condoms."

303. To confirm a suspected diagnosis of gonorrhea in a 16-year-old male who has come to the clinic with a complaint of a thick urethral discharge, the nurse should:
    1. Get a sexual history
    2. Draw blood for a VDRL
    3. Obtain a urethral culture
    4. Collect a urine specimen

304. The nurse in an adolescent clinic is aware that an early diagnosis of syphilis is important and its presence is often determined by:
    1. Evidence of a rash
    2. A lesion on the penis
    3. A discharge from the penis
    4. Multiple gummatous lesions

GASTROINTESTINAL

305. Immediate nursing for a neonate born with a cleft lip is directed primarily toward:
    1. Modifying feeding methods
    2. Keeping the baby from crying
    3. Minimizing handling by parents
    4. Preventing the occurrence of infection

306. A newborn with a cleft lip is fed with a special nipple. To minimize regurgitation of the feedings the nurse instructs the mother to:

1. Give the baby the thickened formula as ordered
2. Hold and burp the baby frequently while feeding
3. Lay the baby on the side with the bottle firmly propped
4. Feed the baby while sitting the baby up in an infant seat

307. The parents of a neonate born with a cleft lip ask when the cleft lip will be repaired. The nurse responds:
1. "Not until the baby has teeth."
2. "Usually at about 18 months of age."
3. "When the baby is 8 to 12 weeks old."
4. "As soon as the baby starts to lose weight."

308. After the repair of a cleft lip, the nurse will provide nutrition for the baby via:
1. A plastic teaspoon
2. Intravenous feedings
3. A rubber-tipped syringe
4. Nasogastric tube feedings

309. The first action following each feeding of a newborn with a fresh surgical repair of a cleft lip should be to:
1. Burp the infant several times
2. Place the infant on the abdomen
3. Cuddle the infant for a few minutes
4. Clean and rinse the suture line of the lip

310. A priority nursing measure for an infant during the immediate postoperative period following a surgical repair of a cleft lip is to:
1. Minimize the infant's crying
2. Restrain the infant at all times
3. Oxygenate the infant frequently
4. Handle the infant as little as possible

311. When assessing an infant with a suspected diagnosis of hypertrophic pyloric stenosis, the nurse would expect to find:
1. Visible peristaltic waves across the lower abdomen
2. A palpable mass in the epigastrium to the right of the umbilicus
3. Tenderness over the epigastric region not relieved by heat application
4. Lower abdominal distention with vomiting of bile-stained gastric contents

312. A 25-day-old infant is admitted after 3 days of vomiting and pyloric stenosis is diagnosed. The most important nursing assessment at the time of admission is the:
1. Character, amount, and times when baby vomited
2. Time of last feeding, type of formula, and amount taken
3. Presence of an olive-shaped mass in the upper abdomen
4. Amount and color of last voiding, skin turgor, and respiratory status

313. The nurse explains to the parents of an infant with pyloric stenosis that the type of surgery scheduled for this problem has a high success rate when:
1. The fluid and electrolyte imbalances are corrected preoperatively
2. Gastric decompression is monitored for amount and type of drainage
3. It is performed before the infant's vomiting becomes severe and projectile
4. The infant receives small, frequent feedings of thickened formula preoperatively

314. The mother of an infant with pyloric stenosis asks the nurse many questions about the problem. When answering these questions the nurse should convey the idea that:
1. It is unlikely that surgery will be necessary
2. This is a condition with an excellent prognosis
3. This condition results from an inborn error of metabolism
4. Special feedings and handling will be needed for a few months

315. A 10-week-old is diagnosed as having a pyloric stenosis and is scheduled for surgery. Oral feedings are usually initiated a few hours after surgery. The nurse expects that initially the baby will receive:
1. Clear liquids
2. Half-strength formula
3. Thickened formula with cereal
4. Oral electrolyte feedings (Pedialyte)

316. An infant is to be discharged following surgery for pyloric stenosis. The mother should be instructed to:
1. Give the baby creamy cereal at each feeding followed by the regular formula
2. Continue the regular formula, hold the baby during all feedings, feed the baby slowly, and bubble frequently
3. Feed the regular formula while the baby is in the crib positioned on the right side; handle the baby as little as possible for 2 hours after each feeding
4. Give the baby about 1 ounce of regular formula per hour for the next 2 weeks; progressing slowly, as tolerated, to larger amounts

317. A mother whose 20-month-old infant has just developed diarrhea calls the pediatric clinic and asks what she should do. The nurse practitioner tells the mother to:
1. Keep the child in bed, hold all oral feedings, observe carefully, and call back in four hours
2. Wrap the child snugly, give sugar water, and bring the child to see the physician immediately
3. Allow the child to continue normal activities, hold all feedings for 24 hours, and call back tomorrow
4. Continue to feed the child as usual, make an appointment with the receptionist, and bring the child to the clinic tomorrow

318. The priority nursing action to be initiated for a child admitted with a diagnosis of salmonellosis should be to:
1. Weigh the child
2. Set up enteric isolation
3. Obtain a recent food history
4. Establish a skin care routine

319. The parents of an infant admitted with gastroenteritis and dehydration want to be involved with the baby's care. The nurse recognizes that they understand the teaching about the maintenance of enteric precautions when they state, "We should:

1. Wear a mask when we are holding the baby."
2. Weigh the diaper each time we change the baby."
3. Wear gloves each time we change the baby's diaper."
4. Keep the door to the baby's room closed most of the time."

320. After receiving and tolerating a water and electrolyte formula (Pedialyte) because of dehydration from diarrhea, a child, 20 months old, improves and is advanced to soft foods. The nurse understands that a food that would be contraindicated is:
1. Creamed soup
2. Strained carrots
3. Animal crackers
4. Mashed bananas

321. To help a child retain tube feedings and avoid aspiration, the nurse should place the child in the:
1. Prone position
2. Left side-lying position
3. Semi-Fowler's position
4. Supine position with head turned

322. The food choice that would ensure maintenance of nitrogen balance after surgery in a 5-year-old child would be:
1. Chicken soup
2. A bacon sandwich
3. Cut up orange slices
4. A hamburger on a bun

323. The nurse is aware that thiamine, which helps to produce more energy for both children and adults, is found in foods such as:
1. Eggs
2. Fruits
3. Green vegetables
4. Whole or enriched grains

324. The nurse recognizes that the diagnosis of celiac disease can be confirmed when a peroral jejunal biopsy reveals:
1. Small areas of fatty plaques
2. Atrophic changes in the mucosal wall
3. Irregular areas of superficial ulcerations
4. Diffuse degenerative fibrosis of the acini

325. When taking the health history and assessing a 6-year-old child with celiac disease, the nurse would expect to find:
    1. Diarrhea, malnutrition, rickets, anemia, steatorrhea
    2. Constipation, abdominal distention, flatulence, rickets
    3. Diarrhea, muscle wasting, anemia, osteomalacia, steatorrhea
    4. Constipation, abdominal distention, peripheral edema, decreased clotting time

326. The nurse explains to the mother of a child with celiac disease who has been placed on a low-gluten diet that this type of diet will mainly restrict:
    1. Milk and dairy products
    2. The grains of corn and rice
    3. Saturated and unsaturated fats
    4. The grains of wheat, rye, oat, and barley

327. The nurse goes over dietary instructions with the mother of a 9-month-old who has a diagnosis of gluten-induced enteropathy. The nurse feels that the teaching has been understood when the mother states, "In planning my child's diet I will avoid:
    1. Beef, pork, chicken."
    2. Corn, spinach, cheese."
    3. Eggs, milk, Rice Krispies."
    4. Chocolate milk, whole wheat toast, fruit."

328. The effectiveness of a gluten-restricted diet in a child with celiac disease can be assessed on the second day by having the nurse and mother evaluate the child for:
    1. Decreased irritability
    2. Maintenance of weight
    3. Normal bowel movements
    4. Disappearance of steatorrhea

329. The nurse recognizes that anemia in a child with celiac disease is caused by:
    1. The poor absorption of iron and folic acid
    2. An inadequate amount of the intrinsic factor
    3. The small amount of iron included in the diet
    4. A low food intake and the child's minimal appetite

330. The nurse teaches the mother of a malnourished child with celiac disease to:
    1. Provide foods high in folic acid, iron, and vitamin B_{12} to correct the blood dyscrasia
    2. Give foods high in potassium and magnesium to correct the bone growth deficiencies
    3. Encourage a high-calorie diet composed of high-protein and high-fat foods to foster weight gain
    4. Supplement the child's diet with megadoses of vitamins A, D, E, and K to correct the coagulation deficiencies

331. After being on a dietary regimen for celiac disease for 6 months, the child's compliance to the diet can be evaluated by assessing the:
    1. Physical and emotional progress
    2. Ability to handle stressful situations
    3. Understanding of the disease process
    4. Knowledge of foods allowed on the diet

332. After an emergency appendectomy, the nurse should place the child in a semi-Fowler's or right Sims' position because:
    1. The lungs can aerate fully in both of these positions
    2. Drainage is facilitated, preventing subdiaphragmatic abscesses
    3. Movement is easier, thus reducing complications from immobility
    4. Splinting of the wound is accomplished by pressure on the operative site

333. The nurse's charting for a child who has had an appendectomy should include, in addition to "coughing and deep breathing," documentation of:
    1. Intake and output and bowel sounds
    2. Mouth care and frequency of dressing changes
    3. Bowel sounds and teaching about the low-residue diet
    4. Teaching to prevent dumping syndrome and early ambulation

334. The nurse is aware that the parents of a 4-year-old with Hirschsprung's disease understand what their child will require when they tell the nurse that they know care at home will most likely include:
1. A low-protein diet
2. A high-caloric diet
3. Soapsuds enemas
4. Nasogastric feedings

335. The nurse recognizes that the parents of a child with Hirschsprung's disease need further teaching about their child's diet when they indicate that they are going to allow the child to have:
1. Apples
2. Spaghetti
3. Ice cream
4. Ripe bananas

336. The nurse teaches a mother how to obtain a specimen of pinworms from her 5-year-old child by instructing the mother to:
1. Tape a 4 × 4 gauze tightly over the child's anus during the night
2. Give the child a tap water enema and save all returns for testing
3. Make an anal impression on cellophane tape before the child uses the bathroom in the morning
4. Insert a cotton tipped swab into the child's rectum to collect a small amount of stool after a bowel movement

337. A baby is born with an imperforate anus and undergoes a pull-through procedure with an anoplasty. The nurse knows that it is most appropriate postoperatively to place the infant:
1. In Buck's extension
2. In the Trendelenburg position
3. Prone with the head of the crib elevated
4. Supine with the legs suspended at a 90-degree angle to the trunk

338. The nurse, working with infants who were preterm, should be alert to the fact that these infants may later develop intestinal obstruction because of:
1. Meconium ileus
2. Imperforate anus
3. Duodenal atresia
4. Necrotizing enterocolitis

339. After several episodes of abdominal pain and vomiting, a 5-month-old child is brought to the hospital. A diagnosis of intussusception is made. To assist in confirming the diagnosis the priority assessment should be:
1. Noting frequency of crying
2. Listening for bowel sounds
3. Measuring fluid intake and output
4. Observing characteristics of stools

DRUG RELATED RESPONSES

340. Ferrous fumerate (Feostat) 30 mg is ordered for an infant. The solution contains 45 mg/0.6 ml. The nurse should administer:
1. 0.6 ml
2. 0.9 ml
3. 6.0 minims
4. 13.0 minims

341. Cough syrup ½ tsp is ordered for a 4-year-old. Each teaspoonful contains dextromethorphan hydrobromide 7.5 mg. When administering the cough syrup the nurse should provide:
1. 0.5 ml
2. 2.5 ml
3. 3.75 ml
4. 7.5 ml

342. After taking levothyroxine sodium (Synthroid) for 3 months for congenital hypothyroidism, an infant returns to the clinic for a checkup. The nurse evaluates that the drug is effective when the mother states that the infant's:
1. Activity level has decreased
2. Fine tremors have decreased
3. Skin is cool and dry to the touch
4. Bowel movements have increased to two soft stools daily

343. A 10-year-old is newly diagnosed with diabetes mellitus and is started on insulin therapy. The child and the family are taught how to give the injections. The child dislikes the injections and asks the nurse why the insulin cannot be taken by mouth. The nurse explains that insulin:
1. Is a protein and would be inactivated by digestion
2. Would irritate the stomach lining and lose its potency

3. Has a carbohydrate portion that would add to blood glucose
4. Is alkaline and would be neutralized by gastric hydrochloric acid

344. Screening for hearing loss should be planned for the child who is receiving:
1. Penicillin
2. Tetracycline
3. Streptomycin
4. Chloramphenicol

345. The nurse would know that the teaching about administration of tetracyline was effective when a teenaged client says that the drug should be taken:
1. Just before meals
2. With meals or milk
3. At least 1 hour before meals
4. Approximately 30 minutes after meals

346. The nurse explains to a teenager who is receiving penicillin G and probenecid for syphilis that the rationale for both drugs being used is:
1. Each drug attacks the organism during different stages of cell multiplication
2. The penicillin treats the syphilis while the probenecid relieves the severe urethritis
3. Probenecid delays excretion of penicillin by the kidneys to maintain effective blood levels for longer periods
4. Probenecid decreases the potential for an allergic reaction developing to the penicillin which treats the syphilis

347. The initial medications that the nurse anticipates that the physician would order for a child admitted with acute glomerulonephritis with hypertension would include:
1. Digitalis and hydralazine
2. Reserpine and hydralazine
3. Reserpine and phenobarbital
4. Furosemide and phenobarbital

348. The nurse would determine that the teaching about the side effects of tetracyline was understood when the client says that the medication could cause:

1. Vertigo
2. Tinnitus
3. Diarrhea
4. Constipation

349. When caring for a child receiving prednisone, it is important for the nurse to know that adrenocorticosteroid therapy:
1. May produce hyperkalemia
2. Accelerates wound healing
3. Increases production of antibodies by the blood
4. Suppresses the inflammatory symptoms of infection

350. The alkylating agent, cyclophosphamide (Cytoxan) is ordered for a child with cancer. When the child is receiving this drug the nurse should assess for:
1. Extent of hydration
2. Increased irritability
3. Unexpected nausea
4. Hyperplasia of gums

351. An 8-year-old girl, in the hospital to receive methotrexate and cranial radiation, is very weak and her mother asks the nurse whether her daughter could receive some vitamin therapy to give her strength. The nurse's best response would be:
1. "That is an excellent idea; I'll ask the doctor to order some for her."
2. "Some vitamins contain folic acid which interferes with methotrexate."
3. "Unfortunately, vitamin supplements won't make her feel any better now."
4. "Your daughter will benefit from vitamins and will be receiving them soon."

352. When assessing a child with leukemia for the possible side effects of vincristine (Oncovin), the nurse should be aware that a sign of toxicity is:
1. Diarrhea
2. Alopecia
3. Hemorrhagic cystitis
4. Peripheral neuropathy

353. When assessing the status of a child with leukemia who is receiving vincristine (Oncovin), the nurse would know that the fluid intake should be increased when the child's:
1. Temperature is 99.8°F
2. Uric acid level is elevated
3. Urine's specific gravity is 1.026
4. Output for the last 24 hours totaled 1700 ml

354. An adolescent who is receiving prednisone and vincristine for leukemia complains of constipation. The nurse is aware that the constipation is most probably caused by:
1. A side effect of the vinicristine
2. A toxic effect of the prednisone
3. An enlarged spleen compressing the bowel
4. An obstruction of the bowel by a leukemic mass

355. An adolescent with acute lymphoblastic leukemia (ALL) completes parenteral chemotherapy and is discharged home with a prescription for mercaptopurine (6-MP) 1 tablet daily by mouth. The statement by the adolescent that indicates an understanding of the reason for this therapy is:
1. "These pills prepare me for additional IV drugs."
2. "Taking pills will be better than having brain radiation."
3. "This medication should help prevent another relapse of my disease."
4. "This medication should prevent the cancer from spreading to my stomach."

356. When considering the side effects of dactinomycin (Cosmegen) and doxorubicin (Adriamycin) therapy, the nurse can suggest to the parents of a child receiving these drugs that the child:
1. Avoid dairy products
2. Wear a baseball cap
3. Dress in light clothing
4. Eat three large meals

357. A 1-year-old is in the pediatric unit for management of AIDS. The child is receiving zidovudine (AZT) every 6 hours around the clock. The nurse evaluates that the child is in life-threatening AZT toxicity when the child manifests:

1. Fatigue and lethargy
2. A progressive weight loss
3. An increased urine output
4. Multiple bruises on the limbs and trunk

358. Priority nursing care for children on chelation therapy for lead poisoning should include:
1. Scrupulous care of the skin
2. Providing a high protein diet
3. Careful monitoring of intake and output
4. Drawing blood daily for liver function tests

359. In addition to removing lead from the blood, chelation therapy with calcium disodium edetate (EDTA) predisposes the child to:
1. Anemia
2. Hyperkalemia
3. Hypocalcemia
4. Hypoglycemia

360. The nurse teaches the parents of a child on long-term phenytoin (Dilantin) therapy about care pertinent to this medication. The nurse recognizes that the teaching is effective when they say, "We should:
1. Give our child the medication 2 hours after breakfast and dinner."
2. Supplement the diet with high-caloric foods and encourage fluids."
3. Provide oral hygiene, especially gum massage and flossing of teeth."
4. Observe our child's urine for the complication of a reddish brown discoloration."

361. The nurse is aware that in children the most common reason for status epilepticus is that the prescribed dosage of phenytoin (Dilantin) is:
1. Toxic to the child
2. At the therapeutic level
3. Probably not taken consistently
4. Insufficient to cover child's activities

362. The side effect that the nurse should expect after administering a preoperative dose of scopolamine to a child undergoing surgery is:
1. Decreased heartbeat
2. Postural hypotension
3. Confusion and hallucinations
4. Hyperpnea and hyperventilation

363. The nurse explains to the parents of a child who is receiving mannitol (Osmitrol) after a craniotomy that the medication is being given to:
1. Increase the filtration rate of the bladder
2. Decrease the peripheral retention of fluid
3. Reduce the amount of glucose in the urine
4. Relieve cerebral pressure following surgery

364. A chelating agent that the nurse would expect to be ordered for a toddler with lead poisoning is:
1. Calcium gluconate
2. Lomustine (CeeNU)
3. Calcium disodium edetate (EDTA)
4. Sodium polystyrene sulfonate (Kayexalate)

365. The nurse tells a 13-year-old with hay fever that the ordered phenylephrine HCl nasal spray must be used exactly as directed to avoid the development of:
1. Nasal polyps
2. Bleeding tendencies
3. Tinnitus and diplopia
4. Increased nasal congestion

366. When reviewing medication instructions with the parents of an infant who is receiving digoxin (Lanoxin) and spironolactone (Aldactone), the nurse would know that the parents understood the instructions when they indicate:
1. Their infant must have orange juice daily
2. Any vomiting should be reported to the physician
3. Their infant's activity should be carefully restricted
4. Aspirin should be avoided while the infant is taking Aldactone

367. The pediatric nurse is aware that digoxin (Lanoxin) toxicity in children is most commonly manifested by:
1. Oliguria
2. Tachypnea
3. Bradycardia
4. Splenomegaly

368. A child is having a cardiac arrest. The physician orders epinephrine as a cardiac stimulant. The nurse is aware that the one factor that would still permit administration of an epinephrine solution that is on hand would be that the reconstituted solution:
1. Is slightly discolored
2. Has been exposed to light
3. Is no more than 72 hours old
4. Contains only slight sediment

369. When assessing a child after the administration of epinephrine, a side effect the nurse should be aware of is:
1. Tachycardia
2. Hypoglycemia
3. Constricted pupils
4. Decreased blood pressure

370. When a 5-year-old child is receiving dactinomycin (Cosmegen) and doxorubicin (Adriamycin) therapy following a nephrectomy for a Wilms' tumor, nursing care should include:
1. Administering aspirin for pain
2. Serving citrus juices with meals
3. Using an anesthetic mouthwash
4. Providing age-appropriate books

371. An important nursing intervention for a child who has been receiving long-term prednisone therapy for nephrotic syndrome would be:
1. Daily checking of pulse for irregularities
2. Frequent checking of stools for occult blood
3. Regular checking of urine for mucus threads
4. Daily checking of the oral mucous membrane for ulcers

372. When a child with acute glomerulonephritis is found to be hypertensive, the nurse would expect the physician to order:
1. Digoxin (Lanoxin)
2. Diazepam (Valium)
3. Phenytoin (Dilantin)
4. Hydralazine (Apresoline)

373. After the severe effects of dehydration are under control in a three-month-old infant, the physician orders Lactinex granules (lactobacilli) to:
1. Diminish inflammatory mucosal edema
2. Relieve the pain caused by gastric hyperacidity
3. Relieve the pain of gas in the gastointestinal tract
4. Recolonize the normal flora of the gastointestinal tract

374. Mebendazole (Vermox) is prescribed for a child with pinworms. When teaching about the medication, the nurse tells the mother and child that:
1. The drug may precipitate transient diarrhea
2. Rectal itching will be relieved rapidly once the drug is started
3. Only the child and no other family member will need treatment
4. A single course of treatment is all that is needed to control the problem

375. The nurse evaluates that pancreatic enzyme replacement being taken by a child with cystic fibrosis is inadequate when the child complains of:
1. Anorexia
2. Constipation
3. Sudden weight gain
4. Abdominal cramping

Answers and Rationales for Pediatric Nursing Questions

GROWTH AND DEVELOPMENT

1. 2 With each age-group, there are different means of communication; the approach used with a school-age child should differ from that used with a toddler or a teenager. (1) (PE; AS; ED; GD)
    1 This might modify the approach, but knowing the child's developmental level is the most important factor.
    3 This would be related to the child's developmental level that should be assessed first.
    4 Although children may fear authoritarian figures, this is only one aspect included in the assessment of developmental level, a more inclusive assessment.

2. 3 This follows the normal course of growth and development skills and is no different with a child who is mentally retarded. (2) (PE; PL; ED; GD)
    1 This would not be taught before self-feeding.
    2 Same as answer 1.
    4 Same as answer 1.

3. 2 The 3-month-old infant is interested in self-recognition and playing with the baby in the mirror. (3) (PE; IM; ED; GD)
    1 This is appropriate for a toddler.
    3 Same as answer 1.
    4 Same as answer 1.

4. 1 During the oral stage, infants tend to complete the exploration of all objects by putting the objects in the mouth as a final step. (2) (PE; AS; ED; GD)
    2 Nine- to 10-month-olds play this way as they learn that objects continue to exist even though they are not visible.

3 These are the random reflexive movements of 1- to 2-month-olds whose voluntary control of distal extremities has not developed.
4 This is the momentary grasp reflex of neonates before the development of eye-hand-mouth coordination.

5. 1 Eight-month-old infants have the ability to use their fingers and thumbs in opposition (pincer grasp); this enables them to pick up small objects and put them in their mouths and aspirate them. (1) (PE; AN; TC; GD)
    2 Although this statement is true, the major concern is preventing infants from putting foreign objects in their mouths where they can be aspirated.
    3 It is not a health hazard if the floor is clean and the object is large enough so that there is no danger of the child aspirating it and obstructing the airway.
    4 The danger is not that the items would be hidden but that they would be put into the mouth and aspirated.

6. 3 Brief messages, with only essential words included (telegraphic speech), are a normal pattern for a child 18 months to $2\frac{1}{2}$ years of age. (2) (PE; AN; ED; GD)
    1 A child with a severe developmental lag would have no obvious recognizable speech pattern and would only make a few sounds.
    2 A child slow for this age would have a smaller vocabulary and would use only single words to identify familiar objects.
    4 A child advanced for this age would have a larger vocabulary and would use 3- to 4-word sentences rather than telegraphic speech.

7. 3 Preschoolers generally have learned to cope with parents' absence; however, emotions associated with separation and perhaps anger at being left are difficult to hide when parents arrive or leave. (2) (PE; IM; ED; GD)

1 Preschoolers usually are quite docile and cooperative because they are afraid of being totally abandoned.

2 The child would demonstrate despair long before the week was over.

4 The presence of other children's parents would be unrelated to their relationship with peers.

8. 3 In the toddler, two- and three-word phrases are used with an increased vocabulary; attributing lifelike qualities to inanimate objects is also associated with preconceptual thought. (3) (PE; EV; PS; GD)

1 This is related to school-age children.

2 This is a phase of concrete operations seen in school-age children.

4 This is related to infants.

9. 2 Although none of the choices is always indicative of pain, a change in behavior is the indicator that occurs most often in children. (2) (PE; AS; PS; GD)

1 Many things can cause crying, including pain, fear, separation, and unhappiness; crying does not always indicate pain.

3 Vital signs are often normal in children, even in the presence of pain.

4 Children often hide their pain; they may perceive it as punishment, or they may fear the injection that would be given to relieve the pain.

10. 1 The external auditory canal curves downward and forward in a child older than 3 years of age and is approximately 1 inch long; to adequately view the tympanic membrane in a child this age, the pinna must be pulled up and back; in a child younger than 3 years of age the pinna should be pulled down and back. (3) (PE; AS; PA; GD)

2 This positioning would impede visualization of the tympanic membrane; the pinna should be pulled backward, not forward.

3 This is how the pinna of a child younger than 3 years of age should be positioned for otoscopic examination.

4 This positioning would impede visualization of the tympanic membrane; it is exactly the opposite of what should be done in a child older than the age of 3 years.

11. 3 A child this age loves to collect and manipulate; this meets the need to develop fine motor skills. (2) (PE; IM; ED; GD)

1 This is more appropriate for an infant.

2 This is below the child's developmental level.

4 The child is too young for scissors and fragile toys.

12. 4 At this age the phallus is large enough for surgical repair and the child has not reached the age at which fear of mutilation develops. (3) (PE; IM; ED; GD)

1 The phallus is not developed enough for surgery to be done at this age.

2 Same as answer 1.

3 The child is in the oedipal stage of development, which is accompanied by fear of mutilation; surgery is inadvisable.

13. 1 This is the most accurate and age-appropriate response to the question. (3) (PE; IM; ED; GD)

2 This is inaccurate; not being truthful interferes with the development of trust.

3 This is inaccurate and may instill more fear.

4 This response is insensitive to the question and does not provide any explanation.

14. 2 The infant has not yet recognized boundaries between herself and her mother and is not particular about who meets and resolves needs. (1) (PE; EV; ED; GD)

1 The infant does not yet differentiate familiar faces from those of strangers.

3 This behavior is that of a younger infant and does not indicate recognition of a specific person but only a human face.

4 Because the concept of self-boundaries has not yet developed, the infant does not really know or fear separation from the mother.

15. 2 This is inappropriate for an 8-month-old; this is appropriate for a toddler to promote imitative play. (3) (PE; EV; ED; GD)

1 A stuffed animal is appropriate; it promotes manipulative play.

3 A hanging mobile is appropriate; it promotes visual stimulation.

4 A textured book is appropriate; it promotes tactile stimulation and touch discrimination.

16. 4 Changes in the daily routines in the home and anxiety expressed by family members lead to anxiety in toddlers. (2) (PE; IM; PS; GD)

1 This is incorrect because the toddler has no reality-based concept of death.

2 This may be true, but the primary motivation for the behavior is a response to the upheaval in the family.

3 This is false reassurance.

17. 2 Stuttering occurs because the child's advancing mental ability and level of comprehension exceed the vocabulary acquisitions in the preschool years. (2) (PE; AN; PA; GD)

1 This is not true; stuttering is common in the preschool years.

3 Same as answer 1.

4 Same as answer 1.

18. 3 A stuffed animal is the most appropriate toy for the 6-month-old because it is safe and cuddly and requires only gross motor movement. (1) (PE; PL; ED; GD)

1 A push-pull toy is appropriate for the older infant (9 to 12 months) and the toddler because it encourages walking.

2 These are inappropriate; a child at this age puts toys in the mouth; playing with blocks requires motor development beyond this age.

4 Shape-matching toys require intellectual and motor development beyond that of this age-group.

19. 4 Lips and teeth closed around the finger create suction and can move permanent teeth forward, causing malocclusions. (1) (PE; IM; PA; GD)

1 If thumb-sucking is practiced only in relation to sleep, no treatment is necessary because it involves only a short period of time.

2 The pacifier will also cause malocclusions when permanent teeth appear.

3 There is no indication that the first teeth are loosened by thumb-sucking.

20. 4 This is appropriate for the child's age and suited to the child's limited motion. (1) (PE; AN; ED; GD)

1 The child will not have enough mobility to engage in this type of play and is too young for this activity.

2 The child is too young for this activity; children of 7 or older are able to play checkers.

3 Because of the spica cast, the child will not have enough mobility to play with this type of toy.

21. 3 This usually occurs by age 8 months. (1) (PE; AS; ED; GD)

1 A two- to three-word vocabulary is an expectation of a 12-month-old child.

2 This is accomplished by the 2-year-old, not the 9-month-old.

4 Whereas the posterior fontanel is closed by age 2 months, the anterior fontanel closes between ages 18 to 24 months.

22. 4 The child with abdominal pain may assume the side-lying position with the knees flexed to the abdomen and/or may self-splint when moving. (1) (PE; AS; PA; GD)

1 A 4-year-old may be unable to define the exact location of the pain; in addition, the pain may be generalized rather than localized.

2 This might be included in the physical assessment, but it is not specific to the assessment of pain.

3 This might be included in the health history, but it is not specific to the assessment of pain.

23. 1 These easily digested foods have usually been introduced by 6 months of age; breast milk or formula is recommended for the first year of life. (2) (PE; PL; PA; GD)

2 Whole milk makes this incorrect; breast milk or formula, rather than cow's milk, is recommended for the first year of life.

3 Ham makes this incorrect; it is too high in fat content for a 6-month-old.

4 Corn is too difficult for a child this age to digest; formula is recommended for the first year of life.

24. 2 Because of expanded experiences and developing cognitive ability the 4-year-old should have a vocabulary of approximately 1500 words. (2) (PE; AS; ED; GD)

1 At 5 years of age, children ask the definitions of new words.

3 At $2\frac{1}{2}$ to 3 years of age, children can name colors.

4 At 3 years of age, children use 3- or 4-word sentences.

25. 4 The canal curves upward in children, and this straightens the canal so that medication will reach the inflamed eardrum. (3) (PE; IM; ED; GD)

1 This is an incorrect technique; the auditory canal must be pulled down and back to straighten it and facilitate cleansing.

2 This is not advised; it can only add more pressure within the ear and prevent the drops from reaching the tympanic membrane.

3 This is an incorrect technique for children under 3 years of age because it will not straighten the ear canal.

26. 4 This explanation illustrates that the child can understand cause-effect relationships and offers information to increase the child's understanding of the illness. (2) (PE; IM; ED; GD)

1 This is too general and does not explain why the child will feel better.

2 This is too authoritarian; the child needs information that will increase understanding and compliance with the regimen.

3 Same as answer 2.

27. 2 The Babinski reflex, present at birth, should remain positive throughout the first 12 months of life. (2) (PE; AS; PA; GD)

1 This reflex, present at birth, disappears by 4 months of age.

3 Same as answer 1.

4 Same as answer 1.

28. 3 Young children have an increased propensity for putting things in their mouths; this age-group uses this as a means of exploring the environment. (1) (PE; AN; ED; GD)

1 Although this may be true in older homes or in the inner city, it is the activity of putting things into the mouth that is the primary cause.

2 This is untrue; toddlers do not have a fragile vascular system; children with a fragile vascular system are severely compromised.

4 This is not true; although gas fumes in areas of heavy traffic have increased pollution, most gasoline used today does not contain lead.

29. 4 A visual display, which simulates a suture holding the testes to the thigh, aids in explanation and understanding; it may help the child express feelings about surgery. (3) (PE; PL; ED; GD)

1 This is used to explain IVs, but it is not specific to this surgery.

2 A binder will not be used after this surgery.

3 This is used to explain abdominal surgery such as an appendectomy; it would not apply to this situation.

30. 2 A 5-year-old is able to negotiate and use make believe to play. (3) (PE; AS; ED; GD)

1 Children in the middle childhood years need conformity and rituals, whether they play games or amass collections; rules to games are fixed, unvarying and rigid; knowing the rules means belonging.

3 The use of a pacifier for oral satisfaction is normal for infants.

4 Parallel play occurs in children ages 2 to 3 years.

31. 3   These are typical behaviors of an 8-month-old. (2) (PE; AS; ED; GD)

1   These are typical behaviors of a 12-month-old.

2   These are typical behaviors of a 3-month-old.

4   These are typical behaviors of an 18-month-old.

32. 2   Intrusive procedures threaten the developing body image of the preschooler. (2) (PE; PL; PS; GD)

1   The preschooler is more tolerant of strangers than is a younger child.

3   Routines are still important to the preschooler, but some deviations in structure of activities can be tolerated.

4   The preschooler can tolerate short periods of separation from parents.

33. 1   This would give the child the opportunity for free expression; its free-form nature can give the child a sense of mobility. (3) (PE; PL; PS; GD)

2   This is less than optimal because coloring within lines of pictures in a coloring book requires more skill than most 4-year-olds possess; also this does not allow freedom of expression or movement.

3   Checkers is a game with too many rules for a 4-year-old to comprehend.

4   Playing dominoes requires the ability to count and conserve numbers, which most 4-year-olds do not possess.

34. 2   The teenage child is concerned with body image and fears change or mutilation of body parts; in sickle cell anemia, bones weakened because of hyperplasia and congestion of the marrow can cause lordosis and kyphosis. (1) (PE; AN; PS; GD)

1   Restriction of movement is not a major problem because when the pain is relieved and the crisis is over, activity can be resumed; for the teenager, the change in body image produces greater anxiety.

3   Teenagers can easily tolerate extended periods of separation from the family.

4   Although this could be a concern at this time for a teenager, altered body image is a more fearful threat.

35. 4   A plastic toy that squeaks provides auditory, tactile, and visual stimulation. (3) (PE; EV; ED; GD)

1   A 1-year-old child is too young for a book.

2   The potential for injury is too great for a 1-year-old on a rocking horse.

3   A stuffed animal would not be kept in a playroom because it could not be washed between use by different children.

36. 1   A 4-year-old can manage large buttons on a shirt. (1) (PE; AS; ED; GD)

2   A child of 4 years can put on shoes but is usually unable to tie them until age 5.

3   A child of 4 years will be able to comb but not part the hair.

4   A child of 4 can handle a fork and spoon but cannot hold the meat with the fork to cut it with the knife; the child is usually 7 years old before this can be managed.

37. 2   Death is viewed as a separation and preschoolers believe they will return to life and former activity; this is part of the fantasy world of the child. (2) (PE; AN; PS; GD)

1   At about 9 or 10 years of age, the child develops an adult concept of death and views it as inevitable, irreversible, and universal.

3   This is true for all age groups.

4   This is true of the 6- to 7-year-old child.

38. 3   The 15-year-old is normally preoccupied with appearance; the side effects of the antineoplastics and prednisone will result in the client's feeling different and may cause a poor body image. (1) (PE; AN; PS; GD)

1   A normal 15-year-old enjoys and strives for independence; the sick role would force the client to be dependent.

2   This may be a possible concern but is not likely to be the outstanding concern or feeling.

4   Same as answer 2.

39. 4 These abilities are age appropriate for the 6-month-old. (2) (PE; PL; PA; GD)
1 These abilities should be developed by 10 months of age.
2 Same as answer 1.
3 Same as answer 1.

40. 2 The eustachian tube in young children is shorter, lacks tone, and opens inappropriately, allowing a reflux of nasopharyngeal secretions. (3) (PE; IM; ED; GD)
1 Immunologic differences are not a factor in the development of otitis media.
3 The size of the middle ear does not play a role in the frequent occurrence of otitis media in very young children.
4 There is no difference in the purpose of the eustachian tube among age-groups.

41. 1 Children feel pain and should receive analgesics when needed. (3) (PE; AN; TC; GD)
2 This is a myth; it may be difficult for children to communicate pain.
3 This is a common, but unsound, belief; addiction and respiratory depression are rare.
4 Some sources suggest this may be a child's way of coping with unrelieved pain; however, it is no reason to withhold medication.

42. 1 This is appropriate for an 11-year-old who sees dying as loss of control over every aspect of living; the child may convey this meaning by physically attempting to run away or by pushing others away by rude behavior; it is a plea for some self-control and power. (3) (PE; AS; PS; GD)
2 This is characteristic of the toddler who is egocentric and has a vague separation of fact and fantasy, which makes it impossible to understand the absence of life.
3 This is characteristic of the preschooler who does not have logical thinking.
4 This is more typical of the adolescent who sees deviation from accepted behavior as the reason for becoming ill.

43. 4 Six-month-olds are capable of holding their bottles. (2) (PE; AS; ED; GD)
1 This is a skill of older infants.
2 Same as answer 1.
3 Same as answer 1.

44. 3 A toddler's increasing mobility and growing independence in behavior, including food behavior, are normal aspects of psychologic development; slowed physical growth at this age requires relatively less caloric intake. (3) (PE; IM; ED; GD)
1 A toddler's growth rate and energy requirements decrease in comparison to the first year of life.
2 Same as answer 1.
4 Nutritious snacks between meals should be encouraged if the child is not eating adequate meals.

45. 4 This type of play is characteristic of 5-year-olds. (2) (PE; AN; ED; GD)
1 This type of play is characteristic of 2-year-olds.
2 This is a type of behavior, not a type of play.
3 Same as answer 2.

46. 3 These age-appropriate games help the infant's social development by fostering a sense of object constancy and object permanency. (2) (PE; PL; ED; GD)
1 This is age-appropriate play for the toddler; it promotes gross and fine motor development, not social development.
2 This is age-appropriate play for preschoolers; it helps develop motor, not social, skills.
4 This is age-appropriate play for an older child; it promotes psychomotor, not social, development.

47. 2 A vocabulary consisting of a minimum of six words with telegraphic-type speech is normal for this age child. (2) (PE; AS; PA; GD)
1 The child with a hearing impairment communicates in this way because the child has not acquired the rudiments of language.

3 Babbling is normal communication for an 8-month-old infant, even one with a moderate hearing loss.
4 This language skill is seen in the 5-year-old child.

48. 4 As part of the maturation process, adolescents need to be made to accept the consequences of their actions. (1) (PE; IM; PS; GD)
1 This is false reassurance; there is no way to predict what will be the outcome of her friends' behavior in the future.
2 The focus should be on pointing out that the girl should be accountable for her own behavior, not that her friends should also be punished.
3 The focus should be on the girl's actions and not those of her friends' parents.

49. 2 Toddlers play individually, although side by side (parallel play). (1) (PE; AN; ED; GD)
1 This kind of play is characteristic of older children.
3 Dramatic play or acting is characteristic of older children; they assume and act out roles.
4 Same as answer 1.

50. 4 This provides a 6-year-old, who is of school age, an appropriate way to express feelings, either by writing or drawing pictures. (3) (PE; PL; ED; GD)
1 This would be appropriate for preschoolers whose imaginations are unlimited.
2 This would be appropriate for preschoolers who enjoy experimenting with different textures.
3 This would be appropriate for preschoolers who like repetition.

51. 2 Adolescents are very aware of their changing bodies and become especially concerned with any alteration due to illness or injury. (3) (PE; IM; ED; GD)
1 This does not educate the mother about concepts concerning the developing adolescent; a discussion about hypochondriasis may reinforce mother's concern.

3 This does not address concepts related to growth and development of the adolescent and could cause unnecessary concern about the daughter's physical condition.
4 This could reinforce the mother's concern as well as promote feelings of guilt; it does not include concepts about growth and development of the adolescent.

52. 3 Striving to attain identity and independence is a task of the adolescent, and rebellion against established norms may be exhibited. (3) (PE; AN; ED; GD)
1 This behavior is not a bid for attention, rather it is an attempt to establish an identity which is a normal developmental task of the adolescent.
2 Although the adolescent may be using denial, denial is not developmentally related to adolescence.
4 This behavior is not regression; it is an attempt to attain identity by rebellion against established norms.

EMOTIONAL NEEDS RELATED TO HEALTH PROBLEMS

53. 2 The child is old enough to be asked a direct question. (2) (PE; IM; PS; EH)
1 The parents are too emotionally involved with the child and may not be trained in principles of mental health and therapeutic communication.
3 A younger child, about 8 to 10 years old, would benefit from this.
4 This may be productive with a younger child.

54. 3 This is a truthful statement; the nurse recognizes the fact that this might hurt and requests expected behavior. (2) (PE; IM; PS; EH)
1 This puts unrealistic expectations on the child.
2 This puts a thought in the mind of the child.
4 This would be too threatening for the child.

55. 2 Children with diabetes mellitus need to be treated normally; they need discipline and should have limits set for their behavior. (1) (PE; EV; PS; EH)

1 This is correct; parents should foster independence in the child with diabetes mellitus.

3 This statement is correct; it is realistic to think that the family will have ups and downs.

4 This is correct; the child with diabetes mellitus should be encouraged to maintain normal interests and activities.

56. 3 These behaviors are associated with separation anxiety; parental contact should be encouraged. (1) (PE; PL; PS; GD)

1 Separation anxiety can be minimized by increasing contact with parents, not peers.

2 Separation anxiety can be minimized by increasing contact with parents, not by distraction with toys.

4 This would increase feelings of anxiety; the same nurse should care for the child to promote consistency, continuity, and the development of trust.

57. 4 The child learned to think and solve problems in a very different culture and used a different language and may feel helpless in the new classroom. (1) (PE; AN; PS; EH)

1 There are not enough data to substantiate this.

2 This is untrue; 5-year-olds are inquisitive and adapt well to school.

3 Most 5-year-olds adapt well to kindergarten.

58. 3 The parents need to recognize that their child must be taught responsibility for self-care. (2) (PE; IM; ED; EH)

1 This supports the parents' need to keep the child totally dependent.

2 This demeans the child and inhibits the parents from expressing additional feelings.

4 This denigrates the parents and does not allow for further expression of feelings.

59. 1 This child needs help adjusting; focusing on feelings and abilities promotes effective coping and raises self-esteem. (2) (PE; PL; PS; EH)

2 In general, the diet is limited to simple carbohydrates; bowel inflammation necessitates avoidance of high-roughage foods.

3 Teaching the relationship of diet to the disease process does not ensure compliance with the diet.

4 Occasional noncompliance is not permitted; it eventually causes a relapse.

60. 4 Life-long adherence to dietary restrictions prevents complications and celiac crisis. (2) (PE; PL; PS; EH)

1 Celiac crisis usually develops as a result of nonadherence to the diet, so adherence would be a primary goal.

2 Respiratory involvement is not a primary problem in celiac disease.

3 Regardless of adherence to the diet, there is an interference with normal growth.

61. 1 Colostomy care may seem overwhelming to the parents, and it may reassure them to know that a therapist is available. (1) (PE; PL; ED; EH)

2 Mealtime should be a pleasant time; also, this assumes that eating habits are poor.

3 Increased fluids are often needed to compensate for fecal fluid loss.

4 This is untrue; physical activity will probably not be limited.

62. 3 The parents need assistance in exploring their feelings and their family relationships with a professional. (1) (PE; EV; PS; EH)

1 The gifts are attempts to relieve guilt feelings; the parent still feels responsible.

2 This is a gift to the child that helps the parents relieve their guilt feelings.

4 The parent is assuming the martyr role and accepting the responsibility for the child's illness.

63. 4 The nurse must emphasize that everything possible is being done because the outcome cannot be predicted. (3) (PE; IM; PS; EH)

1 The outcome is still in doubt; encouraging the parent's positive interpretation of the child's reflexive behavior raises false hope.

2 Same as answer 1.
3 The outcome is still in doubt; this response by the nurse may raise false hope; the parent's statement did not ask for the nurse's religious viewpoint.

64. 3 This response identifies concern and presents an appropriate protective intervention; regular and prompt removal of ticks decreases the chances of the spread of Lyme disease to humans. (2) (PE; IM; ED; EH)
1 The response centers on camping, not on the fear of ticks.
2 This response belittles the child's feelings.
4 This is an inappropriate response because it focuses on the wrong fear.

65. 3 Regardless of age, parenthood confers the rights of an adult on the teenager. (2) (PE; PL; ED; GD)
1 It is unnecessary and not legal for the grandmother to sign the consent; the father is present.
2 This would be done only if neither parent was available to give consent in an emergency.
4 The mother has a legal right to give consent but is not available.

66. 1 People living in poverty have long-term feelings of powerlessness because they do not have buying power or social status to influence change. (1) (PE; AN; PS; EH)
2 The opposite is true; they are focused on the present, not the future.
3 Their anger is covert and not direct; in addition, the anger rarely resolves their situation, resulting in feelings of powerlessness and hopelessness.
4 People in poverty tend to focus on today; health recommendations may not be delivered under optimal circumstances or may be misunderstood, confusing, or of little value.

67. 2 Family strengths must be identified and utilized by the nurse. (3) (PE; AN; PS; EH)
1 The family members and their problems must be viewed as a whole.
3 The opposite is true.
4 This is untrue; values, beliefs, and attitudes greatly influence perceptions.

68. 3 The parents will probably be anxious and will benefit most from short teaching sessions and written material to review at their leisure. (1) (PE; PL; ED; EH)
1 This would be overwhelming, and the parents would not be able to retain everything presented.
2 The nurse could recommend, but not insist, that both parents attend the teaching sessions.
4 The most effective teaching and learning sessions occur in an area with minimal distractions; being in the room with their child at this time would present a major distraction to the parents.

69. 4 In most states, the age of majority is 18 years; however, mothers under 18 years of age are considered emancipated minors and can sign consents for themselves and their children. (2) (PE; AN; ED; EH)
1 The grandmother has no legal right to give consent; the 16-year-old mother is present and can legally give consent.
2 This is unnecessary; the client is an emancipated minor, and this confers adult status.
3 Consent is always needed; the 16-year-old mother is present and can legally give consent.

70. 4 All parents initially grieve over the loss of health in their children. (1) (PE; AN; PS; EH)
1 Many parents have excellent support systems.
2 This may be true of some, not all, parents.
3 At least one-third of the children with cerebral palsy are not mentally retarded.

71. 2 This allows the client to volunteer information first and thus, feel in control; the nurse can ask validating questions later. (1) (PE; AS; PS; EH)
1 This focuses the assessment on vomiting, thus predisposing the client to vomiting during this treatment.
3 This is an unfeeling response; it reminds the child and mother of the many sessions remaining and brings little consolation to the child for the discomfort or the mother for her worry about the prognosis.
4 This response is flippant.

72. 3 This is a truthful answer that offers some hope without false reassurance. (2) (PE; IM; PS; EH)

1 Although true, this response shuts off communication and discourages further ventilation of feelings.

2 This response produces guilt and denies the adolescent's realistic fears.

4 This response denies the adolescent's feelings.

73. 3 This child experienced trauma; the child's reactions to this experience will influence every aspect of the rest of the nurse's care plan. (1) (PE; PL; PS; EH)

1 This is a nursing diagnosis related to the parents of the child, not the child.

2 Although this is an appropriate nursing diagnosis for this child, the child's post-traumatic response is primary and will most profoundly permeate all aspects of care.

4 There is no evidence in the data given that the child's vision is impaired.

74. 2 A private room will provide a secure environment for the child and the family to get to know one another. (2) (PE; PL; PS; EH)

1 This is not therapeutic because it may make the child feel guilty about leaving the biologic family.

3 Same as answer 1.

4 Although some information may be given, too much information about the family may promote preconceived ideas which may be inaccurate.

75. 4 This response is accepting of the individual and communicates concern. (3) (PE; IM; PS; EH)

1 This is the nurse's responsibility and should not be transferred immediately to the client's family.

2 There is no indication that the injuries were deliberate abuse.

3 This response interprets the client's statement as guilt, which may or may not be the true interpretation.

76. 2 Abusers lack personal strengths and adequate support systems, which could help them handle stress and frustration. (1) (PE; AN; PS; EH)

1 Abusers tend to be young, immature, and dependent.

3 Abusers have an incorrect concept of what the small child can do; their expectations are unrealistic.

4 Most abusers were abused as children; physical discipline was probably excessive.

77. 2 Because parents are trying to hide the fact of abuse, the explanations are fabricated and vague. (2) (PE; AS; PS; EH)

1 This is expected; the parents are unable to provide emotional support.

3 The child behaves in this manner because in past experiences adults have inflicted pain rather than provided comfort.

4 This is no surprise; parents do not discuss them because this would be an admission of child abuse.

78. 4 Going to a stranger without protest usually indicates the lack of a meaningful relationship with the mother. (1) (PE; AS; PS; EH)

1 This is a healthy, normal reaction to strangers that is uncommon in children with failure to thrive syndrome.

2 Same as answer 1.

3 Children who fail to thrive avoid eye contact with their mothers and do not prefer them over others.

FLUIDS AND ELECTROLYTES

79. 1 With renal disease a large proportion of the child's body weight is composed of retained fluid; the loss of fluid would be readily reflected by a loss of weight. (3) (PE; AS; TC; FE)

2 It is very difficult to get an accurate recording of output in a young child, especially if vomiting and diarrhea also occur.

3 With renal disease it would be difficult to evaluate return to fluid balance in this way because the edema is generalized, not concentrated in the abdomen.

4 Osmolality reflects kidney activity, not the reduction in edema.

80. 4 This allows the child to get a full cup (1 oz medicine cup) without long waits; a full cup, even if it is a small cup, creates the illusion of receiving more. (3) (PE; PL; TC; FE)

1 When fluid is limited, a smaller amount should be apportioned to sleeping hours.

2 If the child were allowed to drink as much as desired until the limit is reached, 15 to 20 hours might elapse before any fluid would be permitted again.

3 Although fluids can be limited more easily during sleeping hours, 12 hours is too long for a young child to tolerate.

81. 2 KCl is always restricted in the presence of oliguria to prevent cardiac dysrhythmias associated with hyperkalemia. (3) (PE; PL; TC; FE)

1 Glucose and fat are not restricted; they are usually prime sources of calories.

3 Protein restriction is used only when severe azotemia with prolonged oliguria is present.

4 Same as answer 1.

82. 2 The degree of dehydration is correlated with weight loss; continued fever aggravates fluid losses through evaporation. (2) (PE; AS; PA; FE)

1 Poor skin turgor may not occur after only 48 hours of vomiting.

3 This is not relevant; the neurologic status is not altered; the urinary output may show signs of decreasing.

4 This is not relevant because the child has been vomiting and will most likely be npo to rest the gastrointestinal tract.

83. 4 Loss of weight is the best way to evaluate the magnitude of fluid loss in the infant; 1 liter of fluid weighs 2.2 pounds. (2) (PE; AS; PA; FE)

1 This is a subjective assessment; measurement of weight is an objective assessment.

2 Although this would indicate dehydration, it is not an effective monitoring method for assessing fluid loss.

3 This is a subjective and inaccurate assessment.

84. 4 This is a normal adaptation to a state of dehydration; the urine will be concentrated. (2) (PE; AS; PA; FE)

1 There is no indication of celiac disease.

2 The initial response to decreased circulating fluids would be an increased pulse rate.

3 One of the signs of dehydration in an infant is a sunken, not a bulging, fontanel.

85. 4 A decreased urinary output is expected with dehydration in a young infant because of decreased circulating fluid volume. (2) (PE; AS; PA; FE)

1 This is associated with increased intracranial pressure, not dehydration; the fontanel would be depressed with dehydration.

2 This is associated with an adequate fluid balance.

3 Because of loss of fluid and electrolytes the infant would be lethargic, not restless.

86. 3 This is a classic sign of fluid volume deficit in infants. (1) (PE; AS; PA; FE)

1 This is within the normal limits of 1.010 to 1.030.

2 This indicates adequate hydration; the urinary output would be decreased in dehydration.

4 This is unrelated to allergies.

87. 2 Infants have a higher fluid to body mass ratio than do older children or adults; severe dehydration can occur more rapidly and the correction of fluid loss problems is more difficult; early, immediate medical intervention is necessary. (2) (PE; PL; ED; FE)

1 Unrelated, since data do not indicate any administration of antibiotics.

3 Important at all times, but priority at this time is to make the mother understand how serious diarrhea can be.

4 Related but not the priority; diarrhea can be contracted despite cleanliness.

88. 1 Normal arterial blood gas values are pH 7.35 to 7.45; P_{O_2} 83 to 108 mmHg; P_{CO_2} 35 to 45 mmHg; base excess −3 to +3. (2) (PE; AS; PA; FE)
2 The pH is alkalotic.
3 The pH is acidotic, the P_{O_2} is low, the P_{CO_2} is high, and the base excess is outside the normal range.
4 The P_{O_2} is low (hypoxic); the P_{CO_2} is low (hypocapnic); the base excess is high.

89. 3 Respiratory compensation to acidosis involves increased CO_2 elimination through hyperventilation, with a resulting increase in pH to normal limits. (2) (PE; AN; PA; FE)
1 Hypoventilation would not increase expiration of CO_2 with the ultimate increase in pH.
2 If the client is hypoventilating, blood H^+ ions would increase because of CO_2 retention; pH would decrease.
4 With hyperventilation there would be an increase in CO_2 elimination, not a decrease; the pH would increase, not decrease.

90. 4 Metabolic acidosis results from an excess concentration of hydrogen cations; potassium increases; the kidneys cannot convert ammonium (NH_3) to ammonia (NH_4); there is inadequate base bicarbonate to maintain an appropriate acid-base balance. (3) (PE; AN; PA; FE)
1 This child will have an excess of hydrogen ions, resulting in metabolic acidosis; carbonic acid blown off as CO_2 results in respiratory alkalosis.
2 This child has an excess of hydrogen ions from a metabolic problem rather than an excess of carbonic acid due to retained CO_2.
3 This child will have an excess of hydrogen ions, the opposite of an excess of base bicarbonate.

91. 4 In metabolic acidosis the lungs try to compensate by blowing off excess carbonic acid in the form of carbon dioxide. (3) (PE; AN; PA; FE)
1 This is a compensatory mechanism to reduce fever by evaporation.

2 This indicates renal compensation for alkalosis.
3 This is not an adaptation to metabolic acidosis; fever with dehydration results from inadequate fluid for perspiration and cooling.

92. 2 A low blood pH in the presence of severe dehydration indicates metabolic acidosis. (3) (PE; AS; PA; FE)
1 These findings indicate metabolic alkalosis.
3 These findings indicate respiratory acidosis.
4 Same as answer 1.

93. 3 Sodium lactate is converted to sodium bicarbonate; it helps correct the sodium deficit and the metabolic acidosis. (3) (PE; PL; TC; FE)
1 Plasmanate is a colloid used as a substitute when plasma is needed; it is not used in the treatment of metabolic acidosis.
2 Saline results in the chloride combining with the hydrogen ion, intensifying the acidosis.
4 Potassium is not administered until urinary function is restored.

94. 1 The pH indicates acidosis; the HCO_3 level is further from normal than the P_{CO_2} level indicating a metabolic origin (losses from diarrhea). (3) (PE; AS; PA; FE)
2 The pH indicates acidosis, not alkalosis.
3 The HCO_3 level is further from normal than the P_{CO_2} level indicating a metabolic origin to the acidosis.
4 The pH indicates an acidotic, not an alkalotic, state; also, it is of metabolic origin.

95. 4 The symptoms indicate ketoacidosis so both these values would be expected; the pH indicates acidosis (metabolic or ketoacidosis) and the blood glucose, elevated above the normal range of 70 to 105 mg/dl, indicates severe hyperglycemia. (3) (PE; AS; TC; FE)
1 Although the blood pH indicates acidosis, the blood glucose is below the normal range of 70 to 105 mg/dl; with ketoacidosis the client would be hyperglycemic.

2   Both values would be unexpected with keto-acidosis; with ketoacidosis the pH would be lowered and blood glucose elevated.

3   Although the blood glucose would be elevated with ketoacidosis, the pH would be lowered, not elevated; a pH of 7.50 indicates alkalosis.

96. 3   The extremities need to be restrained because the child will use all extremities in an attempt to dislodge the needle. (2) (PE; IM; TC; FE)

1   Pupillary responses are unrelated to dehydration and fluid replacement.

2   Scalp veins used for IVs are not located in these areas.

4   The parents can be taught how to hold a child with an IV infusing via a scalp vein.

97. 4   These are classic signs of dehydration and hyponatremia; a physician's order to increase fluids is needed. (2) (PE; EV; TC; FE)

1   The nurse must have a physician's order for this; also, dehydration can be corrected with fluids via IV or feeding tube.

2   It is not common for the condition of these infants to continue to deteriorate once therapy is implemented.

3   The symptoms indicate dehydration, not undernutrition.

98. 3   One liter of fluid weighs 2.2 pounds; this is the most objective and accurate way to assess fluid loss or gain; weights measured at the same time each day provide for daily comparisons. (2) (PE; EV; TC; FE)

1   This would be appropriate for assessing the progression of ascites, not for assessing rehydration.

2   Color of stools is unrelated to fluid balance; noting consistency would be more important, although subjective.

4   Although this would be done, it is subjective and inaccurate.

99. 4   Safety is a priority; the infant may inadvertently dislodge the circulatory access. (2) (PE; IM; TC; FE)

1   This is contraindicated; oral fluids will not be administered until peristalsis returns.

2   Parent-infant contact should be encouraged.

3   This is unnecessary; the number of voidings should be assessed.

100. 2   To prevent fluid overload, the IV infusion should be maintained at the slowest rate possible to keep the circulatory access patent until the physician can be reached to verify the correct rate. (2) (PE; IM; TC; FE)

1   This is unsafe; after surgery all previous orders are cancelled and new orders must be written by the physician.

3   This is unsafe; the administration of intravenous fluids requires a physician's order.

4   Same as answer 3.

101. 3   The present caloric intake for a 24 hour period is 8 oz × 20 calories × 6 feedings = 960 calories; the recommended intake is 108 calories × 8.52 kg = 920 calories. (3) (PE; EV; PA; FE)

1   The data indicated can be used to calculate the child's daily caloric intake (oz × calories × number of feedings) which can be compared to the recommended caloric intake (108 calories × kg of body weight).

2   The present caloric intake exceeds the daily recommended requirements by 40 calories.

4   Same as answer 2.

102. 3   2.2 lb = 1 kg; 13 lb = 5.9 kg; 150 × 5.9 = 885 ml. (2) (PE; AN; TC; FE)

1   This is inaccurate; this is less than the ordered amount of fluid.

2   Same as answer 1.

4   This is inaccurate; this exceeds the ordered amount of fluid.

103. 3   Use ratio and proportion: multiply the amount to be infused (500 ml) by the drop factor (60) and divide the result by the amount of time in minutes (18 hours × 60 minutes). (2) (PE; AN; TC; FE)

1   It is impossible to deliver a half of a drop.

2   This rate is too slow; less than the ordered amount would infuse.

4   This is too fast; the fluid would be delivered in a shorter period of time than ordered.

104. 3 This is the correct flow rate; multiply the amount to be infused (700 ml) by the drop factor (60) and divide the result by the amount of time in minutes (24 hr × 60 min). (2) (PE; AN; TC; FE)

1 This rate is too slow; less than the ordered amount would be infused.

2 Same as answer 1.

4 This is too fast; the fluid would be administered in a shorter period of time than ordered.

105. 3 This is the correct flow rate; multiply the sum of all IV fluid to be infused for the period (750 ml) by the drop factor (60); divide the results by the amount of time in minutes (24 hr × 60 min); thus, 45,000 ÷ 1440 = 31 gtt/min. (2) (PE; AN; TC; FE)

1 This rate of flow is too slow to deliver the required amount of fluid in 24 hours.

2 Same as answer 1.

4 This rate of flow is too fast; the fluid will be infused before 24 hours.

BLOOD AND IMMUNITY

106. 4 Previously formed antibodies, acquired through active immunity, offer some resistance to infection; adults have higher levels of antibodies than children because over time they have been exposed to more pathogens. (1) (PE; AN; PA; BI)

1 The immune systems of children are as capable of producing antibodies as are those of adults.

2 The pathophysiology of AIDS is the same in both children and adults.

3 Exposure to pathogens in the environment does not differ significantly between children and adults.

107. 4 The passive antibodies received from the mother would be diminished by age 8 weeks and would not interfere with the development of active immunity after this time. (2) (PE; AN; ED; BI)

1 The spleen does not produce antibodies.

2 This is untrue; infants are often exposed to infectious diseases; passive immunity from the mother offers some protection.

3 This is untrue; these immunizations are attenuated; they may cause irritability and fever, but they will not cause the related disease.

108. 2 Mild reactions are redness and induration at the injection site, slight fever, and irritability. (2) (PE; EV; PA; BI)

1 Serious reactions are not common.

3 Occasionally a DTP injection may precipitate a febrile seizure, but it does not cause permanent brain damage.

4 Induration at the site of injection may occur, but deep ulceration does not.

109. 3 Fever is a common reaction to the immunizations; Tylenol helps to reduce fever; both loss of consciousness and convulsions are rare, but serious, complications of the pertussis vaccine. (2) (PE; IM; TC; BI)

1 Heat would cause an extension of the inflammatory response and should be avoided.

2 Infants do not respond well to the application of ice; fever is expected and requires no intervention other than administration of Tylenol.

4 Aspirin should not be given to children because it is associated with Reye's syndrome.

110. 3 The schedule for active immunization is 3 doses of DTP at 2-month intervals beginning at 2 months of age. (2) (PE; AN; PA; BI)

1 Measles vaccine is not given until 12 to 15 months because maternal antibodies block the formation of the infant's antibodies.

2 OPV booster is due at 18 months; it is given at the same time as the DTP booster dose.

4 This is given at 18 months, or approximately 1 year after the third dose that is given at 6 months of age.

111. 3   The American Academy of Pediatrics recommends that infants be given the MMR combination vaccine at 12 to 15 months of age. (1) (PE; PL; TC; BI)
1   The infant should have received this immunization at 2 months, 4 months, and 6 months of age; the next booster will be at 18 months.
2   Same as answer 1.
4   Same as answer 1.

112. 4   Hepatitis B vaccine (Recombivax HB, Engerix B) is not given routinely to all children; if a mother is hepatitis B surface antigen (HB$_s$Ag) positive when the child is born, the child will receive Recombivax at birth and at 1 and 6 months of age. (1) (PE; PL; PA; BI)
1   In the first 6 months, OPV is given to infants at 2, 4, and 6 months of age.
2   This is part of the DTP vaccine; in the first 6 months, it is given at 2, 4, and 6 months of age.
3   Same as answer 2.

113. 1   Children with leukemia are immunosuppressed; the chickenpox virus can cause death in the individual without an intact immune system. (2) (PE; PL; TC; BI)
2   There is no immunization against chickenpox.
3   Prednisone does not confer immunity to the chickenpox virus.
4   This would be unsafe; chickenpox can be spread by airborne droplets in the prodromal stage and by fomites that have come in contact with pox that are oozing.

114. 4   This supplies some iron and protein; it can be eaten with a spoon, encouraging mastery of fine motor muscles. (1) (PE; PL; TC; BI)
1   This provides some protein and iron but has a spicy taste that is not generally a favorite of this age-group.
2   This is low in protein and iron.
3   Same as answer 2.

115. 4   Potatoes and whole milk are not adequate sources of iron; at age 8 months, fetal iron stores are depleted. (2) (PE; AN; PA; BI)
1   Potatoes are a rich source of potassium.
2   The infant is receiving Poly Vi-Sol, which contains vitamins but no iron; Poly Vi-Sol with iron exists, but the data indicate plain Poly Vi-Sol is being used.
3   There are some amino acids in the foods that are being eaten.

116. 4   The physician will probably use a local anesthetic which can hurt; however, there will also be pain as the aspiration needle is inserted through the bone to the periosteum as well as pain and pressure when the bone marrow is withdrawn. (3) (PE; EV; TC; BI)
1   This is true; although the site may be sore and the child may prefer to remain quiet, activity is not usually restricted.
2   This is true; this is done to prevent bleeding from the puncture site.
3   This is true; the anterior or posterior iliac crest is the site most often used for a bone marrow aspiration in children.

117. 2   Before the sex of the unborn child is known, the odds are 25%; 50% of pregnancies will result in boys and each has a 50% chance of having hemophilia. (3) (PE; AN; ED; BI)
1   Because the disease is genetically transmitted, this is not likely.
3   This is too high; there is only a 25% chance that the baby will be affected.
4   Same as answer 3.

118. 2   Joints are the most commonly involved areas, probably because of weight bearing and constant movement of joints. (3) (PE; AS; PA; BI)
1   This is not the most common site; however, bleeding can occur here.
3   Same as answer 1.
4   Same as answer 1.

119. 2   During sickle cell crisis, the RBCs are sickled and clumped and the hemoglobin is ineffective in providing oxygen; therefore fluids to liquify the clumping cells and additional oxygen are necessary. (3) (PE; PL; TC; BI)

1   Neither one of these is required during sickle cell crisis.

3   Hydration is important at this time; even if counseling were needed, it would not be done until the client was out of crisis.

4   Oxygenation is needed; factor VIII is used in hemophilia.

120. 2   Thalassemia is a hemolytic anemia that is not communicable; roommates with infectious diseases should be avoided because a child with sickle cell anemia is susceptible to infections. (2) (PE; PL; TC; BI)

1   The child with sickle cell anemia is susceptible to infection; pneumonia is an infection of the lung.

3   The child with sickle cell anemia is susceptible to infection; osteomyelitis is an infection of the bone.

4   The child with sickle cell anemia is susceptible to infection; pharyngitis is an upper respiratory infection.

121. 2   Hemolysis of RBCs, which carry the heme component, leads to anemia. (2) (PE; AN; PA; BI)

1   It is not the iron intake but ineffective hemoglobin which causes the anemia.

3   The WBCs are not increased unless infection is present.

4   There is no electrolyte imbalance; more fluid is given to decrease the hypertonicity of the blood plasma, thus reversing the sickling process; when the client is adequately hydrated and oxygenated, RBCs tend to appear normal.

122. 1   To prevent crises, the child and family must be taught to prevent sickling by maintaining hydration, promoting adequate oxygenation, and avoiding strenuous exercise. (1) (PE; IM; ED; BI)

2   It is the lack of oxygen that contributes to sickling.

3   Blood transfusions are given more often than occassionally.

4   There are no prophylactic medications used.

123. 4   Widespread petechiae appear first as a result of the low platelet count. (2) (PE; AS; PA; BI)

1   This often occurs from chemotherapy for ALL.

2   These often occur from chemotherapy for ALL.

3   This occurs later, with anemia resulting from erythropoietic failure and blood loss.

124. 1   The platelet count is reduced as a result of the bone marrow depression associated with leukemia. (3) (PE; IM; TC; BI)

2   The uric acid level affects urinary output, not blood clotting.

3   Prothrombin time is influenced by vitamin K factors, not lack of platelets.

4   The red blood cell count will indicate the hematocrit and hemoglobin levels, which would neither provide the reason for nor cause the bleeding.

125. 2   Good nutrition is extremely important to the child's overall health; best results are attained when a child receiving chemotherapy is allowed to eat as desired. (2) (PE; EV; ED; BI)

1   The child should be isolated only from other children with known or possible infections.

3   Mouthwashes can irritate the fragile mucosa, so saline should be used; nutrition is the priority.

4   Although activities are important to the child's health, these should be provided according to the child's interest and should not always be structured.

126. 3   Blood tests indicate response to therapy; if the WBC count drops severely, therapy may be temporarily halted. (2) (PE; PL; TC; BI)

1   These children receive therapy for extended periods, and prolonged isolation from their peers may lead to destructive social isolation.

2   This is a very painful procedure and is not done weekly.

4   Nausea commonly occurs with this therapy; although antiemetic measures are instituted, the drug is not withdrawn.

127. 3   Unless the child has an episode of acute illness, the home is the best place for the child; this prevents nosocomial infection and promotes family interaction. (2) (PE; PL; TC; BI)

1   This is required only for episodes of acute illness that cannot be handled at home.

2   This is not required unless the illness exacerbates.

4   This should be used only if a home environment is not available.

128. 4   HIV has been isolated from blood and other body secretions; the Centers for Disease Control recommend body secretion isolation or universal precautions. (1) (PE; IM; TC; BI)

1   This is unnecessary; HIV is not known to spread by droplets, and masks, which are part of strict isolation, are not required.

2   This type of isolation protects the child from others; its purpose is not the protection of staff; it might be used if the child were severely immunosuppressed.

3   Enteric precautions will not protect others from blood or other body fluids, only feces.

129. 2   Children with AIDS have a dysfunction of the immune system (depressed or ineffective T cells, B cells, and immunoglobulins) and are susceptible to opportunistic infections. (1) (PE; AN; TC; BI)

1   All children have a high risk for injury because of their curiosity, inexperience, and lack of judgment.

3   Although children with AIDS are most likely small for their ages, altered growth and development is not as life-threatening as an infection.

4   Although this can occur in children with AIDS, the prevention of infection is the priority.

INTEGUMENTARY

130. 3   Air-drying promotes healing; moisture macerates the skin and provides a medium for the growth of microorganisms. (1) (PE; IM; PA; IT)

1   Although this statement is true it is not the reason for leaving the baby without a diaper.

2   This is not the reason for leaving the baby exposed; body heat effectively leaves the body through the head; also, the situation does not convey that the baby has a fever.

4   Same as answer 1.

131. 2   White spots (Koplik's spots) and the rash with coryza are very indicative of measles (rubeola). (3) (PE; EV; PA; IT)

1   Rubella (German measles) does not cause Koplik's spots.

3   Varicella (chickenpox) has skin lesions rather than a rash and lesions in the mouth.

4   Scarlet fever does not cause Koplik's spots but a strawberry-red tongue.

132. 3   It is most often found in infants at about 2 to 4 months of age. (1) (PE; AN; PA; IT)

1   The age of the child, the elusive causative factor, and the multifaceted modalities used for therapy make it very difficult to treat.

2   It is not contagious.

4   It is not associated with any respiratory infections.

133. 4   The skin integrity of these children is highly compromised because of their constant scratching; they are prone to streptococcal and staphylococcal infections. (1) (PE; PL; TC; IT)

1   This is always important for infants, but the priority is prevention of secondary infections.

2   Same as answer 1.

3   This is the physician's, not the nurse's, responsibility.

134. 2 All of these contain protein to which the eczematous child is allergic. (2) (PE; AN; PA; IT)

1 Fruit does not contain protein, the food element to which the child is allergic.

3 Woolens provoke itching but do not cause the child to break out.

4 Environmental inhalants cause eczema in the older child; in infants, protein is the offender.

135. 1 The baby's nails should be cut very short to minimize injury from scratching. (1) (PE; EV; TC; IT)

2 This statement is correct; woolens tend to further irritate the eczematous rash.

3 This is a correct statement; infants with eczema should avoid milk.

4 This is a correct statement; this kind of clothing seems to be less irritating.

136. 4 Lymphadenopathy and the development of a rash after a day of fever, sneezing, and coughing characterize rubella. (2) (PE; AS; PA; IT)

1 These are symptoms of rubeola, not rubella.

2 These are symptoms associated with meningitis and encephalitis, not rubella.

3 The spots in the mucous membrane of the soft palate in rubella are called Forschheimer spots; Koplik's spots are present with measles.

137. 4 An unimmunized woman who is exposed to the rubella virus may contract the disease and transmit it to the fetus; there is a potential for pregnancy in this cousin. (1) (PE; PL; TC; IT)

1 There is less risk if a young male adult contracts rubella than if a young adult female, who may be pregnant, does.

2 If the playmate should contract the rubella from the child, the disease would probably be mild and confer immunity.

3 Rubeola has no relationship to rubella; the sister would be at risk only if she were pregnant.

138. 2 Eschar is rigid and may restrict circulation and lead to loss of limb perfusion. (3) (PE; AS; TC; IT)

1 This is not the role of the nurse; blisters are a protective adaptation.

3 Although this would be done, adequate arterial perfusion is the priority.

4 This is unnecessary.

139. 2 The child's burn injury totals 31.5% burned (9% right arm, 4.5% left arm, 18% anterior chest); the "rule of nines" adult chart is applicable for a 12-year-old. (1) (PE; AS; TC; IT)

1 This is too little; (9% right arm, 4.5% left arm, 18% anterior chest = 31.5% burned); the "rule of nines" adult chart is applicable for a 12-year-old.

3 This is too much; (9% right arm, 4.5% left arm, 18% anterior chest = 31.5%). the "rule of nines" adult chart is applicable for a 12-year-old.

4 Same as answer 3.

140. 3 Once a sterile object comes into contact with any object that is not sterile, it is no longer considered sterile. (1) (PE; AN; TC; IT)

1 This is untrue; a 1-inch border around the sterile field is considered contaminated.

2 This is untrue; the object is considered contaminated.

4 This is untrue; dry wounds are considered clean.

141. 1 When all vesicles are dried, chickenpox is no longer transmissible; dried vesicles do not harbor the varicella virus. (2) (PE; IM; ED; IT)

2 This is not true; dry scabs do not transmit the virus.

3 Chickenpox is not associated with a high fever unless a bacterial complication such as pneumonia is present.

4 These vesicles are mature vesicles that occur in successive crops; these vesicles contain the varicella virus.

142. 3 Individuals taking steroids have lowered resistance and may become fatally ill if exposed to the varicella virus. (1) (PE; IM; ED; IT)

1 This does not lower body resistance; therefore it does not increase susceptibility.

2 This does not affect body resistance because topical antibiotics do not have a systemic effect.

4 This may increase resistance rather than decrease it.

143. 4   Patting the lesions will not disturb them, and baking soda is an effective drying agent. (1) (PE; IM; ED; IT)

1   This may tear off the vesicles and lead to scar formation.

2   This may prevent secondary infection but has no drying effect.

3   This may minimize scratching but will not relieve pruritus.

144. 1   Radiation, or the transferring of heat from a warm object to the atmosphere, is prevented by reducing the surface and covering the child with a blanket. (2) (PE; AN; TC; IT)

2   Conduction is the transfer of heat from one molecule to another with contact between the two; very little body heat is lost by conduction.

3   Active transport is not related to loss of heat; this is a process that moves ions or molecules across a cell membrane against a concentration gradient.

4   Vaporization is the conversion of liquid or solid into a vapor; it would occur if a person were perspiring.

145. 4   Foam is soft, so it will not damage the oral mucosa. (1) (PE; EV; ED; IT)

1   A toothbrush will injure the oral mucosa.

2   Hydrogen peroxide will irritate the mucosa and has an offensive taste.

3   Mouthwash may irritate the oral mucosa and should always be diluted.

146. 4   Chemotherapy causes severe alteration in mucous membranes; a rectal thermometer may damage delicate rectal tissue. (2) (PE; AN; TC; IT)

1   Although this may be true, it is not the primary reason to avoid taking rectal temperatures in children receiving chemotherapy for leukemia.

2   Oral temperatures are accurate, provided the child can hold the thermometer in the mouth correctly.

3   This is incorrect; ear temperatures are accurate.

147. 1   Measles is another name for rubeola. (1) (PE; AN; PA; IT)

2   This is known as varicella.

3   This is pertussis.

4   This is rubella.

148. 1   Measles starts with a discrete maculopapular rash on the face and spreads downward, eventually becoming confluent. (2) (PE; AN; PA; IT)

2   This occurs with whooping cough.

3   This occurs with mumps.

4   This occurs with chickenpox.

149. 3   Impetigo may develop as a secondary bacterial infection because of breaks in the skin from scratching. (3) (PE; AN; PA; IT)

1   Eczema is an allergic response, not an infection.

2   This is an extended inflammation that is not commonly found in children with pediculosis.

4   This is a fungal infection of the scalp; it usually occurs by itself, not as a secondary infection to pediculosis.

150. 1   The nurse needs to gather information regarding the symptoms because they can be related to many factors. (2) (PE; AS; PA; IT)

2   A developmental screening is not necessary in an acute situation.

3   This is unnecessary; this information is not related to the situation.

4   A child in good health would not be in a high-risk group and receive an influenza vaccination; a rash is unusual after a sunburn.

151. 4   This is a straightforward, truthful answer at a level that a 12-year-old would comprehend. (2) (PE; IM; ED; IT)

1   The answer is full of medical jargon that the child might not understand.

2   This identifies a feeling but avoids answering the question.

3   This identifies a feeling but disregards the fact that the child has already asked a question.

152. 2   The tick must be carefully removed with tweezers or forceps so that the tick does not further inoculate the individual. (1) (PE; IM; ED; IT)

1   This is an unsafe method of removing a tick; the tick may further inoculate the individual, and the method may hurt the child.

3   Same as answer 1.

4   Same as answer 1.

SKELETAL

153. 3 Cool fingers are a sign of circulatory impairment caused by the pressure of the cast; however, if both hands feel cool it indicates some factor other than circulatory impairment is responsible. (1) (PE; EV; TC; SK)
1 Further assessment to determine the cause of temperature change is indicated before taking immediate remedial action.
2 This should not be done without a physician's order.
4 Further assessment should be done before informing the physician.

154. 2 A damp cloth will remove surface soil but will not damage the plaster cast. (1) (PE; IM; ED; SK)
1 Plastic will cause condensation and wetness, which would soften the cast.
3 Excessive water would soften and damage the cast; cleansing agents could injure the skin.
4 Same as answer 3.

155. 3 The legs must be kept perpendicular to the trunk in order for the child's body weight to serve as countertraction. (2) (PE; AS; TC; SK)
1 In this position, the child's body weight and the angle of pull would be insufficient to supply traction.
2 Same as answer 1.
4 Same as answer 1.

156. 4 Because elastic bandages affix the apparatus to the limbs, the danger of circulatory impairment is always present. (2) (PE; AS; TC; SK)
1 The child in Byrant's traction does not have pins in place; skin traction is utilized.
2 The skin is not punctured, so topical or antibiotic ointment would not be ordered.
3 Removing the bandages would discontinue the traction and would never be done without a physician's order.

157. 1 Injuries in various stages of healing are the classic sign of child abuse. (1) (PE; AS; TC; SK)
2 This can be evaluated after child abuse has been ruled out.

3 Same as answer 2.
4 Same as answer 2.

158. 3 The palm of the hand provides a wide base of support for the casted extremity and prevents indentation of the cast; this preserves the integrity of the cast and prevents neurovascular injury to the lower extremity. (1) (PE; IM; TC; SK)
1 This could cause indentations in the cast that would put pressure on the lower extremity which could compromise the skin and /or neurovascular functioning.
2 This could injure the infant and could compromise the integrity of the cast; the lower extremity and cast must be supported.
4 Same as answer 2.

159. 3 Rough cast edges can cause skin irritation and breakdown; the skin at the edges of the cast should be assessed for edema, signs of pressure, and evidence of skin breakdown. (1) (PE; EV; TC; SK)
1 Adhesive petals will not adhere to a damp cast.
2 Lotions applied to the skin at the edges of a cast can promote skin breakdown.
4 This is contraindicated; plaster casts should be kept dry to maintain their shape; the skin under the cast may become macerated from inadequate drying after water immersion.

160. 4 With specific manipulation, an audible click may be heard or felt as the femoral head slips into the acetabulum. (1) (PE; AS; PA; SK)
1 This is Trendelenburg's sign; it is associated with weight bearing.
2 This is not Ortolani's sign; this is associated with bilateral dislocation.
3 This is Allis' sign.

161. 1 The affected leg appears to be shorter because the femoral head is displaced upward. (2) (PE; AS; PA; SK)
2 There is a limited ability to abduct, not adduct, the affected leg.
3 This does not occur with congenital hip dysplasia.
4 When the femoral head slips out of the acetabulum, it is easily palpable.

162. 3 Difficulty with abduction may indicate a congenital hip problem. (1) (PE; AS; PA; SK)
1 Flexion of extremities is the normal position for a young infant.
2 This is a normal finding in a young infant.
4 Same as answer 2.

163. 3 This is the basis for abduction devices and spica casts when the infant is very young. (1) (PE; AN; PA; SK)
1 This may be true, but the easy moldability of the bones at this age favors corrective devices.
2 Congenital hip dysplasia usually is not painful and does not limit ambulation for the young child.
4 This is incidental; other forms of traction can be used if necessary.

164. 1 This position promotes hip abduction and flexion. (1) (PE; PL; ED; SK)
2 This practice limits hip abduction and puts stress on the hip joint; if mild dysplasia is present, it will be aggravated.
3 Same as answer 2.
4 This allows free movement in the flexed position but does not promote abduction.

165. 4 This is the preferred method of protecting the cast from soiling by excreta. (2) (PE; PL; ED; SK)
1 Special precautions are definitely required to keep the cast clean.
2 Plaster needs to "breathe" and should not be completely covered with occlusive material.
3 They should not be used together because clumping of powder, with resultant irritation, may occur.

166. 3 The palms will not damage the cast; using fingertips on a wet cast may leave impressions and alter the configuration of the cast. (1) (PE; IM; TC; SK)
1 The child may get burned with a hair dryer; also, the outside of the cast dries, leaving the inside wet and weakened; the cast should be permitted to air dry.

2 The crossbar of a spica cast functions only as an abduction bar; it may break if used for turning.
4 The child must be turned every 2 hours.

167. 2 Priority care for any cast application includes checking the color and the temperature of the area surrounding the cast; this ensures that the cast is not too tight, impairing circulation. (1) (PE; PL; TC; SK)
1 The child has had general anesthesia; fluid will be given later to avoid any vomiting and aspiration.
3 This is important, but priority intervention in the immediate postoperative period is checking circulation.
4 If a trapeze is to be used, this teaching would have been done preoperatively or delayed until the child is stabilized and the cast is dry.

168. 2 This may be indicative of an infection under the cast and would probably cause a fever. (1) (PE; EV; TC; SK)
1 Respirations may increase but do not become irregular with a fever.
3 This would not cause a fever; it may indicate neurovascular impairment.
4 This would not cause a fever.

169. 2 Alcohol is a drying agent; it may temporarily diminish the stimulation of the itchy areas and inhibit the release of histamine. (2) (PE; EV; ED; SK)
1 Scratching stimulates release of histamine, which makes the area more itchy; scratching may also break the skin and open up an avenue for infection.
3 Antihistamines are generally not given unless all other measures fail.
4 Powder may become caked, slip under the cast, and cause additional discomfort.

170. 1 The child should be rolled as one unit, with shoulders and hips turned at the same time to prevent injury. (1) (PE; IM; ED; SK)
2 The crossbar is not used to turn because it may dislodge and weaken the cast.
3 This would be used for lifting, not turning.
4 The child will not be able to sit up because the cast immobilizes the hips.

NEUROMUSCULAR

171. 2 Children with cerebral palsy are especially prone to muscle tone disorders, including spasticity, which can lead to contractures. (1) (PE; PL; PA; NM)

1 The therapy program must be balanced to promote progress in all areas of growth and development.

3 This is contraindicated because prolonged immobility promotes the development of contractures.

4 In a therapeutic regimen there must be a balance between exercise and rest.

172. 1 Duchenne's muscular dystrophy follows an X-linked recessive inheritance pattern; when the father is unaffected and the mother is a carrier, there is a 50% chance that a son will be affected and there is a 25% chance that a daughter will be affected. (3) (PE; EV; PA; NM)

2 Sex-linked transmission rarely results in females with the condition; males are predominantly affected and females tend to be carriers.

3 This sex-linked condition is transmitted from the recessive gene carried by the mother only.

4 When the father is unaffected and the mother is a carrier, each son has a 50% chance of being affected.

173. 1 Range of motion exercises are essential to help achieve the primary objectives of maintaining optimal muscle function as long as possible and preventing the development of contractures. (1) (PE; IM; ED; NM)

2 A high caloric diet may result in obesity which may accelerate the time when a wheelchair will be necessary.

3 Seizures are not usually associated with Duchenne's muscular dystrophy.

4 Restricting the use of large muscles may result in disuse atrophy and contractures.

174. 4 Muscular degeneration is advanced in the adolescent; the disease process involves the diaphragm; auxiliary muscles of respiration, and the heart resulting in life threatening respiratory infections and heart failure. (3) (PE; AN; PA; NM)

1 Nutritional problems are less of a priority when compared to cardiopulmonary problems.

2 Central nervous system functioning is not affected by Duchenne's muscular dystrophy.

3 Although the musculoskeletal system will exhibit marked degeneration, it is second in priority to the cardiopulmonary changes.

175. 1 Down's syndrome (Trisomy 21) results from an extra chromosome 21. (1) (PE; AN; PA; NM)

2 Down's syndrome is not infectious in origin.

3 Down's syndrome is not related to an X-linked or Y-linked chromosome.

4 This is not a cause of Down's syndrome, although translocation of chromosomes 15 and 21 or 22 is a genetic aberration found in 4% to 6% of the children with Down's syndrome.

176. 3 Forty percent of the children with Down's syndrome have cardiac anomalies. (2) (PE; AN; PA; NM)

1 This is not a characteristic finding in children with Down's syndrome.

2 Same as answer 1.

4 Same as answer 1.

177. 3 Children who are mentally retarded can learn concrete concepts faster than they can learn abstract concepts. (1) (PE; AN; ED; NM)

1 This is an abstract concept that a child begins to learn between the ages of 7 to 11 years.

2 Same as answer 1.

4 Same as answer 1.

178. 1 This prevents placing undue emphasis on the speech pattern, thus preventing inadvertent reinforcement of the pattern. (3) (PE; IM; ED; NM)
2 This is demeaning; it may decrease self-esteem and increase stuttering.
3 Same as answer 2.
4 Same as answer 2.

179. 4 Erb's palsy results from forces that alter the normal position and relationship of the arm, shoulder, and neck; stretching or pulling away of the shoulder from the head during delivery damages the brachial plexus. (3) (PE; AN; PA; NM)
1 Erb's palsy is a birth injury that is acquired during delivery, not in utero.
2 Erb's palsy is a birth injury; it is not an X-linked inherited disease.
3 Erb's palsy is a birth injury involving the brachial plexus, not a tumor.

180. 4 The nerves that have been stretched normally take about 3 months to recover from the trauma sustained during delivery. (3) (PE; EV; PA; NM)
1 The paralysis is not progressive and the prognosis is usually excellent.
2 This is unnecessary; passive range of motion and intermittent splinting performed by a family member is all that is necessary; recovery usually occurs in 3 months.
3 Intermittent splinting and passive range of motion are all that is required; only in rare instances when avulsion of the nerves results in permanent damage is orthopedic or surgical intervention necessary.

181. 2 Lead blocks formation of normal RBCs because it is very toxic to the biosynthesis of heme; this leads to anemia, an initial sign of the disease. (2) (PE; AN; PA; NM)
1 This does not occur; the child usually has anemia and some CNS disturbances.
3 Same as answer 1.
4 Same as answer 1.

182. 4 This is related to lead toxicity or buildup that causes fluid shifts into brain tissue, producing cell ischemia and destruction; this ultimately results in convulsions, mental retardation, and death. (2) (PE; AN; PA; NM)
1 Although abdominal cramps and headache may be symptoms of chronic lead poisoning, these are not the primary problems as lead poisoning progresses and central nervous system symptoms appear.
2 The child is not necessarily malnourished; the child usually eats the paint or plaster chips containing lead (pica) in addition to the diet.
3 This is not related to this disorder; it is related to hemianopia or hemiparesis.

183. 1 This position utilizes gravity to drain fluid from the head and prevent fluid accumulation. (1) (PE; IM; TC; NM)
2 The semi-Fowler's position has no effect on chemicals, but it does reduce subdural pressure.
3 This is true, but it is primarily done to prevent cerebral edema.
4 Cardiac workload is not reduced in the semi-Fowler's position, but it is in the supine position; the semi-Fowler's position does facilitate oxygenation.

184. 3 Pressure on the hypothalamus, the temperature-regulating mechanism of the brain, causes temperature imbalances. (2) (PE; AN; PA; NM)
1 After an operation, a temperature from the inflammatory response rarely exceeds 101°F; this temperature is not slight.
2 This is not true when aseptic technique is observed.
4 These would not cause such a high temperature unless infection were present.

185. 2 A defective development of the spinal cord resulting in lower extremity paralysis is found only in myelomeningocele. (3) (PE; AN; PA; NM)

1 Hydrocephalus results from associated ventricular abnormalities and can occur with either defect.

3 A saclike cyst containing meninges and spinal fluid may be present in either defect.

4 Infection is possible with either defect because of the exposure of the meninges.

186. 1 This sign is indicative of increased intracranial pressure, which is caused by the fluid accumulation associated with hydrocephalus. (1) (PE; AS; PA; NM)

2 This is a normal finding; conjugate gaze does not occur until 3 to 4 months of age when eye muscles are mature.

3 This is a normal finding; a baby does not do this before 1 to $1\frac{1}{2}$ months of age.

4 This is a normal finding; the head is the largest part of the body at this age.

187. 3 Because the infant cannot be readily held, tactile stimulation meets the infant's needs and fosters bonding with the parents. (1) (PE; IM; PS; NM)

1 An infant with an unrepaired myelomeningocele cannot be held in the arms.

2 Demonstration of feeding techniques is helpful, but may not improve parent-child relationships.

4 This intervention will be more beneficial at a later time.

188. 1 This will avoid sudden increases in intracranial pressure. (2) (PE; PL; TC; NM)

2 This is inappropriate; it may be frightening for the parents.

3 Young infants, especially with this health problem, tolerate a demand schedule better, and it may diminish the possibility of vomiting.

4 This is inappropriate for a 1-month-old infant.

189. 4 The side-lying position and use of supports prevent pressure on the valve, which is on the right side; the flat position prevents too rapid drainage of cerebrospinal fluid. (3) (PE; EV; ED; NM)

1 This is inappropriate in the immediate postoperative period; the infant should be kept flat.

2 Neck supports should not be used with infants; they may cause airway occlusion.

3 The support could push the head to the right and exert pressure on the valve, which is on the right side, possibly causing it to close; this would heighten the risk of increased intracranial pressure.

190. 3 Leakage of cerebrospinal fluid indicates incomplete closure of the defect. (1) (PE; PL; TC; NM)

1 The supine position places too much pressure on the operative site.

2 Moist dressings are applied preoperatively to prevent drying out of the sac.

4 Teaching clean catheterization is not appropriate at this time.

191. 3 This may help to reduce the infant's temperature; chilling should be avoided. (2) (PE; IM; TC; NM)

1 Alcohol should never be used with infants or children; it causes severe chilling, which can lead to increased metabolic activity and a higher temperature.

2 This fever requires more frequent readings than every 2 hours.

4 This is not a priority; temperature reduction should be done first; recording can be done later.

192. 3 A bulging fontanel is the most significant sign of increased intracranial pressure in an infant. (3) (PE; EV; TC, NM)

1 This is not a significant indicator of increased intracranial pressure.

2 Same as answer 1.

4 Same as answer 1.

193. 3 Shortened attention span and fussy behavior may indicate a change in intracranial pressure and/or shunt malfunction. (2) (PE; EV; ED; NM)
1 This is normal behavior for a 2½ year old.
2 Same as answer 1.
4 Same as answer 1.

194. 1 Placing the child flat would prevent complications from a too rapid reduction of intracranial fluid; placing the child on the unoperated side would avoid pressure on the shunt valve. (3) (PE; IM; TC; NM)
2 This is contraindicated; placing the child on the affected side would put pressure on the shunt valve which could cause it to become obstructed interfering with the outflow of cerebral spinal fluid.
3 This is contraindicated; raising the head of the bed would allow too rapid a reduction in cerebral spinal fluid which may cause the cerebral cortex to pull away from the dura resulting in a subdural hematoma; placing the child on the affected side would put pressure on the shunt valve.
4 This is contraindicated; elevating the head would permit too rapid a reduction in cerebral spinal fluid.

195. 4 Cranial radiation destroys leukemic cells in the brain because chemotherapeutic agents are poorly absorbed through the blood-brain barrier. (3) (PE; AN; TC; NM)
1 This is not the primary reason for the treatment; it is a curative measure.
2 This is not the reason for cranial radiation.
3 This is inaccurate; ALL is an abnormality of the bone marrow and lymphatic system.

196. 4 Safety is the priority during the seizure. (2) (PE; IM; TC; NM)
1 It would be unsafe to leave the child having the seizure.
2 Attempting to open clenched jaws could result in injury to the child's teeth and jaw.
3 This may cause airway occlusion by forcing the neck onto the chin; a small flat blanket is more effective.

197. 3 The child's status and the progression of the seizure should be monitored; the child will not breathe until the seizure is over and cyanosis should subside at that time. (1) (PE; IM; TC; NM)
1 Attempting to open clenched jaws could result in injury to the child.
2 Oxygen will be useless until the child breathes when the seizure is over.
4 The physician can be notified later; provision of safety and observation are the priorities.

198. 2 Raising the foot of the bed would increase blood flow to the brain and increase intracranial pressure. (2) (PE; PL; PA; NM)
1 Temperature elevations are expected after a craniotomy due to stimulation of the hypothalamus.
3 Fluids should be monitored closely to reduce the possibility of cerebral edema.
4 Vital signs are a major component of the neurological check.

199. 3 This is one of the most prevalent diseases in young children; approximately 70% have otitis media at least once, and one third of the children under the age of 3 have had at least three episodes. (1) (PE; AN; PA; NM)
1 This is not the causative agent.
2 Same as answer 1.
4 Same as answer 1.

200. 1 The incision allows for drainage, which produces relief of pressure and results in immediate relief of pain. (2) (PE; IM; ED; NM)
2 This incision does not leave any scar because healing by primary intention occurs within 24 hours.
3 A myringotomy is performed to prevent the trauma of perforation.
4 This incision is very small and heals spontaneously within 24 hours.

201. 4 Movement by the child will impede the procedure and may cause additional injuries to the surrounding structures. (2) (PE; IM; TC; NM)
1 This is not essential to the accomplishment of the procedure.
2 The child should have had the local anesthetic applied before the procedure.
3 This will not guarantee that the child will keep still during the procedure.

202. 2 This position facilitates drainage by gravity. (1) (PE; IM; ED; NM)
1 This position will not allow for proper drainage.
3 This position will promote pooling of drainage in the operative site and may lead to reinfection.
4 This is rare and should not occur from this tiny incision.

203. 3 These may indicate the need for a repeat myringotomy because of ineffective drainage. (2) (PE; EV; TC; NM)
1 Bleeding is not seen in otitis media or after a myringotomy.
2 This is characteristic of otitis media and does not indicate a complication.
4 These are not expected complications of a myringotomy.

204. 1 This precaution reduces the transmission of infection from client to client (cross-infection). (1) (PE; AN; TC; NM)
2 The act of isolation has no effect on the infectious process.
3 This is protective (reverse) isolation; it is not used for infectious clients but rather to protect clients with lowered resistance, for example, clients receiving chemotherapy.
4 Thorough hand washing and careful aseptic technique limit nosocomial infections.

205. 3 Strict isolation requires a protective gown, gloves, and a mask for all persons entering the room. (1) (PE; EV; ED; NM)
1 This is inadequate; a mask and gloves are also required.
2 This is inadequate; a gown, a mask, and gloves are also necessary.
4 Sterile protective garb is unnecessary; isolation is a form of medical asepsis, not surgical asepsis.

206. 4 The meningococcal organism is rendered inactive after 24 to 72 hours of antibiotic therapy; therefore isolation is required at least for this time. (2) (PE; PL; TC; NM)
1 Meningococcal meningitis is a serious contagious disease; isolation is required for at least 24 to 72 hours after beginning antibiotics.
2 Treatment with antibiotic therapy for 24 to 72 hours will render the microorganism inactive; after that, isolation is usually not required.
3 The disease is not evident in the incubation period; because the disease is undiagnosed during the incubation period, isolation would not have been instituted.

207. 2 There is a high occurrence of Reye's syndrome in children who have just recently recovered from chickenpox. (1) (PE; AS; PA; NM)
1 Reye's syndrome does not occur after rubella (German measles).
3 Reye's syndrome is associated with viral, not bacterial, illnesses.
4 Same as answer 3.

208. 4 These are some of the symptoms that bring the child to the hospital; they reflect central nervous system involvement. (2) (PE; AS; PA; NM)
1 There is no rash or diarrhea with Reye's syndrome.
2 These are not early symptoms; these may occur later in the disease.
3 The fever is usually high.

209. 3 These children are critically ill and need the constant supervision available in an intensive care unit. (1) (PE; IM; TC; NM)
1 Reye's syndrome is not contagious.
2 Surgery is not a treatment used in Reye's syndrome.
4 These children are critically ill and need intensive nursing care.

210. 4 Reye's syndrome affects the liver, causing problems with blood coagulation because the liver-dependent clotting factors such as prothrombin are diminished. (3) (PE; AS; PA; NM)
1 Liver, not bladder, function is impaired.

2   There is no rash with Reye's syndrome.

3   The liver, not the kidneys, is involved in Reye's syndrome.

211. 4   Reye's syndrome is associated with viral infections, such as influenza or varicella, and frequently follows the ingestion of aspirin during the prodromal stage of these diseases. (1) (PE; IM; ED; NM)

1   Alcohol sponge baths are never used with children; the temperature may be decreased too quickly and this may shock the child; in addition, a fever of 101°F is not high enough for sponge bathing.

2   There is no inoculation against Reye's syndrome.

3   The child's metabolism is increased during illness; the child should have a high caloric intake.

ENDOCRINE

212. 1   Most juveniles are insulin-dependent diabetics and have little or no endogenous insulin; dietary control and exercise reduce the amount of exogenous insulin needed. (2) (PE; PL; PA; EN)

2   Those having insulin-dependent diabetes have little or no endogenous insulin and need exogenous insulin; this regimen is for non-insulin dependent diabetics; blood glucose monitoring is usually used.

3   Those having insulin-dependent diabetes need insulin for control because of a lack of endogenous insulin.

4   Oral hypoglycemics are ineffective in stimulating insulin secretion in clients having insulin-dependent diabetes because they have no endogenous insulin.

213. 2   Negotiation of goals precedes and is essential to successful learning; mutual goal setting provides a focus for learning. (3) (PE; AN; ED; EN)

1   A rapport should already be developed before beginning the teaching-learning process.

3   If the client does not identify this need or set this as a goal, there will probably be little motivation to learn this task.

4   Same as answer 3.

214. 1   Because paresthesias may be present and circulation may be compromised, adequate inspection of the feet is necessary and is the quickest and easiest measure to identify pressure sites and prevent infection. (1) (PE; IM; ED; EN)

2   Hot water should never be used because it can cause injury by burning the skin.

3   The feet should be patted dry, not rubbed vigorously; rubbing can cause abrasion and injure the skin.

4   Strong antiseptics are too harsh and should not be used because they can cause injury to the skin.

215. 1   Urine testing is primarily helpful in detecting ketones, which are most likely to be present during illness and hyperglycemia. (3) (PE; AN; ED; EN)

2   Because of the complexity of the medical regimen and the variety of factors that influence serum glucose levels, such as food ingested, exercise, medications, and the stresses of growth and development, serum glucose levels in children can fluctuate and should therefore be measured by monitoring the serum glucose levels before meals and at bedtime.

3   Blood, not urine, is the best specimen to be tested for determining glucose levels.

4   The opposite is true.

216. 4   The glycosylated hemoglobin (GHb) test provides an accurate long-term index of the client's average blood glucose level for the 100- to 120-day period before the test; the more glucose the RBC was exposed to the greater the GHb percentage; the test result is not affected by short-term variations. (3) (PE; AS; PA; EN)

1   The presence of ketones in the urine may indicate only short-term variations and extreme hyperglycemia.

2   Serum protein levels do not reflect the effectiveness of glucose management in diabetes mellitus.

3   Serum glucose levels reflect short-term (hours) variations.

217. 3 The stress of surgery causes the release of epinephrine and glucocorticoids, which raise blood glucose levels. (2) (PE; AN; PA; EN)

1 Urine test results are affected by many variables such as renal threshold, so they are not accurate enough when control is precarious; serum glucose levels are preferred.

2 Hypoglycemia can result because the client has taken nothing by mouth and body fluids are being lost.

4 Most clients with diabetes mellitus who are diet controlled require insulin for a short period after surgery, especially when receiving IV glucose; most children have insulin-dependent diabetes mellitus.

218. 1 Humulin N (NPH) insulin peaks in 8 to 12 hours; a bedtime snack will prevent hypoglycemia during the night. (1) (PE; PL; TC; EN)

2 This is unsafe because it would intensify the hyperglycemia; if hyperglycemia is present the child needs insulin.

3 When hypoglycemia develops the child will be asleep; the snack should be eaten before going to bed.

4 Humulin N (NPH) insulin is an intermediate, not a long-acting insulin for which bedtime snacks are recommended.

219. 4 Frequent episodes of hypoglycemia result from difficulty in balancing food, exercise, and insulin in active children. (1) (PE; AN; PA; EN)

1 The people associated with the school who are interacting with the child need to know about the child's condition but should be asked to keep the information confidential.

2 With increased activity the child will experience episodes of hypoglycemia, not hyperglycemia.

3 This would be a form of discrimination; the child with diabetes mellitus should be allowed to engage in activities as long as the diabetes remains under control.

220. 2 A quick check of the blood glucose level will confirm if the client is hypoglycemic. (2) (PE; AS; TC; EN)

1 This is inaccurate and does not reflect the present status.

3 Although this might be appropriate to counter hypoglycemia, it does not determine if the client is hypoglycemic or is manipulating.

4 Would not elicit enough data.

221. 3 The client's trouble stems from perceptual difficulties; the preset syringe removes the need to differentiate between 24 and 42 units. (2) (PE; PL; TC; EN)

1 This would not solve the transposition of the numbers; the problem is not caused by the inability to see the numbers but by the child's perception of them.

2 This would not solve the transposition of the numbers.

4 Same as answer 2.

222. 4 Humulin N insulin is an intermediate-acting insulin that peaks approximately 6 to 8 hours after administration. (1) (PE; AN; TC; EN)

1 This is the time when a reaction from a long-acting insulin could be expected.

2 This is the time when a reaction from a short-acting insulin could be expected.

3 Same as answer 2.

223. 2 These are the most common signs of hypoglycemia in children. (2) (PE; AS; PA; EN)

1 These are signs of hyperglycemia.

3 Same as answer 1.

4 Same as answer 1.

224. 1 Proper hand washing is the best infection-prevention technique and should always precede preparation of an injection. (1) (PE; PL; ED; EN)

2 Shaking causes air bubbles, which can interfere with preparing the dosage accurately; the bottle should be gently rotated.

3 The injection site should not be rubbed because this affects absorption of the insulin and also causes reactions at the site.

4 The abdomen, not the upper extremities, is the preferred site for self-administration of insulin; sites should be rotated.

225. 2 The child's confidence, readiness, and skill for giving self injections is essential for long-term management of diabetes. (3) (PE; PL; ED; EN)

1 The sites must be rotated at all times.

3 Learning responsibility for injections should be a gradual process with continuous support and guidance.

4 The recommended procedure is to draw up the Humulin R insulin first and then the Humulin N insulin to prevent contamination of the multidose vial of Humulin R by the intermediate-acting Humulin N.

226. 2 Insulin causes potassium to move into the cells along with glucose, thus lowering the serum potassium level. (3) (PE; PL; TC; EN)

1 Insulin does not lead to reduced blood volume.

3 Insulin does not directly alter sodium levels.

4 Insulin does not affect calcium mobilization.

227. 2 This is an attempt by the respiratory system to eliminate the excess carbon dioxide; it is a characteristic compensatory mechanism of metabolic acidosis. (1) (PE; AS; PA; EN)

1 An increased temperature will only occur if an infection is present.

3 Tachycardia, not bradycardia, results from the hypovolemia of dehydration.

4 Hypotension, not hypertension, may result from decreased vascular volume.

228. 4 Normoglycemia decreases the chances of developing long-term complications such as neuropathy, retinopathy, and atherosclerosis. (2) (PE; AN; TC; EN)

1 Blood glucose levels are more accurate than urine glucose levels; this is an unrealistic goal.

2 This is only one part of the regimen; this would be both a short- and a long-term goal.

3 Stress is difficult to control, particularly in the adolescent; a nonstressful life-style would be utopia.

RESPIRATORY

229. 1 Capillary beds are closest to the surface in a finger or earlobe; this proximity allows for more accurate measurement of the arterial oxygen saturation. (1) (PE; IM; TC; CV)

2 The pulse oximeter requires no routine calibration.

3 Capillary beds are closest to the surface in a finger, toe, or earlobe and not on the abdomen or upper thigh.

4 An almost instantaneous accurate readout can be obtained with the pulse oximeter.

230. 1 The medulla oblongata contains the respiratory center, and the neurons that supply the respiratory muscles originate here; they produce the rhythmic pattern of inspiration and expiration. (2) (PE; AN; PA; RE)

2 This is concerned with the control of skeletal muscles.

3 This links the nervous system to the endocrine system and functions as a relay station between the cerebral cortex and the lower autonomic centers.

4 This is unrelated to respirations; this is the thin surface layer of the cerebrum.

231. 1 The gag reflex is elicited by pressing on the posterior pharynx resulting in glossopharyngeal stimulation; inserting the tongue blade on the side of the mouth avoids this stimulation. (1) (PE; IM; TC; RE)

2 Although this is important, it is not the reason for inserting the tongue blade on the side of the tongue.

3 Same as answer 2.

4 Same as answer 2.

232. 3 Orthopnea is shortness of breath in any position but the erect sitting or standing position. (2) (PE; AS; PA; RE)

1 This is a temporary cessation of breathing.

2 This is labored or difficult breathing regardless of the position.

4 This is an increased respiratory rate, not shortness of breath.

233. 3 Because of the drying nature of oxygen, most oxygen is humidified before it is administered. (2) (PE; PL; PA; RE)

1 Oxygen is combustible and supports fire; it does not ignite; it is not flammable.

2 Oxygen is not warmed before administration; it is cool on administration.

4 Oxygen is considered a drug and therefore must be prescribed.

234. 3 This reply addresses the client's concern; CNS depressant effects may diminish or spontaneously disappear after several days. (2) (PE; IM; ED; RE)

1 Administration of medication is a dependent function of the nurse, and the nurse has no legal authority to tell the client to alter the dose.

2 Administration of medication is a dependent function of the nurse, and the nurse has no legal authority to tell the client to omit a dose.

4 This is unnecessary because the side effect of drowsiness should diminish in several days; the client needs teaching about the drug.

235. 3 Antibiotics should be administered with doses equally spaced over 24 hours so that a constant blood level of the drug is maintained. (2) (PE; IM; TC; RE)

1 The twelve hours between the 8 PM and 8 AM doses is too long; the blood level of the drug will drop and the therapy will not be effective.

2 Doses are not equally spaced over 24 hours and the blood level of the drug will not remain constant.

4 Same as answer 2.

236. 2 When performing pulse oximetry on a child or an adult, the index finger is generally used because the probe is easy to apply and an accurate reading can be obtained. (1) (PE; AS; PA; RE)

1 The great toes of most 10-year-olds are too large for the probe; the great toes of infants are used for monitoring pulse oximetry

3 The probe must be placed on tissue away from a pulse point; pulsatile blood flow is the primary physiologic factor that influences accuracy of the pulse oximeter.

4 Same as answer 3.

237. 3 The infectious and mechanical changes narrow the bronchial passages and make it difficult for air to leave the lungs. (2) (PE; AS; PA; RE)

1 As a result of increased respiratory effort and decreased oxygen exchange, tachycardia may develop.

2 Breath sounds may be diminished because of the swelling of the bronchiolar mucosa and filling of the lumina with mucus and exudate.

4 Intercostal retractions are unlikely because of the overinflation of the chest with air and the shallow, rapid breathing.

238. 1 Adequate hydration and high humidity are essential to loosen tenacious secretions and minimize fluid loss. (1) (PE; PL; TC; RE)

2 Corticosteroids are not used because they have not proved effective.

3 Bronchodilators are not used because the bronchial tree is not in spasm.

4 Antibiotics are ineffectual because the etiologic agent is viral.

239. 3 The infant is having difficulty with breathing; disturbing the infant frequently causes an excessive expenditure of energy and increases oxygen demands. (2) (PE; AN; TC; RE)

1 Constant observation, not constant physical disturbance, is important; the infant needs to rest to minimize oxygen demands.

2 Cool mist helps to liquify secretions and keeps the temperature down; cool mist does not maintain hydration.

4 Too frequent auscultation will disturb the infant's rest, causing an excessive expenditure of energy and increased oxygen demands.

240. 2 These observations are vital to assess the child's hydration status. (2) (PE; AS; TC; RE)

1 The child is too ill to be involved in stimulating activities; energy should be conserved and oxygen demands kept at a minimum.

3 The child needs the parents to limit separation anxiety.

4 Strict isolation is not required although a gown may be worn; cap, mask, and gloves are not required.

241. 1 This is below the normal range of 7.35 to 7.45; hypoxia causes hypercapnia, resulting in a fall in the pH. (3) (PE; AS; PA; RE)

2 This is within the normal range of 80 to 100 mmHg.

3   This is within the normal range of 21 to 28 mEq/L.

4   This is within the normal range of 35 to 45 mmHg.

242. 3   Positioning on the side permits flow of oral secretions that could block the child's airway; a patent airway takes precedence; if the client is not able to take air in, all other measures are futile. (1) (PE; AN; TC; RE)

1   This becomes important after a patent airway is established; the client can receive tepid or cool liquids.

2   After airway patency is established, deep breathing can be encouraged; coughing is contraindicated because it could dislodge a clot.

4   Airway patency is of primary importance.

243. 2   Cold liquid promotes vasoconstriction, decreases bleeding, and limits pain. (1) (PE; IM; TC; RE)

1   Ice cream has a milk component which increases the viscosity of mucus.

3   Milk increases the viscosity of mucus.

4   Orange juice will irritate inflamed tissue.

244. 4   With few exceptions males are sterile; failure of normal development of the Wolffian duct structures (vas deferens, epididymis, and seminal vesicles) and blockage of the vas deferens by abnormal secretions result in decreased or absent sperm production. (3) (PE; IM; ED; RG)

1   This does not answer the client's question.

2   Females with CF generally have normal ovaries and fallopian tubes and are fertile; however, fertility can be inhibited by highly viscous cervical secretions.

3   Theoretically, all offspring of couples who are homozygous for a recessive gene will have the disease; however with cystic fibrosis, affected men are usually sterile.

245. 3   This test establishes genotype with the lowest margin of error. (3) (PE; EV; ED; RE)

1   The results of this test will not determine if the individual is a carrier of CF; this may be part of the testing that is conducted when a client is suspected of having CF.

2   The results of these tests will not determine if the individual is a carrier of CF; these may be part of the testing that is conducted when a client is suspected of having CF.

4   Same as answer 2.

246. 4   Cystic fibrosis is a genetic disorder affecting all mucus-secreting (exocrine) glands. (2) (PE; AN; PA; RE)

1   Exocrine glands, not sweat glands (epocrine glands), are involved with cystic fibrosis; children with cystic fibrosis lose excessive amounts of sodium via perspiration.

2   Exocrine, not endocrine, glands are involved in cystic fibrosis.

3   Cilia are not involved in cystic fibrosis.

247. 4   Dysfunction of the exocrine glands leads to an abnormal accumulation of thick mucus, a slower flow rate of mucus, and incomplete expectoration of mucus, all of which contribute to airway obstruction. (1) (PE; AN; PA; RE)

1   This is associated with pneumonia.

2   This is associated with asthma.

3   The endocrine glands are not affected in cystic fibrosis.

248. 1   Males with cystic fibrosis are sterile; therefore the father does not have cystic fibrosis but he could be a carrier; if both parents are heterozygous carriers, the chance of having a child with CF is 25%; when one parent is a heterozygous carrier and the other has 2 normal genes, the chance of having a child that has CF is 0% but the chance of having a child that is a carrier is 50%. (3) (PE; AS; PA; RE)

2   If both parents are heterozygous carriers or if one parent is a heterozygous carrier and one parent has 2 normal genes, the chance of having a child that is a carrier, not a child that is affected, is 50%.

3   This is an inaccurate conclusion when the father's genotype is unknown.

4   With the data provided, the mother is a heterozygous carrier and the father is either a heterozygous carrier or has 2 normal genes; under these circumstances, it is safe to conclude that the chance that their baby will have CF is 25% or less.

249. 4 Because of a failure of normal development of the vas deferens, epididymis, and seminal vesicles and a blockage of the vas deferens with abnormal secretions, there is decreased or absent sperm production. (3) (PE; AN; ED; RE)

1 This is not true; most men with cystic fibrosis are sterile.

2 Cystic fibrosis is inherited as an autosomal-recessive trait; it is not sex linked.

3 Same as answer 1.

250. 2 The chest is barrel-shaped because of the protrusion of abdominal viscera through the defect into the thoracic cavity. (3) (PE; AS; PA; RE)

1 This is not associated with a diaphragmatic hernia; assessments related to the bowel include colicky pain and constipation.

3 There are no breath sounds over the abdomen and there are diminished or an absence of breath sounds on the affected side of the thorax; bowel sounds may be auscultated over the affected thorax.

4 The abdomen is markedly scaphoid (sunken).

251. 2 The presence of abdominal viscera in the thoracic cavity impinges on the lungs limiting the amount of air that can enter. (3) (PE; AN; PA; RE)

1 A medical diagnosis cannot be used as part of a nursing diagnosis.

3 There are no excessive secretions with a diaphragmatic hernia.

4 The basal metabolic rate is not increased with a diaphragmatic hernia.

252. 4 Placing the infant on the operative side promotes gas exchange in the unimpaired lung. (3) (PE; IM; PA; RE)

1 This would not maximally promote aeration of the unaffected lung.

2 Same as answer 1.

3 This would not maximally promote aeration of the unaffected lung; the prone position increases the effort of breathing because respiratory excursion is impeded by the weight of the body.

253. 3 Bilateral lung sounds indicate that the hypoplastic lung has begun functioning. (3) (PE; AS; PA; RE)

1 This is not a reliable indicator that the respiratory status is improving; it could actually indicate that the infant is hypoxic and too fatigued to cry.

2 A normal pH is 7.35 to 7.45; a decreasing pH indicates respiratory acidosis which can be attributed to decreased gas exchange.

4 Retention of formula is unrelated to gas exchange.

254. 3 Maintenance of a patent airway is always the priority. (2) (PE; IM; TC; RE)

1 An IV can be started later; suctioning to ensure airway patency is the priority.

2 The primary focus now is to establish breathing; the child has a pulse of 50, which can be addressed later.

4 The ICU can be called once the child's vital signs are stabilized and a patent airway is ensured.

255. 1 The degree of the hypoxia and asphyxia the child had will determine the extent of the neurologic, liver, and renal damage. (3) (PE; AN; PA; RE)

2 The child is hypothermic, not hyperthermic.

3 Although emotional trauma can be all encompassing, it usually does not influence the ultimate physical prognosis as does hypoxia.

4 Although initially severe, aspiration pneumonia does not result in long-term sequelae as does hypoxia.

256. 3 The chest was opened during surgery for the sternal repair, and air was allowed into the thorax; the air must be removed for the lungs to expand properly. (2) (PE; IM; ED; RE)

1 The chest tube is unrelated to the baby's ability to retain feedings.

2 Chest tubes are uncomfortable; also, this response discounts the importance of the chest tube to the baby's respiratory status.

4 The baby did not have a punctured lung.

CARDIOVASCULAR

257. 4 A discrepancy in blood pressures from the arms to the legs indicates a vascular stenosis. (2) (PE; AS; PA; CV)

1 Projectile vomiting results from a gastrointestinal problem and is usually not manifested immediately after birth.

2 An irregular respiratory rhythm is common and expected in the newborn.

3 Hyperreflexia of the extremities may be indicative of a neurological problem.

258. 4 During a bowel movement the Valsalva maneuver can occasionally initiate a hypercyanotic spell (tet spell, blue spell); the Valsalva maneuver causes increased intrathoracic pressure, slowing of the pulse, decreased return of blood to the heart, and increased venous pressure. (3) (PE; AN; PA; CV)

1 This would not influence cardiovascular functioning.

2 Same as answer 1.

3 Same as answer 1.

259. 2 A positive antistreptolysin titer is present with rheumatic fever because of previous infection with streptococci. (3) (PE; AN; PA; CV)

1 A positive, not a negative, C-reactive protein would be present; this is indicative of an inflammatory process.

3 This is usually related to a decrease in mature RBCs caused by hemorrhage or other blood diseases; it is unrelated to an infectious or inflammatory process.

4 The ESR would be elevated, not decreased, indicating the presence of an inflammatory process.

260. 2 A cardiac catheterization will identify the exact location of the ventricular septal defect as well as assess pulmonary pressures. (1) (PE; AN; PA; CV)

1 This is demonstrated by electrocardiographic and echocardiographic examinations.

3 Murmurs can be heard with a stethoscope placed at the left lower sternal border.

4 Same as answer 1.

261. 1 Children are kept on complete bedrest after a cardiac catheterization to reduce the risk of bleeding or trauma to the insertion site; the order for bathroom privileges should be questioned. (3) (PE; EV; TC; CV)

2 This is an expected part of post catheterization care; a pressure dressing is placed over the insertion site to reduce the possibility of bleeding.

3 This urinary output is within acceptable limits; the child was kept npo before and during the procedure; after the procedure oral fluids need to be encouraged to promote hydration and voiding.

4 Frequent blood pressure checks are part of routine post catheterization care.

262. 1 The catheter insertion site should not be submerged in water; sponge baths limit trauma and infection at the insertion site. (1) (PE; IM; ED; CV)

2 This is contraindicated; ice will cause vasoconstriction and could compromise circulation.

3 Fluids should be encouraged to enhance excretion of the contrast media used during the procedure.

4 The child is not sent home with a pressure dressing.

263. 1 The body responds to the chronic hypoxia caused by the heart defect by increasing the production of red blood cells in an attempt to increase the oxygen carrying capacity of the blood. (3) (PE; AS; PA; CV)

2 This does not result from hypoxia, it occurs in disease processes where the WBCs drop to very low levels and neutropenia becomes pronounced.

3 Thrombocytopenia (low platelet production) does not result from hypoxia; it occurs in disease processes where platelet production is suppressed, as in leukemia.

4 The hematocrit would be elevated because the body increases the production of red blood cells in an attempt to make more cells available to carry oxygen.

264. 2 Small frequent feedings with adequate rest periods in between may improve the child's intake at each feeding; these children become extremely fatigued while sucking. (2) (PE; PL; PA; CV)
1 To reduce cardiac workload, fluids are usually not forced and may sometimes be restricted in clients with congestive heart failure.
3 The head circumference is not a parameter in congenital heart disease; head measurement would be done when infants have hydrocephaly.
4 Positioning with the head elevated facilitates ease in respiration; placing the infant flat on the stomach restricts lung expansion.

265. 2 This defect causes blood to bypass the lungs; surgery increases blood flow to the lungs. (3) (PE; AN; PA; CV)
1 This would not improve the oxygen content of the blood.
3 Same as answer 1.
4 Same as answer 1.

266. 3 A calibrated dropper is the most accurate way to measure the medication. (1) (PE; IM; ED; CV)
1 This is not an accurate way to measure medication.
2 Same as answer 1.
4 If the dose of medication is diluted in 1 oz of water and the infant does not drink the entire oz, the resulting dose will be insufficient.

267. 4 Because the mechanism of CHF is the same in all children, the same basic treatment of a cardiac glycoside (digoxin) and a loop diuretic (Lasix) is used, although the dosage may vary. (1) (PE; AN; TC; CV)
1 CHF in infants is not in itself a congenital defect but results from a congenital defect of the heart.
2 This is untrue; the treatment of CHF is basically the same whether the client is an infant or a senior citizen.
3 Children can develop CHF just as adults can; if there is cardiac decompensation, the treatment is the well-established combination of digoxin and Lasix.

268. 3 The increased blood volume and pressure in the lungs resulting from left ventricular failure cause pulmonary edema; dyspnea, an early sign of failure, is probably caused by the decreased distensibility of the lungs. (3) (PE; AN; PA; CV)
1 Anemia is fairly well tolerated in infants and does not cause dyspnea.
2 Dyspnea, not hypovolemia, is an early sign of pulmonary edema; hypovolemia would cause signs of shock.
4 Respiratory, not metabolic, acidosis could develop; this occurs because of the pulmonary insufficiency resulting in retention of carbon dioxide.

269. 2 Fluid retention is reflected by an excessive weight gain in a short period of time in a child with CHF; inadequate cardiac output decreases blood flow to the kidneys, thus leading to increased intracellular fluid and hypervolemia. (1) (PE; IM; ED; CV)
1 This would be an appropriate answer if renal pathology or hypovolemia were present; however, other assessments such as hourly output, and BUN values would then also be indicated.
3 Weight gain resulting from nutritional intake is gradual and would not vary greatly on a day-to-day basis.
4 Weight is helpful in determining drug dosages but the drug dosage would not need to be recalculated daily according to weight changes.

270. 4 Compromised heart function and inadequate oxygen reserve in the infant often result in feeding problems such as cyanosis and fatigue while sucking and swallowing. (2) (PE; AN; PA; CV)
1 Poor sucking is always significant.
2 This may be true in the first days of life but is not true as the infant grows unless there is a major health problem.
3 Same as answer 2.

271. 1 Hypoxia leads to poor peripheral circulation; clubbing occurs as a result of additional capillary development and tissue hypertrophy of the fingertips. (2) (PE; AS; PA; CV)
2 Respirations will be increased.

3 The child's problems are related to decreased oxygenation, not to a clotting deficit.

4 The body attempts to compensate for the hypoxemia by increased erythropoiesis.

272. 2 This position has the same effect as squatting, which decreases venous return from the legs; the blood returning to the heart and lungs has a higher O_2 content. (1) (PE; IM; TC; CV)

1 Although this would reduce pressure of abdominal organs on the diaphragm, it does not put enough pressure on the femoral veins and vena cava to sufficiently reduce venous return to the heart.

3 This position does not reduce venous return to the heart.

4 Same as answer 1.

273. 2 Postprocedure hemorrhage is a major life-threatening complication following cardiac catheterization because arterial blood is under pressure and an artery has been entered by the catheter. (2) (PE; PL; TC; CV)

1 The child has an oxygen deficit; rest would be encouraged; flexion of the insertion site should be avoided to prevent disturbance of the clot.

3 The blood pressure should not be unstable unless a problem developed; fluids should be administered as ordered.

4 This is unnecessary; the distal pulses would be monitored.

274. 1 The vital signs must be taken first to determine the child's postoperative status and to compare them with the vital signs recorded in the recovery room. (3) (PE; AS; TC; CV)

2 Although this is important, obtaining the vital signs is the priority.

3 Same as answer 2.

4 Same as answer 2.

REPRODUCTIVE AND GENITOURINARY

275. 4 Surgery before school age reduces concerns about body image in relation to peers. (2) (PE; AN; PS; RG)

1 Malignancy may develop with or without surgical correction.

2 Maturation of testes starts about age 5; surgery should be done before maturation to prevent sterility.

3 The puboscrotal ring has nothing to do with the outcome of this surgical procedure.

276. 1 In cryptorchidism, sperm-producing abilities of the testes are destroyed, resulting in sterility. (1) (PE; AN; ED; RG)

2 This is enlargement of the scrotum with fluid; it is not related to cryptorchidism.

3 This is an abnormal dilation and tortuosity of the scrotal veins; it is not caused by undescended testicles.

4 Inflammation of the epididymis may occur whether or not cryptorchidism is corrected.

277. 1 This is the critical period of organogenesis, during which fetal development is most likely to be adversely affected. (1) (PE; IM; ED; RG)

2 The fetus is less vulnerable during this period because development is almost complete.

3 The fetus is less vulnerable to major anomalies during this period because all major organ systems are already formed.

4 At the time of implantation, cellular differentiation has not occurred; the genital bud appears in the seventh week.

278. 3 Circumcisions are never done because the foreskin may be needed for repair and reconstruction of the penis. (2) (PE; PL; ED; RG)

1 The penis does not need to be wrapped in petrolatum gauze because no surgery has been done.

2 A cystostomy tube is not inserted because there is no interference with voiding.

4 Hypospadias is not a genetic disorder although there appears to be some evidence that it may be familial.

279. 3 Arm and leg restraints are necessary to maintain the position of the urethral stent to ensure optimum healing of the newly formed urethra. (3) (PE; PL; TC; RG)
  1 Although this is important, the site must be assessed frequently and safety is the priority.
  2 There is no tension device.
  4 The indwelling catheter is never clamped because back-up pressure may disturb the suture line.

280. 3 The constant seepage of urine from the exposed ureteral orifices makes the area very susceptible to infection; infection must be prevented or controlled because an infection could ultimately lead to renal failure. (1) (PE; AN; TC; RG)
  1 This will not occur because of the constant seepage of urine.
  2 Although this could occur if the infant is not well hydrated, high risk for infection is the priority nursing diagnosis for the infant at this time.
  4 Although this could be a problem when the child reaches puberty or later, it is not the primary nursing diagnosis at this time.

281. 4 These help prevent infection and ulceration of the surrounding skin, as well as prevent the diaper from adhering to the mucosa. (3) (PE; PL; TC; RG)
  1 Seepage of urine would prevent ointments from remaining on the exposed mucosa for more than a few moments; also, ointments may irritate the mucosa and result in bleeding.
  2 Pediatric urine collectors would not adhere because of the moist environment; also, the adhesive backing would be irritating to the skin.
  3 These are contraindicated because they would increase the moisture and temperature in the area, which would enhance the growth of microorganisms and the potential for infection.

282. 3 Kinking or twisting of the tubing, which can result in an obstruction of urine flow, can be easily resolved by the parents. (1) (PE; IM; ED; RG)
  1 This is not the first action; the parents should not call the physician until they have attempted to resolve the problem.
  2 Although it is important to keep the child adequately hydrated, the patency of the tubing should be assessed first.
  4 Although this eventually may be done to assess for distention, the first action should be to determine patency of the tubing.

283. 3 In view of the smoky urine and the other symptoms, the nurse may suspect glomerulonephritis, which usually occurs after a recent streptococcal infection. (2) (PE; AS; PA; RG)
  1 This kind of pain is found in rheumatic fever, which never results in smoky-colored urine.
  2 Weight loss generally occurs with children who have developed diabetes mellitus, not glomerulonephritis.
  4 This rash would be related to scarlet fever, with which there is no smoky-colored urine.

284. 3 These tests would confirm glomerulonephritis mainly because they identify the causative organism and its pathologic effects; also, the ASO titer confirms a past presence of streptococci. (2) (PE; AN; PA; RG)
  1 A urinalysis would be done, but a chest x-ray film, a blood glucose level test, and an IVP would not confirm a diagnosis of glomerulonephritis.
  2 A urinalysis would be done, but a chest x-ray film, an electrocardiogram, and a heterophile antibody test are not specific for the symptoms described.
  4 A blood chemistry and nasopharyngeal culture may be done; an upper GI series and a 24-hour urinalysis are not specific.

285. 3 Acute hypertension, which may occur in these children, must be anticipated and identified early to prevent any unpredictable complications. (2) (PE; PL; TC; RG)
   1 This should be noted, but identifying hypertension is the priority.
   2 This does not occur with glomerulonephritis.
   4 Same as answer 2.

286. 4 The beta-hemolytic streptococcus immune complex becomes trapped in the glomerular capillary loop, causing glomerulonephritis. (2) (PE; AN; ED; RG)
   1 The cause is known; prevention depends on treating infected individuals with antibiotics to eliminate the organism.
   2 This is not an inherited but an acquired disease; incidence in males outnumbers that in females by 2:1.
   3 The precipitating streptococcal infection is usually a localized pharyngitis, and clots do not form in the small renal tubules.

287. 3 Because of glomerular dysfunction, there is decreased filtration of plasma, leading to excessive water accumulation and sodium retention; this leads to congestion and edema. (3) (PE; AS; PA; RG)
   1 This does not occur with glomerulonephritis.
   2 There is usually a decrease in urine volume.
   4 Same as answer 1.

288. 1 All these foods are permitted on low-sodium, low-potassium diets. (1) (PE; PL; TC; RG)
   2 All are fairly high in sodium and/or potassium.
   3 Carrots are high in sodium, a banana is high in potassium, and buttermilk is high in both sodium and potassium.
   4 All but the peach are high in sodium; all but the butter are fairly high in potassium.

289. 4 The glomerular filtration rate is reduced; this results in sodium retention, protein loss, and fluid accumulation, producing these symptoms. (2) (PE; AS; TC; RG)
   1 The blood pressure would be elevated; proteinuria would be greater than 1+; glycosuria is unrelated; anorexia would be present.
   2 The blood pressure would be elevated; proteinuria would be greater than 1+; anorexia and hematuria would be present.
   3 The blood pressure and specific gravity would be elevated; proteinuria would be greater than 1+.

290. 4 Bedrest conserves energy; a diet with no added salt is permitted; the other care monitors the response to therapy. (2) (PE; PL; TC; RG)
   1 Isolation is unnecessary because the disease is not communicable; fluids would not be encouraged but limited or permitted as desired.
   2 The blood pressure is not monitored every hour, and IV therapy is not used unless there is no oral intake or convulsions occur.
   3 Vital signs do not need to be monitored every 2 hours, a no-sodium diet is not possible, and bedrest is maintained to conserve energy.

291. 4 Sodium is usually limited to control or prevent edema and/or hypertension until the child is asymptomatic. (2) (PE; PL; ED; RG)
   1 The child should not be kept active for long periods because rest is needed; the child will not usually need a long convalescence.
   2 The nurse would not give a home phone number; the mother should contact the physician for follow-up care.
   3 Glomerulonephritis does not cause such severe kidney damage that a kidney transplant would be necessary.

292. 1 Protein (albumin) is present in the urine in nephrotic syndrome and is evidence of kidney injury or disease; if the urine is gently shaken, it will foam if protein is present. (2) (PE; AS; PA; RG)

2 Crystals are not found in the urine of clients with nephrotic syndrome.

3 A large amount of protein in the urine would result in a high specific gravity.

4 Only rarely do RBCs or RBC casts get through the glomerular basement membrane in nephrotic syndrome.

293. 3 This is characteristic of a child in nephrotic syndrome; large amounts of protein in the urine cause it to have a dark, frothy appearance. (2) (PE; AS; PA; RG)

1 The child may be somewhat lethargic but usually not severely.

2 Blood pressure is normal or decreased; hypertension is associated with glomerulonephritis.

4 These children are usually pale.

294. 4 In children with nephrotic syndrome, infection is always a threat because of anemia and lowered resistance; the child with a fractured femur is noninfectious so is appropriate as a roommate; in addition, the closeness of age will provide for preschool socialization. (3) (PE; IM; TC; RG)

1 This disorder is caused by a pathogen; it exposes the client to infection.

2 Same as answer 1.

3 Same as answer 1.

295. 1 The massive edema predisposes to skin breakdown. (3) (PE; PL; TC; RG)

2 Carbohydrates are not restricted; proteins may be limited.

3 This is far too much fluid; the damaged kidneys would not be able to handle this amount.

4 These children usually do not receive blood transfusions.

296. 4 With nephrotic syndrome the child's blood pressure will be normal or slightly decreased; with glomerulonephritis the child's blood pressure will be elevated. (3) (PE; AS; PA; RG)

1 This occurs in both nephrotic syndrome and glomerulonephritis.

2 Same as answer 1.

3 Same as answer 1.

297. 1 This is incorrect; weight gain must be monitored carefully because it could be indicative of an accumulation of fluid. (1) (PE; EV; ED; RG)

2 This is a correct statement; the child should be monitored for edema.

3 This is a correct statement; this is to determine if kidney functioning is impaired.

4 This is a correct statement; steroids are given with milk or food to prevent gastric irritation.

298. 2 This is correct; this is an indication that kidney function is impaired. (1) (PE; EV; ED; RG)

1 A 5-year-old is not old enough to reliably test the urine.

3 Acetone in the urine is associated with diabetes mellitus, not nephrotic syndrome.

4 A cloudy urine is indicative of the presence of protein; this is actually a positive, not a false-positive result.

299. 3 This is contraindicated because the pressure of the inflated cuff could disrupt the integrity of the arteriovenous fistula. (1) (PE; EV; ED; RG)

1 This would be desirable because vomiting or diarrhea could lead to dehydration and an acid-base imbalance.

2 Not only should this be done to assess vascular functioning distal to the arteriovenous fistula, but this assessment should be done bilaterally and the results compared.

4 This would be desirable because an inadequate fluid intake could result in dehydration and an acid-base imbalance.

300. 2 Because the child has only 1 kidney, efforts to prevent urinary tract infections, which can compromise kidney function, must be on-going. (3) (PE; AN; TC; RG)

1 Fluids are not restricted; adequate fluid is encouraged to prevent urinary tract infections.

3 After surgery sodium is usually not restricted.

4 With a unilateral tumor a kidney transplant is not necessary because the child still has 1 kidney.

301. 4 The presence of a chordee can affect the child's future reproductive capabilities related to the inability to inseminate directly. (3) (PE; AN; PA; RG)

1 Kidney function is not affected.

2 The risk of testicular torsion is not increased.

3 The incidence of testicular cancer is not increased.

302. 4 This response indicates that the teenager understands that she can have sexual intercourse even though she has cystic fibrosis; also, other than abstinence, condoms offer the best protection from sexually transmitted diseases. (3) (PE; EV; ED; RG)

1 Although fertility can be inhibited by highly viscous cervical secretions, which act as a plug blocking sperm entry, pregnancy is possible; in vitro fertilization also makes pregnancy possible.

2 A female with cystic fibrosis can have sex.

3 A diaphragm provides protection against pregnancy but it does not protect the individual from sexually transmitted diseases.

303. 3 The *Gonococcus* organism is present in the genitourinary tract of males and is easy to identify with a culture. (1) (PE; IM; PA; RG)

1 This does not confirm the diagnosis; it may identify sexual activity and partners.

2 The *Gonococcus* organism is in the genitourinary tract, not the blood; VDRL is a test for syphilis, not for gonorrhea.

4 Although urine may contain *Gonococcus* organisms, the urine would dilute the concentration; the organisms are more concentrated in the urethral discharge.

304. 2 A chancre is the earliest symptom of syphilis; a dark-field examination of the scraping will reveal the *Treponema* organism. (3) (PE; AS; PA; RG)

1 A rash is found in the secondary stage of syphilis; if a rash is found, it is too late for early diagnosis.

3 This is associated with gonorrhea.

4 These are late manifestations of syphilis.

GASTROINTESTINAL

305. 1 Because of the anomalous structure of the upper lip, the neonate may have difficulty sucking on a nipple; duckbill nipples and other modifying devices may have to be used. (1) (PE; PL; TC; GI)

2 This is not an immediate concern before surgery; it is necessary after surgery to prevent tension on the suture line.

3 The infant should be cuddled like any newborn.

4 The cleft lip does not predispose the neonate to infection; difficulty in feeding is the main problem.

306. 2 Because of the cleft (opening) in the lip the infant tends to suck in more air than usual; burping will prevent frequent regurgitation of formula. (1) (PE; PL; ED; GI)

1 Thickened formula is given to an infant with reflux problems such as vomiting after each feeding.

3 The infant's bottle should never be propped; the infant can aspirate.

4 The baby should be held while being fed.

307. 3 Surgeons prefer to do surgery as soon as possible; if the infant is in good health it can be done right after delivery or at 6 to 12 weeks of age. (2) (PE; IM; ED; GI)

1 This is incorrect; surgery is done much earlier; babies begin to have teeth at about 7 to 8 months of age.

2 This is incorrect; cleft palates, not cleft lips, are repaired at this time.

4 This would indicate a health problem because the infant should not lose weight; the infant's weight should be stabilized before surgery.

308. 3 Feeding the infant this way does not put any stress or pressure on the suture line. (1) (PE; IM; TC; GI)

1 A plastic spoon may be too hard against the lip; also, it is inflexible and it may be difficult to get formula into the side of the infant's mouth.

2 This is unnecessary and nonnutritious; the infant can be fed formula with a rubber-tipped syringe as soon as it can be tolerated.

4 A nasogastric tube may be uncomfortable and cause the infant to cry; the infant can be fed with a rubber-tipped syringe.

309. 4 Meticulous care of the suture line is necessary because inflammation and sloughing of tissue disrupt healing. (1) (PE; IM; TC; GI)

1 This would be done throughout the feeding; the priority care after a feeding is cleansing the suture line.

2 This is contraindicated; the infant may rub the face on the sheet and irritate the suture line.

3 The infant can be cuddled at all times; priority care after feeding is cleansing the suture line.

310. 1 This is important; crying would put tension on the suture line. (2) (PE; PL; TC; GI)

2 The infant should be out of restraints periodically.

3 This is unnecessary; the infant should have no respiratory difficulty.

4 The infant needs to be cuddled frequently; parents are encouraged to pick the baby up as much as possible.

311. 2 Hypertrophy of the circular muscle of the pylorus forms this palpable mass. (1) (PE; AS; PA; GI)

1 There are visible peristaltic waves that move from left to right across the epigastric area, not the lower abdomen.

3 Discomfort is felt because of hunger, but there is no pain or tenderness.

4 Abdominal distention is not seen; food never reaches the intestines because of the gastric obstruction.

312. 4 When a baby has scanty dark urine, poor skin turgor, and increased depth of respirations, it is likely that dehydration and metabolic alkalosis are present; these occur because of the fluid and hydrochloric acid loss and the potassium depletion; immediate intervention is necessary. (2) (PE; AS; TC; GI)

1 This would be difficult to determine accurately; it is far more important to assess the infant for signs of dehydration and metabolic alkalosis.

2 These are not indicators of immediate needs; assessment for signs of dehydration and metabolic alkalosis is more important.

3 Although this might help to confirm the diagnosis, the most important concern at this time is to assess for dehydration and metabolic alkalosis.

313. 1 This corrects the metabolic alkalosis; fluid and electrolytes should be in balance when the child is undergoing the stress of anesthesia and surgery. (2) (PE; IM; ED; GI)

2 This does not include the necessary fluid replacement.

3 Conservative treatment rather than surgery would be used if vomiting were not severe and projectile.

4 This may help restore protein, but it will not balance fluids and electrolytes.

314. 2 In the absence of severe dehydration and malnutrition the mortality rate is very low; immediate fluid and electrolyte replacement followed by surgery usually results in full recovery of the infant with pyloric stenosis. (1) (PE; IM; ED; GI)

1 The success rate with surgery is extremely high and produces a rapid recovery; surgery is usually necessary.

3 Pyloric stenosis is a congenital structural defect; hypertrophy of the circular muscle of the pylorus causes obstruction at the pyloric sphincter; it is not caused by an inborn error of metabolism.

4 The infant will be feeding normally within a week following surgery.

315. 1 Initial feedings postoperatively consist of clear fluids until tolerance for feeding is determined. (2) (PE; PL; TC; GI)
2 An increase in feeding osmolarity is attempted after the tolerance for clear liquids is assessed.
3 Thickened formula with cereal is utilized when an infant experiences gastroesophageal reflux.
4 Fluid and electrolyte status is stabilized preoperatively; if necessary MES would be given IV.

316. 2 Without complications, the infant is usually feeding normally within a few days of the surgery. (2) (PE; IM; ED; GI)
1 Within a few days of the surgery the infant will be feeding normally and needs no special dietary modification.
3 Holding the infant should be encouraged because it is an important part of the mother/child relationship at this age.
4 Same as answer 1.

317. 1 This reduces activities, allows the intestines to rest, and provides for early follow up. (1) (PE; IM; ED; GI)
2 Wrapping elevates temperature; sugar water does not include electrolytes and may cause further gastric irritation; there is no emergency.
3 This does not provide for rest nor for more immediate contact with a health professional.
4 Food may increase the diarrhea; the immediate intervention does not support the mother's attempt to manage the situation at home; there is no emergency.

318. 2 Bacteria are spread by contaminated stool; thus to protect others, isolation procedures must be initiated immediately on admission. (2) (PE; AN; TC; GI)
1 This is part of the initial assessment and would have been accomplished before admission.
3 Although this will be done, the priority is to establish appropriate isolation precautions.
4 Same as answer 3.

319. 3 The organisms causing gastroenteritis are eliminated along with the feces; gloves provide a protective barrier and are used for medical asepsis. (2) (PE; EV; ED; GI)
1 This is required in respiratory isolation, not enteric precautions.
2 This is not necessary for enteric precautions; this is necessary for an accurate measure of intake and output.
4 This is required in respiratory and strict isolation, not enteric precautions.

320. 1 This contains milk, which irritates the gastrointestinal tract; milk products are usually withheld for at least 1 week. (2) (PE; PL; TC; GI)
2 These are an appropriate soft food; they also replace the sodium lost in diarrhea.
3 These are an appropriate bland food; they are not irritating to the GI tract.
4 This is an appropriate soft food; it also replaces the potassium lost in diarrhea.

321. 3 This position limits the potential for aspiration; the infant will be partially upright, and fluid is held in the stomach by gravity. (2) (PE; IM; TC; GI)
1 This position allows gastric reflux and may lead to aspiration.
2 Same as answer 1.
4 Same as answer 1.

322. 4 This is the best source of the complete protein that is needed to maintain nitrogen balance. (2) (PE; PL; TC; GI)
1 This is a source of protein, but not the best source.
2 Same as answer 1.
3 This is high in vitamin C, which is needed for healing but not for nitrogen balance.

323. 4 Whole grains, legumes, and meat are excellent sources of thiamine, an essential coenzyme factor in energy metabolism, with an RDA standard of 0.5 mg/1000 kcal intake. (3) (PE; IM; ED; GI)
1 Eggs are only a fair source of thiamine.
2 Fruits do not contain thiamine.
3 Vegetables are only a fair source of thiamine.

324. 2 Celiac disease is a primary defect in which the intestinal mucosal transport system is impaired; the inability to digest gliadin results in an accumulation of glutamine; which is toxic to mucosal cells and causes atrophy of the villi. (3) (PE; AS; PA; GI)
1 This does not occur in celiac disease.
3 Same as answer 1.
4 The pancreatic acini degenerate in cystic fibrosis.

325. 3 These are classic signs of celiac disease caused by pathologic mucous cells and atrophy of intestinal villi, which result in poor absorption of nutrients and increased stools. (2) (PE; AS; PA; GI)
1 Rickets is not seen because bone growth is arrested in celiac disease; the remainder of the symptoms do occur.
2 Constipation leading to fecal impaction is not expected, although this may occur because of decreased peristalsis; rickets is not seen.
4 There is an inability of the villi to absorb vitamin K, with a tendency toward inadequate or prolonged blood coagulation.

326. 4 These grains, mainly wheat, are major dietary sources of gluten, the gliadin fraction of which causes celiac syndrome. (1) (PE; IM; ED; GI)
1 There is no gluten in milk and dairy products.
2 Corn and rice are good substitute grain foods because they contain no gluten.
3 There is no gluten in saturated or unsaturated fats.

327. 4 Primary sources of gluten are wheat, rye, barley, and oats; chocolate and whole wheat bread contain wheat flour or wheat by-products; these foods must be avoided. (2) (PE; EV; PA; GI)
1 Meats, in small to average portions, are allowed on gluten-free diets because their protein is digestible; these foods need not be avoided.
2 Spinach and cheese are gluten-free; corn is a grain that can be tolerated; these foods need not be avoided.
3 Eggs and milk are gluten-free; rice is a grain that can be tolerated; these foods need not be avoided.

328. 1 After the removal of gluten, most children demonstrate a favorable personality change within 48 hours. (2) (PE; EV; TC; GI)
2 Weight is not affected for several days or weeks.
3 Diarrhea usually persists for several days or weeks.
4 Steatorrhea usually persists for several days or weeks.

329. 1 Because mucosal lesions cause diarrhea and limit nutrient absorption, inadequate nutrients required for hemoglobin synthesis (iron and folic acid) cause anemia. (1) (PE; AN; PA; GI)
2 This causes pernicious anemia.
3 This child's anemia is caused by poor absorption rather than the quantity consumed.
4 Same as answer 3.

330. 1 Foods high in folic acid, iron, and vitamin B_{12} promote hemopoiesis. (3) (PE; PL; ED; GI)
2 Potassium and magnesium, necessary elements, are lost during celiac crisis but are not related to bone growth.
3 Fat is not absorbed in celiac disease; therefore a low-fat diet is indicated.
4 Of these supplements, only vitamin K is related to blood coagulation.

331. 1 Weight gain, improved appetite, improved behavior, and the disappearance of diarrhea and steatorrhea should have occurred. (1) (PE; EV; PA; GI)
2 This is not a stress-related disease; it is caused by a basic defect in metabolism or an immunologic response.
3 Even with understanding of the disease process, adherence to the diet may be relaxed; in time, symptoms may recur.
4 It is important to assess this, but it does not guarantee the child will select the foods on the diet.

332. 2 Drainage is promoted by the principle of gravity preventing fluid accumulation and possible abscess formation. (2) (PE; PL; TC; GI)
1 The lungs aerate well in any position if a subdiaphragmatic abscess does not form; with an abscess breathing will be splinted.

3   Deep breathing and coughing, leg exercises, and ambulation must be employed to prevent problems with immobility; maintaining a constant position does not provide mobility.

4   Splinting of an abdominal wound is best accomplished by direct external pressure to the site, not by positional changes.

333. 1   Assessment of fluid balance and peristalsis are important aspects of care after surgery. (1) (PE; PL; TC; GI)

2   Mouth care is not specific, and following appendectomy there is little drainage.

3   A low-residue diet is considered to be one of the factors leading to appendicitis because it tends to decrease peristalsis.

4   Dumping syndrome is a phenomenon associated with a gastrectomy.

334. 2   A high-calorie, low-residue, high-protein diet is important to improve the child's nutritional status. (1) (PE; EV; ED; GI)

1   A high-protein diet is important to promote nutritional status.

3   Isotonic, not soap suds, enemas are given.

4   Because the obstruction is in the large intestine, there is no indication for nasogastric feedings.

335. 1   Most raw fruits are high-residue foods; the colon cannot handle this type of food. (1) (PE; EV; ED; GI)

2   This is a low-residue food.

3   Same as answer 2.

4   Ripe bananas are raw fruit but are not classified as high residue.

336. 3   The impression is made on the sticky side of the tape; the specimen is collected before toileting so the ova deposited in the perianal area during the night have not been removed. (2) (PE; IM; ED; GI)

1   This will prevent the female worm from migrating to the perianal area and laying her eggs.

2   This will wash away the eggs; they must be directly collected from the perianal area.

4   The eggs are deposited in the perianal area, not in the stool.

337. 4   This is one of the preferred positions to prevent pressure on the perineal sutures following this surgery, which is done to correct intermediate anorectal malformations. (3) (PE; IM; PA; GI)

1   Buck's traction is usually applied in the supine position and this would put pressure on the perineal sutures; it would also contribute to prolonged contamination of the operative site by feces.

2   This would not promote healing of the anal area and could impede respiratory excursion.

3   This would increase pressure in the perineal area; the child may be placed in the side-lying prone (Sims') position with the hips elevated, not with the head of the bed elevated.

338. 4   Necrotizing enterocolitis (NEC) is an inflammatory disease of the gastrointestinal mucosa related to several factors including prematurity, hypoxemia, and high-solute feedings; it includes shunting of blood from the GI tract, decreased secretion of mucus, greater permeability of the mucosa, and increased gas-forming bacteria, eventually causing obstruction. (3) (PE; AS; PA; GI)

1   Meconium ileus is not related to the development of NEC; it is a common complication of cystic fibrosis.

2   Imperforate anus is the failure of fetal tissue to connect early in gestation and is present at birth.

3   Duodenal atresia may be a genetic or environmental defect that occurs early in gestation and is present at birth.

339. 4 Because intussusception creates intestinal obstruction where the intestine "telescopes" and becomes trapped, passage of intestinal contents is lessened; stools are red and currant jelly-like from the mixing of stool with blood and mucus. (2) (PE; AS; PA; GI)
 1 This is not as important to assessment as is observable behavior associated with crying.
 2 Bowel sounds would not be significantly affected.
 3 Accurate fluid intake and output records are important, but they are not essential to confirming this diagnosis.

DRUG RELATED RESPONSES

340. 3 This is the correct amount; use ratio and proportion; desired : have = desired : have; no conversion is necessary because desired and available dosage are both in milligrams; it is more accurate to convert less than 1 ml to minims. (2) (PE; AN; TC; DR)
 1 This is too much; 0.6 ml = 9 minims.
 2 This is too much; 0.9 ml = 13.5 minims.
 4 This is too much; the child should receive 6 minims.

341. 2 5 ml = 1 teaspoon; therefore 2.5 ml = ½ (0.5) teaspoon. (2) (PE; AN; TC; DR)
 1 This is too little; 0.5 ml = 0.10 teaspoon.
 3 This is too much; 3.75 ml = 0.75 teaspoon.
 4 This is too much; 7.5 ml = 1.5 teaspoons.

342. 4 Because Synthroid speeds up the basal metabolic rate, an absence of constipation is a therapeutic response to the medication. (3) (PE; EV; PA; DR)
 1 This is a clinical sign of hypothyroidism and is related to a slow basal metabolic rate.
 2 Fine hand tremors are related to hyperthyroidism and would not have been present in an infant with hypothyroidism.
 3 Same as answer 1.

343. 1 Insulin is a hormone and protein; when taken orally it is destroyed by the digestive enzymes, particularly pepsin. (2) (PE; IM; ED; DR)
 2 The potency of insulin is not just reduced, it is totally inactivated.
 3 This is untrue; insulin does not contain a carbohydrate that would raise the blood glucose.
 4 Insulin is not neutralized, it is inactivated by digestive enzymes.

344. 3 Streptomycin is potentially ototoxic and nephrotoxic. (3) (PE; PL; TC; DR)
 1 Penicillin reactions are usually allergic reactions.
 2 Tetracycline causes discoloration of forming teeth.
 4 Chloramphenicol may cause blood dyscrasias.

345. 3 Absorption of tetracycline is enhanced when the stomach is empty. (3) (PE; EV; ED; DR)
 1 Food interferes with absorption.
 2 Same as answer 1.
 4 Same as answer 1.

346. 3 Probenicid results in better utilization of the penicillin by delaying the excretion of the penicillin through the kidneys. (3) (PE; IM; ED; DR)
 1 This is untrue; the penicillin destroys the *Treponema* during all stages of its development; the probenicid delays the excretion of penicillin.
 2 The probenicid does not treat the urethritis, it delays excretion of the penicillin.
 4 Probenicid does not prevent allergic reactions.

347. 2 Reserpine and hydralazine are used to control hypertension. (2) (PE; PL; TC; DR)
 1 Digitalis is not used because there is no cardiac involvement.
 3 Phenobarbital may be used only if hypertensive encephalopathy causes convulsions.
 4 Furosemide is used as a diuretic; phenobarbital would be used only if hypertensive encephalopathy caused convulsions.

348. 3   Diarrhea is initially related to GI irritation; later, overgrowth of drug-resistant microbes can result in superinfection, which also causes diarrhea. (2) (PE; EV; ED; DR)

1   Vertigo is unrelated to tetracycline.

2   Tinnitus is unrelated to tetracycline; this is associated with ASA toxicity.

4   The opposite occurs because GI irritation increases motility.

349. 4   Because of the suppression of the inflammatory symptoms of infection, such as an increase in body temperature, the nurse must be alert to the subtle signs of infection such as changes in appetite, sleep patterns, and behavior. (1) (PE; AS; TC; DR)

1   Adrenocorticosteroid therapy may cause hypokalemia, not hyperkalemia, because of the retention of sodium and fluid.

2   Adrenocorticosteroid therapy delays, not accelerates, wound healing.

3   Adrenocorticosteroid therapy decreases, not increases, the production of antibodies.

350. 1   Cystitis is a potentially serious adverse reaction to Cytoxan, which can sometimes be prevented by increased hydration because the fluid flushes the bladder. (3) (PE; PL; TC; DR)

2   Irritability may be present but is not necessarily a result of Cytoxan administration.

3   This is an expected but not serious side effect of Cytoxan.

4   This is unrelated to Cytoxan administration; it occurs with Dilantin therapy.

351. 2   Many vitamins contain folic acid, which is contraindicated with methotrexate, a folic acid antagonist. (1) (PE; IM; ED; DR)

1   Vitamins would be contraindicated because folic acid interferes with the action of methotrexate.

3   This is true but does not answer the question; it permits vitamin use in the near future, which long-term chemotherapy contraindicates.

4   This is inaccurate; vitamin use is contraindicated.

352. 4   Neurotoxicity is a specific common side effect to this drug; the client can have numbness and ataxia. (3) (PE; AS; PA; DR)

1   Vincristine causes adynamic ileus, resulting in constipation; diarrhea occurs with other antineoplastics and radiation therapy.

2   Alopecia is an expected side effect rather than a toxic response; it is not considered serious, and hair will regrow.

3   This is not a side effect of this drug but a toxic response to Cytoxan.

353. 2   Elevated uric acid levels from destroyed cells may lead to renal problems; increased fluid intake helps dilute urine. (3) (PE; AS; TC; DR)

1   This will have to be monitored, but it is not of primary importance at this time.

3   Same as answer 1.

4   Same as answer 1.

354. 1   Constipation is a common side effect of vincristine because gastric motility is slowed. (3) (PE; EV; TC; DR)

2   This is not a toxic effect of prednisone.

3   An enlarged spleen would put pressure on the stomach and diaphragm, not on the large bowel.

4   This is not likely.

355. 3   The objective of the oral chemotherapy is to achieve a remission and prevent further relapses. (1) (PE; EV; PA; DR)

1   If the oral chemotherapy is effective, additional IV drugs will be unnecessary.

2   Oral chemotherapy is an adjunct to other therapies, not an alternative of other therapies.

4   The prime site of metastasis of ALL is to the central nervous system.

356. 2   Antineoplastic drugs exert their effect on rapidly dividing tissues such as hair follicles, resulting in alopecia. (2) (PE; IM; PS; EH)

1   This is not related to any of the side effects of the antineoplastics that are being used.

3   Same as answer 1.

4   Same as answer 1.

357. 4   AZT can cause life-threatening blood dys-crasias including thrombocytopenia. (3) (PE; EV; TC; DR)
   1   With AZT toxicity the child would demonstrate agitation, restlessness, and insomnia, not fatigue and lethargy.
   2   This is usually a response to the disease rather than the therapy.
   3   Urinary output is unrelated to AZT toxicity; a decreased urinary output can be related to a decreased fluid intake, vomiting, and diaphoresis associated with fever.

358. 3   Kidney function must be adequate to handle the lead being excreted; if kidney function is not adequate, nephrotoxicity or kidney damage may result. (2) (PE; PL; TC; DR)
   1   There is no skin breakdown with chelation therapy.
   2   A normal protein intake is adequate; excessive protein is not lost unless kidney damage is present.
   4   This would not be a nursing function; liver damage does not occur with chelation therapy.

359. 3   EDTA removes calcium along with lead; serum calcium levels need to be monitored periodically. (3) (PE; EV; TC; DR)
   1   This does not happen with chelation therapy.
   2   Same as answer 1.
   4   Same as answer 1.

360. 3   This may reduce the risk of gingival hyperplasia, a common side effect of Dilantin. (2) (PE; EV; ED; DR)
   1   The drug is strongly alkaline and should be administered with meals to avoid gastric irritation.
   2   Avoidance of overeating and of overhydration may result in better seizure control.
   4   A pink, not reddish brown, color may occur during drug excretion; it is not a complication.

361. 3   This behavior is a form of denial that may occur once the seizures are controlled; status epilepticus may occur when the medication is not taken regularly. (2) (PE; EV; PA; DR)
   1   Toxic reactions to Dilantin are not manifested by constant seizures.
   2   This is desired; it should prevent status epilepticus at this level.
   4   The dosage is not based on activity but on the type of seizure.

362. 3   These are side effects of scopolamine that are seen especially in the young and the elderly. (1) (PE; EV; PA; DR)
   1   This a side effect of tranquilizers.
   2   This is a side effect of narcotic analgesics.
   4   Scopolamine can cause respiratory depression, not hyperventilation or rapid respirations.

363. 4   Mannitol is an osmotic diuretic that is used to relieve cerebral edema. (2) (PE; AN; ED; DR)
   1   The bladder is a storage basin and is not involved with filtration; mannitol acts in the kidneys.
   2   Mannitol is an osmotic diuretic that does not reduce peripheral edema.
   3   Mannitol is an osmotic diuretic that has no effect on the body's glucose.

364. 3   This is a chelating agent used to remove lead from the body. (2) (PE; AN; TC; DR)
   1   This is a calcium salt often used as an antidote in magnesium sulfate toxicity.
   2   This is an antineoplastic drug used in cancer chemotherapy.
   4   This is a potassium-removing resin used for the treatment of hyperkalemia.

365. 4   Phenylephrine HCl, with frequent and continued use, can cause rebound congestion of mucous membranes. (2) (PE; IM; TC; DR)
   1   Nasal polyps may be associated with allergies but are unrelated to phenylephrine HCl.

2   Bleeding tendencies are related to inadequate clotting mechanisms; nasal bleeding may be associated with dry mucous membranes, but with rebound congestion the tissues are full of fluid.

3   These symptoms are unrelated to this drug; phenylephrine HCl may cause hypotension, tachycardia, and tingling of the extremities.

366. 2   Vomiting is a classic sign of digoxin toxicity, and the physician must be notified. (3) (PE; EV; ED; DR)

1   This is rarely needed because Aldactone spares potassium.

3   This is rarely necessary except when the defect is severe; infants are usually not overactive.

4   There is no restriction on taking aspirin with Aldactone; however, infants and children are generally not given aspirin because of its association with Reye's syndrome.

367. 3   The chronotropic effect of Lanoxin, a cardiac glycoside, slows the heart rate; when the dose of Lanoxin is excessive the child can develop bradycardia. (3) (PE; EV; TC; DR)

1   This is associated with congestive heart failure, not Lanoxin toxicity.

2   Same as answer 1.

4   This is associated with congestive heart failure, specifically right-ventricular failure.

368. 2   This would not affect the potency of the solution. (3) (PE; AN; TC; DR)

1   The drug should not be used if the solution is discolored.

3   The drug should not be used 24 hours or more after it is reconstituted from its powdered form.

4   The drug should be void of sediment; contamination is indicated if it is present.

369. 1   Epinephrine is a sympathetic nervous system stimulant that causes tachycardia. (1) (PE; EV; PA; DR)

2   Hyperglycemia, not hypoglycemia, may result.

3   The pupils will be dilated, not constricted.

4   Epinephrine is more likely to cause hypertension.

370. 3   This would minimize oral discomfort; ulceration of the oral mucosa occurs as a result of the antineoplastic effect on the rapidly dividing GI epithelium. (2) (PE; PL; TC; DR)

1   Although pain may be present, aspirin would be avoided because doxorubicin is also being used, and a side effect of this medication is thrombocytopenia.

2   These would aggravate the stomatitis that is a common side effect of Cosmegen.

4   This is not related to the administration of Cosmegen.

371. 2   Because steroids are irritating to the gastric mucosa, a peptic ulcer with bleeding may occur; stools should be checked for occult blood. (3) (PE; EV; TC; DR)

1   Steroids do not cause this to occur.

3   Same as answer 1.

4   Same as answer 1.

372. 4   This is an appropriate medication for hypertension because it acts to relax the smooth muscles of the arterioles. (2) (PE; PL; PA; DR)

1   This increases the contractility and output of the heart.

2   Diazepam is inappropriate; this relaxes the skeletal muscles, not the smooth muscles of the arterioles.

3   This is an anticonvulsant that might be prescribed later in the course of the disease if the antihypertensives were not effective and hypertensive encephalopathy caused convulsions.

373. 4   The purpose of administering lactobacilli, normally found in the GI tract, is to help recolonize the normal flora excreted with the diarrheal stools. (1) (PE; AN; PA; DR)

1   This is not the action of this medication.

2   Same as answer 1.

3   Same as answer 1.

374. 1 This is expected; clients should be advised so that they do not become alarmed and can protect clothing and bedding. (1) (PE; PL; ED; DR)
2 The drug will not affect rectal itching; it will eliminate the pinworms, and this takes some time to accomplish.
3 All family members should be treated.
4 Reinfestation is common; the drug may be needed again.

375. 4 Abdominal cramping and distention are associated with inadequate pancreatic enzyme replacement because foods are not being digested. (2) (PE; EV; PA; DR)
1 The opposite is true; they would have a voracious appetite.
2 Diarrhea, not constipation, would result.
3 There would be a weight loss because of decreased digestion and absorption, not a weight gain.

Pediatric Nursing Quiz

1. An 11-month-old injured in a fall has a fractured right femur and is placed in Bryant traction. The nurse should frequently monitor a child in Bryant traction to ensure that the buttocks are:
1. Flat on the bed
2. Slightly elevated
3. Elevated 3 to 4 inches
4. Resting on a small pillow

2. A child is admitted with acute lymphocytic leukemia (ALL). When performing the admission history and physical assessment, the nurse should assess the child for the common early signs of ALL including:
1. Nosebleeds and papilledema
2. Fever and areas of ecchymosis
3. Enlargement of the liver and spleen
4. Abdominal pain and reddened complexion

3. A 5-year-old is admitted to the hospital with a diagnosis of acute glomerulonephritis. A nursing diagnosis of fluid volume excess would be correct if the assessment data included:
1. Dysuria, pruritus, weight loss
2. Diarrhea, polyuria, weight gain
3. Hypotension, tachycardia, hematuria
4. Periorbital edema, smoky urine, headaches

4. An 8-year-old is admitted in sickle cell crisis. Appropriate nursing care during this period includes:
1. Administration of oxygen
2. Cold compresses to painful joints
3. Restricted fluids until crisis is over
4. Active range of motion exercises to all joints

5. The mother of a school-age child asks the school nurse how her child could have gotten head lice. When replying the nurse should remember that:

1. Transmission occurs through household pets
2. Transmission just occurs through direct personal contact
3. Infestation is most common where crowded conditions exist
4. Infestation is more widespread among lower socioeconomic groups

6. One month after abdominal surgery, a 6-month-old infant is brought to the pediatric clinic for a follow-up visit. The nurse observes the child performing all of the following tasks. The task that would be most unusual for a child of this age is:
1. Putting clothespins in a plastic bottle
2. Sitting alone for brief periods in a crib
3. Playing with his toes during examination
4. Showing stranger-anxiety when the nurse approaches

7. A child with iron deficiency anemia is placed on supplemental oral iron therapy. The parents of the child should be prepared to expect that the child may develop:
1. Positive stool guiac
2. Staining of the teeth
3. Orange-colored urine
4. Greenish-black stools

8. When preparing a pre-schooler for a surgical procedure, the best time to tell the child what will happen is:
1. 2 weeks before
2. 3 to 4 days before
3. 1 month in advance
4. Just before it happens

9. To promote growth and development, the nurse instructs the mother of a 4-month-old to provide the infant with:
1. Push-pull type toys
2. Snap beads and strings
3. Nesting blocks and cups
4. Soft squeeze toys with squeakers

10. Acute glomerulonephritis may occur secondary to impetigo. The treatment most beneficial in the prevention of this sequela is the:
    1. Use of an oil-based soap for bathing
    2. Administration of a systemic antibiotic
    3. Application of an antibiotic ointment to the lesions
    4. Removal of crusts with an antimicrobial liquid and water

11. When the nurse is teaching the parents about celiac disease, the mother sighs and states, "My neighbor told me that I would only need to watch the diet until my child is 8 years old. I'm so relieved; you know how kids are about eating!" The nurse's response should be based on the fact that:
    1. The basic defect of celiac disease is life-long
    2. Susceptibility to celiac crisis lessens with age
    3. Though difficult at first, the diet is fairly easy to follow
    4. These children can tolerate small amounts of gluten by age 5

12. A 6-year-old is hospitalized with a diagnosis of nephrotic syndrome and the child's mother asks the nurse what she should bring her child to play with during the hospitalization. Considering the child's age the nurse should suggest that the mother bring:
    1. Action toys such as a hula hoop
    2. Stuffed animals, large puzzles, and large blocks
    3. Table games, checkers, simple card games, and crayons
    4. A record player, transistor radio, and children's magazines

13. A 30-month-old child is brought to the emergency room in acute respiratory distress and a diagnosis of laryngotracheobronchitis (viral croup) is made. Upon admitting this child to the pediatric unit the nurse should anticipate the need for a:
    1. Cot so that a parent can stay
    2. Tracheotomy set at the bedside
    3. Pad for the side rails of the Croupette
    4. Quiet, cool room to facilitate breathing

14. The physician's orders for a child admitted with meningitis include specific isolation. The nurse understands that the child should be placed on:
    1. "Reverse" isolation
    2. Enteric precautions
    3. Respiratory isolation
    4. Syringe and needle precautions

15. An infant is born with talipes equinovarus (club foot) and the physician applies a cast to the lower extremity. The nurse knows that the mother will have to bring the baby back to the physician's office for a cast change:
    1. Each week
    2. Once a month
    3. Every other day
    4. When the cast is soiled

16. A 3-month-old with acute spasmodic bronchitis (spasmodic croup) is admitted in severe dyspnea. The child has a temperature of 104°F. The child is placed in a high-humidity tent with cold mist. The nurse is aware that the main reason cold humidity is preferred to steam is that:
    1. Cold humidity dries up the mucosal secretions
    2. Cold humidity aids in reducing mucosal edema
    3. Cold mist produces a more comfortable environment
    4. Cool water vapor is more readily absorbed by the mucosa

17. A platelet transfusion is ordered for a child with acute lymphocytic leukemia, and an IV is started. The nurse should:
    1. Administer the platelets rapidly
    2. Administer the platelets over 2 hours
    3. Check vital signs 3 hours after the transfusion
    4. Flush the line with 5% dextrose and normal saline

18. Long-range management for children with asthma includes exercise. The nurse should teach the parents to encourage their son who has asthma to participate in the sport of:

1. Soccer
2. Baseball
3. Wrestling
4. Basketball

19. The nurse in a pediatric health clinic would be especially observant for signs of cerebral palsy in a 6-month-old infant who:
1. Weighed less than 1500 g at birth
2. Had a positive Moro reflex at birth
3. Was born by elective cesarean delivery
4. Was born to a mother over 35 years old

20. A $2^1/_2$-year-old child with cystic fibrosis is admitted to the pediatric unit with a severe upper respiratory infection. The nurse assesses that the child is very small for age and attributes the slow growth to:
1. The retention of CO_2
2. Increased salt retention
3. An atrial ventricular defect
4. The absence of pancreatic enzymes

21. A preadolescent brings home a note from the school nurse informing the parents that the child should be evaluated for scoliosis. The mother calls the school nurse to ask what scoliosis is. To answer the question the nurse must understand that it is a:
1. Pathologic process involving the vertebrae
2. Concave lumbar curvature that is very exaggerated
3. Lateral curvature of the spine with a rotary deformity
4. Curvature of the thoracic spine that has an increased convex angulation

22. Following a successful craniotomy for the removal of a brain tumor in a 9-year-old, the nurse notes an area of serosanguinous drainage on the child's dressing about the size of a quarter. The nurse should:
1. Notify the physician immediately
2. Mark the area with nonabsorbable ink
3. Reinforce the dressing with gauze pads
4. Remove the dressing and check the sutures

23. An intravenous is started in the scalp vein of an infant, and the mother asks why the intravenous is not placed in the hand as for an adult. The nurse responds:

1. "Putting the IV in the scalp improves the absorption rate of the IV."
2. "Inserting the IV in the scalp decreases the need to restrain the baby."
3. "The IV solution is too irritating to be introduced through a vein in the hand."
4. "Veins are closer to the surface of the scalp making it easier to insert the IV."

24. A child with a history of swollen lymph nodes, prolonged fever unresponsive to antibiotics, and erythema of the extremities is admitted with a diagnosis of Kawasaki disease. The nurse is aware that this diagnosis was probably based on:
1. An elevated ASO titer
2. A combination of symptoms
3. An elevated sedimentation rate
4. A decreased serum protein level

25. A 3-year-old, who was born prematurely and was a recipient of several blood transfusions while in the neonatal intensive care nursery, is admitted with AIDS and is placed on bedrest with oxygen via a tent. The mother having just been informed that her child has AIDS is visibly upset at the child's bedside. The nurse's most therapeutic statement would be:
1. "You must really feel like screaming."
2. "Let me give you a referral for social service."
3. "Your child will get the best care possible at this hospital."
4. "It is a shame that your child needed so many blood transfusions."

26. A 9-year-old is admitted for treatment of a badly infected wound of the toe. The aunt with whom the child now lives is uncertain if the child has had a tetanus immunization. An immunizing dose of tetanus immune globulin (Hyper-tet) is administered because it:
1. Confers life-long passive immunity
2. Induces longer-lasting active protection
3. Confers immediate passive protection of short duration
4. Immediately stimulates increased production of antibodies

27. A mother brings her child to the physician because the child is constantly scratching the anus. In caring for a child who is suspected of having a pinworm infestation, the initial nursing responsibility would be to:
1. Prevent reinfection
2. Identify the organism
3. Collect a stool specimen
4. Notify the Health Department

28. At 1 AM, a 28-month-old is admitted to the pediatric unit with meningitis. At 3 AM, after the child is settled down, the mother tells the nurse, "I have to leave now, but whenever I try to go my child gets upset and then I start to cry." The nurse should:
1. Walk the mother to the elevator
2. Encourage the mother to spend the night
3. Stay with the child while the mother leaves
4. Tell the mother to wait until the child falls asleep

29. The nurse realizes that lead poisoning affects various organ systems but its irreversible side effects are exerted mainly on the:
1. Urinary system
2. Skeletal system
3. Hematological system
4. Central nervous system

30. In the recovery room, following a tonsillectomy, a child is swallowing frequently. The nurse suspects that the child is:
1. Experiencing pain in the throat
2. Reacting from general anesthesia
3. Hemorrhaging from the operative site
4. In need of suctioning to keep the airway patent

31. A ten-month-old, injured in an automobile accident, is brought to the trauma center. The child, who is quiet but does not appear lethargic, has a large hematoma on the left temporal area. When assessing the child, the nurse should be particularly alert for signs and symptoms that may indicate neurologic involvement such as:
1. Persistent vomiting
2. A positive Babinski reflex
3. The development of a headache
4. A pulse rate of 110 beats per minute

32. The nurse recalls that some of the most common early signs of leukemia are:
1. Pallor, joint pain, anorexia, fever
2. Lethargy, petechia, splenomegaly
3. Fatigue, pallor, alopecia, hemorrhage
4. Fatigue, mouth lesions, hepatomegaly

33. Because of a measles epidemic a 6-month-old infant receives a measles vaccination. The nurse should help the mother understand that to ensure continuous protection against measles, the baby should be revaccinated at approximately:
1. 8 months of age
2. 10 months of age
3. 12 months of age
4. 18 months of age

34. A 6-week-old infant has just had surgery for pyloric stenosis. An immediate postoperative nursing care priority for this infant would be:
1. Giving the oral feedings very slowly
2. Reporting any vomiting to the physician
3. Checking the patency of the nasogastric tube
4. Observing for signs of infection at the incisional site

35. One percent gamma benzene hexachloride (Kwell) is ordered for a 5-year-old with pediculosis capitis (head lice). When teaching the mother about treatment for head lice, the nurse should include the fact that:
1. The shampoo must be repeated within 7 to 10 days
2. The medicated shampoo used has no known side effects
3. Clothing and personal belongings must be boiled or discarded
4. Other children should be kept away from the infected child for 1 week

36. Surgery is scheduled for a 5-month-old infant with intussusception. The physician plans to order a vagolytic agent preoperatively. An example of this type of drug is:
1. Atropine
2. Morphine
3. Phenergan
4. Secobarbital

37. A 4-year-old is admitted for a diagnostic workup for pulmonic stenosis. The nurse understands that pulmonic stenosis is:
1. Narrowing of the valve between the left atrium and left ventricle
2. Hardening of the valve between the right atrium and right ventricle
3. Hardening of the lining of the pulmonary artery at a point close to the lungs
4. Narrowing of the valve between the right ventricle and the pulmonary artery

38. Three siblings are termed accident prone because of frequent incidents. The community health nurse involves the parents in a teaching program and instructs them to lower the risk of accidents by using discipline that emphasizes:
1. Realistic rigidity
2. Rational consistency
3. Guarded indifference
4. Serious overprotection

39. An infant is born with a cleft lip. The nursing care of this newborn, unlike that of other newborns, would include:
1. Changing the infant's position frequently
2. Using modified techniques to feed the infant
3. Keeping the infant's head elevated at all times
4. Maintaining the infant on strict intake and output

40. A nurse teaches a group of mothers in the community how AIDS can be transmitted via blood transfusions. The nurse recognizes that further teaching is necessary when one of the mothers states:
1. "Blood obtained from individuals in high risk groups is discarded."
2. "Once tested for antibodies, negatively tested blood cannot transmit the virus."
3. "The process of donor screening has improved since the AIDS virus was discovered."
4. "Blood that has tested negative for the AIDS virus can develop antibodies at a later time."

41. An 18-month-old with celiac disease is placed on a gluten free diet. A teaching program about the diet is instituted with the child's parents. The nurse knows that the parents understand the teaching about food substances that must be avoided when they state that their child cannot have:
1. Mashed corn
2. Steamed rice
3. Fresh applesauce
4. Grilled frankfurter

42. A 6-year-old is admitted with nephrotic syndrome. The nurse should be aware that the changes in body fluid distribution that occur with this disorder are related to the fact that:
1. The loss of sodium and water through an impaired basement membrane of the glomerulus results in hypovolemia
2. The loss of body protein reduces oncotic pressure so that fluid moves from the intravascular to the interstitial space
3. Hyperproteinemia results in increased oncotic pressure which causes fluid to move from the intravascular to interstitial space
4. The basement membrane of the glomerulus becomes selectively impermeable to water so that fluid is retained in the tissues

43. A 2½-year-old has a pediatric microdrip set up. A 500 ml bottle of D5 1/3NS is hung at 1 AM and is to infuse at 45 ml per hour. At 6 AM, the night nurse notes that the child's IV bottle has 125 ml left. The nurse correctly evaluates that the:
1. IV has infused at the prescribed rate through the night
2. Total amount of fluid infused is less than ordered for the child
3. Total amount of fluid infused is more than the child should have received
4. Amount of fluid infused should be calculated at the change of shift or 7 AM

44. A 3-year-old with chronic lead poisoning must have 60 injections of Ca EDTA before the lead is chelated and removed from the body. The nurse should prepare the child for this painful treatment by:
   1. Rotating the injection sites and adding procaine to the chelating agents to lessen the discomfort
   2. Role playing with puppets dressed as physicians and nurses to minimize the child's fear of unfamiliar adults
   3. Allowing the child to play with a syringe and a doll before the therapy is initiated and after receiving each injection
   4. Carefully explaining the rationale for the injections so that the child does not feel punished for eating paint chips

45. For a child with the diagnosis of lead poisoning (plumbism), initial care should focus on the nursing diagnosis of:
   1. Constipation related to the excretion of lead
   2. High risk for injury related to the ingestion of lead
   3. Altered growth and development related to parental neglect
   4. Altered nutrition, less than body requirements related to decreased iron intake

Pediatric Nursing Quiz Rationales

Pediatric Nursing Quiz Rationales

1. 2 The buttocks should be elevated just enough to slip a hand underneath; this permits the weight of the body to act as countertraction. (1) (PE; PL; TC; SK)

   1 This is counterproductive because it eliminates the use of the child's weight for countertraction.

   3 This is too high.

   4 Same as answer 1.

2. 2 These symptoms are caused by unrestricted white blood cell proliferation and resultant decreased platelet production. (1) (PE; AS; PA; BI)

   1 Papilledema is not a common presenting symptom because the blood-brain barrier is an initial deterrent.

   3 These are not the presenting symptoms; these occur through infiltration of the vascular organs of the reticuloendothelial system by immature WBCs.

   4 Pain is not an early symptom; the skin will be pale.

3. 4 Periorbital edema is indicative of excess fluid; the kidneys are inflamed and the output of urine is lessened; hematuria can occur. (2) (PE; EV; PA; RG)

   1 These symptoms do not indicate excess fluid.

   2 Diarrhea and polyuria would lead to fluid deficit and, perhaps, weight loss.

   3 Same as answer 1.

4. 1 Oxygen limits further sickling and compensates for compromised oxygen transportation capacity of hemoglobin. (1) (PE; IM; TC; BI)

   2 Cold will constrict blood vessels, further depleting oxygenation to affected parts; warmth is preferable.

   3 Increased hydration is necessary to promote hemodilution, improve circulation, and reverse sickling.

   4 There is too much swelling and pain in the joints during a crisis for this intervention.

5. 3 Transmission occurs through direct contact with infected individuals and indirect contact with contaminated articles; crowded conditions aid transmission. (1) (PE; IM; ED; IT)

   1 Lice are not carried or transmitted by household pets.

   2 Pediculosis can also be transmitted by contact with infested clothing, personal articles, or bedding.

   4 All socioeconomic groups are equally affected.

6. 1 This is a behavior seen in 9- to 12-month-olds; this is the most advanced behavior listed, and is the most unusual for this age. (2) (PE; AS; ED; GD)

   2 This is a coordination ability seen in 5- to 7-month-olds.

   3 This is a coordination ability seen in 3- to 5-month-olds.

   4 This is a behavior seen in 6- to 8-month-olds.

7. 4 Iron is excreted in the feces, and the change in color results from the insoluble iron compound in the stool. (1) (PE; AS; ED; DR)

   1 This is associated with GI bleeding, not iron administration.

   2 This should not occur with proper administration of the iron; iron elixir should be diluted in fluid and administered with a straw; the teeth should immediately be brushed after administration.

   3 This is not associated with iron; it occurs with pyridium administration.

8. 2 This will give the child adequate time to adjust and prepare for the surgery without presenting it too far in advance. (2) (PE; PL; ED; GD)

   1 This is too far in advance; the child will forget or build up a great deal of fear.

   3 Same as answer 1.

   4 This is appropriate for a toddler.

9. 4 This is appropriate for a 4-month-old; the child enjoys squeezing and hearing the sound of the squeaker. (1) (PE; PL; ED; GD)

1 This is appropriate for a child 12 to 24 months of age.

2 This is appropriate for a child 10 to 12 months of age.

3 This is appropriate for a child 16 months of age.

10. 2 Systemic antibiotics are necessary to eradicate the streptococcal organism, which caused the primary infection, impetigo. (2) (PE; PL; TC; RG)

1 This would not prevent glomerulonephritis, a sequela of streptococcal infections.

3 This would not prevent glomerulonephritis; this is part of the local therapy for impetigo.

4 Same as answer 3.

11. 1 The diet must be followed forever because there will always be an absence of peptidase; some variations to this diet may be allowed, but this should not be promised. (2) (PE; IM; ED; GI)

2 This is untrue; each phase of child development may have problems related to dietary management; follow-up care is needed to prevent crises.

3 This is untrue; a restricted diet is never easy to follow, especially for a growing child.

4 This is untrue; gluten must be avoided for a prolonged period of time and usually indefinitely.

12. 3 School-age children enjoy competition, have manipulative skills, and are creative. (1) (PE; IM; ED; GD)

1 This activity is inappropriate during the acute phase of nephrotic syndrome because it requires too much energy.

2 These are appropriate for the toddler who is developing fine motor skills.

4 Magazines would interest an older child who would be more proficient in reading.

13. 2 A patent airway is the first priority, and the necessary equipment must be immediately available. (1) (PE; PL; TC; RE)

1 Although helpful, this is not the priority.

3 This would be appropriate for convulsions, which are not associated with croup; respiratory promotion is the priority.

4 Same as answer 1.

14. 3 Respiratory isolation is necessary because meningitis is most commonly spread by droplet infection, which is carried by airborne microorganisms. (3) (PE; IM; TC; NM)

1 This is an outdated term; the client's immune system is not affected; others must be protected from the client's infection.

2 This is unnecessary; meningitis is not transmitted via the feces.

4 Meningitis is not a bloodborne disease; syringe and needle precautions are observed for all clients under universal precautions.

15. 1 Casts are changed weekly to accommodate the rapid growth in early infancy. (2) (PE; PL; TC; SK)

2 This is not frequent enough in early infancy; the cast could become too tight because of rapid growth of the infant.

3 This is too frequent; muscles and tendons would not be stretched and relaxed enough between cast changes to affect foot position.

4 Soiling is not usually a problem because casts for clubfoot do not extend to the perineal area.

16. 2 Cold causes vasoconstriction and reduces edema; it may also help to reduce fever. (2) (PE; AN; PA; RE)

1 Heat dries secretions.

3 Cold mist is less comfortable, because the environment is cold and damp.

4 Absorption via the mucosa is insignificant and cannot be considered fluid intake.

17. 1 Platelets are rapidly administered to avoid destruction after hanging the IV. (2) (PE; IM; TC; BI)

2 Platelets should not hang for a long time because of their fragility.

3 This is too long an interval; during infusion of blood derivatives, vital signs are more closely monitored.

4 Dextrose solution is not appropriate for flushing a blood derivative line because it may become clogged.

18. 2 Moderate exercise, including baseball and skiing, that involves starting and stopping does not overtax the respiratory mechanism; endurance exercise such as basketball, soccer, and wrestling is not well tolerated. (3) (PE; PL; ED; RE)

1 Endurance exercise overtaxes the respiratory mechanism.

3 Same as answer 1.

4 Same as answer 1.

19. 1 Studies indicate that a large percentage of children with cerebral palsy had birth weights below 1500 g. (2) (PE; AS; PA; NM)

2 The Moro reflex is normally present at birth.

3 There is no greater incidence of cerebral palsy in children born by a cesarean delivery that is not done for fetal distress.

4 Studies do not indicate any greater incidence of cerebral palsy in children born to women older than 35 years of age.

20. 4 Nutrients such as protein, carbohydrates, and fats are not digested and are not properly absorbed by the intestinal mucosa. (2) (PE; AN; PA; EN)

1 It is not the retention of carbon dioxide, but the deprivation of nutrients and oxygen to all body cells that retards physical growth.

2 These children lose high concentrations of sodium and chloride in perspiration.

3 There is no evidence that the child has an atrial ventricular defect.

21. 3 This is the correct definition. (1) (PE; AN; PA; SK)

1 There are no pathologic changes in the vertebrae.

2 This is a description of lordosis.

4 This is a description of kyphosis.

22. 2 If the drainage progresses beyond the markings, it would enable the nurse to determine whether an abnormal amount of drainage was occurring. (1) (PE; IM; TC; NM)

1 This is not an emergency; some drainage is expected.

3 This would not enable the nurse to monitor progression of the drainage.

4 In the immediate postoperative period, the dressing is to be removed only by the neurosurgeon.

23. 4 This provides an accurate statement of why scalp veins are used in infants; other veins are not well developed for IV therapy. (2) (PE; IM; ED; CV)

1 The absorption rate through a peripheral vein is the same regardless of placement.

2 The infant will still need to be restrained to prevent pulling out the IV or rolling over on it.

3 Placement of the needle is not related to whether the solution is irritating.

24. 2 The diagnosis is based on the presence of five out of six specific symptoms including fever, trunk rash, enlarged cervical lymph nodes, bilateral congestion of the conjunctiva, edema, and redness of the extremities. (3) (PE; AS; PA; NM)

1 An elevated ASO titer may be seen with a streptococcal infection.

3 This is non-specific to Kawasaki disease; the sedimentation rate is elevated in the presence of inflammation with many disorders.

4 This is not present in Kawasaki disease.

25. 1 This statement acknowledges the mother's feelings. (3) (PE; IM; PS; EH)

2 This statement does not address the mother's feelings.

3 Although this statement may be true, it gives false hope for recovery.

4 Same as answer 2.

26. 3 Tetanus immunoglobulin (TIG) contains ready-made antibodies and only confers short-term passive immunity. (2) (PE; AN; TC; BI)
1 Passive immunity is temporary.
2 Immune globulins confer passive artificial immunity.
4 Immune globulins are antibodies and do not stimulate the formation of antibodies.

27. 3 A specimen must be obtained and analyzed before the physician can prescribe treatment. (1) (PE; PL; TC; GI)
1 The priority is identifying the organism, then handwashing techniques can be taught.
2 The organism can be identified only by laboratory analysis of a stool specimen.
4 This is not a reportable communicable disease.

28. 3 This action would encourage the mother to leave and reassure her that someone will be with and will comfort the child. (2) (PE; IM; PS; EH)
1 The mother has indicated she is upset when the child is upset; the mother knows the way to the elevator; this intervention meets no one's needs.
2 The mother has said she must leave; convincing her to stay will make her feel guilty about having to leave.
4 Same as answer 2.

29. 4 Damaged nerve cells do not regenerate; once mental retardation has occurred, it is not reversible. (1) (PE; AN; PA; NM)
1 Changes in this system are reversible with treatment.
2 Same as answer 1.
3 Same as answer 1.

30. 3 If there is a trickle of blood from the operative site, the child will swallow frequently; this is usually the first sign of hemorrhage. (2) (PE; EV PA; RE)
1 The child with a sore throat tries to minimize the frequency of swallowing.
2 Swallowing frequently is not a specific reaction to general anesthesia.
4 The child may need suctioning, but the presenting symptoms for this intervention would be restlessness or a color change, such as cyanosis.

31. 1 Vomiting frequently accompanies a head injury because of increased intracranial pressure and stimulation of the vomiting reflex. (1) (PE; AS; PA; NM)
2 A positive Babinski reflex is normal and expected in a 10-month-old child.
3 A 10-month-old child would not complain of a headache; persistent vomiting is an objective sign.
4 This would be within the normal range for a child this age.

32. 1 Vague symptoms frequently prolong the accurate diagnosis of the leukemic process; all of these are early signs related to the leukocyte alteration. (1) (PE; AS; PA; BI)
2 Splenomegaly is not a common sign of early leukemia; the symptoms are usually vague and nonspecific.
3 Alopecia is not a common sign of early leukemia; the early symptoms are usually vague and nonspecific.
4 Mouth lesions and an enlarged liver are not common symptoms of early leukemia; the early symptoms are usually vague and nonspecific.

33. 3 The optimum age for measles vaccination is between 12 to 15 months; if a vaccination is given earlier than this because of exposure to a person with measles, it is not counted as one of the 2 required doses. (1) (PE; IM; PA; BI)
1 This is too early; the baby would still have antibodies from the previous vaccination.
2 Same as answer 1.
4 This is not the optimal time; the measles immunization should be given between 12 to 15 months of age.

34. 3 A nasogastric tube is used postoperatively to decompress the stomach and limit tension on the suture line. (2) (PE; IM; TC; GI)
1 To limit pressure on the suture line, oral feedings should not be used in the immediate postoperative period when the gastric tube is in place.
2 Vomiting indicates obstruction of the nasogastric tube; the initial action should be to check the patency of the nasogastric tube.
4 This is too soon for signs of infection to occur.

35. 1 Reapplication destroys any surviving ova (nits) which eventually become lice. (1) (PE; IM; ED; IT)
   2 This is untrue; excessive use can cause an eczematous rash and central nervous system disturbances.
   3 Personal items can be soaked in pediculicidal solution; clothing and linen should be laundered in hot water and dried in a hot drier.
   4 Once the hair has been shampooed, there is no reason to isolate the child.

36. 1 Atropine is a vagolytic and drying agent used preoperatively. (1) (PE; AN; TC; DR)
   2 This is a narcotic analgesic.
   3 This is a tranquilizer.
   4 This is a sedative.

37. 4 The cusps of the valves may be fused or the infundibulum below may be hypertrophied, thus restricting blood flow to the lungs. (3) (PE; AN; PA; CV)
   1 The mitral valve is not involved in pulmonic stenosis.
   2 The tricuspid valve is not involved in pulmonic stenosis.
   3 This is untrue; pulmonic stenosis is a congenital condition that results from the failure of tissues to develop normally in utero.

38. 2 Unwavering adherence to the same principles and regulations promotes safe, firm limits. (1) (PE; PL; ED; GD)
   1 This stifles the child's natural development in learning to explore.
   3 Injuries are promoted when there is lack of care.
   4 This hinders the child's freedom to explore and enjoy the surroundings.

39. 2 With a cleft in the lip the baby will be unable to suck like other newborns. (1) (PE; PL; PA; GI)
   1 This is common for all newborns, not just a baby with a cleft lip.
   3 This is contraindicated in a newborn because the normal alignment of the spine will be interfered with if the head is elevated at all times.
   4 This is not necessary because intake and output will be normal once a feeding method is established.

40. 2 This statement is not true because the virus could still be transmitted if the result was a false negative. (3) (PE; EV; ED; BI)
   1 This is a true statement; members of high-risk groups are more apt to be HIV positive.
   3 Blood screening has improved and has reduced the incidence of transmission, but it is still not perfect.
   4 Blood that tests negatively can seroconvert at a later time.

41. 4 Frankfurter has grain filler; parents should read labels and unless they are sure of ingredients, should not feed the food to the child. (2) (PE; EV; ED; GI)
   1 This does not contain gluten; this is a substitute for grain foods.
   2 Same as answer 1.
   3 This does not contain gluten.

42. 2 The basement membrane of the glomerulus becomes permeable to protein that is lost in the urine; decreased serum protein reduces the oncotic pressure in the capillaries, which normally helps to hold fluid within the vascular system. (3) (PE; AN; PA; FE)
   1 Hypoproteinemia causes decreased oncotic pressure, which results in hypovolemia; sodium and water are retained to counter the hypovolemia.
   3 Increased oncotic pressure pulls fluid from the interstitial space into the intravascular compartment; nephrosis is characterized by hypoproteinemia and therefore, the opposite is true.
   4 The basement membrane becomes permeable to protein, not impermeable to water.

43. 3 If the IV infused at the prescribed rate of 45 ml/hr for 5 hrs, 225 ml would have infused, leaving 275 ml in the bottle. (2) (PE; EV; TC; FE)
   1 This is incorrect; an excessive amount of fluid has been infused.
   2 Same as answer 1.
   4 This is untrue; the IV should be delivered at 45 ml/hr and should be monitored continually.

44. 3 The child should be given an outlet for tension, and playing with a syringe and doll is the most appropriate in this situation. (1) (PE; PL; PS; EH)

1 This may ease some of the discomfort, but an outlet for feelings should be provided.

2 The child's fear is not caused by unfamiliar adults but by the painful treatments.

4 This is part of the preparation, but not the most important; the child must be allowed to express feelings; the child is too young to comprehend too much.

45. 2 The most serious and irreversible effects of lead intoxication are on the nervous system; lead encephalopathy causes convulsions, mental retardation, paralysis, blindness, and ultimately coma and death. (2) (PE; AN; TC; NM)

1 Although constipation can occur it is not caused by the excretion of lead; lead is excreted via the urinary tract.

3 Although some studies have identified that some children with plumbism have received less than adequate child care, a cause and effect relationship between plumbism and parental neglect has not been established.

4 Altered nutrition less than body requirements is not caused by a decrease in the intake of iron; high serum blood levels of lead interfere with the biosynthesis of heme preventing the formation of hemoglobin, resulting in anemia.

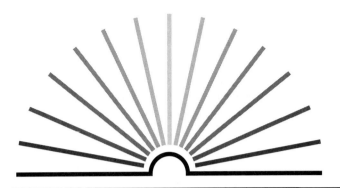

CHAPTER 5

Mental Health Nursing Review Questions

PERSONALITY DEVELOPMENT

1. One afternoon the nurse overhears a young female client having an argument with her boyfriend. A while later the client complains to the nurse that dinner is always late and the meals are terrible. The nurse recognizes that the defense mechanism the client is using is:
   1. Projection
   2. Dissociation
   3. Displacement
   4. Intellectualization

2. Although upset by a young client's continuous complaints about all aspects of care, the nurse ignores them and attempts to divert the conversation. Immediately following this exchange with the client, the nurse discusses with a friend the various stages of development of young adults. The defense mechanism the nurse is using is:
   1. Substitution
   2. Sublimation
   3. Identification
   4. Intellectualization

3. During an interview with the parents of an adolescent female, the nurse notices that her father continually defends and makes excuses for all of his daughter's actions while her mother seems to feel her daughter is just lazy and that there is nothing wrong with her that she couldn't fight with some effort. The nurse recognizes that this family probably relates by using the mechanism known as:
   1. Coalitions
   2. Resignation
   3. Scapegoating
   4. Reaction formation

4. The nurse is aware that according to Erikson, a young child's increased vulnerability to anxiety in response to separations or pending separations from significant others results from failure to complete the developmental task called:
   1. Trust
   2. Identity
   3. Initiative
   4. Autonomy

5. The nurse knows that Erikson identified the developmental tasks of the school-aged child from 6 to 12 years as:
   1. Initiative vs guilt
   2. Industry vs inferiority
   3. Breaking away vs staying at home
   4. Psychosexual impulses vs psychosexual development

6. According to Erikson, a young adult must accomplish the tasks associated with the stage known as:
   1. Initiative vs. Guilt
   2. Intimacy vs Isolation
   3. Industry vs. Inferiority
   4. Generativity vs. Stagnation

7. A 65-year-old who immigrated from Cuba 25 years ago is admitted with a history of depression. The client who speaks little English and has few outside interests since retiring states, "I feel useless and unneeded." According to Erikson, the client is in the developmental stage of:
   1. Initiative vs guilt
   2. Integrity vs despair
   3. Intimacy vs isolation
   4. Identity vs role confusion

8. A 7-year-old boy wakes up crying because he has wet his bed. It would be most appropriate for the nurse to:
   1. Allow him to change his own bed and pajamas
   2. Change his bed while he changes his pajamas
   3. Take him to the bathroom and change his pajamas
   4. Remind him that he must call for the nurse the next time

9. The mother of an 18-year-old comes to the clinic at the local mental health center. She is extremely upset because her son has returned from his freshman year at college and is uncontrollable. He takes his brother's clothing, comes in at all hours, and refuses to get a job. Sometimes he is happy and outgoing and other times he is withdrawn. The mother asks why her son is like this and speculates that college has done this to him. While contemplating this situation, the nurse understands that adolescents are usually:
   1. Anxious and unhappy
   2. Angry and irresponsible
   3. Impulsive and self-centered
   4. Hyperactive and self-destructive

10. According to Erikson, an individual who fails to master the maturational crisis of adolescence will most often:
    1. Experience role confusion
    2. Be interpersonally isolated
    3. Rebel at all parental orders
    4. Use drugs and alcohol to escape

11. A constructive and lengthy method of confronting the stress of adolescence and preventing a negative and unhealthy developmental outcome is:
    1. Role experimentation
    2. Adherence to all peer standards
    3. Sublimation through school work
    4. Development of dependency on parents

12. The parents of an overweight adolescent female tell the nurse that they are concerned that their daughter feels inferior to her sister who is an attractive, successful college senior. They ask the nurse what they can do about this problem. The nurse should:
    1. Suggest that they seem to be creating a problem where none exists
    2. Tell them to avoid talking about their older daughter's accomplishments
    3. Suggest that they give this adolescent recognition for her own strong points
    4. Advise them to tell the adolescent to view her sister's success as a challenge

13. The nurse, along with an adolescent and the adolescent's parents, set bolstering the adolescent's self-esteem as a high-priority goal. The nursing action that would contribute to the achievement of this goal would be:
    1. Urging the adolescent to join a neighborhood social group
    2. Supporting the adolescent's interest in getting a newspaper route
    3. Suggesting that the mother give the adolescent lots of hugs and cuddling
    4. Encouraging the adolescent to talk about feelings of pride in successful siblings

14. The nurse would evaluate that the plan for bolstering an overweight adolescent's self-esteem was effective when, three months later, the adolescent's mother reports that the adolescent:
    1. Asks her to prepare a favorite dessert
    2. Seems to be doing average work in school
    3. Has joined a dirt bicycle club that meets at the school
    4. Imitates an older sibling's manner of speech and dress

15. According to Erikson, a person's adjustment to the period of senescence will depend largely on the adjustment the individual made to the developmental stage of:
    1. Intimacy vs Isolation
    2. Industry vs Inferiority
    3. Generativity vs Stagnation
    4. Identity vs Identity confusion

16. When helping the older adult (65 to 75) successfully complete Erikson's tasks of this stage, the nurse should assist the client to:
    1. Invest creative energies in promoting social welfare
    2. Redefine a role in society and offer something of value
    3. Look to recapture opportunities that were not started or completed
    4. Feel a sense of satisfaction when reflecting back on past achievements

17. The nurse's role in maintaining or promoting the health of the older adult should be based on the principle that:
    1. There is a strong correlation between successful retirement and good health
    2. Some of the physiologic changes that occur as a result of aging are reversible
    3. Thoughts of impending death are frequent and depressing to most older adults
    4. Older adults can better accept the dependent state chronic illness often causes

18. When planning care for an older adult the nurse is aware that normal aging has little effect on a client's:
    1. Sense of taste or smell
    2. Gastrointestinal motility
    3. Muscle or motor strength
    4. Ability to handle life's stresses

DISORDERS FIRST EVIDENT BEFORE ADULTHOOD

19. The nurse is aware that a child's emotional symptoms usually occur as a result of:
    1. Family pathology
    2. Rejection by the parents
    3. Authoritarian parenting style
    4. Overbearing overprotectiveness

20. The nurse is aware that a child experiencing emotional problems would probably exhibit:
    1. Impaired ability to reality test
    2. Passive and deliberate behavior
    3. Overinvolvement with peer group
    4. A mild to moderate level of anxiety

21. When assessing disturbed children, the clue that the nurse would find most indicative of severe emotional problems would be the child's:
    1. Physical complaints
    2. Behavioral outbursts
    3. Poor school performance
    4. Lack of response to the environment

22. A young school-age child is brought to the clinic by the mother who states, "Something is very wrong. My child never seems happy and refuses to play." When assessing this child for depressed behavior the nurse should initially begin with the statement:
    1. "Tell me about yourself."
    2. "Let's talk about what you do after school."
    3. "Can you tell me what is making you so unhappy?"
    4. "Why does your mother think that you are unhappy?"

23. When implementing a tertiary preventive program in mental retardation, the nurse should:
    1. Teach mentally retarded children how to feed themselves
    2. Refer children for evaluation if they fail to meet developmental milestones
    3. Encourage the use of birth control methods by women who are mentally retarded
    4. Utilize the Denver Developmental Screening Test to evaluate children attending well-child clinics

24. A young child has a history of frequent temper tantrums. The mother asks how to limit this acting-out behavior. The nurse's most therapeutic response would focus on:
    1. Restraining the child whenever a tantrum begins
    2. Moving the child to a quiet area before the tantrum begins
    3. Telling the mother to ignore the tantrum whenever possible
    4. Asking the physician to order medication for behavioral control

25. With the diagnosis of a possible pervasive developmental autistic disorder, the nurse would find it most unusual for a 3-year-old to demonstrate:
1. Ritualistic behavior
2. An interest in music
3. An attachment to odd objects
4. A responsiveness to the parents

26. A 7-year-old third grader is brought to the clinic by her mother who tells the nurse that her child has been having trouble in school, has difficulty concentrating, and is falling behind in her school work since she and her husband separated 6 months ago. The mother reports that lately her daughter has not been eating her dinner and she often hears her crying in her room. The nurse realizes that the child:
1. Feels different from her classmates
2. Is working through her feelings of loss
3. Would probably be happier living with her father
4. Probably blames herself for her parents' breakup

27. When assessing mental status in a 7- or 8-year-old child it is most important for the nurse to:
1. Engage the child in a discussion about feelings
2. Listen to the parent's description of the child's behavior
3. Compare the child's functioning from one time to another
4. Use direct questions to determine the child's mental ability

28. An only child, who lives with the mother, begins demonstrating school and emotional problems after the parents' marital breakup. It is decided that the child would probably benefit most from family therapy. The nurse plans that the first group session will include:
1. The parents
2. The mother and the child
3. The parents and the child
4. The mother, the child, and the child's teacher

29. A 10-year-old child, who has a history of school failure and destructive acting out, is admitted to a child psychiatric unit with the diagnosis of attention deficit disorder with hyperactivity. The youngest of 3 children, the child is identified by both the parents and the siblings as the family problem. The parents tell the nurse that the child's behavior has resulted in severe marital problems. The nurse would be correct in identifying the family's pattern of relating to the child as:
1. Controlling
2. Patronizing
3. Scapegoating
4. Overburdening

30. To help a disturbed, acting-out child develop a trusting relationship the nurse should:
1. Inquire as to child's feelings about the parents
2. Implement daily 30-minute one-to-one interactions
3. Offer support and emphasize safety in play activities
4. Initiate limit setting and explain the rules that must be followed

31. An acting-out, hyperactive 9-year-old boy is started on a behavior modification program. One day he is playing a game with his peers and becomes frustrated when he begins to lose. He begins to kick the other children under the table and call them names. The nurse, using the most appropriate behavior modification technique, should:
1. Require the child to have a time-out and regain control
2. Negatively reinforce the child by taking two of his tokens
3. Ignore the child's behavior with the intent of extinguishing it
4. Engage the child in a conversation about good sportsmanship

32. After 1 month in a special school, a hyperactive 10-year-old is asked to leave the group therapy session because of disruptiveness. The child begins to cry when being led out. The nurse's best approach at this time would be to:

1. Send the child for a time-out in a quiet room
2. Engage the child in a talk about the school day
3. Offer an interpretation of the child's self-defeating behavior
4. Provide nurturance by sharing a snack and a glass of milk with the child

33. A hyperactive, self-destructive child is to be discharged from an inpatient setting in a couple of weeks. In preparation for the child's discharge it is most important for the nurse to plan to:
    1. Establish, maintain, and/or enforce limits on behavior
    2. Meet with the child's teacher to review the child's needs
    3. Help the child begin to terminate relationships with the staff
    4. Schedule a home visit and a community trip with the child's family

EATING DISORDERS

34. A young adolescent is diagnosed as having anorexia nervosa. The nurse is aware that anorexia nervosa is usually precipitated by:
    1. The acting out of aggressive impulses, which results in feelings of hopelessness
    2. An unconscious wish to punish a parent who tries to dominate the adolescent's life
    3. The inability to deal with being the center of attention in the family and a desire for independence
    4. An inaccurate perception of hunger stimuli and a struggle between dependence and independence

35. The nurse interviews a young female client with anorexia nervosa to obtain information for the nursing history. The client's history is likely to reveal:
    1. A strong desire to improve her self-image
    2. A close, supportive mother-daughter relationship
    3. Low achievement in school, with little concern for grades
    4. Satisfaction with and a desire to maintain her present weight

36. The nursing intervention that should receive the highest priority in the period immediately following an emaciated 13-year-old's admission for starvation secondary to anorexia nervosa would be:
    1. Providing adequate rest and nutrition
    2. Monitoring the client's fluid and electrolyte balance
    3. Completing an assessment of the client's mental status
    4. Obtaining more data about the client's diet and exercise program

37. The nurse is aware that a major health problem associated with severe anorexia nervosa is:
    1. Protein depletion resulting in muscle wasting
    2. Endocrine imbalance resulting in amenorrhea
    3. Glucose intolerance resulting in hypoglycemia
    4. Cardiac dysrhythmias resulting in cardiac arrest

38. While admitting a young client with severe anorexia nervosa to the unit, the nurse finds a bottle of assorted pills in the client's luggage. The client tells the nurse they are antacids for stomach pains. The best initial response by the nurse would be:
    1. "Let's talk about your drug use."
    2. "These pills don't look like antacids."
    3. "Tell me more about these stomach pains."
    4. "Some adolescents take pills to lose weight."

39. The parents of an adolescent female are very upset about their daughter's diagnosis of anorexia nervosa and the treatment plan proposed. The best intervention by the nurse when the client's parents ask to bring food in for the client is to state:
    1. "Your concerns about food contribute to her problem."
    2. "While in the hospital she should eat the hospital food."
    3. "For now, allow the hospital staff to handle her food needs."
    4. "It is important that you bring in whatever you think she'll eat."

40. When interacting with an adolescent client with the diagnosis of anorexia nervosa, the nurse should:
    1. Show empathy
    2. Maintain control
    3. Set and maintain limits
    4. Focus on dietary nutrition

41. The multidisciplinary team decides to employ a behavior modification approach to a young female's problem with anorexia nervosa. A planned nursing intervention that would follow this approach would be:
    1. Have the client role play interactions with her parents
    2. Provide the client with a high-caloric, high-protein diet
    3. Restrict the client to her room until she gains 2 pounds
    4. Force the client to talk about her favorite foods for 1 hour a day

42. When an adolescent female client with the diagnosis of anorexia nervosa starts to discuss food and eating, the nurse should plan to:
    1. Tell her gently but firmly to direct all discussion of food to the dietician
    2. Use her current interest in food to encourage her to increase her intake
    3. Listen closely to determine her favorite foods and secure these foods for her
    4. Let her talk about food as long as she wants, but limit discussion about her eating

43. When talking with one of the day nurses, a client with the diagnosis of anorexia nervosa states that the day nurses give better care and are nicer than the night nurses. The client also asks a question that the day nurse is aware was answered by one of the night nurses. The nurse should recognize that the client:
    1. Needs assistance in exploring and verbalizing feelings about the night nurses
    2. Is trying to develop a bond of trust with a staff member that should be encouraged
    3. Is attempting to divide the staff and the behavior should be reported to the other staff members
    4. Has negative feelings about the night nurses and the nurses should be informed of these feelings

44. The nurse notes that a young female with anorexia nervosa telephones home just before each mealtime. She ignores reminders to eat and continues talking until the other clients are finished eating. She then refuses to eat "cold food." The nurse should:
    1. Insist that the client eat the cold food
    2. Remove the client's telephone privileges
    3. Hang the telephone up when meals are served
    4. Schedule a family meeting to discuss the problem

45. A young female client with anorexia nervosa telephones home just before mealtime. The client uses the phone calls to avoid eating. The nurse could evaluate that the nursing plan to set limits on this avoidance behavior was effective when the client:
    1. Organizes an aerobic group for the clients
    2. Arrives on time for meals without being called
    3. Begins reading and clipping recipes from magazines
    4. Contacts her family frequently by telephone between meals

EMOTIONAL PROBLEMS RELATED TO PHYSICAL HEALTH AND CHILDBEARING

46. A three-year-old's parents have been unable to visit since the child was admitted to the hospital. The toddler has become quiet and withdrawn. To best help the child at this time the nurse should:
    1. Bring the child a doll or stuffed animal to cuddle
    2. Encourage the child to play games with the other children
    3. Assign the same nurse to care for the child whenever possible
    4. Contact the child's parents and tell them to come immediately to visit

47. A 3½-year-old begins screaming and kicking when the laboratory technician comes to draw blood. The nurse recognizes that this reaction is due primarily to the child's:

1. Fear of loss of control
2. Inability to localize pain
3. Fear of intrusive procedures
4. Past experience with this procedure

48. Just prior to having a physical examination by the physician, the nurse can best meet an eight-year-old's developmental needs by:
1. Allowing the child to handle the examination equipment
2. Explaining exactly what will happen during the examination
3. Having the child talk to a child who has recently had an examination
4. Arranging to have one of the child's parents present during the examination

49. A 9-year-old boy, admitted with a fractured femur, has just been told he must stay in the hospital in traction for at least a month. The nurse finds him crying and unwilling to talk. At this time, the nurse should give the highest priority to:
1. Giving him privacy and allowing him to cry
2. Telling him that his injury will not be permanent
3. Trying to distract him to prevent embarrassment
4. Arranging for him to have a tutor begin immediately

50. A client with a history of hypertension comes to the clinic where the intake physical reveals a blood pressure of 180/102. When the nurse asks if the client has been taking any medications the client replies, "I took the pills the doctor prescribed for a few weeks, but I didn't feel any different. So, I decided I'd just take them if I felt sick." The best initial response by the nurse would be:
1. "I'm glad to hear you felt well enough to stop the medication."
2. "You must be quite frightened about having high blood pressure."
3. "You really should try to take your medication, the doctor felt it was needed."
4. "I think we should talk to the physician about a plan of treatment you can follow."

51. A male client with a history of ulcerative colitis, who is admitted with severe rectal bleeding, appears to be an angry demanding person. One day the nursing assistant tells the nurse, "I've had it with that client and all his demands. I'm not going in there again." The nurse's best response to this statement would be:
1. "You need to try to be patient with him. He's going through a lot right now."
2. "I'll talk with him and see if I can figure out the best way for us to handle this."
3. "He's frightened and taking it out on the staff. Let's think how we can approach him."
4. "Just ignore him and get on with the rest of your work. Let someone else take a turn."

52. A client calls out to every nursing staff member who passes by the door and asks them to do something or get something. The nurse can best manage this behavior by:
1. Closing the door to the room so the client cannot see the staff members as they pass by
2. Assigning one staff member to approach the client regularly and spend time talking with the client
3. Informing the client that one staff member will come in frequently to see if the client has any requests
4. Arranging for a variety of staff members to take turns going into the room to see if the client has any requests

53. One day a client admitted for testing prior to a possible colon resection and colostomy says to the nurse, "If I have to have this surgery, I know my husband will never come near me." The nurse's best initial response would be, "You're:
1. Probably underestimating his love for you."
2. Concerned that your husband will reject you."
3. Wondering about the effect on your sexual relations."
4. Worried that the surgery will change how others see you."

54. A client requiring surgery because of mitral valve incompetence is admitted to the hospital and states, "I need a new valve and do an oil change too!" The most therapeutic response by the nurse would be:
    1. "You really don't need to hide your anxieties."
    2. "You sure came to the right place for a valve job."
    3. "I'm glad to see you're handling the situation so well."
    4. "I'm sure you have a great deal to ask about your surgery."

55. A female client who has been told by her physician that she has untreatable metastatic carcinoma tells the nurse that she believes the physician has made an error and that she does not have cancer and is not going to die. The nurse evaluates that the client is experiencing the stage of death and dying known as:
    1. Anger
    2. Shock
    3. Bargaining
    4. Acceptance

56. A 68-year-old has metastatic carcinoma and has been told by the physician that death will occur within a month or two. The nurse enters the client's room after the physician leaves and finds the client crying. The nurse's action should take into consideration that:
    1. Crying relieves depression and helps the client face reality
    2. Crying releases tension which frees psychic energy for coping
    3. Nurses should not interfere with a client's behavior and defenses
    4. Accepting a client's crying maintains and strengthens the nurse-client bond

57. A terminally ill 76-year-old client is very quiet, not talking much, and unwilling to have visitors. During the initial contact with the client, the nurse should:

1. Attempt to understand what the death and dying process means to the client
2. Avoid talking about the client's condition unless the client initiates the discussion
3. Ascertain how much pain the client is experiencing and what medications have been ordered
4. Explore the extent to which the client is aware of the prognosis and the client's feelings about the situation

58. A female client terminally ill with cancer says to the nurse, "My husband is avoiding me. He doesn't love me anymore because of this damn tumor!" The nurse's most appropriate response would be:
    1. "What makes you think he doesn't love you?"
    2. "Avoidance is a defense; he needs your help to cope."
    3. "He is probably having difficulty dealing with your illness."
    4. "You seem very upset. Tell me how your husband is avoiding you."

ANXIETY, SOMATOFORM, AND DISSOCIATIVE DISORDERS

59. An elderly client who lives alone tells the nurse at the community health center, "I really don't need anyone to talk to, the TV is my best friend." The nurse recognizes that the client is using the defense mechanism known as:
    1. Denial
    2. Projection
    3. Sublimation
    4. Displacement

60. The symptoms that distinguish posttraumatic stress disorders from other anxiety disorders are:
    1. Lack of interest in family and others
    2. Reexperiencing the trauma in dreams or flashbacks
    3. Avoidance of situations and certain activities that resemble the stress
    4. Depression and a blunted affect when discussing the traumatic situation

61. A client with an anxiety disorder is hospitalized. The nurse realizes that an environment
conducive to reducing emotional stress and
providing psychologic safety is one in which:
    1. All the client's needs are met
    2. Needs are a primary concern
    3. Realistic limits and controls are set
    4. The physical environment is kept in order

62. A client comes to the hospital because of intense feelings of unrest, inability to sleep,
and frequent episodes of panic. The client
tells the nurse, "I admitted myself because I
think I'm going crazy." The nurse should recognize the client's remark as a:
    1. Plea for support
    2. Symptom of depression
    3. Reflection of insightfulness
    4. Test of the nurse's trustworthiness

63. A nurse is accompanying a client with a diagnosis of anxiety disorder, who is pacing the
halls and crying. When the client's pacing and
crying increase, the nurse suddenly feels uncomfortable and experiences a strong desire to
leave. The probable reason for this feeling is:
    1. An empathic communication of anxiety
    2. A desire to go off duty after a busy day
    3. A fear of the client's becoming assaultive
    4. An inability to tolerate any more bizarre
behavior

64. The nurse is aware that nursing intervention for
clients with anxiety disorders should include:
    1. Promoting the verbalization of feelings by
the client
    2. Promoting the suppression of anger/hos-
tility by the client
    3. Insisting that the client accept the role of
psychological factors
    4. Limiting the involvement of the client's
family during the acute phase

65. A client is pacing the floor and appears extremely anxious. The nurse approaches in an
attempt to alleviate the client's anxious feelings. The most therapeutic question by the
nurse would be:

1. "Are you feeling upset right now?"
2. "Would you like me to walk with you?"
3. "Shall we sit and talk about your feelings?"
4. "Would you like to go to the gym and
work out?"

66. Without knocking, the nurse enters the room
of a young male client with the diagnosis of
panic disorder and observes him masturbat-
ing. The nurse should:
    1. Say "Excuse me" and leave the room
    2. Tactfully assess why he needs to masturbate
    3. Pretend nothing was seen and carry out
whatever task needs to be done
    4. Explain in a calm, quiet manner that his
behavior is inappropriate in the hospital

67. A 15-year-old client with the diagnosis of
panic disorder jumps when spoken to, complains of feeling uneasy, and states, "It's as
though something bad is going to happen." It
would be most therapeutic for the nurse to:
    1. Be physically present in the room
    2. Encourage the client to communicate
with the staff
    3. Allow the client to set the parameters for
the interaction
    4. Help the client to understand the cause
of the feelings described

68. A client with a diagnosis of panic disorder, who
had a panic attack on the previous day, says to
the nurse, "That was a terrible feeling I had yesterday. I'm so afraid to talk about it." The
nurse's most therapeutic response would be:
    1. "It's best that you try to talk about it."
    2. "Okay, we don't have to talk about it."
    3. "What were you doing yesterday when
you first noticed the feeling?"
    4. "I understand but don't be concerned;
that feeling probably won't come back."

69. The nurse plans to teach a client to use more
healthy coping behaviors which can be consciously used to reduce anxiety including:
    1. Eating, dissociation, fantasy
    2. Sublimation, fantasy, rationalization
    3. Repression, intellectualization, smoking
    4. Exercise, talking to friends, suppression

70. A male client asks one of the female staff members for a date. It is most likely that:
1. The staff member may have led the client on
2. The client misinterpreted the staff member's friendliness
3. The client may be trying to protect a threatened sexual identity
4. The staff member may have been acting unprofessionally toward the client

71. The nurse could evaluate that the staff's approach to setting limits for a demanding, angry client was effective if the client:
1. No longer calls the nursing staff for assistance
2. Understands the reasons why frequent calls to the staff were made
3. Apologizes for disrupting the unit's routine when something is needed
4. Discusses concerns about the physical condition that required hospitalization

72. The change in an elderly client's behavior that would indicate that the nurse should reassess the client's needs and current plan of care, which was attempting to maintain the client's independent living style, would be the development of:
1. Confusion
2. Hypochondriasis
3. Additional complaints
4. Increased socialization

73. During the first meeting of a therapy group, the members become quite uncomfortable. The nurse notes frequent periods of silence, tense laughter, and a good deal of nervous movement in the group. The nurse would assess that these responses:
1. Require active leader intervention to relieve symptoms of obvious stress
2. Indicate unhealthy group processes with an unwillingness to relate openly
3. Are expected group behaviors because relationships are not yet established
4. Should be pointed out and discussed so members will not become too uncomfortable

74. During the working phase, a female group member becomes tearful after being told by another member that she needs to change her behavior. The nurse evaluates that the client:
1. Has had her feelings hurt by this response
2. Feels too fragile to be challenged at this time
3. Is angry about the confrontation with another member
4. Has been depressed about this aspect of her behavior

CRISIS SITUATIONS

75. A crisis can best be defined as:
1. An imbalance of life
2. A threat to homeostasis
3. The perception of the problem by the client
4. A situation requiring help other than personal resources

76. When working with families encountering problems, it is most important that the nurse has a:
1. Good memory for details
2. Common social background
3. Warm nature and loving personality
4. Sense of self and empathy for others

77. An adolescent client seeks help at a crisis intervention clinic. The client relates, "I dropped out of college because the instructors were dumb and the kids acted like babies. I was a psychiatric aide for 6 weeks. I got into trouble because the staff's thinking was archaic. I tried waiting on tables but got fired. The boss said I was nasty to the customers. They were the nasty ones. Now I can't even pay my rent. If people were nicer, I wouldn't be in this mess." In relation to crisis theory, this client's stressful events can be seen as:
1. Experiential
2. Age-related and frequent
3. Situational and maturational
4. Usually noncrisis-producing

78. A 60-year-old client complains of headaches, restlessness, and insomnia. During an interview, the nurse learns that the symptoms began three months ago after the client was forced into early retirement. The nurse recognizes that the client is probably experiencing a:
1. Social crisis
2. Economic crisis
3. Situational crisis
4. Developmental crisis

79. Situational crises are usually resolved in a time period of:
1. 1 to 4 days
2. 2 to 3 weeks
3. 1 to 2 months
4. 2 to 6 months

80. According to crisis theory, the minimal long-term goal in crisis intervention is:
1. Relief of acute symptoms
2. Relief of panic level anxiety
3. Restoration of the original functioning level
4. Reorganization and reordering of the personality

81. The most critical factor for the nurse to determine during crisis intervention is the client's:
1. Developmental history
2. Available situational supports
3. Underlying unconscious conflict
4. Willingness to restructure the personality

82. When intervening in a crisis situation, the initial concern of the nurse is:
1. What was the precipitating factor
2. How is the individual affecting others
3. How will the client deal with successive crises
4. Whether the individual can go back to daily activities

83. The nurse suggests a crisis intervention group to a client experiencing a developmental crisis. These groups are successful because the:

1. Client is encouraged to talk about personal problems
2. Crisis group supplies a workable solution to the client's problems
3. Crisis intervention worker is a psychologist and understands behavior patterns
4. Client is assisted to investigate alternative approaches to solving the identified problem

84. When talking with a client in crisis, the crisis intervention nurse should:
1. Restate the problem, putting it in the proper perspective
2. Respect the client and involve the client in deciding what will be done and how it will be done
3. Explain to the client that the center has helped many other people with the same problem
4. Explore the client's religious and cultural beliefs so the instructions are within the client's value system

85. A young college student tells the nurse in the school's health service that his girlfriend's period is late and they both think she is pregnant. The client, with a broad smile on his face, states loudly and angrily, "If she is pregnant I will drop out of school, marry her, and get a full-time job." The nurse's best initial assessment of the client's verbal and nonverbal behavior would be that they are:
1. Uniform
2. Consistent
3. Appropriate
4. Incongruent

86. When talking to the nurse about his decision to drop out of school and marry his girlfriend who is pregnant, a young college student says, "It's really the best decision. It is important for a child to have two parents." The nurse recognizes that the client is using the defense mechanism known as:
1. Projection
2. Introspection
3. Displacement
4. Intellectualization

87. A 24-year-old secretary, pregnant for the first time, receives a letter from her boyfriend with a check for $500 and the news that he has left. The client is very upset, feels at the end of her rope, and calls the crisis intervention center for help. The nurse recognizes that the client is experiencing a crisis because:
1. The client is under a great deal of stress
2. The client is going to have to raise her child alone
3. The client's boyfriend left her when she was pregnant
4. The client's past methods of adapting are ineffective for this situation

88. A single, pregnant client, attending a crisis intervention group, has decided to go through with the pregnancy and keep the baby. Now the crisis intervention nurse's primary responsibility is to:
1. Support the client for making a wise decision
2. Explore other problems the client may be experiencing
3. Make an appointment for the client to see a physician for prenatal care
4. Provide information about other health resources where the client may receive additional assistance

89. A single, pregnant client, who has been attending a crisis intervention clinic, has decided to keep the baby and is looking forward to motherhood. The nurse recognizes the decision to attend prenatal child care classes is an example of:
1. Intrinsic motivation
2. Extrinsic motivation
3. Operant conditioning
4. Behavior modification

90. A couple in their late twenties are very happy to be expecting a child. After the client delivers, she is disappointed that the baby is a boy but the husband is pleased. On the second day after delivery, when the baby is brought to the client, she seems far away as though she is daydreaming. The nurse calls the client's name and the client states, "I don't have a baby. I have sinned." She proceeds to rock her empty arms. The nurse recognizes that the precipitating factor for the client's emotional reaction is probably her:

1. Alteration in role
2. Husband's behavior
3. Religious upbringing
4. Desire for a baby girl

91. If it is doubtful that a retarded adult resident of a community home, who has had 4 pregnancies in 2 years, is able to exercise informed consent for sterilization, the nurse should be aware that the procedure cannot be performed without approval from the:
1. Court
2. Next of kin
3. Legal guardian
4. Court and legal guardian

92. When obtaining informed consent for sterilization from a mentally retarded adult client, the nurse must be sure that the:
1. Parent or guardian signs the permit
2. Client comprehends the outcome of the procedure
3. Client is fully able to explain what the procedure entails
4. Parent or guardian has encouraged the client to make the decision

93. Child abuse is suspected in a 3-year-old girl admitted with many poorly explained injuries. During a conversation, the statement by the mother that would further this suspicion would be:
1. "When I get angry, I take her for a walk."
2. "I send her to her room alone when she misbehaves."
3. "I make her stand in the corner when she doesn't eat her dinner."
4. "The other children were no problem; this one is stubborn and whiney."

94. A mother of four is remanded to the psychiatric unit by the court for observation. She was arrested and charged with abusing her 2-year-old son, who is in the pediatric intensive care unit in critical condition with a fractured skull and other injuries from a beating. When approaching the client, the nurse should expect the client to:
1. Deny beating her son
2. Express concern for her son
3. Ask where her three other children are
4. Avoid talking about the situation completely

95. When speaking with a mother accused of child abuse the nurse should expect her to:
1. Attempt to rationalize and explain her behavior
2. Offer a detailed explanation of how her child was injured
3. Reveal an overwhelming feeling that her children are worthless
4. Ask how she may get permission to visit her child on the pediatric unit

96. One morning before work a nurse becomes very angry with her daughter, and both mother and daughter end the argument in tears. At the hospital the nurse is assigned to care for a mother accused of severely beating her young child. The nurse has difficulty spending time with the client and tells another nurse about the argument and states, "This client makes me feel very uncomfortable today." The best explanation of what is happening with the nurse is that she:
1. Has identified with a client of the same sex
2. Would have difficulty caring for any client today
3. Is beginning to question her own potential for abuse
4. Is experiencing guilt that is causing her to be ineffective

97. The nurse may best assist an abusing parent to alter behavior toward an abused 2-year-old child by helping the client to:
1. Learn what behavior is appropriate for a 2-year-old child
2. Learn appropriate ways of punishing the child's inappropriate behavior
3. Identify the specific ways in which the child's behavior provokes frustration
4. Ignore the child's negative, nondestructive behavior and support acceptable behavior

98. A nurse on the pediatric unit is assigned to care for a 2-year-old child with a history of abuse. The nurse should expect the child to:
1. Smile readily at anyone who enters the room
2. Be wary of physical contact initiated by anyone
3. Pay little attention to the nurse standing at the bedside
4. Begin to cry and scream as the nurse nears the bedside

99. When the physician examines the genital area of a child suspected of being abused, the nurse can be most therapeutic by:
1. Explaining the procedure and remaining with the child during the examination
2. Telling the child that the doctor wants to see if there is "anything wrong down there"
3. Helping the mother explain the examination and the findings in terms the child will understand
4. Asking if the child would prefer the nurse or the mother to be present during the examination

100. A young child suspected of being sexually abused says to the nurse, "Did I do something bad?" The nurse's most therapeutic reply would be:
1. "Who said you did something bad?"
2. "What do you mean, something bad?"
3. "Do you think that you did something bad?"
4. "I'm not sure I would say it was something bad."

101. A recently married 22-year-old is brought to the trauma center by the police. She had been robbed, beaten, raped, and sodomized. The client, although very anxious and tearful, appears in control. The physician orders diazepam (Valium) 5 mg po prn for agitation. The nurse should administer this medication when the:
1. Client requests something to calm her
2. Client's crying and trembling seem to increase
3. Physician is ready to do a vaginal examination
4. Nurse determines the client's anxiety is increasing

102. The husband of a rape victim arrives at the hospital after being called by the police. After reassuring him about his wife's condition, the nurse should give priority to:
1. Discussing with him his own feelings about the situation
2. Calling the rape counselor in to immediately meet with the wife
3. Helping him to understand how his wife feels about the situation
4. Making him comfortable until the physician has completed examining his wife

103. The nurse is at the rape intervention clinic when a rape victim comes in saying, "I've got to talk to someone or I'll go crazy. I should not have dated him." When assessing the client's condition, it is important for the nurse to identify the client's:
1. Support network
2. Sexual background
3. Ability to relate the facts
4. Knowledge of rape victimology

104. The biggest problem for an elderly female client to deal with right after the death of her husband will probably be her:
1. Anger
2. Finances
3. Loneliness
4. Estrangement

105. A male client is brought to the psychiatric emergency room after attempting to jump off a bridge. The client's wife states that he lost his job several months ago and has been unable to get another job. The primary nursing intervention at this time would be to assess for:
1. A past history of depression
2. Feelings of excessive failure
3. Current plans to commit suicide
4. The presence of marital difficulties

106. In response to a parent's question about childhood suicide, the nurse's most appropriate response would be:
1. "Children do not have readily available means to kill themselves."
2. "Suicide threats and gestures in children should be taken seriously."
3. "Children under the age of 6 may threaten but do not attempt suicide."
4. "Suicide in young children is manipulative rather than self-destructive acting out."

107. A 7-year-old has been diagnosed as having acute myelogenous leukemia. The physician has discussed the diagnosis and prognosis with the parents. While the parents are sitting in the lounge after visiting their child they have a severe argument over something trivial. The nurse should help them recognize that they are using the defense mechanism of:

1. Denial
2. Projection
3. Displacement
4. Compensation

108. An 8-year-old with a terminal illness is demanding of the staff. The child asks for many privileges the other children on the unit do not have, such as staying up later to watch TV and eating candy. The staff knows the child does not have long to live. The nurse can best help the staff cope with the child's demands by encouraging them to:
1. Give as many extra treats as possible since the child is dying
2. Give the child some extra treats so they will feel less anxiety after the child dies
3. Set reasonable limits to help the child and the family become more secure and content
4. Recognize that the dying child has unique needs and special privileges can provide the necessary security

109. When the parents visit their hospitalized child, the child continues to play and ignores their presence. The parents are extremely disturbed by the child's reaction to them. The nurse informs them that this behavior is common among hospitalized children and tells them this is called:
1. Denial
2. Undoing
3. Repression
4. Sublimation

110. A 7-year-old child dies after an explosion at school. The parents arrive at the hospital a few minutes later and are told what had happened. The parents ask the nurse if they can see their child. The best response by the nurse would be:
1. "It's best to wait a while."
2. "I will take you in to see your child now."
3. "Would you like to wait until the physician can be with you?"
4. "It will be less traumatic if you wait to see your child at the funeral home."

111. A mother whose daughter is killed in a school bus accident tells the nurse that her daughter was just getting over the chicken-pox and did not want to go to school but she insisted that she go. The mother cries bitterly and says her child's death is her fault. The nurse should realize that perceiving a death as preventable will most often influence the grieving process in that:
    1. The loss may be easier to understand and to accept
    2. Bereavement may be of greater intensity and duration
    3. The grieving process may progress to a psychiatric illness
    4. It causes the mourner to experience a pathological grief reaction

112. The initial nursing intervention for the significant others during the shock phase of a grief reaction should be focused on:
    1. Staying with the individuals involved
    2. Mobilizing the individuals' support systems
    3. Directing the individuals' activities at this time
    4. Presenting full reality of the loss to the individuals

113. Shortly after the death of her husband following a long illness, the wife visits the mental health clinic complaining of malaise, lethargy, and insomnia. The nurse, knowing that it is most important to help the wife cope with her husband's death, should attempt to determine the:
    1. Age of the wife
    2. Timing of the husband's death
    3. Socioeconomic status of the husband
    4. Adequacy of the wife's support system

114. The nurse understands that an individual will probably have the greatest difficulty with the grieving process if the relationship with the significant other was:
    1. Loving
    2. Long-term
    3. Ambivalent
    4. Domineering

115. When an individual successfully completes the grieving process after the death of a significant other, the individual will be able to:

    1. Accept the inevitability of death
    2. Go on with life and forget the past
    3. Remember the significant other realistically
    4. Focus mainly on the good qualities of the person who died

116. A male client is brought to the psychiatric unit by family members who state, "He's just not himself since his wife died 2 years ago. He has no interests and doesn't care for himself any more, just sitting alone at home when he's not working." The nurse completes a history and physical assessment, particularly noting that the client has lost a significant amount of weight, has poor eye contact, and appears sad. The most important assessment for the nurse to explore with the client at this time is:
    1. Feelings about his wife's death
    2. What seems to be making him sad
    3. His relationship with his deceased wife
    4. Whether he has considered suicide recently

117. The nurse discusses the plan of care with a depressed client whose husband has recently died. The nurse recognizes it would be most helpful to:
    1. Involve the client in group outdoor games each morning
    2. Encourage the client to talk about and plan for the future
    3. Encourage the client to interact with male clients and staff
    4. Talk with the client about her husband and the details of his death

118. A client, whose spouse recently died, attends a group therapy session in which a nurse is a co-leader. Toward the end of the session another client talks about being divorced and the resulting feelings of abandonment. As the members are leaving the session, the nurse notices that tears are running down the depressed client's face. Considering this client's depressed state the nurse should:
    1. Ask another client to stay and spend time talking with the client
    2. Ask the group members to return and discuss this client's feelings
    3. Observe the client's behavior carefully during the next several hours
    4. Go to the client's room and encourage a discussion of thoughts and feelings

119. A male client has been hospitalized on a medical unit for various aches and pains he has been experiencing for several weeks. The client appears depressed and tense. When talking with the client, the nurse finds that his wife died 3 months ago and he has not adjusted to the loss. When caring for the client the nurse should:
    1. Continue the discussion of the death of his wife
    2. Focus on teaching the client relaxation techniques
    3. Ask the internist for a psychiatric consult for the client as soon as possible
    4. Explain to the client why he needs to recognize his ambivalence toward his wife

120. An elderly female comes to the mental health clinic. Assessment reveals the client feels depressed and vaguely anxious and is unable to sleep at night. The client states, "I haven't felt right since my husband died 8 months ago." The nurse makes the nursing diagnosis of dysfunctional grieving related to the loss of the husband. The nurse uses this diagnosis because of the client's:
    1. Inability to talk about her loss
    2. Difficulty in expressing her loss
    3. Inability to sleep and the presence of symptoms of depression
    4. Prolonged period of grief and mourning after her husband's death

121. A client with an inoperable occipital lobe tumor has been experiencing rather frightening visual hallucinations especially when alone. The nurse can best help the client cope with these hallucinations by planning to:
    1. Move the client to a four-bed room closer to the nurse's station
    2. Suggest that the client turn on the radio or television when alone
    3. Have family or friends remain with the client until the hallucinations stop
    4. Suggest that the client not be alone and work out a schedule for visitors

122. The nurse recognizes that a characteristic behavior often demonstrated in the initial stage of a client's coping with dying often includes:
    1. Criticizing medical care
    2. Sleeping for long periods
    3. Asking for additional medical consultation
    4. Ringing the call light as soon as the nurse leaves

123. The wife of a client who is dying tells the nurse that, although she wants to visit her husband daily, she can only visit twice a week because she works and has to take care of the house and their cat and dog. The nurse assesses that the wife's statement demonstrates the use of the defense mechanism known as:
    1. Projection
    2. Sublimation
    3. Compensation
    4. Rationalization

124. The husband of a client who is dying tells the nurse that he knows that his wife is asking the nurses to leave her pain medication on her bedside table and fears she is saving it up for a suicide attempt. The nurse knows that many of the staff members have mixed feelings about the client's terminal status and prolonged pain. The nurse uses an approach which is ethically sound by:
    1. Speaking to all of the nurses and telling them not to leave the medication at the bedside
    2. Reporting the information and concern to the supervisor and letting the supervisor handle it
    3. Asking the head nurse to handle the problems of the client's medication and the staffs' feelings
    4. Suggesting a nursing conference be held to discuss staff feelings as well as the medication problem

125. The nurse recognizes that at this time to assist a couple to deal with their feelings about the husband's terminal illness, it would be important to:

1. Assist the couple to express their feelings about his terminal illness to each other
2. Place the couple in a couple's therapy group that deals with the terminal illness of one partner
3. Refer the husband to the psychotherapist for assistance in dealing with his anger about death
4. Encourage the couple to verbalize their feelings to a therapist during their individual therapy sessions

126. An elderly female client, whose husband had been ill for a prolonged period of time, is visited by her husband's hospice nurse following the funeral for her husband. The nurse recognizes that the wife's biggest problem at this time will probably be her:
1. Loneliness and feelings of isolation
2. Anger at the husband for abandoning her
3. Financial worries about maintaining her life-style
4. Guilt over feelings of relief that her husband has died

127. The grieving wife of a client who has just died says to the nurse, "We should have spent more time together. I always felt the children's needs came first." The nurse recognizes that the wife is experiencing:
1. Displaced anger
2. Normal feelings of guilt
3. Shame for past behaviors
4. Ambivalent feelings about him

128. The nurse is aware that tranquilizers are rarely ordered for individuals undergoing acute grief because they:
1. Magnify depression and increase the risk of suicide
2. Suppress the brain activity needed to prevent depression
3. Extend the period of denial and suppress normal mourning
4. Cause lethargy and prevent the return to interpersonal activity

129. A female client is readmitted to the hospital in the terminal stage of cancer. When talking with the nurse the client states, "I don't understand why my husband won't tell me what's going on at home. His telling me not to worry, everything is being taken care of, doesn't help." The most realistic interpretation of the husband's behavior is that he is:
1. Attempting to stop the client from worrying
2. Expressing his unacknowledged anger with her dying
3. Acting out his need for dominance in their relationship
4. Attempting to deal with his own needs and trying to cope without her input

130. A female client with a history of depression tells the nurse that she is planning to retire from her job next year. The nurse can best respond to the client by recognizing that retirement is:
1. A developmental task of tremendous significance
2. Damaging to both the self-image and self-esteem
3. Eagerly anticipated by the majority of older people
4. Always emotionally associated with the concept of aging

DISORDERS OF MOOD

131. A client's methods of coping are maladaptive. The nurse can best help the client develop healthier coping mechanisms by:
1. Promoting interpersonal relationships with peers
2. Providing a stress-free environment for the client
3. Allowing the client to assume responsibility for decisions
4. Setting realistic limits on the client's maladaptive behavior

132. The nurse can minimize agitation in a disturbed client by:
1. Ensuring constant client and staff contact
2. Increasing appropriate sensory stimulation
3. Discussing the reasons for suspicious beliefs
4. Limiting unnecessary interactions with the client

133. When caring for the depressed client the nurse usually has the most difficulty dealing with the:
1. Client's lack of energy
2. Negative non-verbal responses
3. Client's psychomotor retardation
4. Contagious quality of depression

134. When working with a client who is depressed, the nurse should initially:
1. Accept what the client says
2. Attempt to keep the client occupied
3. Try to keep the client from talking too much
4. Keep the client's surroundings bright and gay

135. When planning continuing care for the depressed client, the nurse should include:
1. Offering the client the opportunity to make some decisions
2. Encouraging the client to decide how to spend leisure time
3. Making all decisions to relieve the client of this responsibility
4. Allowing the client time to be alone to decide in which activities to engage

136. The nurse identifies establishing trust as a major nursing goal for a depressed client. This goal can best be accomplished by:
1. Spending the day with the client
2. Asking the client at least one question daily
3. Waiting for the client to initiate conversation
4. Spending short periods of time with the client every day

137. One day, the nurse sits by a depressed client's bed and states, "I will be spending some time with you today." The client responds angrily, "Go talk to someone else. They need you more." The most therapeutic response by the nurse would be:

1. "Why are you angry with me?"
2. "I'll go, but I will be back tomorrow."
3. "Don't say that. You are important too."
4. "I will be spending the next 15 minutes with you."

138. One morning a client with the diagnosis of acute depression states to the nurse, "God is punishing me for my past sins." The nurse's best response would be:
1. "Why do you think that?"
2. "God is punishing you for your sins?"
3. "You really must feel upset about this."
4. "If you feel this way, you should talk to your clergyman."

139. When the nurse sees a client who is depressed sitting alone in the day room, the best action would be to approach the client and say:
1. "May I sit with you for a while?"
2. "Call me if you would like to talk."
3. "Do you mind if I sit and talk to you?"
4. "I'll be sitting with you for a while today."

140. On the fifth hospital day, the nurse observes that a depressed client remains lying on the bed when the clients are called to the dining room for lunch. To encourage the client to eat the nurse should:
1. Simply state, "I will accompany you to the dining room."
2. Bring a tray to the client's room and leave it without comment
3. Provide information about the importance of eating to maintain health
4. Simply state, "All clients are expected to go to the dining room for meals."

141. When taking a history from a client with the diagnosis of a major depressive episode, melancholic type, the nurse should expect to find that the client's premorbid behavioral characteristics would include:
1. No clear boundaries to the client's lifestyle
2. A narrow range of interest and overmeticulousness
3. A history of jealousy and abrupt onset of symptoms
4. The presence of nervous hypermanic and depressive symptoms

142. A 50-year-old homemaker is brought to the hospital with a history of loss of weight, crying spells, restlessness, early morning insomnia, sitting in one place just staring into space, and picking at her skin. During the last 6 months her husband of 30 years has been made president of his company and their children have both married. From the history, the nurse should realize the client is demonstrating the classic symptoms associated with:
1. Bipolar mood disorders
2. Involutional induced reactions
3. Mood-incongruent manic disorders
4. Major depression-melancholic types

143. When assessing the premorbid personality characteristics of a client with a major depression, it would be unusual for the nurse to find that this client demonstrated:
1. Rigidity
2. Stubbornness
3. Diverse interests
4. Overmeticulousness

144. A depressed client is very resistive and complains about inabilities and worthlessness. The best approach by the nurse would be to:
1. Listen to the client and delay any planned activity for another time
2. Schedule activities for the client that can be implemented independently
3. Involve the client in activities in which success can be ensured
4. Encourage the client to select an activity in which there is some interest

145. A woman who attempted suicide is brought to the hospital by her husband. During the admission interview the woman says, "I do not deserve to live. I am a bad mother and have mistreated my child." The husband later indicates that his wife has been a good mother and never hurt their child. He states that their marital relationship has deteriorated since the birth of their child 2 years ago and that he plans to get a divorce. The nurse should recognize that the most probable basis for the client's depression is her:

1. Use of withdrawal as a defense in an attempt to survive in a relationship with a man who wishes to desert her
2. Child-abusing behavior that has resulted in feelings of guilt and shame that are being relieved by self-punishment
3. Unmet dependency needs that have aroused unacceptable, hostile feelings that are turned inward against the self
4. Basic feeling of loneliness that has resulted in the use of self-abasement to evoke love, sympathy, and compliments from others

146. A depressed client is admitted after being found bleeding from a self-inflicted superficial gunshot wound. The client does not respond to any of the nurse's questions. To assess the client's current potential for suicide, the nurse should:
1. Ask the client why suicide was attempted
2. Determine if there is a family history of suicide
3. Ask the family about any previous suicidal attempts or threats by the client
4. Observe the client for scars on the wrists or other signs of previous suicide attempts

147. To further assess a client's suicidal potential the nurse should be especially alert to the client's expression of:
1. Anger and resentment
2. Anxiety and loneliness
3. Frustration and fear of death
4. Helplessness and hopelessness

148. A client whose wife recently died appears extremely depressed. The client states, "What's the use in talking? I'd rather be dead. I can't go on without my wife." The best response by the nurse would be:
1. "You'd rather be dead?"
2. "Are you thinking about killing yourself?"
3. "I can understand why you feel that way."
4. "Tell me, what does death mean to you?"

149. The nurse should recognize that there is an increased suicidal potential when a client exhibits:
1. Severe depression and a preoccupation with religion
2. Withdrawal from reality with a history of suicidal threats
3. Persistent severe anxiety and increased somatic complaints
4. Sleep and appetite disturbances with a history of suicidal ideation

150. A female client has been hospitalized for three weeks while receiving a tricyclic medication for a severe depression. One day the client states to the nurse, "I'm really feeling better, my energy level is up. Did the nurse's aide tell you I gave her my designer purse?" The nurse recognizes that this statement may indicate:
1. An increased risk of suicide
2. An improved socialization level
3. A marked improvement in mood
4. A decreased need for continued observation

151. The nurse becomes aware of an elderly client's feeling of loneliness when the client states, "I only have a few friends. My daughter lives in another state and couldn't care whether I live or die. She doesn't even know I'm hospitalized." The nurse recognizes that the client's communication is probably a:
1. Call for help to prevent acting out of suicidal thoughts
2. Clue to depression that is blocking the motivation for self-care
3. Manipulative attempt to persuade the nurse to call the daughter
4. Request for information about community social support groups

152. A female client, who was admitted to the hospital because she attempted suicide, reveals that her desire for sex has diminished since her child's birth 3 years ago. The most accurate nursing diagnosis would probably be sexual dysfunction related to:

1. Decreased sexual desire associated with depression
2. Decreased sexual desire associated with dependency
3. Inadequate sexual desire associated with marital stress
4. Inadequate sexual desire associated with identity confusion

153. A depressed, suicidal client is placed on one-to-one observation. A short-term goal specific for this client's nursing care needs is that within:
1. Two days the client will go for a walk on the grounds with other clients
2. Two days the client will understand why there was a desire for suicide
3. Three days the client will verbally accept responsibility for own actions
4. Three days the client will understand the continued presence of a staff member

154. The nurse recognizes that the suicidal risk for depressed clients is greatest:
1. As their depression begins to improve
2. When their depression is most severe
3. Before any type of treatment is started
4. As they lose interest in the environment

155. During individual sessions with a depressed, suicidal client, the nurse should listen to the client's verbalizations for the themes of:
1. Control and betrayal
2. Power and dominance
3. Anger and indecisiveness
4. Fear of aloneness and hopelessness

156. A client has been severely depressed and suicidal for almost two months. As the client becomes more energized and communicative the nurse should:
1. Continue to check on the client at regular intervals
2. Encourage the client's participation in group activities
3. Increase the vigilance of the client's suicidal precautions
4. Recognize that the client's suicidal potential has decreased

157. The nurse enters a depressed client's room on the evening of admission and sees the client sitting in a chair crying. An appropriate response by the nurse would be:
1. "You're crying. Let's talk about it"
2. "Let me get a cup of coffee and we can talk."
3. "Your visitors will be here soon. You better go get ready."
4. "You will feel better soon. Come to the sitting room with me."

158. When talking with a depressed client who has recently lost a spouse the client states, "I really see no purpose to life and sometimes feel like ending it all." The nurse's best response should be:
1. "How much consideration have you given to the method you would use to kill yourself?"
2. "Death is hard on everyone, but people make it through every day. You'll see, things will get better."
3. "Even though you feel that way now, you still have your whole life ahead of you. Make a new start!"
4. "It must be hard to lose someone you care about so much; it makes life seem not worth living right now."

159. A client who has been forced into early retirement is admitted with severe depression. The client states, "I feel useless and have nothing to do." The best initial response by the nurse would be:
1. "Tell me what you would like to do."
2. "Your illness is adding to you feelings."
3. "Have you thought about volunteering?"
4. "You feel useless; tell me more about that."

160. When assessing a client with a diagnosis of mood disorder-manic episode, the nurse is aware that the manic episode is in reality an:
1. Exaggerated response to an elating situation
2. Uncontrolled acting out of uncensored id drives
3. Incorrect interpretation of environmental stimuli
4. Attempt to block unconscious feelings of depression

161. When caring for clients demonstrating manic behavior the nurse must be aware of these clients' physical needs. This is particularly important because:
1. Left alone, these clients will withdraw to their rooms
2. These clients have difficulty making their needs known
3. These clients may gain too much weight from overeating
4. The danger of exhaustion is always present for these clients

162. A client is admitted to the psychiatric unit wearing evening clothes and bright facial makeup. During the first 24 hours the client paces continually and laughs loudly. When approached by the nurse, the client refuses to cooperate with any requests, shouting, "I am in charge. I give the orders!" The nurse recognizes that the client's manic symptoms are:
1. The fulfillment of innate desires
2. An uncontrollable urge to relate
3. A response to an imagined loss
4. An attempt to ward off depression

163. A nursing care plan for a client with a bipolar disorder should include:
1. Providing a structured environment
2. Touching the client to provide reassurance
3. Engaging the client in conversation about current affairs
4. Designing activities that will require the client to maintain contact with reality

164. A client demonstrating manic-type behavior is demanding and active. The nurse's major objective should be to:
1. Maintain a supportive, structured environment
2. Point out reality through continued communication
3. Help lessen the client's feelings of guilt and rejection
4. Broaden the client's contacts with other clients and staff

165. The nurse realizes that when caring for a client with a diagnosis of mood disorder-manic episode the environment is very important. The nurse should therefore:
    1. Put bright drapes in the client's room to help cheer the client up
    2. Place the client in a private room to provide a quiet atmosphere
    3. Assign the client to a room with other clients to provide company
    4. Assign the client to a room near the day room to provide access to activities

166. A client demonstrating manic behavior is elated and sarcastic. The client is constantly cursing and using foul language and has the other clients on the unit terrified. The nurse should:
    1. Firmly tell the client that the behavior is unacceptable
    2. Demand that the client stop the behavior immediately
    3. Ask the client to identify what is precipitating the behavior
    4. Increase the client's medication or get additional medication ordered

167. Encouragement and praise should be given to hyperactive clients to help them increase their feelings of self-esteem. When they have behaved well, the best way to let them know the staff is aware of their improvement is for the nurse to say:
    1. "You behaved well today."
    2. "I knew you could behave."
    3. "Everyone likes you better when you behave like this."
    4. "Your behavior today was much better than yesterday."

DISORDERS OF PERSONALITY

168. The desensitization method that has been used successfully with clients experiencing phobias focuses on:
    1. Imagery
    2. Role-playing
    3. Modeling or imitation
    4. Assertiveness training

169. The mother of a 17-year-old female, hospitalized for extremely disturbed acting-out behavior, leaves a shopping bag at the desk saying, "This is for my daughter's birthday. I'm too busy to visit today." The gift is an unwrapped expensive pocketbook with the price tags attached. The daughter becomes extremely upset and tearful after being given the message and opening the package. The mother's behavior is an example of:
    1. Maternal rejection
    2. Projective behavior
    3. A double-bind message
    4. Passive-aggressive behavior

170. A nurse on a mental health unit has developed a therapeutic relationship with an acting-out, manipulative client. One day as the nurse is leaving, the client says, "Please stay, I'm afraid the evening staff doesn't like me. They often punish me." The nurse can best assist this client by saying:
    1. "I'll ask the staff not to punish you."
    2. "Tell me more about what you're feeling now."
    3. "Don't worry, I told you that you would be all right."
    4. "You know I leave at this time. We'll talk about this in the morning."

171. To maintain a therapeutic relationship with a client diagnosed as having a borderline personality disorder the nurse on the psychiatric unit should:
    1. Be firm, consistent, and understanding and focus on specific behaviors
    2. Provide an unstructured environment for the client to promote self expression
    3. Use an authoritarian approach because this type of client needs to learn to conform to rules of society
    4. Record but ignore marked shifts in mood, suicidal threats, and temper displays because they last only a few hours

172. After a conference with the psychiatrist, a client with a borderline personality disorder cries bitterly, pounds the bed in frustration, and threatens suicide. It would be most helpful for the nurse to:

1. Leave the client for a short period until the client regains control
2. Pat the client reassuringly on the back and say, "I know it is hard to bear."
3. Sit down and listen attentively if the client wishes to talk about the situation
4. Ask about the client's troubles and point out that other people also have problems

173. A client is exhibiting withdrawn patterns of behavior. The nurse is aware that this type of behavior eventually produces feelings of:
1. Anger
2. Paranoia
3. Loneliness
4. Repression

174. The nurse recognizes that a client's withdrawn behavior may temporarily provide a:
1. Defense against anxiety
2. Basis for emotional growth
3. Time for internal problem solving
4. Time to collect personal resources

175. For 2 weeks prior to admission a client spent hours each day performing a complicated handwashing ritual. The client's hands are raw and bloody. The nurse recognizes that the client's ritual represents a conflict with dirt, which is often associated with:
1. Aggression, with the ritual done to control rage
2. Freedom, with the ritual done to stay dependent
3. Initiative, with the ritual done to rebel against autonomy
4. Gender identity, with the ritual done to avoid homosexual panic

176. A client misses breakfast because of an elaborate handwashing ritual. During the early period of the client's hospitalization it would be most therapeutic for the nurse to:
1. Prevent the client from beginning the ritual until after breakfast is served
2. Encourage the client to interrupt the ritual for meals at the scheduled times
3. Allow the client to choose between eating breakfast or completing the ritual
4. Wake the client early so the ritual can be completed before breakfast is served

177. An executive secretary experiences an overwhelming impulse to count and arrange the rubber bands and paper clips in the desk. The client feels something dreadful will occur if the ritual is not carried out. In regard to the client's symptoms, the nurse is aware that:
1. Compulsive rituals are useful in our society as long as they can be controlled
2. Compulsive rituals serve to control anxiety resulting from unconscious impulses
3. The client is able to consciously control the symptoms although this raises anxiety
4. The symptoms are a displacement of general anxiety onto an unrelated specific fear

178. A client who uses a time consuming counting ritual tells the nurse, "I am spending 30 minutes counting each time and my boss is getting very upset. What should I do?" The nurse could best suggest that the client:
1. Limit the counting activity to only 20 minutes each time
2. Arrive at work thirty minutes early each morning for counting
3. Substitute another activity at home such as counting shoes or other objects
4. Talk with the boss and ask for tolerance until the psychiatric treatments help

179. A client who uses a complex ritual says to the nurse, "I feel so guilty. None of this makes any sense. Everyone must really think I'm crazy." The most therapeutic response by the nurse would be:
1. "Your behavior is bizarre, but it serves a useful purpose in your life."
2. "You are concerned about what other people are thinking about you."
3. "Guilt serves no useful purpose. It just helps you stay stuck where you are."
4. "I am sure people understand that you cannot help this behavior right now."

180. When attempts are made to prevent a client from carrying out ritualistic behavior, the nurse would expect that the client's response would be one of:
1. Relief
2. Anger
3. Gratitude
4. Embarrassment

181. An adolescent with a long history of drug abuse, stealing, refusal to comply with rules, and an inability to get along in any setting is admitted to an adolescent unit for evaluation. The most appropriate plan of care for the adolescent at this time would be for the nurse to:
   1. Allow as much freedom as possible, setting few rules and minimum structure
   2. Provide activities that ensure immediate gratification as well as social stimulation
   3. Act as a role model for mature behavior while providing a very structured setting
   4. Behave in a moralistic, punitive manner toward the adolescent when rules are not followed

182. A male adolescent with the diagnosis of antisocial personality disorder spends a great deal of time with a female adolescent client on the unit. One day the nursing assistant enters the female client's room and finds them in her bed. Later the nursing assistant reports the incident to the nurse. The nurse should:
   1. Arrange a discussion with both adolescents
   2. Lock the bedroom doors to keep clients within view of the staff
   3. Assign a staff member to observe both clients every 15 minutes
   4. Call a ward meeting to talk about sexual activity among all the clients

183. An adolescent female with an antisocial personality disorder plans to live with her parents after discharge. The parents request advice on how to respond to their daughter's behavior. The nurse tells them it would be most therapeutic for them to:
   1. Discuss her behavior with her and encourage her to develop self-control
   2. Avoid setting expectations for her behavior and react to each situation as it arises
   3. Help her find new friends and encourage her to get a job and assume responsibility for herself
   4. Set clear limits, explain the consequences of disregarding them, and firmly and consistently apply them

184. Windows in the recreation room of the adolescent unit have been found broken on numerous occasions, and, after group discussion, one of the adolescents indicates another male adolescent client has broken them. The nurse, using assertive intervention instead of aggressive confrontation, should:
   1. Knock on the door of the adolescent's room and ask if he would like to come out and talk about the situation
   2. Confront the adolescent openly in the group, using a controlled voice and maintaining direct eye contact with him
   3. Approach the adolescent when he is alone and, after making eye contact, inquire about his involvement in these incidents
   4. Use a trusting approach to the adolescent, implying that the staff doubts his involvement but requests his denial for the record

185. An 18-year-old is admitted to the hospital after taking 20 tablets of diazepan (Valium). The client's diagnosis is antisocial personality disorder. When obtaining the history the nurse learns that the client had been arrested for drugs and is out on bail. During visiting hours, the nurse discovers the client and visitors smoking. By the odor, the nurse knows they are smoking marijuana. When confronted, the client responds, "I'm celebrating. Didn't you hear? I went to trial today and just got put on probation." The nurse's best response would be:
   1. "You were lucky you just got probation, so don't get right back into trouble."
   2. "I understand your relief about the trial, but pot smoking is against the rules."
   3. "Why don't you and your friends come out and join the other clients and their visitors."
   4. "If you can't follow the rules against pot smoking, your visiting privileges will be cancelled."

186. An adolescent client, with an antisocial personality disorder, was admitted to the hospital because of drug abuse and repeated sexual acting-out behavior. The nurse could evaluate that nursing actions directed toward modifying the behavior of this client had been successful when the client:
1. Promises never to take drugs again
2. Discusses the need to seduce other adolescents
3. Recognizes the need to conform to society's norms
4. Identifies the feeling underlying the acting-out behavior

187. A nursing diagnosis for a client with a multiple personality disorder is, "Disturbance in self-esteem probably related to childhood abuse." The most appropriate short-term client outcome would be:
1. Engaging in object-oriented activities
2. Recognizing each existing personality
3. Eliminating defense mechanisms and fears
4. Verbalizing the need for antianxiety medications

188. A client with a multiple personality disorder is to be discharged after a 2 week hospitalization. The nurse evaluating the effectiveness of the short-term therapy would expect the client to verbalize:
1. That many of the personalities can be ignored
2. The ability to deal openly with feelings and fears
3. The need for long-term outpatient psychotherapy
4. That the personalities now serve no protective purpose

SUBSTANCE ABUSE

189. The defense mechanism commonly used by clients who are alcoholics is:
1. Denial
2. Projection
3. Displacement
4. Compensation

190. A client who has been drinking heavily since the death of a child 3 years ago is brought to the mental health unit in a stupor by the spouse. Taking the client's history into consideration, the nurse makes a tentative nursing diagnosis of:
1. Dysfunctional grieving
2. Substance abuse, alcohol
3. Personal identity disturbance
4. Ineffective family coping: disabling

191. Within a few hours of alcohol withdrawal the nurse should assess a client for the presence of:
1. Yawning, anxiety, convulsions
2. Tremors, fever, profuse diaphoresis
3. Disorientation, paranoia, tachycardia
4. Irritability, heightened alertness, jerky movements

192. A 42-year-old with a long history of alcohol abuse seeks help with the problem in one of the local hospitals. The nurse is aware that the major underlying factor for success in an alcohol treatment program will be the client's:
1. Family
2. Motivation
3. Psychiatrist
4. Self-esteem

193. The nurse understands that clients with a history of alcohol abuse ingest alcohol primarily because they:
1. Are dependent upon it
2. Lack the motivation to stop
3. Have no other coping mechanism
4. Enjoy the associated socialization

194. On the third hospital day after being admitted for alcoholism, a client is confused, disoriented, and delusional. The nurse should be aware that the client may be developing alcoholic:
1. Amnesia
2. Dementia
3. Hallucinosis
4. Withdrawal delirium

195. A male client who has a long history of alcohol abuse is informed that he has extensive liver damage. The client, whose father was an alcoholic who died of cirrhosis, lives with his mother. The client when told that he has approximately one year to live if alcohol abuse persists becomes intensely depressed and one evening leaves the hospital and returns drunk. The nurse is aware that the client's behavior suggests that he:
1. Wants to punish his mother for his physical and emotional discomfort and cause her pain
2. Does not trust the judgment of the health professionals because he feels well physically
3. Cannot associate his increasing depression and lack of fulfillment to his heavy use of alcohol
4. Believes that he inherited the disease of alcoholism from his father and cannot stop drinking

196. When dealing with a client who is in an alcohol detoxification program, it would be most important for the nurse to:
1. Accept the client as a worthwhile person
2. Provide nurturing since the client needs it
3. Discuss the ill effects of alcohol with the client
4. Promote compliance by gently prodding the client

197. To give clients with long histories of alcohol abuse greater responsibility for self-control, the nurse should initially plan to:
1. Tell them about detoxification programs
2. Confront them with their substance abuse
3. Assist them to identify and adopt more healthful coping patterns
4. Administer their medications according to the prescribed schedule

198. Two days after admission to the detoxification program, a client with a long history of alcohol abuse tells the nurse, "I don't know why I came here." The nurse's best response would be:

1. "You feel you don't need this program."
2. "You did admit yourself into the program."
3. "You realize you are trying to avoid your problem."
4. "Don't you remember why you decided to come here?"

199. On the third day of hospitalization a client with a history of heavy drinking develops delirium tremens. When the client is experiencing hallucinations it would be most appropriate for the nurse to:
1. Do nothing because the client may just be having vivid dreams or nightmares
2. Pretend to see the imaginary things the client is talking about and do what the client asks
3. Tell the client that others do not sense or perceive the same things that seem to be so frightening
4. Ask the client to describe the sensation, then assure the client that the sensation is caused by the alcohol

200. A client has been in the alcohol detoxification unit for 5 days. One evening the client complains of numbness and tingling in the feet and legs. At this time it would be most appropriate for the nurse to:
1. Gently massage the client's lower extremities with lotion
2. Emphasize the need to rest and to keep the lower extremities elevated
3. Use mechanical aids to keep bed sheets off the client's lower extremities
4. Observe for the progression of symptoms and monitor the pedal pulses frequently

201. The family of a client who has completed alcohol detoxification relates that they are concerned about the client's behavior if drinking occurs. They state, "When the drinking starts it really disrupts family life and we're not sure how to handle it." The nurse's best response would be:

1. "Try to maintain a normal home environment for your family."
2. "Include the client in the family's activities even when drinking has occurred."
3. "Search the house regularly for hidden alcohol and accompany the client outside."
4. "Help avoid embarrassment by making excuses for the client when functioning is impossible."

202. With a tentative diagnosis of opiate addiction, the nurse should assess a recently hospitalized client for signs of opiate withdrawal. These signs would include:
1. Lacrimation, vomiting, drowsiness
2. Nausea, dilated pupils, constipation
3. Muscle aches, pupillary constriction, yawning
4. Rhinorrhea, convulsions, sub-normal temperature

203. After a visit from several friends the nurse finds a client with a known history of opiate addiction in a deep sleep and unresponsive to attempts at arousal. The nurse assesses the client's vital signs and would evaluate that an overdose of opiates had occurred if the findings showed a:
1. Blood pressure of 70/40, a pulse of 120, and respirations of 10
2. Blood pressure of 120/80, a pulse of 84, and respirations of 20
3. Blood pressure of 140/90, a pulse of 76, and respirations of 28
4. Blood pressure of 180/100, a pulse of 72, and respirations of 18

204. The nurse, when planning care for a client recovering from an opiate overdose, should take into consideration that the client's underlying problem is probably a feeling of:
1. Guilt with a rejection of reality
2. Hostility with a need for acceptance
3. Inferiority with strong dependency needs
4. Anger with an overwhelming need for independence

205. The nurse is aware that opiates are most frequently used because the individual:
1. Desires to become independent
2. Wants to fit in with the peer group
3. Attempts to blur reality and reduce stress
4. Enjoys the social interrelationships that occur

206. A client with a known history of opiate addiction is treated for multiple stab wounds to the abdomen. After surgical repair the nurse notes that the client's pain does not seem to be relieved by the prescribed IM meperidine hydrochloride (Demerol) injections. The nurse recognizes that the failure to achieve pain relief from the Demerol injections indicates that the client is probably experiencing the phenomenon of:
1. Tolerance
2. Habituation
3. Physical addiction
4. Psychological addiction

207. Addicted clients frequently expect prejudice and hostility from psychiatric personnel. The nurse can best overcome their expectation by using:
1. Acceptance and consistency in the approach
2. Reassurance that non-judgmental attitudes exist
3. Self-disclosure to promote a therapeutic relationship
4. Confrontation of these judgmental attitudes in the client

208. At a staff meeting the question of a staff nurse returning to work after a drug rehabilitation program is discussed. The nursing supervisor helps the staff to decide that the best way to handle the nurse's return would be to:
1. Offer the nurse support in a direct straight-forward manner
2. Avoid mentioning the problem unless the nurse brings up the topic
3. Assign another staff member to keep the nurse under close observation
4. Make certain the nurse is assigned to administer only non-narcotic medications

209. It is determined that a staff nurse has a drug abuse problem. As an initial intervention the staff nurse should be:
1. Counseled by the staff psychiatrist
2. Dismissed from the job immediately
3. Forced to promise to abstain from drugs
4. Referred to the employee assistance program

210. The nursing care coordinator in the surgical intensive care unit notes that a number of clients do not seem to be responding to meperidine hydrochloride (Demerol) that has been administered for pain. Later that evening the coordinator finds a staff nurse in the nurses' lounge dozing. On being awakened the staff nurse appears somewhat uncoordinated and drugged with slurred speech. The coordinator should:
1. Ask the other staff members if they have noticed anything unusual
2. Tell the staff nurse that everyone now knows who has been stealing the Demerol
3. Call the nursing director and have the director present before confronting the staff nurse
4. Arrange to secretly observe the staff nurse the next time the staff nurse administers Demerol

211. A client with the dual diagnosis of major depression and polysubstance abuse has been attending group therapy. One day the client tells the nurse, "The things they talk about in group don't really pertain to me." At this time it would be most appropriate for the nurse to:
1. Confront the client with realistic feedback
2. Identify the client's stress-coping tolerance
3. Question what the client means by the statement
4. Communicate that the client needs to get involved

212. A client with a long history of alcohol abuse is placed on a diet high in vitamin B_1 (thiamine). The nurse would know that the diet is understood when the client states, "I will select something for each meal from among:

1. Fish, aged cheese, and breads."
2. Poultry, milk products, and eggs."
3. Lean pork, organ meat, and nuts."
4. Leafy and green vegetables and citrus fruits."

213. A client with a long history of alcohol abuse who has been in the hospital for a week tells the nurse, "I feel much better and will probably not require any further treatment." When evaluating the client's progress the nurse should recognize that:
1. The client has accepted the illness and now needs to use willpower to resist the alcohol
2. As long as the client's family remains supportive, the client will probably not use alcohol again
3. The client lacks insight about the emotional aspects of the illness and most likely needs continued supervision
4. The physician must be notified of the client's statement so that aversion therapy can be started before the client's discharge

SCHIZOPHRENIC DISORDERS

214. When working in a psychiatric setting, it is imperative that the nurse prevent clients from:
1. Breaking contracts
2. Using delusional thinking
3. Harming themselves or others
4. Increasing hallucinatory behaviors

215. When the rights of a client on a mental health unit are suspended, the nurse has the specific responsibility to:
1. Inform the client's family or guardian
2. Carefully monitor all pharmacological intervention
3. Complete a rights denial form and forward it to the administrative officer
4. Document the client's behavior and the reason why the specific right was denied

216. A newly delivered client continues to be apathetic and exhibits an inappropriate affect. A diagnosis of acute schizophrenic reaction is made. Considering the diagnosis, a characteristic symptom the nurse would expect to observe in the client's communication or behavior is:

1. Suicidal preoccupation
2. Autistic magical thinking
3. Absence of self-criticism
4. Abstract and logical deductions

217. When a client's acting-out behavior becomes increasingly bizarre, the client is transferred to a psychiatric unit. When obtaining a history from the client's family, the nurse would expect to find that the premorbid behavior included:
1. Depression and anxiety
2. Irritability and circumstantiality
3. Suspiciousness and introversion
4. Extroversion and inflated self-esteem

218. When assessing a client with the diagnosis of an acute schizophrenic reaction the nurse recognizes that the potential for recovery is better in a client whose history reveals the:
1. Occurrence of a precipitating event
2. Slow and insidious onset of the illness
3. Presence of a family history of schizophrenia
4. Presence of many poorly defined prepsychotic symptoms

219. When asking the family about the onset of problems in a young client with the diagnosis of acute schizophrenia, the nurse would expect that they would relate the client's difficulties began in:
1. Puberty
2. Adolescence
3. Late childhood
4. Early childhood

220. A female client, recently admitted to the hospital, is pacing the floor, acting aloof and suspicious. According to her husband she laughed in a silly manner when told her father was critically injured, and she has had difficulty with her colleagues at work, accusing them of sabotage. The client has stated that she is being controlled by others. The nurse, to be most helpful, should first:
1. Obtain a complete copy of the client's history
2. Review a textbook description of the schizophrenic client
3. Meet with the client's husband to learn why she was admitted
4. Observe and evaluate the behavior in terms of the client's needs

221. When making an assessment of a client's hallucinatory behavior, the nurse realizes that the most common type of hallucination is:
1. Visual
2. Tactile
3. Auditory
4. Olfactory

222. A client with the diagnosis of schizophrenia repeatedly says to the nurse, "No moley, jandu!" The statement "No moley, jandu" is an example of:
1. Echolalia
2. Concretism
3. A neologism
4. Paleologic thinking

223. A young client is admitted with a diagnosis of acute schizophrenia. The family relates that one day the client looked at a linen sheet on a clothesline and thought it was a ghost. The nurse recognizes that this was:
1. An illusion
2. A delusion
3. A confabulation
4. An hallucination

224. A young male client with the diagnosis of schizophrenia states that he cannot eat because someone has taken his stomach. The nurse recognizes this as an example of:
1. An illusion
2. An hallucination
3. Depersonalization
4. A somatic delusion

225. Many clients with schizophrenia often experience opposing emotions simultaneously. The nurse recognizes this phenomenon as:
1. Double bind
2. Ambivalence
3. Loose associations
4. Inappropriate affect

226. Breaks with reality, such as those experienced by clients with schizophrenia, necessitate that the nurse first realize that:
1. Extended institutional care is a necessary part of the treatment modality
2. Clients believe what they feel they have undergone and are experiencing
3. Electroconvulsive therapy produces remission in most clients with schizophrenia
4. The clients' families must cooperate in the maintenance of the psychotherapeutic plan

227. While the nurse is assisting a client with the diagnosis of schizophrenia with morning care, the client suddenly throws off the covers and starts shouting, "My body is disintegrating; I am being pinched." The term that best describes the client's behavior is:
1. Paranoid ideation
2. Depersonalization
3. Loose association
4. Ideas of reference

228. The nurse is aware that a common nursing diagnosis for clients with a schizophrenic disorder is:
1. Social isolation related to impaired ability to trust
2. Sleep disturbances related to impaired thinking ability
3. Potential for violence directed at others related to hallucinations
4. Impaired mobility related to fear of loss of control of hostile impulses

229. A disturbed female client refuses to remove her clothing on admission for psychiatric evaluation. To best meet the client's needs the nurse should:
1. Provide her with two outfits to assist the client to make a simple decision
2. Get assistance and remove her clothing to meet her basic hygiene needs
3. Tell her she will look more attractive in clean clothes to increase her self-esteem
4. Wait and allow her to undress when she is ready, to help the client maintain her identity

230. The central problem the nurse might face with a disturbed schizophrenic client is the client's:
1. Continuous pacing
2. Relationship with the family
3. Concern about working with others
4. High anxiety and suspicious feelings

231. A long-term client goal for a paranoid male client who has unjustifiably accused his wife of having many extramarital affairs would be to help the client develop:
1. Faith in his wife
2. Better self-control
3. Feelings of self-worth
4. Insight into his behavior

232. The most appropriate intervention for the nurse to take after finding an acting-out, disturbed client in the fetal position would be to:
1. Tap the client gently on the shoulder and say, "I'm here to spend time with you."
2. Sit down beside the client on the floor and say, "I'm here to spend time with you."
3. Go to the client and say, "I'll be waiting for you by the table and chairs so please get up and join me."
4. Leave the client alone because the behavior demonstrates the client is too regressed to benefit from talking with the nurse

233. The nurse believes an emotionally disturbed client is ready to begin participating in therapeutic activities. The nurse should initially suggest:
1. Participating on the softball team
2. Attending a class on medications
3. Drawing or painting with the nurse
4. Watching television in the dayroom

234. To deal with a client's hallucinations therapeutically the nurse plans to:
1. Reinforce the perceptual distortions until the client develops new defenses
2. Provide an unstructured environment and assign the client to a private room
3. Avoid helping the client make connections between anxiety-producing situations and hallucinations
4. Distract the client's attention by providing a competing stimulus that is stronger than the hallucination

235. When planning activities for a withdrawn, hallucinatory client, the nurse should recognize that it would be most therapeutic for the client to:
1. Go for a walk with the nurse
2. Watch a movie with other clients
3. Play cards with a group of clients
4. Play solitaire alone in the dayroom

236. To plan care for a client with undifferentiated schizophrenia, the nurse should recognize that the client's delusions are a defense against underlying feelings of:
1. Guilt
2. Inferiority
3. Aggression
4. Persecution

237. A male client claims the voices he hears are clearly telling him what actions and decisions to make. It would be most therapeutic for the nurse to:
1. Play soft music when the client starts hearing voices
2. Begin talking to the client when he is hearing the voices
3. Demonstrate to the client that his perceptions are wrong
4. Recognize that the client must be frightened by the voices

238. When a client with the diagnosis of schizophrenia talks about being controlled by others, the nurse should:
1. Express disbelief about the client's delusion
2. Arrange an interesting daily schedule for the client
3. Respond to the verbal content of the client's delusion
4. Respond to the feeling tone or theme of the client's delusion

239. A client on the psychiatric unit sits alone most of the day. No other clients ever seem to go near the client. The nurse, deciding to establish a relationship, approaches the client. As the nurse gets approximately three feet away the client lets out a string of profanity and says, "Leave me alone; I don't want to talk to you!" The most appropriate response for the nurse to make at this time would be:

1. "I'll leave for now, but I'll be back later."
2. "Why do you feel the need to greet me in this way?"
3. "Do not talk to me like that. I am here to spend time with you."
4. "I don't like it when you talk like that. Are you trying to push me away?"

240. One afternoon the nurse notes a male client rushing down the hall of the unit, rapidly hitting his fist against the wall as he goes. The best nursing action at this time would be to:
1. Forcefully use additional staff members to subdue the client and stop his acting-out behavior
2. Observe the client to see if this behavior escalates and may involve harm to other clients or staff
3. Attempt to approach the client in a non-threatening manner to determine the basis for his agitation
4. Immediately summon staff assistance to enable administration of medication prescribed for the client's agitation

241. When helping a client with the diagnosis of an acute schizophrenic reaction select foods for breakfast, the most therapeutic question by the nurse would be:
1. "What kind of foods do you like?"
2. "Which of these foods do you want?"
3. "Do you want boiled or scrambled eggs?"
4. "How do you want your eggs fixed today?"

242. A client, with the diagnosis of schizophrenia, watching the nurse pour juice for the morning medication from an almost empty pitcher, screams, "That juice is no good. It's poisoned." The nurse should:
1. Remark, "You sound frightened."
2. Assure the client that the juice is not poisoned
3. Pour the client a glass of juice from a full pitcher
4. Take a drink of the juice to show the client that it is okay

243. A disturbed client is scheduled to begin group therapy. The client refuses to attend. The nurse should:
1. Accept the client's decision without discussion
2. Have another client ask the client to reconsider
3. Tell the client that attendance at the meeting is required
4. Insist that the client join to help the socialization process

244. When a disturbed acting-out client's condition improves, the physician suggests giving a one-day pass. The client's family is very nervous about the pass and is worried about what they will do if the client starts to act up. The nurse's best intervention at this time would be to:
1. Have the social worker talk with the family
2. Cancel the pass until the family is reassured
3. Have the client promise the family that acting out will not occur
4. Discuss this concern at a meeting with the client and the family present

245. One morning the nurse finds a disturbed client curled up in the fetal position in the corner of the dayroom. The most accurate initial evaluation of the behavior would be that the client is:
1. Feeling more anxious today
2. Attempting to hide from the staff
3. Tired and probably did not sleep well last night
4. Physically ill and experiencing abdominal discomfort

246. An extremely agitated male client hospitalized in a mental health unit begins to pace around the dayroom. The nurse should:
1. Lock the client in his room to limit external stimuli
2. Let the client pace in the hall away from other clients
3. Get the client involved in a card game to distract his thoughts
4. Encourage the client to work with another client on a unit task

247. The nurse should be aware that the defense mechanism a client with the diagnosis of schizophrenia, undifferentiated type, would most probably exhibit is:
1. Projection
2. Repression
3. Regression
4. Rationalization

248. The nurse notices a male client sitting alone in the corner smiling and talking to himself. Realizing that the client is hallucinating, the nurse should:
1. Ask the client why he is smiling
2. Leave the client alone until he stops talking
3. Invite the client to join in watching television
4. Tell the client it is not good for him to talk to himself

249. A male client tells the nurse he hears a man speaking to him from the corner of the room. He asks whether the nurse hears him too. The nurse should respond:
1. "What is he saying to you? Does it make any sense?"
2. "No one is in the corner of the room. Can't you see that?"
3. "Yes, I hear him, but I can't understand what he is saying."
4. "No, I don't hear him, but it must make you uncomfortable to hear him."

250. One morning a client tells the nurse, "My legs are turning to rubber because I have an incurable disease called schizophrenia." The nurse recognizes that this is an example of:
1. An hallucination
2. Paranoid thinking
3. Depersonalization
4. Autistic verbalization

251. A college student is admitted to the hospital with the diagnosis of schizophrenic disorder, paranoid type. The client is very guarded and suspicious and states, "My professors are trying to fail me because of my controversial ideas." A few hours after admission, another client sits down beside this client. The client jumps up and runs down the hall angrily shouting, "Leave me alone! Don't you touch me!" The most accurate assessment of this behavior is that the client:

1. Fears close contact with people
2. Is responding to delusional thoughts
3. Is having an hallucinatory experience
4. Has confused the other client with a professor

252. A client presents at emergency services stating, "The FBI is trying to kill me." The client is dressed in soiled clothes, wears no shoes, has on a pair of sunglasses, and has body odor. The client's symptoms are most typical of:
1. Shared paranoia
2. Paranoid disorder
3. Paranoid schizophrenia
4. Paranoid personality disorder

253. A male client's statement about a microcomputer implanted in his ear by a foreign agent would help the nurse recognize that the client is experiencing:
1. Illusions
2. Hallucinations
3. Neologistic thinking
4. Delusional thoughts

254. In establishing a nursing care plan the nurse should understand that a male client's delusion that he is an important government advisor is most likely related to:
1. A psychotic loss of touch with his real identity
2. An attempt at wish fulfillment created to manipulate others
3. A need to feel a sense of importance and control over his environment
4. An attempt to compensate for feelings of depression about his problems

255. During the admission procedure, a client who has paranoid ideation refuses to answer the nurse's questions stating, "You are in a conspiracy to kill me." The nurse understands these feelings are related to the client's:
1. Low self-esteem
2. Need to be alone
3. Need for attention
4. Lack of acceptance

256. The nurse recognizes that a paranoid client's accusations are an example of:

1. A delusion
2. A neologism
3. An hallucination
4. An idea of reference

257. In planning care for a client using paranoid ideation, the nurse should realize the importance of:
1. Reducing all stress so the client can relax
2. Not placing any demands on the client at all
3. Giving the client difficult tasks to provide stimulation
4. Providing the client with activities in which success can be achieved

258. A disturbed client is admitted for psychiatric evaluation. In taking the nursing history, the nurse asks why the client came to the hospital. The client states, "They lied about me. They said I murdered my mother. You killed her. She died before I was born." The nurse recognizes that the client is experiencing:
1. Ideas of grandeur
2. Confusing illusions
3. Persecutory delusions
4. Auditory hallucinations

259. The nurse who is planning to establish a trusting relationship with a client using paranoid ideation should begin by:
1. Seeking the client out frequently to spend long blocks of time together
2. Sitting on the unit and observing the client's behavior throughout the day
3. Being available on the unit frequently but waiting for the client to approach
4. Calling the client into the office to establish a contract for regular therapy sessions

260. A disturbed client states, "The voices are saying I killed my husband." The nurse could best respond:
1. "I just saw your husband and he is doing fine."
2. "Tell me more about your concerns for your husband."
3. "You are having very frightening thoughts at this time."
4. "We'll put you in a private room where you will be safe."

261. A client refuses to eat stating, "The food is poisoned." The nurse should:
    1. Ask the client what foods are desired so they can be ordered
    2. Encourage the client's family to bring favorite foods from home
    3. Go with the client to the cafeteria and taste the food to show that it is not poisoned
    4. Suggest going to the cafeteria and selecting those foods the client feels safe eating

262. A disturbed male client tells the nurse that the voices have told him that he is in danger. He states, "They told me I would only be safe if I stay in this room, wear these clothes, and avoid stepping on the cracks between the floor tiles." The nurse's best initial response to this statement would be:
    1. "Don't worry. You're safe here. The door is locked. I won't let anyone hurt you."
    2. "I know these voices are real to you, but I want you to know that I do not hear them."
    3. "You need to leave this room and get your mind occupied so the voices don't bother you."
    4. "Tell me more about the voices. Are they men or women? How many voices are there?"

263. A client using paranoid ideation tells the nurse, "Foreign agents are conspiring against me. They're out to get me at every turn." It would be most therapeutic for the nurse to respond:
    1. "These people you call foreign agents are out to do you in. What else is happening?"
    2. "It must be frightening to believe that people are out to trick you at every opportunity."
    3. "What's happened to make you believe these people you call foreign agents are after you?"
    4. "I can understand how frightening your thoughts are; however, your thoughts do not seem factual to me."

264. During a team conference a family member suggests that a relative, who has the diagnosis of schizophrenia, paranoid type, be assigned to group therapy. The nurse understands that:

    1. Individuals with schizophrenia, paranoid type respond well to small therapeutic groups
    2. Therapeutic group work tends to be threatening to individuals who are very suspicious
    3. Compliance with unit rules and medication regimens increases as the client's group involvement increases
    4. Involvement in small therapeutic groups prevents the regression and dependency associated with institutionalization

DELIRIUM, DEMENTIA, AND OTHER COGNITIVE DISORDERS

265. When the nurse is communicating with a client with substance-induced persisting dementia, the client cannot remember facts and fills in the facts with imaginary information. The nurse is aware that this is typical of:
    1. Concretism
    2. Confabulation
    3. Flight of ideas
    4. Associative looseness

266. When taking a health history from a client with moderate dementia, the nurse would expect to note the presence of
    1. Hypervigilance
    2. Increased inhibition
    3. Enhanced intelligence
    4. Accentuated premorbid traits

267. In planning activities for an elderly nursing home resident with a diagnosis of vascular dementia, the nurse should:
    1. Plan varied activities that will keep the resident occupied
    2. Provide familiar activities that the resident can successfully complete
    3. Offer challenging activities to maintain the resident's contact with reality
    4. Make sure that the resident actively participates in the unit's daily activities

268. An elderly client's family tells the nurse that the client has suffered some memory loss in the last few years. They say that the client is sensitive about not being able to remember and tries to cover up this loss to avoid embarrassment. When attempting to increase the client's self-esteem the nurse should try to avoid discussing events that require memory of the client's:

1. Married life
2. Work years
3. Recent days
4. Young adulthood

269. During the first month in a nursing home an elderly client demonstrates numerous behaviors related to disorientation and cognitive impairment. The nurse's plan for care should continue to take into consideration the:
1. Assessment of the client's orientation to time, place, and person
2. Realistic ability of the client to perform without becoming frustrated
3. Identification of stressors which appear to precipitate the client's disruptive behavior
4. Fact that the client's cognitive impairment will increase until adjustment to the home is accomplished

270. An elderly female client, who is quite confused and often does not recognize her children, is admitted to a nursing home. The client appears slovenly in attire, often soiling her clothing with excreta or urine. The nurse can best manage this problem by:
1. Putting the client into orientation therapy
2. Toileting the client at least once every two hours
3. Supervising the client's bathroom activities closely
4. Explaining to the client how offensive her behavior is to others

271. To assess orientation to place in a client suspected of having dementia of the Alzheimer's type, the nurse should ask:
1. "Where are you?"
2. "Who brought you here?"
3. "Do you know where you are?"
4. "Do you know the day you arrived?"

272. An elderly nursing home resident with the diagnosis of dementia of the Alzheimer's type likes to talk about olden days and at times has a tendency to confabulate. The nurse should recognize that this behavior serves to:
1. Prevent regression
2. Increase self-esteem

3. Attract the attention of others
4. Reminisce about achievements

273. A priority of care for a client with a dementia due to HIV disease would be:
1. Maintaining adequate nutrition
2. Planning for remotivational therapy
3. Arranging for long-term custodial care
4. Providing basic intellectual stimulation

274. When planning care for a 72-year-old client who has been admitted because of bizarre behavior, forgetfulness, and confusion, the nurse should give priority to:
1. Preserving the dignity of the client
2. Promoting a structured environment
3. Limiting the acceleration of symptomatology
4. Determining or ruling out an organic etiology

275. An elderly nursing home resident, with the diagnosis of Alzheimer's type dementia, hoards leftover food from the meal tray and other seemingly valueless articles and stuffs them into pockets "so the others won't steal them." The nurse should plan to:
1. Remove unsafe and soiled articles from the resident's belongings during the night
2. Give the resident a small bag in which to place selected personal articles and food
3. Explain to the resident why the nursing home's policy for cleanliness and safety must be followed
4. Tell the resident that the staff is required to keep harmful objects out of reach in the resident's closet

276. The nursing diagnosis that would be most appropriate for a client with vascular dementia would be:
1. Loss of remote memory related to anoxia
2. Loss of abstract thinking related to emotional state
3. Inability to concentrate related to decreased stimuli
4. Disturbance in recalling recent events related to cerebral hypoxia

277. A 54-year-old client has demonstrated increasing forgetfulness, irritability, and antisocial behavior. After being found disoriented and semi-naked walking down a street, the client is admitted and a diagnosis of Alzheimer's disease is made. The client expresses fear and anxiety. Considering the client's diagnosis, the best approach would be for the nurse to:
1. Initiate a program of planned interaction and activity
2. Reassure the client by the frequent presence of staff
3. Explore in-depth the reasons for the client's concerns
4. Explain the purpose of the unit and why admission was necessary

278. Nursing management of a forgetful disoriented client with the diagnosis of Alzheimer's disease should be directed toward:
1. Rechanneling the client's excessive energies
2. Managing the client's somewhat bizarre behaviors
3. Restricting all gross motor activity to prevent injury
4. Preventing further deterioration in the client's condition

279. An elderly resident with the diagnosis of dementia of the Alzheimer's type frequently talks about the good old days at the ranch as a child. On the basis of an understanding of the resident's diagnosis, the nurse's most appropriate action at this time would be to:
1. Involve the resident in interesting diversional activities in a small group
2. Allow the resident to reminisce about the past and listen with interest to the stories
3. Gently remind the resident that those "good old days" are past and thinking should focus on the present
4. Introduce the resident to other residents of the same age so that they can mutually share their past experiences

280. An elderly female client is admitted to a nursing home from the general hospital with a diagnosis of dementia of the Alzheimer's type. One morning, after being in the nursing home for several days, the client is going to join a group of residents in recreational therapy. The nurse notes that the client has laid out several dresses on her bed but has not changed from her night clothes. It would be most helpful for the nurse to:
1. Remind the client to dress more quickly to avoid delaying the other residents
2. Help the client select appropriate attire and offer her assistance in getting dressed
3. Help the client dress and tell her what time the residents are expected at the activity
4. Allow the client as much time as she needs but explain that she is too late to attend this activity

DRUG-RELATED RESPONSES

281. A client's family ask about the treatment of schizophrenia. The nurse, before responding, recalls that:
1. Electroconvulsive therapy is more effective in treating schizophrenia than mood disorders
2. Family therapy has not proven to be effective in the treatment of clients with schizophrenia
3. Insight therapy has proven to be highly successful in the treatment of clients with schizophrenia
4. Drug therapy, while not treating the underlying problem, reduces the symptoms of acute schizophrenia

282. Nurses should be aware that the use of opiates creates:
1. Psychologic addiction, tolerance, and physical addiction
2. Physical addiction, psychologic addiction, but no tolerance
3. Physical addiction, tolerance, but no psychologic addiction
4. Psychologic addiction, tolerance, but no physical addiction

283. To prevent life-threatening complications from the administration of chlorpromazine (Thorazine) to a client with delirium tremens, it is important that the nurse:
1. Provide adequate restraint
2. Monitor the client's vital signs
3. Protect against exposure to direct sunlight
4. Watch the client for extrapyramidal side effects

284. In addition to hydration during delirium tremens, the physician prescribes parenteral administration of chlorpromazine (Thorazine) for the client. The nurse understands that chlorpromazine is given during detoxification primarily to:
1. Prevent physical injury to the client when convulsions occur
2. Enable the client to sleep and eat better during periods of agitation
3. Quiet the client and encourage cooperation and acceptance of treatment
4. Reduce the anxiety-tremor state and prevent more serious withdrawal symptoms

285. When lithium levels are scheduled to be done the nurse should remember that a client's serum lithium concentration is more stable:
1. 2 to 4 hours after the last dose
2. 4 to 6 hours after the last dose
3. 6 to 8 hours after the last dose
4. 8 to 12 hours after the last dose

286. After a client has been receiving chlorpromazine (Thorazine), the nurse observes extrapyramidal symptoms and anticipates that the physician will limit these side effects by prescribing:
1. Hydroxyzine (Atarax)
2. Benztropine mesylate (Cogentin)
3. Sodium amobarbital (Sodium Amytal)
4. Acetaminophen chlorzoxazone (Parafon Forte)

287. The nurse is aware that haloperidol (Haldol) is most effective for clients who exhibit:
1. Manic-assaultive behavior
2. Excited-overactive behavior
3. Excited-depressed behavior
4. Withdrawn-secretive behavior

288. A client is receiving lithium for the treatment of a bipolar disorder, manic phase. When planning client teaching about this medication, the nurse understands that it is important for the client to know that:
1. A low-sodium diet must be followed every day
2. It will be necessary to take a diuretic with the lithium
3. Lithium will need to be taken for the rest of the client's life
4. Lithium blood levels must be checked every 2 to 3 months

289. The immediate treatment for a client who has ingested a tricyclic antidepressant in an amount that is 20 to 30 times the daily recommended dose would include:
1. Dialysis or forced diuresis
2. Administration of physostigmine salicylate
3. IM or IV administration of an anticholinergic
4. Closer monitoring to prevent further suicide attempts

290. A client is started on fluphenazine decanoate (Prolixin Decanoate). When teaching about this drug, the nurse should emphasize that:
1. Driving is forbidden while taking this drug
2. There will be a feeling of increased energy while on this drug
3. A sunscreen must be used for all outdoor activity on a year-round basis
4. The client's essential hypertension will indirectly be controlled by this drug

291. In a client suspected of and demonstrating the symptoms associated with opiate overdose, the nurse would expect the physician to prescribe:
1. Naloxone
2. Methadone
3. Epinephrine
4. Amphetamine

292. The nurse should teach a client receiving tranylcypromine sulfate (Parnate) that failure to adhere to the dietary restrictions can result in:
1. Syncope
2. Bradycardia
3. Hypertensive crisis
4. Hyperglycemic episodes

293. Therapy has helped a client with a long history of alcohol abuse make a fairly satisfactory adjustment while in the hospital. The client will continue to receive therapy on an outpatient basis and will be discharged with the drug disulfiram (Antabuse). The nurse should caution the client to avoid using:
1. Elixirs and liniments
2. Suntan lotions and oils
3. White sugars and all vinegars
4. Undecaffeinated coffee and strong tea

294. A client is to be discharged on a regimen of lithium carbonate. In the teaching plan for discharge the nurse should include:
1. Advising the client to watch the diet carefully
2. Suggesting that the client take the pills with milk
3. Reminding the client that a CBC must be done once a month
4. Encouraging the client to have blood levels checked as ordered

295. A client who is going home on a weekend pass has been receiving chlorpromazine hydrochloride (Thorazine) 75 mg tid. The nurse should inform the client that:
1. The dosage of the medication can be reduced if feeling better at home
2. The medication does not need to be taken during the time spent at home
3. No alcoholic beverages should be consumed while taking this medication
4. All the medication should be taken early in the day to be sure it is not forgotten

296. After talking with a client about the tricyclic antidepressant medication that has been prescribed, the nurse diagnoses the presence of a knowledge deficit when the client states:
1. "I notice I'm a little drowsy in the mornings."
2. "I'm expecting to feel somewhat better in 3 weeks."
3. "I've been on the medication for 8 days now and I don't feel any better."
4. "I know I will probably have to take this medication for at least a few months."

297. A client with vascular dementia becomes increasingly agitated and abusive. The physician orders haloperidol (Haldol). The nurse should assess the client for untoward effects including:
1. Jaundice and vomiting
2. Tardive dyskinesia and nausea
3. Hiccups and postural hypotension
4. Parkinsonism and agranulocytosis

298. A client with the diagnosis of schizophrenia is given one of the antipsychotic drugs. The nurse is aware that of all the extrapyramidal effects associated with these drugs the one causing the most concern would be:
1. Akathisia
2. Tardive dyskinesia
3. Parkinsonian syndrome
4. An acute dystonic reaction

299. The nurse should continually assess a client receiving lithium for an early sign of lithium toxicity which would be:
1. Tinnitus
2. Diarrhea
3. Akathisia
4. Torticollis

300. The nurse understands that after starting administration of diazepam (Valium) it is important to assess for potential side effects. Initially the nurse should:
1. Monitor the client's blood pressure
2. Measure the client's urinary output
3. Assess the client for abdominal distention
4. Check the client's pupil size every 4 hours

301. The physician orders haloperidol (Haldol) concentrate 10 mg po bid for a client who is also receiving phenytoin (Dilantin) for control of epilepsy. In planning the client's care, the nurse should be aware that anticonvulsants may interact with Haldol to:
1. Mask its therapeutic effect
2. Interfere with its absorption
3. Enhance its rate of metabolism
4. Potentiate its CNS depressant effect

302. A client is extremely depressed, and the physician orders a tricyclic antidepressant, imipramine hydrochloride (Tofranil). The client asks the nurse what the medication will do. The nurse's best response would be:
1. "This medication will help you forget why you are depressed."
2. "The medication will help increase your appetite and make you feel better."
3. "You will really begin to feel much better after taking this medication for 2 to 3 days."
4. "When you take this along with phenelzine sulfate (Nardil) you'll feel less depressed."

303. A client with a mood disorder-manic episode is receiving lithium carbonate. The client complains of diarrhea, tremors, and drowsiness. The nurse should:
1. Withhold the medication
2. Get an order for a stimulant
3. Make certain the client stays on the special diet
4. Decrease the client's fluid intake to 2000 ml daily

304. A depressed client is placed on amitriptyline hydrochloride (Elavil) twice a day. The nurse would expect to observe a therapeutic response to this medication in:
1. 1 to 3 days
2. 1 to 3 weeks
3. 12 to 24 hours
4. 30 minutes to 2 hours

305. A client is receiving haloperidol (Haldol) for agitation. When observing the client for side effects, the nurse would recognize that the side effect that is unrelated to extrapyramidal tract symptoms would be:
1. Akathisia
2. Opisthotonos
3. Oculogyric crisis
4. Hypertensive crisis

306. A client receiving buspirone hydrochloride (BuSpar) is admitted to the hospital with the diagnosis of possible hepatitis. The nurse notices that the client's sclera looks yellow. The nurse's initial action regarding this medication should be to:

1. Omit the BuSpar
2. Give the BuSpar with milk
3. Reduce the dosage of the BuSpar
4. Assure the client that the BuSpar can be given parenterally

307. A female client who is taking clozapine (Clozaril) calls the nurse to say she has suddenly developed a sore throat and has a high fever. The nurse, recognizing the drug's effects, evaluates the client's complaints and tells her to:
1. Stay in bed, force fluids, take aspirin, and skip the next two scheduled doses of Clozaril
2. Stop the medication immediately and see her physician when an appointment is available
3. Skip the medication and, if her physician cannot see her today, go to the emergency room for evaluation
4. Continue the medication, drink fluids, take aspirin, and see her physician if not improved in a few days

308. The physician plans to have a client continue on lithium after discharge. The nurse would recognize that the teaching about the medication plan was understood when the client states, "I know that this medication:
1. Should be stopped if illness is suspected."
2. May need to be taken for the rest of my life."
3. Must be increased at the first sign of a manic episode."
4. Rarely causes serious side effects when taken correctly."

309. The psychiatrist orders lithium carbonate 600 mg po tid for a client. The nurse would be aware that the teaching about the side effects of this drug were understood when the client states, "I will call my doctor immediately if I notice any:
1. Sensitivity to bright light or sun."
2. Fine hand tremors or slurred speech."
3. Sexual dysfunction or breast enlargement."
4. Inability to urinate or difficulty when urinating."

310. A client is admitted to the hospital with a diagnosis of depression that has not responded to tricyclic antidepressants or outpatient ECT. The physician orders tranylcypromine sulfate (Parnate). The nurse would be aware that the teaching about the drug was understood when the client states, "While taking this medicine I should avoid eating:
1. Fish."
2. Chocolate"
3. Red meat."
4. Citrus fruit."

311. Forty-eight hours after starting on haloperidol (Haldol) a male client is observed standing by the nurse's station with his head arched sharply backward. The nurse should recognize that the client:
1. Needs to have the dosage increased as his psychotic behavior is not lessening
2. Is experiencing temporary side effects that usually disappear after several days
3. Is having pseudoparkinsonian side effects and needs to have his medication adjusted
4. Needs immediate treatment because he is experiencing an acute dystonic reaction to the drug

THERAPEUTIC RELATIONSHIPS

312. An elderly female who has been a widow for 20 years comes to the community health center with a vague list of complaints. Her only child, a son, died at birth. She has lived alone since her husband's death and performs all of her own daily tasks of living. She has had a very active social life in the past but has outlived many of her friends and family members. When taking this client's health history, it is important for the nurse to ask:
1. "Do you feel all alone?"
2. "Do you still miss your husband?"
3. "What unfulfilled hopes do you have?"
4. "How did you feel when your son died?"

313. A client with the diagnosis of panic disorder is placed on alprazolam (Xanax) which the client refuses to take because of fear of addiction. Initially the nurse should:

1. Provide the client with information about Xanax
2. Further assess the client's knowledge and feelings about Xanax
3. Have the physician speak to the client about the safety of this drug
4. Speak with the physician regarding a change in the client's medication

314. In addition to hallucinating, a client yells and curses throughout the day. The nurse should:
1. Isolate the client until the behavior stops
2. Ignore the behavior exhibited by the client
3. Become aware of what the behavior means to the client
4. Be willing to explain the meaning of the behavior to the client

315. The head nurse gives permission to the hospital's inservice division to use a child's chart in a nursing seminar on the care of children with leukemia. The nurse believes releasing the information will help other nurses give better care to children with this illness. The legal right of the client that was violated is the right to:
1. Privacy
2. Freedom
3. Respectful care
4. Informed consent

316. At times a client's anxiety level is so high it blocks attempts at communication and the nurse is unsure of what is being said. To clarify understanding, the nurse states, "Let's see whether we both mean the same thing." This is an example of the technique of:
1. Reflecting feelings
2. Making observations
3. Seeking consensual validation
4. Attempting to place events in sequence

317. When a nurse revises a client's nursing care plan based on the client's responses that show evidence that goals were not attained, the phase of the nursing process being applied is:

1. Planning
2. Evaluation
3. Assessment
4. Implementation

318. The psychotherapeutic theory that uses hypnosis, dream interpretation, and free association as methods to release repressed feelings is the:
1. Behaviorist model
2. Psychoanalytic model
3. Psychobiologic model
4. Social-interpersonal model

319. The nurse is aware that the phase of the nurse-client relationship where most of the problem solving occurs is called the:
1. Initial stage
2. Working stage
3. Planning stage
4. Evaluation/termination stage

320. A staff nurse on a medical-surgical unit has been assigned to have daily one-to-one interactions with a number of clients. Before making an initial contact with the clients, the nurse decides to review their individual medical records. This phase of the nurse-client relationship could best be referred to as the:
1. Working phase
2. Orientation phase
3. Termination phase
4. Preinteraction phase

321. The nurse is aware that in the working phase of the nurse-client relationship, clients:
1. Often focus the conversation on the nurse
2. Accept limits and initiate topics for discussion
3. Frequently exhibit testing behaviors such as flirtation and lateness
4. May repress emotionally charged material to avoid shocking the nurse

322. Three days after a stressful incident a client can no longer remember what there was to worry about. The inability to recall the situation is an example of the defense mechanism of:
1. Denial
2. Repression
3. Regression
4. Dissociation

323. An environment conducive to psychologic safety is one in which:
1. There is passive acceptance
2. All the client's needs are met
3. Realistic limits and controls are set
4. The physical environment is kept in order

324. A goal for a client with the nursing diagnosis, "Impaired verbal communication related to psychologic barriers" would be, the client will:
1. Be free of injury
2. Demonstrate decreased acting-out behavior
3. Interact with others in the external environment
4. Identify the consequences of acting-out behavior

325. A 15-year-old is admitted to an adolescent unit for evaluation. The adolescent has a long history of drug abuse, stealing, refusal to comply with rules, and an inability to get along in any setting. When collecting data related to the adolescent's life-style, the nurse may be prevented from accurately listening to what the client is saying by:
1. Personal cultural beliefs
2. The client's disease process
3. The pressure of time to complete care
4. A personal need to secure information

326. The condition of a child dying from leukemia deteriorates and the child becomes comatose. The parents state that a relative said they should not allow the child to be resuscitated but that they are unsure about this. The response by the nurse that would best demonstrate a recognition of the ethical issues involved is:
1. "Let me tell you about the implications of a DNR, then you can decide."
2. "Have you talked to your doctor about this yet? I'll be happy to page him."
3. "You should discuss this thoroughly with your doctor and then with your religious advisor."
4. "The final decision must be made by you and your physician, but it is important to talk about it."

327. Before effectively responding to a rape victim on the phone, it is essential that the nurse in the rape intervention center:
   1. Get the client's full name and address
   2. Call for assistance from the psychiatrist
   3. Know some myths and facts about rape
   4. Be aware of any personal bias about rape

328. The nurse is aware that value clarification is a technique useful in therapeutic communication in that it helps:
   1. Make clients aware of their personal values
   2. Provide information related to clients' needs
   3. Assist clients in making correct decisions related to their health
   4. Alter clients' poor values to make them more socially acceptable

329. A reasonable short-term goal for clients who are functioning below the optimum level of mental health would be to help them become better able to:
   1. Understand the dynamics behind their inadequate interpersonal relations
   2. Discuss their feelings regarding significant others and their life experiences
   3. Confront their inadequacies in interpersonal relations and be more sociable
   4. Take actions which will increase their satisfaction with their relationships with others

330. The nurse recognizes that the past life of clients who have immigrated to this country:
   1. Affects all of their inherited traits
   2. Has little impact on their lives today
   3. Is important in assessing their values
   4. Established forever how they would interact

331. A client who is dying tells the nurse, "I would love to learn to speak German before I die." The nurse's response to the client's desire to learn a foreign language should be based on an awareness of the fact that:
   1. Activities that support the client's denial should not be encouraged
   2. Conversations and activities should focus on pleasant experiences
   3. Clients should be encouraged to set meaningful goals for themselves
   4. The energies expended on such an activity would not justify the outcome

332. It is most helpful to the nurse who is attempting to apply the principles of positive mental health to understand that:
   1. Emotionally ill people can empathize easily with others
   2. Emotionally healthy people function optimally in all settings
   3. A sense of mastery of self and environment is crucial to emotional health
   4. Mental illness is always characterized by observable signs or socially inappropriate behavior

333. An inexperienced nurse assigned to a mental health day-care setting elects to have a one-to-one therapeutic relationship with an elderly, depressed, withdrawn, female client. The nurse's selection was most likely based on the fear of being:
   1. Hurt by a more active client
   2. Rejected by a more alert client
   3. Useless and then saying the wrong thing to a more alert client
   4. Overly concerned for a younger client's well-being and mental status

334. The nurse should always take the time to keep a client's family informed about what is happening to the client. The main reason for this action is that informed families:
   1. Decrease the client's anxiety
   2. Frequently cause less nursing problems
   3. Are more relaxed and at ease with the client
   4. Are better equipped to undertake necessary family role changes

335. The nurse must recognize that when a client is a member of an ethnic community it is important to:

1. Ensure that the nurse's biases are understood by the family
2. Offer a therapeutic regimen compatible to the lifestyle of the family
3. Recognize that the client's responses will be different than other client's
4. Make plans to counteract both the client's and family's misconceptions of family practice

336. After working with an elderly male client for a period of time the client tells the nurse he always enjoyed working and playing with children. During discharge planning the nurse recommends that the client look into the volunteer Foster Grandparent Program in his area. The nurse recognizes that this type of activity may help the client to:
1. Be able to find new acquaintances with similar interests
2. Forget his problems when he sees the problems of others
3. Take better care of himself if he feels needed by someone
4. Become motivated to become involved with younger people

337. The nurse is scheduled to be the co-leader of a therapy group to be formed in the mental health clinic. When planning for the first meeting, it is of primary importance that the nurse first consider the:
1. Number of clients in the group
2. Needs of the clients being included
3. Diagnoses of the clients being included
4. Socioeconomic status of the clients in the group

338. To further develop trust among members in a therapy group the nurse plans to:
1. Reveal some personal data as a role model for trusting behavior
2. Remind group members about the need for confidentiality in the group
3. Have group members reveal some personal information about themselves
4. Bring up for discussion the need for and the importance of trusting each other

339. During the first session of a therapy group one of the clients asks, "What is supposed to happen in this group?" The most appropriate response by the nurse leader would be:
1. "Before I answer that, I'd like for you to tell me what you want to happen."
2. "This is your group and your participation will largely determine what happens."
3. "The purpose of this group is to examine the way each of you interacts with the other."
4. "You and the others are supposed to discuss any reality-based concerns you have about your illness."

340. Increased socialization and verbalization of reality-based concerns are the nurse's primary goals for a therapy group of clients with the diagnosis of schizophrenia. At the first session of the group, after introductions, the nurse could best begin by:
1. Asking the clients what they hope to gain from the meetings
2. Allowing the clients to discuss anything they wish to bring up
3. Having each of the clients identify a concern to be discussed
4. Sharing with the clients the purpose of the meetings and explaining the rules of behavior

341. The best initial approach to take with a self-accusatory, guilt-ridden client is to:
1. Contradict the client's persecutory delusions
2. Accept the client's statements as the client's beliefs
3. Medicate the client when these thoughts are expressed
4. Redirect the client whenever a negative topic is mentioned

342. The initial intervention strategy that is of primary importance in counseling an elderly female client who desires to remain independent and who is having increased difficulty in maintaining her independent living status is:
1. Maintaining her routine and supporting her usual habits
2. Helping her to secure assistance with cleaning and shopping
3. Writing down and repeating important information for her use
4. Setting clear goals and time limitations for visits with the nurse

343. The nurse plans to use family therapy as a means of assisting a family to cope with their child's terminal illness. The nurse's basis for this choice is that:
1. It is more time-efficient to deal with the whole family together
2. The entire family is involved, since they can be perceived as victims
3. The nurse can control manipulation and alliances better by using this mode of intervention
4. It will prevent the parents from deceiving each other about the true nature of their child's condition

344. A male client with advanced AIDS tells the nurse that all he wants is to pass his high school equivalency test before he dies. He asks the nurse if this is possible. The nurse's best approach would be to:
1. Attempt to get the client to see that his wish is too taxing and somewhat unrealistic
2. Refocus the conversation on the things the client has already accomplished in his life
3. Set up a study schedule with the client and offer to work with him in preparing for the test
4. Suggest to the client that he use this energy to work through his unexpressed anger at dying

345. The parents of an autistic child begin family therapy with a nurse therapist. The father states that the family wish to share their religion with the therapist. The nurse should:

1. Limit the father's discussion of religion
2. Invite the family's minister to a therapy session
3. Plan for a mutual discussion of religious beliefs
4. Keep the sessions focused on the family's concerns

346. A 17-year-old, admitted to the hospital because of loss of weight and malnutrition, is diagnosed as having anorexia nervosa. After the client's physical condition is stabilized, the psychiatrist, in conjunction with the client and the parents, decides to institute a behavior modification program. The nurse is aware that a major component of behavior modification is that it:
1. Rewards positive behavior
2. Deconditions fear of weight gain
3. Decreases necessary restrictions
4. Reduces anxiety-producing situations

347. When caring for a client with a bipolar disorder-depressive episode, the nurse's first priority should be to help the client to:
1. Feel comfortable with the nurse
2. Investigate new leisure activities
3. Participate in small group activities
4. Initiate conversations about feelings

348. After treatment a young male adolescent with a history of schizophrenia improves and is to go home on a weekend pass. The client's parents tell the nurse they are concerned about how to respond if "Our son starts to act crazy." It would be most therapeutic for the nurse to:
1. Teach the parents how to respond to the client's bizarre behavior
2. Reassure the parents that the client is improved and is unlikely to act out
3. Refer the parents to a self-help group for the parents of schizophrenic clients
4. Meet with the parents and the client together to discuss their mutual concerns

349. The nurse is planning a discharge conference with a psychiatric client and the client's family. The priority nursing action that should be included in the discharge plan is:

1. Obtaining a more complete family history
2. Teaching the client about the medication to be taken
3. Discussing new issues that could be worked on at home
4. Exploring what has been learned from this hospitalization

350. The most basic therapeutic tool used by the nurse to assist a client's psychological coping is the:
1. Self
2. Milieu
3. Client's intellect
4. Helping process

351. In an attempt to remain objective and support a client during a crisis, the nurse uses imagination and determination to project the self into the client's emotions. The nurse accomplishes this by using the technique known as:
1. Empathy
2. Sympathy
3. Projection
4. Acceptance

352. Following a traumatic event a client is extremely upset and exhibits pressured and rambling speech. A therapeutic technique that the nurse can use when a client's communication rambles is:
1. Touch
2. Silence
3. Focusing
4. Summarizing

353. When a client with paranoid ideation tells the nurse about people coming through the doors to commit murder the nurse should:
1. Listen to what the client is saying
2. Refuse to listen to the client's stories
3. Tell the client that no one can get through the door
4. Ask the client to explain where this information came from

354. In communicating with a client with a psychiatric diagnosis the nurse uses silence. When using silence in therapeutic communication, clients should feel:
1. It is their turn to talk
2. Unhurried to answer
3. The nurse is thinking
4. There is nothing more to say

355. After speaking with the parents of a child dying from leukemia, the physician gives a verbal DNR order but refuses to put it in writing. The nurse should:
1. Follow the order as given by the physician
2. Refuse to follow the order, unless the nursing supervisor okays it
3. Ask the physician to write the order in pencil on the client's Kardex before leaving
4. Determine whether the family is in accord with the physician and follow hospital policy

356. When speaking with an emotionally disturbed client the nurse notices that the client keeps interjecting sentences that have nothing to do with the main thoughts being expressed. The client asks whether the nurse understands. The nurse should reply:
1. "You aren't making any sense; let's talk about something else."
2. "I'd like to understand what you are saying, but you are too confused now."
3. "Why don't you take a rest and then we can talk again later this afternoon."
4. "I'd like to understand what you are saying, but I'm having difficulty following you."

357. In responding to a confused, hallucinating male client's statement that his head is turning to stone it would be most appropriate for the nurse to state:
1. "Your head looks fine to me."
2. "When did this feeling first start?"
3. "That's a rather unusual sensation."
4. "That must be a frightening way to feel."

358. A mother, visiting her hospitalized teenage daughter, gets into an argument with her. Leaving her daughter's room in tears, the mother meets the nurse and relates the argument stating, "I can't believe I got so angry I could have hit her." The most therapeutic response by the nurse would be:
1. "Sometimes we find it difficult to live up to our own expectations of ourselves."
2. "Why don't you bring a surprise for your daughter. It will make you both feel better."
3. "You can't compare yourself to an abusing parent. After all, you didn't beat your child."
4. "You're a wonderful mother. Everything will be okay. Teenagers can really drive you to distraction."

359. A husband is upset that his wife's delirium tremens have persisted for the second day. The initial response by the nurse that would be most appropriate is:
1. "I see that you are very worried. Medications are being used to lessen your wife's discomforts."
2. "This is totally normal. I suggest that you go home because there is nothing you can do to help at this time."
3. "Are you afraid that your wife may die? I assure you that very few alcoholics die during the detoxification process."
4. "The staff is making your wife comfortable while she is undergoing the withdrawal process. Your wife will not feel pain."

360. At a staff meeting discussing the return of one of the staff nurses from a drug rehabilitation program one nurse states, "I don't know why we are wasting time on this. We all know that those people go back to using drugs as soon as the pressures increase." The nursing care coordinator's best response would be:
1. "It's important for us to share our feelings about staff members with problems."
2. "I know it's hard, but it's our professional obligation to work with these individuals."
3. "I guess you feel somewhat guilty that you failed to recognize that this nurse was addicted."
4. "Since you have such strong negative feelings, I don't think you should be assigned to work with this staff member."

361. A female nurse on the mental health unit has been assigned to work with a young male college student who was admitted the previous night. The client has never used any mental health services before. The nurse's most appropriate initial approach to this client would be to:
1. Address the client as Mr., saying, "Hello," and giving her first and last name.
2. Address the client by his first name and state, "I've been assigned to care for you today."
3. Say good morning, addressing the client by his first name, stating, "I see you were admitted last night. Tell me what brought you to our unit."
4. Say good morning, addressing the client as Mr., using his last name, and introducing herself by her first and last name, stating, "I am a registered nurse assigned to the mental health unit."

362. A newly admitted client looks at but does not respond to a nurse's greeting. The nurse's most appropriate action would be to state:
1. "I guess you would rather be alone for now; I will return later so we can talk."
2. "I am talking to you. Are you having trouble understanding what I am saying?"
3. "I am here to tell you about the services available to you on the mental health unit and to offer you my help."
4. "This is the mental health unit of the hospital. We have many services to offer. Let me tell you about them."

363. A newly admitted client quietly listens to a nurse's explanation of the services and activities available on the mental health unit. When the nurse is finished, the client looks around and states, "So this is where they keep the crazies." The nurse's most appropriate initial response would be:
1. "These people are sick. They are not crazy."
2. "Some people feel that way. Let's talk about mental health."
3. "No, that is not correct. Let me explain the purpose of a mental health unit."
4. "Are you feeling that a person has to be crazy to need mental health services?"

364. The nurse tells a client that talking with staff is part of the therapy program. The client responds, "I don't see how talking to you can possibly help." The nurse's most appropriate response would be:
1. "You will never know if it is helpful or not unless you are willing to give it a try."
2. "I can see how you would feel that way now, but hopefully you'll change your mind."
3. "The one-to-one relationship has proven itself very helpful for others. Why don't you give it a try?"
4. "Hopefully, I can help you sort out your thoughts and feelings so you can better understand them."

365. The nurse can best handle the answering of personal questions asked by a client in any phase of the nurse-client relationship by:
1. Reviewing the positive and negative aspects of the subject
2. Providing brief, truthful answers and redirecting the focus of conversation
3. Offering an honest, brief expression of personal views on the subject raised
4. Gently reminding the client that the nurse's feelings are not the client's concern

366. The wife of a client, ultimately hospitalized with the diagnosis of Alzheimer's disease, appears tired and angry on her first visit with her husband. As she is leaving she says to the unit nurse in a sarcastic tone, "Let's see what you can do with him." The nurse's most therapeutic response would be:
1. "It must have been very difficult to care for him."
2. "I don't understand what you mean by that comment."
3. "It's too bad you didn't realize you needed help to care for him."
4. "We have experience in caring for clients such as your husband."

367. An overweight, 12-year-old male is brought to the clinic by his parents. The father states, "You've got to do something to help him. Just look at his size." The child tells the nurse that he dislikes school because his classmates tease him about his weight. He states rather sadly, "I'm always last when they choose up sides in gym." The nurse's most therapeutic response would be:
1. "That hurts a lot when you want to be liked."
2. "Not everybody's a great athlete. You have other strengths."
3. "Have you tried letting them know how that makes you feel?"
4. "Won't it be great when you lose weight and can do better in gym?"

368. During the meetings of a therapy group one member tends to monopolize the group discussions and no one has confronted this behavior. The nurse could best handle this situation by:
1. Saying to the client, "You use too much of the time in our sessions."
2. Ignoring the behavior because the client may become upset if confronted
3. Encouraging other members of the group to do more talking by calling on various silent members
4. Saying to the group, "I'm wondering why the group is so willing to let this client do so much of the talking."

369. At a therapy group session a group member, using a teasing manner, makes several negative remarks about the nurse's appearance and behavior. The nurse could best respond by saying to:
1. The group, "What do you think this client is trying to tell me?"
2. The group, "Do you think this client's behavior is appropriate today?"
3. The client, "You seem very interested in my appearance and behavior. What's this all about?"
4. The client, "I cannot just sit here and let you talk about me this way. What have I done to make you angry?"

370. At a therapy group session a female client tearfully tells the other members that she lost her job as a receptionist during the past week. It would be most appropriate for the nurse to:
1. Ask her to look at the reasons this may have occurred
2. Quietly observe how the group responds to her statement
3. Suggest she check the help wanted advertisements in the local paper
4. Request that the group help her see how she may have precipitated the dismissal

371. At a therapy group session, after a client tearfully tells the other members about losing a job during the past week, another member states with a smile, "Things haven't gone well in my life this week either." It would be most appropriate for the nurse to:
    1. Ask the client to share what has been happening during this week
    2. Make a note of the incongruity of the client's message but remain silent
    3. Say to the client, "You say things have been bad this week, yet you are smiling."
    4. Comment, "This seems to have been a bad week for a number of group members."

372. As a young male client is receiving a dialysis treatment, the nurse notes he is not talking with the other clients and his eyes are lowered and his jaw is clenched. The nurse states, "You look discouraged." The client replies, "I'm a bother. Not much good to anyone anymore. My wife would at least get some insurance money if I died." The nurse's most therapeutic response would be:
    1. "I can understand how you feel."
    2. "You feel so bad you wish you were dead."
    3. "We all have days we feel like that. Let's talk about your diet."
    4. "I know it's hard, but don't let it get you down or let your wife hear you."

373. When the behavior of a visiting family member agitates a client who is extremely disturbed, the nurse should:
    1. Take the client to the coffee shop for a treat
    2. Distract the client by providing another activity
    3. Limit the client's contact with the family member
    4. Discuss the family member's behavior with the client

374. The staff could interpret that a client has established some trust in the nurse who has been regularly working with a small group of clients if the client:
    1. Attends morning meeting every day for one week
    2. Plays bingo with the nurse and some other clients each day
    3. Demonstrates decreased muscle tension and is able to maintain direct eye contact
    4. Acts out until seclusion is required on each day that the particular nurse is not available

375. The nurse would be aware that a therapy group had reached the working stage when the members:
    1. Appear happy in their group interactions
    2. Focus on a wide variety of needs and concerns
    3. Show concern for the feelings of the group leaders
    4. Say and do what is expected and wanted by the others

Answers and Rationales for Mental Health Nursing Questions

PERSONALITY DEVELOPMENT

1. 3 Displacement reduces anxiety by transferring the emotions associated with an object or person to another emotionally safer object or person. (2) (MH; AS; PS; PD)

1 In projection, the individual attempts to deal with unacceptable feelings by attributing them to another.

2 Dissociation is an attempt by the person to detach emotional involvement or the self from an interaction or the environment.

4 Intellectualization is the use of facts or other logical reasoning rather than feelings to deal with the emotional impact of a problem; a form of denial.

2. 4 The nurse is using facts and knowledge to detach the self from the emotional impact of the client's problem and decrease the anxiety it is causing. (3) (MH; AS; PS; PD)

1 Substitution is similar to displacement; this reduces anxiety by transferring the emotions associated with an object or person to another, safer object or person.

2 Sublimation is the channeling of unacceptable thoughts or feelings into acceptable activity.

3 This is trying to unconsciously imitate the behavior of another who is considered important in an attempt to incorporate this important other into the self.

3. 1 The father is siding with his daughter and supports her when the mother accuses her of negative behavior; this is an example of coalitions or alliances; in this instance the mother may also be in denial. (3) (MH; AS; PS; PD)

2 Resignation is evident when someone gives up.

3 Scapegoating is when an individual is labeled or blamed by other family members as the cause of the family's problems.

4 Reaction formation is consciously behaving in a manner that is exactly opposite to what one really feels.

4. 1 Without the development of trust the child has little confidence that the significant other will return; separation is considered abandonment by the child. (1) (MH; AN; ED; PD)

2 Without identity, the individual will have a problem in forming a social role and a sense of self; this results in identity diffusion and confusion.

3 Without initiative, the individual will experience the development of guilt when curiosity and fantasies about sexual roles occur.

4 Without autonomy, the individual has little self-confidence, develops a deep sense of shame and doubt, and learns to expect defeat.

5. 2 This is the developmental task of the school-aged child; the child will feel inferior if recognition is not given. (2) (MH; AN; ED; PD)

1 This is the task of the preschool child.

3 This is not a developmental task identified by Erikson.

4 Same as answer 3.

6. 2 The major tasks of young adulthood are centered around human closeness and sexual fulfillment; lack of love results in isolation. (1) (MH; AN; ED; PD)

1 This stage is associated with early childhood.

3 This stage is associated with middle childhood.

4 This stage is associated with middle adulthood.

7. 2 This is the task of the older adult; this client has not adapted to triumphs and disappointments, so there is no acceptance of what life is and was, and this results in feelings of despair and disgust. (2) (MH; AN; ED; PD)

1 This is the task of the preschool period.

3 This is the task of the young adult.

4 This is the task of the adolescent.

8. 2 This action would not call attention to the accident and would minimize the child's embarrassment. (2) (MH; IM; PS; PD)

1 The child would probably be unable to accomplish this task without assistance; failure to complete the task would add to embarrassment.

3 This would add to the child's embarrassment.

4 Same as answer 3.

9. 3 Adolescence is a time of great upheaval and maturation; before this maturational process is completed, adolescents act without thinking things through and are most concerned with their own needs, rather than the needs of others. (1) (MH; AN; PS; PD)

1 The rapid and complex biological, social, and emotional changes during adolescence do not necessarily lead to these psychological conflicts.

2 Same as answer 1.

4 Same as answer 1.

10. 1 According to Erikson, adolescents are struggling with identity versus role confusion. (2) (MH; AN; PS; PD)

2 Adolescents tend to be group oriented, not isolated; they struggle to belong, not to escape.

3 This reflects part of the struggle for independence; it does not indicate failure to achieve the developmental task of adolescence; "all" is too inclusive.

4 This is untrue; most adolescents do not use drugs and alcohol to escape.

11. 1 Adolescents learn about who they are by assuming and experiencing a variety of roles; experimentation results in the retention or rejection of behavior and roles. (2) (MH; EV; PS; PD)

2 This is not constructive; this would not allow for experimentation with a variety of roles.

3 Continuous sublimation would not be constructive; this would delay and interfere with the successful completion of the struggle to formulate one's identity.

4 This is not constructive; it does not allow for the development of independence.

12. 3 This action would foster the development of an improved self-image. (2) (MH; IM; PS; PD)

1 A problem does exist; their child is unhappy.

2 Parents cannot avoid talking about the sibling but should avoid any comparisons.

4 The child already is doing this, and the measure has diminished self-esteem.

13. 2 This is an achievable goal that will bolster the child's self-esteem. (2) (MH; AN; PS; PD)

1 This would not improve the child's self-esteem.

3 Same as answer 1.

4 Same as answer 1.

14. 3 This would demonstrate a movement toward peer group activity and interests; exercise would also demonstrate an interest in an improved physical condition. (2) (MH; EV; PS; PD)

1 This would not demonstrate an increase in self-esteem.

2 No data to indicate that there was a change.

4 Same as answer 1.

15. 3 Erikson theorized that how well people adapt to the present stage depends on how well they adapted to the stage immediately preceding it, in this instance adulthood. (2) (MH; AN; ED; PD)
  1 These are the developmental tasks of an earlier stage of development; although Erikson believed that the strengths and weaknesses of each stage are present in some form in all succeeding stages, their influence decreases with time.
  2 Same as answer 1.
  4 Same as answer 1.

16. 4 This allows the client to accept what life is or was and helps avoid feelings of despair. (3) (MH; AN; ED; PD)
  1 This could require a reversal in the client's past lifestyle; this is unlikely, if not impossible, for the client at this age.
  2 This would be impossible to accomplish and denies the reality of what was or is in life.
  3 Same as answer 2.

17. 1 The individual who can reflect back on life and accept it for what it was and is and who can adjust and enjoy the changes retirement brings is less likely to develop health problems, especially stress-related health problems. (2) (MH; AN; ED; PD)
  2 These changes are usually not reversible.
  3 This is untrue; most emotionally healthy older individuals do not focus on these thoughts.
  4 This is not true; dependency is often more threatening to this age-group.

18. 4 An individual's ability to handle stress develops through experience with life; aging does not reduce this ability but often strengthens it. (1) (MH; PL; ED; PD)
  1 The senses of taste and/or smell are often diminished in the aged individual.
  2 Gastrointestinal motility is slowed in the aged individual.
  3 Muscle or motor strength is diminished in the aged individual.

DISORDERS FIRST EVIDENT BEFORE ADULTHOOD

19. 1 A child usually assumes a role in the family and the child's symptoms reflect the pathology that develops to fill that role. (3) (MH; AN; PS; BA)
  2 This may create problems, but these problems usually develop later in life.
  3 Same as answer 2.
  4 Same as answer 2.

20. 1 Children with emotional problems usually have difficulty dealing with reality and tend to withdraw; they are afraid to use reality testing. (2) (MH; AS; ED; BA)
  2 Behavior is more often disorganized rather than deliberate, and aggressive rather than passive.
  3 There is usually a withdrawal from the peer group.
  4 The anxiety level is usually severe, often approaching the panic level.

21. 4 Unresponsiveness to the environment may be a serious indicator of childhood depression, autism, or possibly schizophrenia; all three are serious disorders. (3) (MH; AS; PS; BA)
  1 This may be seen in children without emotional problems as well as in those with emotional problems; this behavior alone would not indicate severe emotional problems.
  2 Same as answer 1.
  3 Same as answer 1.

22. 2 This structured but nonthreatening statement avoids beginning with problems and may put the child at some ease, producing information that may be useful. (3) (MH; AS; PS; BA)
  1 This statement is too open and global; the child would probably not know how to answer this question or know where to begin.
  3 This question can produce a "yes" or "no" answer; also, the child may not know the answer to this question.
  4 This question would probably produce an "I don't know" response; the focus should be on the child, not the mother.

23. 1 Tertiary prevention focuses on interventions that prevent complete disability or reduce the severity of a disorder or its associated disabilities. (3) (MH; PL; TC; BA)

2 This would be secondary prevention aimed at case finding and early intervention.

3 This would be primary prevention.

4 Same as answer 2.

24. 2 This helps the child gain control by reducing stimuli while helping limit and prevent the use of tantrums by the child as an attention-getting behavior. (3) (MH; IM; TC; BA)

1 This would probably increase the behavior associated with the tantrum.

3 Although ignoring the temper tantrum may sometimes help, it often forces the child to act out further; using time-out is more successful because the child is removed and both the parent and child have a "cooling off" period.

4 Medication is not the treatment of choice.

25. 4 One of the symptoms an autistic child displays is a lack of responsiveness to others; there is little or no extension to the external environment. (2) (MH; AS; PS; BA)

1 Repetitive behavior provides comfort.

2 Music is nonthreatening, comforting, and soothing.

3 Repetitive visual stimuli, such as a spinning top, are nonthreatening and soothing.

26. 4 Children usually blame themselves for their parents' marital problems, believing that they are the reason one parent leaves. (2) (MH; AN; ED; BA)

1 No data are presented to lead to this conclusion.

2 The child's response is not typical of grief work.

3 Same as answer 1.

27. 3 Comparison over time is the only way for the nurse to accurately assess the mental status of a child. (2) (MH; AS; ED; BA)

1 This would not be an accurate method because a child's ability to discuss feelings is limited.

2 This may be unrealistic and biased; the nurse should take the parents' description of behavior into consideration but should mainly rely on personal assessment and observation over time.

4 This would be threatening and may increase the child's anxiety.

28. 2 This is the family constellation as it is now constructed; without prior discussion and permission, an invitation to anyone else would be an intrusion of privacy. (3) (MH; AN; ED; BA)

1 In addition to needing the mother's permission to invite the father, the nurse must also include the child in family therapy.

3 The father cannot be invited without prior discussion with and permission of the mother.

4 The teacher is not part of the family constellation.

29. 3 When all the members of a family blame one member for all their problems, scapegoating is occurring. (2) (MH; AN; PS; BA)

1 There are no data to support identifying this pattern of relating.

2 Same as answer 1.

4 Same as answer 1.

30. 3 This action would set a foundation for trust because it allows the child to see that the nurse cares. (2) (MH; IM; PS; BA)

1 This would be threatening at this stage of a relationship.

2 This would be too infrequent to develop trust.

4 Although this is necessary, limit setting really does not support the development of a trusting relationship.

31. 1 This response would be most successful because it provides a time period for the hyperactive child to regain control; it is neither a positive nor a negative reinforcement of acting-out behavior. (3) (MH; IM; TC; BA)
2 The child would interpret removal of tokens as a punishment.
3 Ignoring behavior can force the child to act out even more to gain attention.
4 This action would reward acting-out behavior by providing special attention.

32. 3 This would help the child develop insight into reasons for acting-out behavior. (3) (MH; IM; PS; BA)
1 This denies that the child's problem behavior is continuing and does not help the child develop insight.
2 Same as answer 1.
4 Same as answer 1.

33. 4 This would provide a trial opportunity for the client and the family to reunite outside the confines of the hospital. (2) (MH; PL; PS; BA)
1 It is too late; this should have been done much earlier.
2 This is not the responsibility of the nurse.
3 Same as answer 1.

EATING DISORDERS

34. 4 This is a theoretical explanation for the development of anorexia nervosa. (2) (MH; AN; PA; EA)
1 This does not play a role in the development of anorexia nervosa.
2 Same as answer 1.
3 The basis is the struggle between dependence and independence, not a desire for independence alone.

35. 1 Clients with anorexia nervosa have a disturbed self-image and always see themselves as fat and needing further reducing. (2) (MH; AS; PS; EA)
2 The relationship is usually not supportive, it is disturbed.

3 There is usually high achievement and great concern about grades.
4 There is usually dissatisfaction with weight and a desire to lose weight.

36. 2 These clients are usually severely malnourished and have severe fluid and electrolyte imbalances; unless these imbalances are corrected, cardiac irregularities and death can occur. (2) (MH; PL; PA; EA)
1 This is important, but it is not the highest priority at this time.
3 Same as answer 1.
4 Same as answer 1.

37. 4 These clients have severely depleted levels of potassium and sodium because of their starvation diet and energy expenditure; these electrolytes are necessary for proper cardiac functioning. (2) (MH; AN; PA; EA)
1 Although this may occur, it is not immediately life threatening.
2 Same as answer 1.
3 Same as answer 1.

38. 3 This is a nonthreatening, open-ended response that focuses discussion and leaves channels of communication open. (2) (MH; IM; PS; EA)
1 Although this does not quite accuse the client of lying, it is a threatening response that questions the client's truthfulness.
2 Same as answer 1.
4 Same as answer 1.

39. 3 It is most therapeutic for the staff to control food needs, thus removing the parents from the struggle. (3) (MH; IM; TC; EA)
1 This may be interpreted as accusatory and increase the parents' guilt.
2 This is nontherapeutic; it cuts off the parents from future involvement.
4 This is nontherapeutic; it only continues the struggle between the parents and the client.

40. 3 The client's security is increased by limit setting; guidelines remove responsibility for behavior from the client and increase compliance with the regimen. (2) (MH; PL; PS; EA)
1 The client needs control, not empathy.
2 Simply maintaining control is not therapeutic and increases the power struggle.
4 Emphasis on dietary intake increases the power struggle between the client and the staff.

41. 3 This action would be neither a positive nor negative reinforcement of specific behavior; it would provide rewards for achievement of specific goals. (2) (MH; PL; TC; EA)
1 This would not be included in a behavior modification program.
2 Same as answer 1.
4 Clients talk freely about food; the problem is with ingestion not discussion.

42. 1 All food issues should be discussed with the dietician, thus removing a potential source of conflict between nurse and client. (2) (MH; PL; PS; EA)
2 This would increase the conflict between the nurse and client.
3 This would accomplish little because the client's failure to eat is not based on likes or dislikes.
4 This may be self-defeating because discussion of food would be the major focus of all nurse-client interactions.

43. 3 Clients with anorexia nervosa use manipulation to divide the nursing staff; sharing this knowledge alerts health team members. (3) (MH; AN; PS; EA)
1 This would be counterproductive because it supports the client's manipulative behavior.
2 The client is attempting to manipulate the staff; this is not how trust is established.
4 Same as answer 1.

44. 4 By talking to the client on the telephone at mealtimes, the family is enabling the client to continue destructive behavior; the client and family must be included in discussion of and possible solutions to the problem. (2) (MH; PL; PS; EA)
1 This would be a punitive approach that would not deal with the underlying problem.
2 Same as answer 1.
3 Same as answer 1.

45. 2 This would demonstrate a change in behavior, as well as a positive approach to meals. (2) (MH; EV; PS; EA)
1 This would be typical behavior of a client with anorexia nervosa.
3 The problem is not a lack of interest about food but a deliberate failure to ingest food.
4 This behavior is unrelated to the behavior that needed to be changed.

EMOTIONAL PROBLEMS RELATED TO PHYSICAL HEALTH AND CHILDBEARING

46. 3 This action would provide the child with a constant caregiver with whom the child could relate. (1) (MH; IM; TC; EP)
1 Although this may provide some comfort, the child needs to receive love and attention from an adult.
2 Same as answer 1.
4 This would increase the parents' guilt and anxiety; data given assume parents have been unable, not unwilling, to visit the child.

47. 3 The preschooler is terrified by intrusive procedures and views them as a punishment for curiosity and fantasies. (2) (MH; AN; ED; EP)
1 This age child does not fear loss of control.
2 This age child may be able to localize pain even if unable to express it.
4 This age child would be unlikely to recall the procedure merely by the appearance of the technicians.

48. 1 This would permit the 8-year-old to investigate and become familiar with the equipment to be used. (2) (MH; IM; ED; EP)

2 This would be beyond the comprehension of the average 8-year-old and would do little to reduce anxiety.

3 This is beyond the ability of an 8-year-old and would do little to reduce anxiety.

4 This would be supportive but is not always possible; even with the parent present the child should be given an opportunity to handle the equipment.

49. 1 The 9-year-old needs an opportunity to express emotions in private; talking about feelings after the child has regained control would be therapeutic. (2) (MH; AN; PS; EP)

2 This is not of great concern to the child at this moment.

3 This action would give the child a feeling that crying was wrong.

4 Same as answer 2.

50. 4 This is a nonjudgmental response that does not pressure the client but does clearly indicate that treatment is necessary. (2) (MH; IM; TC; EP)

1 This is an unrealistic response that gives approval to the client's behavior.

2 This is an unrealistic response that is unsupported by any data.

3 This nonsupportive response tells the client that the physician knows best.

51. 3 This response interprets the client's behavior without belittling the nursing assistant's feelings; it encourages the assistant to get involved with plans for future care. (3) (MH; IM; ED; EP)

1 Although this response recognizes the client's feelings, it does nothing to assist the nursing assistant in dealing with the client.

2 This assumes the nursing assistant has nothing to contribute and only the nurse can deal with the problem.

4 This statement does not help the nursing assistant with the situation or demonstrate any understanding of the client's feelings.

52. 2 This action provides continuity and demonstrates to the client that the nursing staff is concerned; frequent contact reduces client's need to call staff in. (2) (MH; PL; TC; EP)

1 This would increase the client's anxiety and need for contact with staff.

3 Telling the client is not the same as doing it; the client would not believe staff would come in frequently.

4 This would not provide continuity of care.

53. 4 This is an open-ended response that encourages further discussion without focusing on an area that the nurse, not the client, feels is the problem. (3) (MH; IM; PS; EP)

1 This response denies the client's feeling and can cause feelings of guilt for questioning the partner's love.

2 This is too specific; the nurse does not have enough information to come to this conclusion.

3 Same as answer 2.

54. 4 This response fosters open lines of communication with the client. (2) (MH; IM; PS; EP)

1 This response would put the client on the defensive because it exposes the defensive behavior being used.

2 This response does not recognize the client's concern and cuts off further communication.

3 This could be interpreted as a sarcastic response that may cut off further communication.

55. 2 The client has difficulty accepting the inevitability of death and attempts to deny the reality of it. (1) (MH; AN; PS; EP)

1 In the anger stage the client strikes out with the "why me" and the "how could God do this" type of statements; the client is angry at life and still angrier to be removed from it by death.

3 In this stage the client attempts to bargain for more time; the reality of death is no longer denied, but the client attempts to manipulate and extend the remaining time.

4 In the acceptance stage the client accepts the inevitability of death and peaceably awaits it.

56. 2 Crying is an expression of an emotion that, if not expressed, increases anxiety and tension; the increased anxiety and tension use additional psychic energy and hinder coping. (2) (MH; AN; PS; EP)

1 Crying does not relieve depression, nor does it help a client face reality.

3 This is not universally true; in most instances the client's defenses should not be taken away until they can be replaced by more healthful defenses; the nurse must always interfere with behavior and defenses that may place the client in danger; the client's current behavior creates no threat to the client.

4 This is not always true; many clients are embarrassed by what they consider to be a "show of weakness" and have difficulty relating to the individual who witnessed it; the nurse must do more than just accept the crying to strengthen the nurse-client relationship.

57. 4 A starting point for working with all clients is ascertaining what is known, their understanding of their particular situation, and its meaning to them. (2) (MH; AS; PS; EP)

1 It is not merely understanding what death and the dying process means, which is a philosophical discussion, but how the individual feels about the situation.

2 Encouraging conversation about the situation tends to decrease anxiety.

3 This may be part of the care plan but it is not the most important piece of information during the initial contact.

58. 4 This response recognizes the client's feelings and encourages the client to look at the basis or reality of the expressed concern. (2) (MH; IM; PS; EP)

1 This response goes in circles; the client has already told the nurse the basis for her feelings.

2 This puts the responsibility for the husband's behavior on the client who may not be able to handle it.

3 This is a weak excuse for the behavior of the husband and may or may not be true.

ANXIETY, SOMATOFORM, AND DISSOCIATIVE DISORDERS

59. 1 The client's statement is an example of the use of denial, a defense that blocks problems by unconsciously refusing to admit they exist. (2) (MH; AS; PS; AX)

2 The client is not using projection, a defense that is used to deny unacceptable feelings and emotions and attribute them to others.

3 The client is not using sublimation, a defense that is used to substitute socially acceptable behavior for unacceptable instincts.

4 The client is not using displacement, a defense mechanism that is used to allow the shifting of feeling from an emotionally charged person or object to a safe substitute person or object.

60. 2 Reexperiencing the actual trauma in dreams or flashbacks is the major symptom that distinguishes post-traumatic stress disorders from other anxiety disorders. (2) (MH; AN; PS; AX)

1 This symptom is not usually associated with anxiety disorders.

3 This symptom would be more common in phobic disorders.

4 Although depression may be generated by discussion of the traumatic situation, the affect is usually exaggerated, not blunted.

61. 3 These actions make the environment as emotionally unthreatening as realistically possible. (2) (MH; PL; TC; AX)

1 It is not possible or realistic to meet all of a person's needs.

2 All needs are not realistic; the person must learn how to deal with delaying gratification.

4 Order in the environment is of less importance; providing a nonthreatening environment is the priority action.

62. 1 Anxiety is a threat to the identity of the individual; the client is seeking assurance that the fear and panic being experienced will not mean loss of control. (2) (MH; AN; PS; AX)

2 The client is not exhibiting depression but severe anxiety and panic.

3 This is not evidence of insightfulness but a plea for help in reducing the anxiety.

4 The client is not testing the nurse; the client is asking for help.

63. 1 Because anxiety can be an interpersonal experience, it is contagious; the nurse then has a strong urge to get away. (2) (MH; AN; PS; AX)

2 The desire to go off duty would not suddenly make the nurse uncomfortable.

3 This is possible, but not probable; the client is exhibiting anxiety, not hostility, at this time.

4 There is no indication that this or any other behavior encountered has been bizarre.

64. 1 Freedom to ventilate feelings acts as a safety valve to reduce the anxiety. (1) (MH; PL; PS; AX)

2 The suppression of anger or hostility would add to the client's anxiety.

3 This would not be therapeutic; it might add to the anxiety the client is feeling.

4 This may or may not be helpful; the client's family may provide support to the client.

65. 2 The nurse's presence may provide the client with support and feelings of control. (2) (MH; IM; TC; AX)

1 It is evident that the client is upset; this question is not therapeutic and may lead to anger, which would interfere with the development of a therapeutic nurse-client relationship.

3 The client is too distraught to sit; to be therapeutic the nurse would have to be where the client is.

4 The client is in a panic; anger is not primary; there is no need to work off aggression.

66. 1 The client has the right to privacy; his behavior is acceptable in the privacy of his room. (3) (MH; IM; PS; AX)

2 Masturbation is a normal sexual outlet; assessment is unnecessary unless the act is practiced to excess.

3 This can cause needless embarrassment to the client and may close off further communication.

4 His behavior is not inappropriate because he was in the privacy of his own room.

67. 1 Fear can be overwhelming; the staff's presence provides protection from possible danger. (2) (MH; IM; PS; AX)

2 The client's anxiety level is interfering with the ability to communicate; anxiety must be reduced first.

3 The client's anxiety level is so high that sufficient emotional energy to set parameters would not be available.

4 This would only add to the client's anxiety at this time.

68. 3 This response helps the client focus on situations that precipitate frightening feelings. (2) (MH; AS; PS; AX)

1 This response would not help the client to focus on feelings.

2 The nurse cannot be certain what the client means about being afraid to talk about it; this response would not help the client to focus on feelings.

4 This is false reassurance; the nurse cannot guarantee that the feelings will not come back.

69. 4 These are positive coping behaviors that can consciously be used to promote mental health. (1) (MH; PL; TC; AX)
1 These are not healthy coping behaviors, and their frequent use can lead to distortions of reality.
2 Same as answer 1.
3 Same as answer 1.

70. 3 Clients frequently respond in this manner when they feel threatened; this behavior supports the client's ego integrity. (2) (MH; AN; TC; AX)
1 The nurse's actions play only a minor role in these situations.
2 This is not true; the client's feelings, not the situation, precipitate this response.
4 Same as answer 1.

71. 4 This would document that the client feels comfortable enough to discuss the problems that have motivated the behavior. (3) (MH; EV; TC; AX)
1 This does not demonstrate a resolution of problems underlying the behavior.
2 Without discussion of the problems underlying the behavior, little would be accomplished.
3 Same as answer 1.

72. 1 The development of confusion would indicate that the client's ability to maintain equilibrium has not been achieved and that further disequilibrium was occurring. (2) (MH; EV; TC; AX)
2 This would not indicate the plan needed to be changed unless the client's history demonstrates no prior use of this defense.
3 Same as answer 2.
4 This would be a positive response to any plan of care but is not directly related to independence.

73. 3 Members have not established trust and are hesitant to discuss problems; the behaviors observed reflect anxiety and insecurity. (2) (MH; AS; PS; AX)
1 This would add to the anxiety and insecurity of group members.
2 These behaviors are expected in the early stage of the group.
4 Same as answer 1.

74. 2 The client's response demonstrates an inability to deal with the other member's confrontive approach at this time. (2) (MH; EV; PS; AX)
1 The group has reached the working stage and, if the client was able to deal with this area, the nurse would expect the client to state the feeling generated by the statement.
3 Same as answer 1.
4 There is not enough information to make this evaluation.

CRISIS SITUATIONS

75. 2 Caplan's theory states that a crisis is an internal disturbance caused by a stressful event that alters the usual way of coping with a threat to the self; this temporarily disturbs the homeostasis of the person involved. (3) (MH; AN; PS; CS)
1 This is not the definition of a crisis.
3 This is not the definition of a crisis, but the assessment the nurse must make in the first phase of crisis intervention.
4 This is not the definition of a crisis, but is how a crisis is resolved.

76. 4 Awareness of limitations and the ability to place oneself in another's situation are essential to be able to intervene effectively. (1) (MH; AN; PS; CS)
1 This is not a necessary characteristic to help families with problems and many times would be impossible to achieve; this is not a prerequisite for understanding.
2 Although this may be helpful it is not a priority.
3 Same as answer 2.

77. 3 The data presented indicate developmentally related struggles and specific situations that are extremely stressful; multiple stresses can produce a crisis situation for the individual when past coping mechanisms are ineffective. (1) (MH; AS; TC; CS)
1 It is not the experience, but the individual's response to the experience, that determines a crisis.

2   A crisis is not an age-related problem; a crisis results when the individual's past coping mechanisms are no longer effective for dealing with a present stressful situation.

4   The extent of the stress, although a factor, is not the most significant factor in identifying the presence of a crisis; the individual's inability to cope indicates a crisis.

78. 3   A situational crisis occurs when a specific external event upsets an individual's psychological equilibrium. (2) (MH; AN; PS; CS)

1   A social crisis occurs when a person feels discomfort with others or has a fear of being observed or scrutinized.

2   There are insufficient data to come to this conclusion; the client may or may not be facing a financial crisis.

4   Adjustment to retirement is a developmental task of later adulthood; the client was forced into early retirement, it was not a choice.

79. 4   A situational crisis is a sudden unexpected event with which the individual is unable to cope using past coping behaviors; this time frame provides an opportunity for the individual to learn new coping behaviors. (2) (MH; AN; PS; CS)

1   This would be too short a period of time for the individual to develop new successful coping mechanisms.

2   Same as answer 1.

3   Same as answer 1.

80. 3   The major goal of crisis intervention is to resolve the present crisis and return the client to the pre-crisis level of functioning. (1) (MH; AN; PS; CS)

1   This would be a short-term goal.

2   Same as answer 1.

4   This is a goal of psychotherapy, not crisis intervention.

81. 2   Personal internal strengths and supportive individuals are critical factors that can be employed to assist the individual to cope with a crisis (2) (MH; AS; TC; CS)

1   Although this information may be helpful, it is not essential; factors concerning the present situation are paramount.

3   This is unrealistic; identifying unconscious conflicts takes a long time and is inappropriate for crisis intervention.

4   This is a goal of psychotherapy, not crisis intervention; it is usually not necessary to restructure the personality to resolve a crisis.

82. 4   The assessment of the client's present status and ability to perform ADL is the priority because it will influence the choice of an appropriate therapeutic regimen. (3) (MH; AS; TC; CS)

1   Although significant, it is not the priority.

2   Concern now is for the client, not how the client's behavior affects others.

3   The present crisis must be dealt with first.

83. 4   A crisis intervention group helps clients reestablish psychologic equilibrium by assisting them to explore new alternatives to coping; it considers realistic situations using rational and flexible problem-solving methods. (1) (MH; AN; TC; CS)

1   This is not an immediate goal of crisis intervention.

2   Clients are never given a solution; they are assisted in arriving at their own acceptable, workable solutions.

3   It is not necessary for crisis intervention workers to be psychologists.

84. 2   Behavior that reflects the recognition of the intrinsic worth of each individual is essential in all supportive relationships; problem-solving potential is increased when clients are involved in exploring alternatives that will affect the direction of their own lives. (1) (MH; PL; PS; CS)

1   The client, not the worker, is encouraged to identify the problem.

3   This is useless; the client is unable to empathize with others at this time.

4   This is impossible during the immediate intervention period; the client needs to find direction immediately.

85. 4 Although the client's facial expression suggests happiness, the client's tone of voice gives the message of anger; the behaviors do not go together. (1) (MH; AS; PS; CS)
1 The data given do not support this assessment.
2 Same as answer 1.
3 Same as answer 1.

86. 4 The client is using intellectual reasoning to block confronting the unconscious conflict and the stress of having to deal with his girlfriend's pregnancy. (2) (MH; AS; PS; CS)
1 No data demonstrate that the client is projecting blame on anyone else.
2 No data demonstrate that the client is concentrating thoughts and emotions on his inner self.
3 No data demonstrate the shifting of emotions from an emotionally charged object or person to a neutral one.

87. 4 A crisis is defined as a situation in which the client's previous methods of adaptation are inadequate to meet present needs. (2) (MH; AN; PS; CS)
1 A crisis is not necessarily related to the degree of stress; it occurs when past coping mechanisms are ineffective.
2 This is not the immediate stress for which the client has no coping mechanism.
3 This is not causing the crisis; the client's lack of coping mechanisms is.

88. 4 The crisis center nurse's main responsibility is to assist the client in utilizing the problem-solving process; the client will be helped in exploring alternative solutions to a situation and will be given information regarding other agencies, facilities, and services. (2) (MH; PL TC; CS)
1 This is part of the general interaction with the client; it is not a specific primary responsibility.
2 This is not part of the immediate goal during the crisis; the client may be encouraged to seek help later for other problems.
3 This is one of many instructions for which the client must take primary responsibility.

89. 1 Intrinsic motivation is motivation that is stimulated from within the learner; it is most effective because the learner recognizes the need to know, is self-directed, and is ready to learn. (2) (MH; EV; ED; CS)
2 This is stimulation from without and is very often ineffective; desire must come from within.
3 There is no external reward for attending classes.
4 This is a new behavior based on a new situation; there is no external reward for attending classes.

90. 1 Emotionally immature individuals are often unable to deal with the role changes associated with parenthood. (2) (MH; AN; PS; CS)
2 This may have contributed to the crisis but did not precipitate it.
3 Same as answer 2.
4 Same as answer 2.

91. 4 According to the Guidelines for Sterilization of the American Association on Mental Deficiency, consent for sterilization in most states must be obtained from the court and legal guardian if the client is mentally incompetent and unable to give informed consent. (3) (MH; PL; TC; CS)
1 The court alone cannot decide the issue; a legal guardian must be involved.
2 The next of kin may place pressure on the client; therefore, permission should also be obtained from the court and legal guardian.
3 Legal guardians (who may be next of kin) may exert undue influence; therefore, they alone cannot sign the consent.

92. 2 The client must be intellectually competent, that is, able to comprehend the outcome of the procedure in order to give informed consent. (2) (MH; PL; TC; CS)
1 Informed consent can only be obtained from a client who is intellectually competent to understand the outcome of the procedure.

3   This is unrealistic; a mentally retarded client would be unable to fully explain what the procedure entails; it is more important for the client to understand the outcome of the procedure.

4   The client should be free from the influence of a parent, legal guardian, or any others who might press to have the procedure performed.

93. 4   If one child in the family is identified as being different by the parents or siblings, coupled with other signs of abuse, abuse should be suspected and the situation warrants further investigation. (1) (MH; AS; PS; CS)

1   Taking a walk would be helpful for both the mother and the child and would not indicate abuse.

2   This is an acceptable punishment for misbehaviors.

3   Although this is demeaning, it is not abuse.

94. 4   In most instances, the abusing parent attempts to avoid talking about the situation as a means of reducing guilt and repressing the action. (2) (MH; AS; PS; CS)

1   Denying the beating requires the parent to fabricate a story about how the obvious physical injury occurred.

2   Little concern is expressed for the child because this would require verbal expression and acceptance of the action.

3   A parent's concern for the unabused children without the expression of concern about the abused child would document a different feeling about the abused child, which the parent would try to avoid.

95. 3   These underlying feelings frequently precipitate trying to improve the child's behavior by the beating. (2) (MH; AS; PS; CS)

1   These parents usually do not admit their behavior, so they do not have a need to rationalize it.

2   These parents offer many vague explanations of how the child was injured; rarely is the explanation detailed.

4   This would be an unusual request because abusing parents do not usually ask to see their children.

96. 3   The nurse feels that an inability to deal with the daughter could have resulted in a loss of control, leading to possible abuse. (3) (MH; AN; PS; CS)

1   The nurse is uncomfortable because the client's situation probably resulted from similar feelings.

2   Same as answer 1.

4   Nothing in the data presented leads to this conclusion; the argument could have been justified.

97. 3   By learning how the child's behavior provokes frustration, parents may develop more acceptable ways of responding. (3) (MH; IM; ED; CS)

1   Although these parents need to learn what behavior is appropriate for a given age level, they must also learn how to respond correctly to less appropriate behavior.

2   Punishment of a child for behavior is usually futile; it is an act of retribution, not an act of discipline.

4   The abusing parent responds to both negative and acceptable behavior with abuse.

98. 2   This child would distrust any approach because approaches frequently result in pain; abused children remain alert in an attempt to ward off an attack. (2) (MH; AS; PA; CS)

1   This child would not be open to an approach by a stranger; basic trust of others has not developed in abused children.

3   This child would be acutely aware of anyone coming near; abused children attempt to defend themselves by keeping alert to the possibility of attack.

4   This child would usually not cry out; abused children learn not to expect comforting or soothing of pain by others.

99. 1 This would provide reassurance and support for the child (2) (MH; IM; PS; CS)

2 Using the phrase "anything wrong down there" could cause the child to have negative feelings about the self.

3 Depending upon the mother's involvement in the situation, the mother's involvement might be threatening rather than supportive to the child.

4 Asking the child to make this decision at this time would be nontherapeutic and may be threatening.

100. 2 This response would elicit further clarification of what the child means by "bad." (3) (MH; AS; PS; CS)

1 This would not be helpful; it would do nothing to clarify the child's idea of what "bad" means or the child's feelings about what happened.

3 The nurse needs to determine what the child means by the word "bad" before reflecting the term back to the child.

4 This would be a nontherapeutic response because the uncertainty implied by the nurse would increase the child's feelings of guilt.

101. 1 Because rape is a threat to the sense of control over one's life, some control should be given back to the client as soon as possible. (3) (MH; PL; TC; CS)

2 This is a normal form of ventilating emotions; the client should be told that medication is available if desired.

3 This takes control away from the client; the client could view this as an additional assault on the body that increases feelings of vulnerability and anxiety and does not restore control.

4 Same as answer 3.

102. 1 Partners may themselves feel angry and abused; these feelings should be rapidly and openly discussed. (3) (MH; AN; TC; CS)

2 This should not be done yet; rape counselors deal with the victim and partner together.

3 The partner's feelings must be resolved before the partner can really help the client.

4 This may be reassuring, but it leaves the partner alone to deal with feelings.

103. 1 Identification of support networks and relationships is a priority if the victim is to be helped after the immediate crisis is over. (3) (MH; AS; PS; CS)

2 This may eventually be of value, but at this time it is irrelevant to assessing the client's condition or needs.

3 Same as answer 2.

4 This is not necessary for evaluation of the client's condition or support network.

104. 1 Her anger at her husband for leaving her will make her feel guilty for having these feelings. (3) (MH; AS; PS; CS)

2 Money may or may not be a problem for this client.

3 Loneliness will be something she will have to deal with later depending on her support system; it is not an immediate problem.

4 Estrangement may be something she will have to deal with later; it is not an immediate problem.

105. 3 Whether or not there is a suicide plan is a major criterion in assessing the client's determination to make another attempt. (1) (MH; AS; TC; CS)

1 Although this may be important for planning future therapeutic approaches, this does not explore the potential for suicide, the priority at this time.

2 Same as answer 1.

4 Same as answer 1.

106. 2 Suicide threats and gestures are a means of communicating anger, frustration, hopelessness, and despair to significant others and should always be taken seriously. (1) (MH; IM; ED; CS)

1 Children have many means readily available; many means of suicide are common objects around the home and playground.

3 Although suicide is the second leading cause of death in the 15- to 24-year-old age group, children under the age of 6 do attempt suicide and some succeed.

4 A suicide gesture is usually a cry for help but a suicide attempt is usually self-destructive; a suicide attempt is usually carried out with the belief that death will result; neither a suicidal gesture nor a suicide attempt is manipulative; an impulsive act that is a rage response designed to punish others may be manipulative.

107. 3 The parents are focusing their feelings about their child's prognosis on someone or something else, in this case each other. (1) (MH; IM; PS; CS)

1 Denial is ignoring, avoiding, or refusing to recognize painful realities.

2 Projection is the attribution of one's own feelings to another person.

4 Compensation is a defense in which one makes up for a perceived deficiency by emphasizing another feature perceived as an asset.

108. 3 Reasonable limits are necessary because they provide security and help to keep the child's behavior in acceptable bounds. (3) (MH; PL; ED; CS)

1 This is an unrealistic approach that allows the child to manipulate the total situation.

2 Care should be directed to help the child, not the staff.

4 Relationships, not special privileges, should provide the necessary security.

109. 1 Children frequently use denial of parents as a stage of coping with separation; they avoid the fact that separation is real. (1) (MH; IM; ED; CS)

2 Undoing is a behavior or communication technique calculated to neutralize earlier behavior or communication.

3 Repression is the involuntary exclusion of painful thoughts, impulses, or memories; this child's behavior is voluntary.

4 Sublimation is the act of substituting socially acceptable behavior for an unacceptable feeling or drive.

110. 2 Seeing their child as soon as possible will validate the death for them and initiate the grieving process. (2) (MH; IM; PS; CS)

1 This will delay and prolong the grieving process; the response offers no explanation for waiting.

3 This is unnecessary; the parents have asked to see their child now.

4 This is untrue; it would be more traumatic to wait and delay the reality of the death.

111. 2 Deaths that are perceived as preventable cause more guilt for the mourners and therefore increase the intensity and length of the grieving process. (2) (MH; AN; PS; CS)

1 This is untrue; it is usually more difficult.

3 It may prolong and intensify the mourning process but will not necessarily result in a pathologic reaction.

4 Same as answer 3.

112. 1 This provides support until the individuals' coping mechanisms and personal support systems can be mobilized. (3) (MH; IM; PS; CS)

2 The individuals, not the nurse, must mobilize their support systems.

3 This is not the role of the nurse.

4 The individuals need time before the full reality of the death can be accepted.

113. 4 Support is most important when dealing with the crisis of death; the support system must be relied on for coping with the loss. (2) (MH; AS; PS; CS)

1 The client's age may play a role in coping but it is not the most important factor.

2 The timing may be important if death is just one of a multiplicity of stresses, but it is not the most important factor in helping a client cope.

3 The socioeconomic status may be important in long term planning but it is not the most important factor in the grieving process.

114. 3 When the relationship was ambivalent there is both anger and guilt to work through. (1) (MH; AN; PS; CS)

1 A loving relationship evokes less feelings of guilt and a less complicated grieving process.

2 The length of the relationship seems to have little to do with the ease or difficulty in completing the grieving process.

4 The individual in the subservient role has usually learned to accept directions and either finds a new director or else is relieved to have a chance to express own feelings.

115. 3 Successful resolution means being able to remember the good as well as the bad qualities of the deceased and accepting them as part of being human. (1) (MH; EV; PS; CS)

1 Resolution involves working through feelings not just accepting what occurred.

2 Resolution does not mean forgetting but rather realistically remembering what was.

4 This is an unhealthy response that can become pathological because of the unresolved feelings about the other person's qualities.

116. 4 It is important to know if the client is considering suicide so that the nurse can provide a safe environment and therapeutic care. (3) (MH; AS; PS; CS)

1 Concern for the client's safety takes priority at this time over present feelings or past relationships.

2 Same as answer 1.

3 Same as answer 1.

117. 4 Discussing the partner and the partner's death will help the client work through the grief process. (3) (MH; PL; PS; CS)

1 This would refocus the client's attention away from dealing with feelings; the client would probably not have the physical or emotional energy to get involved with group activities.

2 The client must deal with the past and present before dealing with the future.

3 Same as answer 1.

118. 4 Helping a client deal with unresolved grief involves assisting the client to express thoughts and feelings about the lost object or person as a necessary part of grief work. (1) (MH; IM; PS; CS)

1 This is the responsibility of the nurse; another client would not have the expertise to help the client.

2 This would be too threatening; at this point the client needs a therapeutic one-to-one interaction.

3 The current nonverbal behavior indicates that the client is dealing with feelings; an opportunity should be provided for a verbal exploration.

119. 1 This will enable the client to begin speaking about the spouse and resolve the loss. (2) (MH; IM; PS; CS)

2 Although this may be beneficial, the primary focus should be on the expression of feelings.

3 A psychiatric consultation is not indicated by the data at this time.

4 The data does not indicate ambivalence toward the spouse.

120. 3 These are the defining characteristics of dysfunctional grieving. (3) (MH; AS; PS; CS)

1 The client's communication does not lead to this conclusion.

2 Same as answer 1.

4 Eight months does not constitute a prolonged period of mourning.

121. 2 Such stimuli encourage the client to remain reality oriented; research has shown that competing stimuli are useful in controlling hallucinations. (2) (MH; PL; ED; CS)

1 This does not ensure that the client's needs will be met.

3 This is not very realistic and fosters greater dependency; it focuses on the client's inability to deal with the problem and increases the client's fear of being alone.

4 Same as answer 3.

122. 3 Denial may be handled by seeking other opinions in an attempt to prove an unacceptable one incorrect. (1) (MH; AS; PA; CS)
   1 This occurs during the stage of anger, which is a later stage.
   2 This occurs during the stage of depression, which is a later stage.
   4 This is not associated with the initial stage; this behavior usually occurs after the client recognizes the inevitable outcome and is fearful of being alone.

123. 4 Rationalization is offering a socially acceptable or logical explanation to justify an unacceptable feeling or behavior. (1) (MH; AS; PA; CS)
   1 Projection is the denial of emotionally unacceptable feelings and the attribution of the traits to another person.
   2 Sublimation is the substitution of a socially acceptable behavior for an unacceptable feeling or drive.
   3 Compensation is making up for a perceived deficiency by emphasizing another feature perceived as an asset.

124. 4 This approach is positive because it attempts to deal with the staff's feelings and the problem without singling out people for blame; the nurse therefore is taking ethically sound action without being moralistic or authoritarian. (1) (MH; PL; TC; CS)
   1 This abdicates the nurse's responsibility and may create anger and guilt in the staff.
   2 Same as answer 1.
   3 Same as answer 1.

125. 1 It is important for the couple to discuss their feelings to maintain open communication and support each other. (2) (MH; PL; ED; CS)
   2 This may be useful in the future but is most likely premature; they need to deal with their own feelings first.

   3 This action would not meet the needs of this couple; it focuses only on the client's needs and ignores the partner's; in addition, psychotherapy is a long-term process.
   4 This may elicit feelings but will not improve communication; this is a rather long-term goal.

126. 1 The client has lost a companion and a purpose in life and these feelings can be overwhelming until new activities are developed. (2) (MH; AS; PS; CS)
   2 Anger should not be a major problem for this client; data do not address any problem in the husband-wife relationship.
   3 Data do not address the financial status of this client.
   4 If there is guilt over feelings of relief about the husband's death they would be transitory and not a major problem.

127. 2 The spouse is expressing the normal feelings of guilt associated with the death of a loved one; there is always initial guilt over what might have been. (1) (MH; AN; PS; CS)
   1 No evidence supports this conclusion.
   3 The spouse is expressing guilt, not shame.
   4 Same as answer 1.

128. 3 With the medication the individual does not face the reality of the loss and merely delays the onset of the pain associated with it; because most support is available at the time of the death and the funeral, tranquilizers at this time deny the individual the opportunity to use this assistance. (2) (MH; AN; PS; CS)
   1 This is untrue; tranquilizers do not magnify the risk of suicide.
   2 Brain activity does not cause depression.
   4 Although tranquilizers may initially cause some lethargy, this is not the reason they are not ordered.

129. 4 The nurse should recognize that the behavior represents anticipatory grieving. (3) (MH; AN; PS; CS)

1 Although this may be true, the husband is extremely involved with his own needs at this time.

2 The husband is beginning the grieving process; the husband's actions do not appear to be an expression of anger, but rather an attempt to cope with the situation.

3 There are no data to substantiate this conclusion.

130. 1 Because of the individuality of people, the response to retirement may vary, but it is a task representing a developmental milestone for all people. (2) (MH; AN; ED; CS)

2 This may or may not be true; it depends on the individual and the circumstances.

3 Same as answer 2.

4 Same as answer 2.

DISORDERS OF MOOD

131. 4 This provides structure and helps the client learn acceptable behavior. (2) (MH; PL; TC; MO)

1 The client may not be ready for this at the present time.

2 No environment will be stress free.

3 Same as answer 1.

132. 4 Limiting unnecessary interactions will decrease stimulation and, thus, agitation. (2) (MH; PL; TC; MO)

1 Constant client and staff contact increases stimulation and, thus, agitation.

2 This bombards the client's sensorium and increases agitation.

3 Not all disturbed clients are suspicious.

133. 4 Depression is contagious; it affects the nurse as well as the client. (2) (MH; AN; PS; MO)

1 The client's lack of energy really does not make nursing care difficult.

2 These clients usually do not offer negative responses; they offer no responses.

3 Same as answer 1.

134. 1 Because clients cannot be argued out of their feelings, it is best to initially accept them; it also encourages communication. (2) (MH; PL; PS; MO)

2 This delays discussing the client's feelings and has little value.

3 The depressed client does very little talking and needs to be encouraged to communicate.

4 This has little effect on the depressed client; it can increase depression.

135. 1 Allowing the client to make those decisions that can be handled helps improve confidence. (2) (MH; PL; TC; MO)

2 The client is depressed, and this would probably result in total inactivity.

3 This action would demoralize the client; also, it is impossible for one individual to make all the decisions for another.

4 Same as answer 2.

136. 4 This action demonstrates to the client that the nurse feels the client is worth spending time with, and it helps restore and build trust. (2) (MH; PL; TC; MO)

1 This action would be impossible to carry out on a regular basis unless the client was potentially suicidal.

2 This action does little to establish communication between the nurse and client and might be threatening.

3 The depressed client may never get around to speaking to the nurse and, left alone, will withdraw even further.

137. 4 The fact that the nurse spends time with the client conveys a feeling of importance and helps build the client's self-esteem. (3) (MH; IM; TC; MO)

1 This places the client on the defensive and does not respond to the feelings of worthlessness communicated by the client.

2 This infers agreement with the client's statement that the client is not worthy; the nurse should stay to convey a sense of self-worth to the client.

3 This response cuts off communication; the client responds better to actions than to words.

138. 3 This response focuses on the client's feelings rather than the statement, and it serves to open channels of communication. (2) (MH; IM; PS; MO)
   1 This response asks the client to decide what is causing feelings; most people are unable to answer why they feel as they do.
   2 Such a response simply echoes the client's statement and does not reflect feelings or stimulate therapeutic communication.
   4 This response does nothing to stimulate further communication; in fact, it tells the client to talk about feelings with someone else.

139. 4 This removes the necessity of making the decision from the client and demonstrates that the client is worth spending time with. (2) (MH; IM; TC; MO)
   1 This requires the client to make a decision the client may be unable to make; if the client says "no," communication is blocked.
   2 This requires an action the client may be unable to take.
   3 Same as answer 1.

140. 1 The client will be most likely to eat if accompanied and encouraged by an individual with whom a trusting relationship has been established. (1) (MH; IM; PS; MO)
   2 This will not encourage the client to eat and will promote isolation.
   3 This is inappropriate at this time; the client is not interested in maintaining health, nor is the client ready for any teaching.
   4 This would be ineffective at this time; the client is too introspective to care.

141. 2 In a melancholic type depressive episode the range of interests becomes increasingly narrow with eventual loss of pleasure in almost all activities; overmeticulousness occurs because the client cannot tolerate any change in the environment. (3) (MH; AS; PS; MO)
   1 The boundaries would be increasingly narrowed because the client cannot tolerate change, which is viewed as a threat.

   3 Jealousy is a symptom that is unrelated to a major depressive episode; the symptoms usually develop slowly over a period of time.
   4 There is nothing to indicate that the client ever had a hypermanic episode in which this behavior would be expected; hypermanic behavior does not occur in a major depressive episode.

142. 4 This is a psychiatric disease in which there is no prior history of depression; it is related to age, changes in life-style, and feelings of not contributing and being worthless. (1) (MH; AS; PS; MO)
   1 In bipolar disorders, depression alternates with periods of extreme restlessness, hyperactivity, and flamboyance in dress and behavior; this is not evident here.
   2 Involutional melancholia, which was usually characterized by depression with agitation, is no longer considered a specific disorder.
   3 There is no inconsistency between the behavior and the mood.

143. 3 Before onset of depression, these clients usually have very narrow, limited interests. (2) (MH; AS; PS; MO)
   1 Many individuals have been conforming, conscientious, and hardworking in an attempt to feel needed; feelings of guilt, anger, worthlessness, and hopelessness occur with the depression.
   2 Same as answer 1.
   4 Same as answer 1.

144. 3 Some success is important to increase the client's self-esteem. (3) (MH; IM; PS; MO)
   1 This would support the client's feelings of uselessness.
   2 The client who is in a major depression would not have the interest or energy to act independently.
   4 Same as answer 2.

145. 3   Caring for a child often refocuses a client's unmet dependency needs resulting in resentment and anger; the feelings cause ambivalence and guilt which are turned inward. (3) (MH; AS; PS; MO)
1   There are no data to support this conclusion.
2   There are no data to support the conclusion that child abuse occurred.
4   Self-destructive behavior does not usually evoke love, sympathy, and compliments from others.

146. 3   Because the client refuses to talk, pertinent data must be obtained from the family. (2) (MH; AS; TC; MO)
1   The client is not responding to questions; the client may not know the reason.
2   This may or may not have influenced current behavior.
4   The presence of scars is an inaccurate way to determine past behavior.

147. 4   The expression of these feelings may indicate that this client is unable to continue the struggle of life. (2) (MH; AS; TC; MO)
1   These are not indications of potential suicide; the client is still responding to the world, not attempting to leave it.
2   These are usually not sufficient to precipitate a suicidal attempt.
3   The client attempting suicide usually sees death as a release.

148. 2   This is the most important assessment to make because suicide is a possibility with every depressed client. (2) (MH; AS; TC; MO)
1   The client has already said this and it responds to only part of the client's statement.
3   The nurse does not have enough information to have this understanding; this response does not encourage communication.
4   This is a philosophic approach that would not encourage discussion of feelings.

149. 4   Sleep and appetite disturbances are clues that the client is anxious; a history of suicidal ideation indicates that the client is thinking about self-harm; the client may attempt suicide to obtain relief from the anxiety. (2) (MH; AS; TC; MO)
1   The severely depressed client would not have the energy to act on a suicidal plan.
2   The client who is out of contact with reality would not have the ability to develop or follow through with a suicide plan.
3   Severe anxiety would interfere with the client's ability to focus energy and act out a suicidal plan.

150. 1   When energy levels improve in the depressed client, the risk of suicide increases; also, the client has given away a personal belonging, which may indicate a plan to commit suicide. (1) (MH; AS; TC; MO)
2   This may be true, but the gift of a personal belonging decreases the possibility that it is simply an improved socialization level.
3   This may be true, but the gift of a personal belonging decreases the possibility that it is simply an improvement in mood.
4   This may be true, but the situation should be explored further; the physician would ultimately make this decision.

151. 2   This statement provides clues that the client feels no one cares, so there is no reason the client should care. (2) (MH; AN; PS; MO)
1   The clues presented do not lead to this conclusion.
3   Same as answer 1.
4   Same as answer 1.

152. 1   Decreased sexual desire is a major symptom of clinical depression. (1) (MH; AN; PS; MO)
2   Although depression is often related to unmet dependency needs, decreased sexual desire is associated with the depression.

3 The sexual difficulties are associated with the depression, and the depression is the major cause of the marital stress.

4 Role confusion, not identity confusion, is associated with the depression.

153. 4 In 3 days the client should understand that the staff cares enough to prevent suicidal acting out. (3) (MH; AN; PS; MO)

1 This is unrealistic within the stated time period.

2 Same as answer 1.

3 Same as answer 1.

154. 1 At this point the client may have enough energy to plan and execute an attempt. (1) (MH; AN; TC; MO)

2 The motor retardation accompanying depression usually limits the client's acting out on impulse.

3 Same as answer 2.

4 Loss of interest in the environment is an early sign of depression, and the client would not have the energy to act out.

155. 4 Although fear of aloneness may play a part, the main factor leading to acting out on suicidal impulses is the feeling of hopelessness. (3) (MH; AS; PS; MO)

1 The struggle for control is a more common theme expressed by clients with bipolar depression; betrayal is a feeling more often verbalized by clients with a diagnosis of a borderline personality disorder.

2 The struggle for power and dominance is a more common theme in the verbalization of clients who are diagnosed with paranoid schizophrenia.

3 Anger and indecisiveness may be associated with depression, but an indecisive individual would usually not make the decision to commit suicide.

156. 3 As the depression lifts and physical energy increases, the increased energy permits the person to act out suicidal thoughts. (1) (MH; PL; TC; MO)

1 This is unsafe; the priority is to protect the client from self-harm.

2 Same as answer 1.

4 The opposite is true.

157. 1 This response addresses the behavior observed and the offer by the nurse to spend time to help the client implies that the client is worthy. (1) (MH; IM; PS; MO)

2 The nurse offers to help but places the client second by stating the desire to have coffee first.

3 The nurse denies the client's feelings by focusing on getting ready for visitors.

4 This response first recognizes the client's feelings and then moves away from discussing them; this response closes off communication.

158. 1 Clients who have a plan are more apt to carry it out; safety is the priority. (2) (MH; IM; PC; MO)

2 This is a noncaring response and may be viewed as false reassurance.

3 This response is too upbeat for a depressed client and provides false reassurance.

4 Although this response is empathic, it does nothing to assist the client and may be viewed as a consent for suicide.

159. 4 This open-ended response encourages further discussion and allows for an exploration of feelings. (2) (MH; IM; PS; MO)

1 This response ignores the client's feelings expressed in the statement.

2 The depression is not adding to the feelings, the feelings are causing the depression.

3 Same as answer 1.

160. 4 The manic phase is the mirror image of the depressed phase; the behavior is an attempt to ward off depression by racing into reality. (2) (MH; AS; PS; MO)

1 It does not have to be an elating situation; the situation itself matters little, and the client responds to any stimuli.

2 It is an attempt to block feelings of depression, not an acting out of innate drives.

3 It is not an incorrect interpretation but an incorrect response to the stimuli.

161. 4 The elated client expends a great deal of energy; dehydration, oxygen deficits, cardiac problems, and death can occur. (2) (MH; AS; PA; MO)
1 The elated person does not withdraw from reality but continues to run headfirst into it.
2 The elated client has little difficulty verbalizing needs.
3 The elated client usually does not take time to eat while expending a great deal of energy, so weight loss is the problem.

162. 4 The client expends a great amount of energy running headlong into reality in an attempt to ward off or avoid facing feelings of depression. (3) (MH; AN; PS; MO)
1 The behavior is not an expression of innate desires but an attempt to avoid feelings of depression.
2 The client has no difficulty relating to others; this behavior is an attempt to avoid feelings of depression.
3 This client is not attempting to compensate for an imagined loss but is trying to avoid feelings of depression.

163. 1 Structure tends to decrease agitation and anxiety and increase the client's feelings of security. (1) (MH; PL; PS; MO)
2 Touching can be threatening for many clients and should not be used indiscriminately.
3 Conversations should be kept simple; the client with a bipolar disorder, either depressed or manic phase, may have difficulty following involved conversations about current affairs.
4 Clients with bipolar disorders are in contact with reality so this activity would serve little purpose.

164. 1 These clients are acutely aware of and sensitive to the environment; they need a structured environment in which stimuli are reduced and a feeling of acceptance and support is present. (1) (MH; PL; TC; MO)
2 This client is acutely aware of reality and does not need to have it clarified.
3 Although important, this can best be achieved by establishing a supportive, structured environment.
4 The client needs reduced, not increased, stimuli.

165. 2 The excited, overactive client needs a calm environment; external stimulation only serves to cause further excitation. (2) (MH; IM; PS; MO)
1 The client needs reduced, not increased, external stimulation.
3 Same as answer 1.
4 Same as answer 1.

166. 1 A firm voice is most effective; the statement tells the client that it is the behavior, not the client, that is upsetting to others. (2) (MH; IM; TC; MO)
2 Demanding that the client stop the current behavior is a useless action; the client is out of control and needs external control.
3 The client does not know what is precipitating the behavior, and the question would be frustrating.
4 This should only be done when there is real danger from exhaustion; external controls must be set.

167. 1 This response simply states a fact and delivers praise without making demands. (3) (MH; IM; PS; MO)
2 This puts the total responsibility for control on a client who needs external controls set.
3 This does not help the client separate the self from the behavior; it tells the client that acting-out behavior will result in rejection.
4 The client may not recall what happened yesterday and would not know why today's behavior was better.

DISORDERS OF PERSONALITY

168. 1 Imagery is a therapeutic approach used to facilitate positive self-talk; mental pictures under the control of and initiated by the client may correct faulty cognitions. (3) (MH; AN; PS; PR)
2 This is a useful general behavioral approach, but is not a specific desensitization technique.
3 These are useful general behavioral approaches, but are not specific desensitization techniques.
4 Same as answer 2.

169. 3   The mother's behavior sends two conflict-ing messages, one says "I care" and the other says "I don't care"; this behavior is often demonstrated by people with per-sonality disorders. (3) (MH; AS; PS; PR)

1   If the mother were rejecting the daughter, she would not have brought a gift.

2   No evidence of a projection of feelings is given.

4   Passive-aggressive behavior is an indirect, rather than direct, expression of angry or hostile feelings.

170. 4   This response demonstrates acceptance of the client and sets limits on the client's manipulative behavior. (3) (MH; IM; TC; PR)

1   This is false reassurance and it assists in the attempt to manipulate the next shift.

2   The nurse would be allowing further manipulation by the client by not leaving when the shift was over.

3   This is false reassurance; the nurse cannot make everything all right.

171. 1   Consistency, limit setting, and supportive confrontation are essential nursing inter-ventions to provide a secure, therapeutic environment for this client (1) (MH; PL; TC; PR)

2   To be therapeutic the environment needs structure and the staff must assist the client to set short-term goals for behav-ioral changes.

3   The use of an authoritarian approach will increase anxiety in this type of client, re-sulting in feelings of rejection and with-drawal.

4   Ignoring the client's behavior would be nontherapeutic and would reinforce the client's underlying fears of abandonment.

172. 3   Sitting with the client indicates accep-tance and demonstrates that the nurse feels the client is worthy of the nurse's time. (2) (MH; IM; PS; PR)

1   It would be better to stay with the client quietly until control is regained; staying prevents a follow-through on the client's threat.

2   This would have the effect of closing off further communication and denying the client's feelings.

4   This would provide little comfort for the client.

173. 3   The withdrawn pattern of behavior pre-vents the individual from reaching out to others for sharing; the isolation produces feelings of loneliness. (2) (MH; AN; PS; PR)

1   Feelings of anger may result in withdraw-al, but withdrawal does not produce feel-ings of anger.

2   Feelings of paranoia may result in with-drawal, but withdrawal does not produce these feelings.

4   Repression is an unconscious defense whereby the individual excludes ideas, feelings, or situations from the conscious level of thought; this is not the result of withdrawal.

174. 1   Withdrawal provides a temporary defense against anxiety because it limits contact with reality and decreases the client's world. (2) (MH; AN; PS; PR)

2   Withdrawal does not accomplish this, be-cause feelings and anxieties are still present and little attempt is made to work through problems.

3   Same as answer 2.

4   Same as answer 2.

175. 1   This ritual is a process of undoing arising from unconscious conflicts from the anal stage in which dirt, or soiling oneself, is associated with an aggressive act against authority; the rage is controlled by rituals such as handwashing. (2) (MH; AN; PS; PR)

2   There is a desire for freedom and indepen-dence; the ritual is an act against authori-ty.

3   There is initiative; the rebellion is against authority, not autonomy.

4   There is usually no problem with gender identity.

176. 4   In the early part of treatment before new defenses are developed, enough time must be allowed for the client to complete the ritual to keep anxiety under control. (2) (MH; IM; PS; PR)

1   The ritual is a defense that cannot be interrupted or delayed; it is used until new defenses are developed.

2   Same as answer 1.

3   Same as answer 1.

177. 2   This is the psychoanalytic explanation for the development of obsessive-compulsive symptomatology. (2) (MH; AN; PS; PR)

1   Compulsive rituals frequently result in interference with activities of daily living and the individual becomes dysfunctional; rituals cannot be controlled.

3   The client is unable to consciously stop the behavior because anxiety would become overwhelming if the defense were not used.

4   This is not related to rituals but rather to phobias.

178. 1   This limits the time and still allows the ritual; until the underlying cause of anxiety can be dealt with, rituals should be allowed as much as possible. (2) (MH; PL; TC; PR)

2   This provides for only one time period and probably would result in increased anxiety.

3   One ritual cannot be substituted for another; this would interfere with the performance of the original ritual and could result in overwhelming anxiety.

4   This is the client's decision; the nurse should not recommend this action.

179. 2   Paraphrasing encourages further ventilation by the client. (2) (MH; IM; PS; PR)

1   This is a negative response that may increase the client's fears about being crazy.

3   This response denies the client's feelings.

4   This provides false reassurance and implies that the client is out of control, which may increase her fears.

180. 2   Clients use ritualistic behavior to control anxiety; when the defense is taken away, the client experiences the anxiety and becomes angry at the one who stopped the defense against it. (2) (MH; EV; PS; PR)

1   Because the anxiety increases discomfort, the client would not feel relief or gratitude when the behavior that controlled the anxiety was interrupted.

3   Same as answer 1.

4   Although these clients recognize that the ritualistic behavior is not necessary, they are unable to stop it and usually are not embarrassed by it.

181. 3   The client is unable to control impulses at this time, so controls must be provided for the client; the nurse's behavior provides a role model. (2) (MH; PL; PS; PR)

1   The client is not able to set controls; freedom could prove frightening to a client who is not in control.

2   This is nontherapeutic; this would probably provoke even more acting-out behavior.

4   Same as answer 2.

182. 1   Both clients must be included in a discussion about this behavior to make certain that limits on future behavior are understood by both of them; this action also places controls on the manipulative behavior often used by clients with an antisocial personality disorder. (2) (MH; PL; PS; PR)

2   This action would merely cause the clients to find another place to meet; the response sets no limits on behavior but only addresses location.

3   This action would not set any limits on behavior but merely put staff in the policing role.

4   Although this may be necessary, the nurse must respond directly to the clients involved in this situation.

183. 4 This would be the most therapeutic thing the parents could do; the client must be made accountable for behavior and must know that manipulation and acting out will not be tolerated. (2) (MH; PL; ED; PR)

1 This would probably be a continuation of the parents' previous response to client and would prove to be of little value.

2 Would probably cause client to continue to act out to test limit of parent's endurance.

3 Same as answer 1.

184. 3 Private confrontation with reported facts provides for verification; a calm, direct manner is most assertive. (2) (MH; IM; PS; PR)

1 This action places control in the hands of the client rather than the nurse, which could lead to aggressive confrontation.

2 This is aggressive confrontation, not assertive intervention.

4 This is not assertive intervention; it is manipulation and is not truthful.

185. 4 This client needs firm, realistic limits set on behavior; this statement permits the client to make the choice and clearly states the consequences of behavior. (2) (MH; IM; TC; PR)

1 This is an unrealistic response; clients with this diagnosis do not learn from past errors.

2 This is an unrealistic response; this client would care very little about rules.

3 This is an unrealistic response; the client and visitors do not want to socialize with other clients and visitors.

186. 4 The expression of feelings by this individual would demonstrate the development of some insight and a willingness to at least begin to look at underlying causes of behavior. (2) (MH; EV; PS; PR)

1 These words would probably have little meaning to the client.

2 Same as answer 1.

3 Same as answer 1.

187. 2 The client must recognize the existence of the subpersonalities so that interpretation can occur. (3) (MH; AN; PS; PR)

1 This is not relevant to clients with multiple personality disorders; this outcome relates to clients with obsessive-compulsive behaviors.

3 This is not realistic; integration of the personalities generates fear and defensiveness in the client and defense mechanisms will be used.

4 This is inappropriate; anxiety serves as a motivator for behavioral change and anti-anxiety medications must be used judiciously.

188. 3 A multiple personality disorder is a complex, multifaceted problem that requires long-term therapy to achieve integration of the personalities. (3) (MH; EV; PS; PR)

1 None of the personalities can be ignored because their presence must be dealt with before integration can occur.

2 Each personality has the ability to deal openly with feelings and fears but the personalities need to be integrated.

4 This is untrue; if they did not serve a protective purpose they would be abandoned.

SUBSTANCE ABUSE

189. 2 In projection a person faults another person for having the unacceptable impulses, thoughts, or behaviors that are too uncomfortable to accept as one's own. (1) (MH; AN; PS; SA)

1 Denial is a method of resolving conflict or escaping unpleasant realities by ignoring their existence.

3 Displacement refers to the transfer of an emotion from one object or situation to another, usually safer, object.

4 In compensation the person makes up for personal inadequacies by emphasizing attributes to gain social approval.

190. 1   The history of the loss of a child and the intensity of the client's drinking since the child's death should lead to this nursing diagnosis. (3) (MH; AN; PS; SA)

2   This is a symptom or a medical diagnosis, not a nursing diagnosis.

3   There is no documentation that the client is unable to distinguish between the self and nonself.

4   There is no documentation that the family has not attempted to provide support; it is the family who has brought the client for help.

191. 4   Alcohol is a central nervous system depressant; these symptoms are the body's neurologic adaptation to the withdrawal of alcohol. (2) (MH; AS; PA; SA)

1   Tonic-clonic seizures are not early signs of alcohol withdrawal; they would not occur before 48 to 72 hours of abstinence.

2   Fever and diaphoresis may be seen during prolonged periods of delirium and are a result of autonomic overactivity.

3   These are late signs of severe withdrawal that occur with delirium tremens; tachycardia results from autonomic overactivity.

192. 2   Motivation is necessary to assist the client in withstanding the pain of giving up a defense; motivation is more influential in facilitating change than any external factor. (2) (MH; AN; PS; SA)

1   Most families of individuals with alcoholism are enablers; enabling behavior does not help the individual to deal with the drinking problem but denies that problems exist.

3   This can be of assistance, but internal factors will have a greater impact on rehabilitation than will external factors.

4   Self-esteem will be useful if it precipitates abstinence behavior; however, people with alcoholism frequently have low self-esteem.

193. 1   Alcohol causes both physical and psychologic dependence; the individual needs and depends on the alcohol to function. (2) (MH; AN; PS; SA)

2   This is untrue; alcoholism is a disease that entails physical and psychologic dependence.

3   This is a myth often associated with alcoholism; the individual needs to learn how to use other coping mechanisms more consistently and effectively.

4   People with alcoholism frequently drink alone or feel alone in a crowd.

194. 4   The data demonstrate the classical symptoms of withdrawal dementia that occur within a week after the cessation or reduction of alcohol intake. (2) (MH; AN; PS; SA)

1   The information does not demonstrate the presence of impaired short-term or long-term memory; this usually develops shortly after a period of prolonged heavy drinking.

2   There are insufficient data to identify dementia; impairment of thought processes, judgment, and intellectual abilities would have to continue for 3 weeks or longer.

3   The information does not demonstrate the presence of hallucinations; these usually develop within 48 hours of cessation or reduction of alcohol intake.

195. 3   This behavior indicates that the client lacks insight and is denying that alcohol is the problem. (1) (MH; AN; PS; SA)

1   There are no data to support this conclusion.

2   Same as answer 1.

4   Same as answer 1.

196. 1   Clients who abuse alcohol characteristically have lowered self-esteem; therefore, it is important for the nurse to accept the person as an individual with value. (1) (MH; PL; PS; SA)

2   Although nurturing is important, this client must learn self-reliance.

3   This would probably be an old story to this client and would have little positive effect.

4   This action would not provide an atmosphere that would help the client withstand the stress of the detoxification program.

197. 3 The client must learn to develop and use more healthful coping mechanisms if drinking is to be stopped; the responsibility is with the client because the client must do the changing. (2) (MH; PL; PS; SA)

1 This would tell the client what to expect but would not instill responsibility for change.

2 This will increase guilt and place the client on the defensive; it usually does not foster the development of a trusting relationship.

4 Medications do not provide the motivation for change; this must come from within the client.

198. 1 This statement recognizes the feeling of ambivalence associated with admitting that a problem with alcohol exists; this occurs early in treatment. (2) (MH; IM; PS; SA)

2 This places the client on the defensive and interferes with communication.

3 Same as answer 2.

4 Same as answer 2.

199. 3 This strengthens the client's link with reality and reassures the client of safety because the hallucinations are usually frightening. (2) (MH; IM; TC; SA)

1 The nurse must respond to the client's behavior by attempting to point out reality and reduce anxiety.

2 Validation reinforces the client's distorted perceptions of reality, is not helpful, and may even be unsafe.

4 It is not helpful to argue or try to explain the hallucinations away because they are real to the client.

200. 3 Peripheral neuropathy is present, and this measure will limit tactile stimulation. (2) (MH; IM; PA; SA)

1 This would do little to relieve discomfort or reduce the occurrence of neurologic symptoms.

2 Same as answer 1.

4 This may be done periodically; however, these symptoms are not caused by impaired circulation but rather by peripheral neuropathy.

201. 1 This supports the family of the addicted individual and allows the family to continue on with life by reducing guilt. (2) (MH; IM; TC; TR)

2 The family has already stated this is impossible when drinking occurs.

3 This places the burden for preventing drinking on the family and will create feelings of resentment and guilt.

4 This is enabling behavior, which does not help the abuser or the family.

202. 3 These symptoms are all associated with opiate withdrawal, which occurs after cessation or reduction of prolonged moderate or heavy use of opiates. (2) (MH; AS; PA; SA)

1 Lacrimation and vomiting are present, but insomnia, not drowsiness, occurs with opiate withdrawal.

2 Nausea is present, but diarrhea not constipation, and constricted pupils rather than dilated pupils, occur with opiate withdrawal.

4 Rhinorrhea is present, but fever, rather than a subnormal temperature, and muscle aches, rather than convulsions, occur with opiate withdrawal.

203. 1 Opiates cause central nervous system depression, resulting in severe respiratory depression, hypotension, and unconsciousness. (2) (MH; AS; PA; SA)

2 These findings, particularly the respirations, are not indicative of an overdose of an opiate.

3 Same as answer 2.

4 Same as answer 2.

204. 3 Addicted individuals usually use a substance to increase their feelings of worth; the substance helps them appear bigger in their own eyes; they usually have strong unmet dependency needs. (2) (MH; AN; PS; SA)

1 Although guilt about breaking society's code may be present, there is no rejection of reality, just an inability to deal with it.

2 Although there is a need for acceptance, there is no underlying feeling of hostility.

4 Although anger is present and internalized, there is no struggle for independence.

205. 3 Individuals usually take drugs because they cannot deal with the pain of reality; the drug blurs the pain. (1) (MH; AN; PS; SA)
1 Drugs increase dependency rather than foster independence.
2 Although this factor may encourage initial use by some adolescents, it is not the most frequent reason for use.
4 The use of drugs fosters social isolation rather than social relationships.

206. 1 Tolerance is a phenomenon that occurs in addicted individuals and increases the amount of drug needed to satisfy their need; because this phenomenon is not permanent and may disappear without warning, overdose frequently occurs. (1) (MH; AN; PA; SA)
2 The problem is not related to dependence and addiction; the failure to respond to an adult dose of an opiate is related to tolerance.
3 Same as answer 2.
4 Same as answer 2.

207. 1 Acceptance and consistency are the best approaches to overcome these clients' expectations; what the nurse does is a better indicator of acceptance than the words that are verbalized. (1) (MH; PL; PS; SA)
2 Behaviors and actions of the nurse over time are better indicators of acceptance than is verbal reassurance.
3 Self-disclosure gets into the realm of a social, rather than a therapeutic, relationship.
4 Confrontational measures would only serve to increase anxiety and heighten dependency needs.

208. 1 This allows the client to use the staff as a support system and removes an opportunity to deny the problem. (3) (MH; PL; ED; SA)
2 This supports and permits denial; both the client and the staff know a problem exists, and the client must admit it.
3 This is a nonprofessional approach that would be nontherapeutic for the client.
4 Same as answer 3.

209. 4 This is a nonpunitive approach that attempts to salvage the nurse as an individual and as a professional. (2) (MH; IM; TC; SA)
1 This may be necessary for long-term therapy but would not be the initial approach.
2 This is a punitive, nontherapeutic response that offers no chance for rehabilitation.
3 The client is addicted; promises will not keep the client from abusing drugs.

210. 3 This is a serious charge, and confrontation should occur in the presence of the supervisor. (3) (MH; IM; PS; SA)
1 This is unnecessary; as a professional the nurse has enough information to confront the other nurse.
2 This is an assumption that may result in an altercation; a witness should be present.
4 This is not a professional approach; the nurse has a legal responsibility to intervene.

211. 1 The client is using denial to separate from the group members and needs realistic feedback to prevent withdrawal. (3) (MH; IM; PS; SA)
2 This would do nothing to help return the client to the group.
3 The client's meaning is clear; questioning the client at this point would be nontherapeutic.
4 This is inadequate; the client first needs to recognize that the problems being discussed are applicable.

212. 3 These provide high levels of thiamine; other sources include legumes, whole and enriched grains, and lean beef. (2) (MH; EV; ED; SA)
1 In this list, only fish is considered a source of thiamine.
2 In this list, only eggs are considered a source of thiamine; this list contains sources of protein.
4 Most vegetables contain only traces of thiamine; citrus fruits provide vitamin C.

213. 3 The client is still denying the illness and has not resolved the basic problem that led to the alcoholism. (2) (MH; EV; PS; SA)

1 This is incorrect because the client is still denying the illness; willpower alone will not keep the client away from alcohol.

2 This may be true, but it does not ensure compliance or successful rehabilitation.

4 This is not helpful unless the basis of the conflicts and the client's role in resolving them are understood by the client.

SCHIZOPHRENIC DISORDERS

214. 3 Physical safety of the client and others is the priority. (1) (MH; PL; TC; SD)

1 Although it is important for the client to live up to contracts, it is not imperative.

2 The nurse cannot prevent or control the client's use of defensive behavior.

4 Same as answer 2.

215. 4 Seclusion or restraints are special procedures for dealing with acting-out, aggressive behavior for the protection of the client or others; clear documentation in the progress notes is essential when suspension of the client's rights is necessary. (1) (MH; IM; TC; SD)

1 This is not necessary because the use of restraints and/or seclusion would be included in the general consent form signed on admission.

2 This monitoring should be done for all clients.

3 There is no such form; however, documentation to justify the need for seclusion or the use of restraints is required.

216. 2 These clients are threatened by reality; withdrawal from reality and the use of magical thinking reduces anxiety. (2) (MH; AS; PS; SD)

1 Clients with schizophrenia are not preoccupied with suicidal thoughts.

3 Clients with schizophrenia have poor self-esteem and a low self-image and usually have feelings of guilt and self-blame.

4 The loosening of associative links that occurs in schizophrenia makes these impossible.

217. 3 These are the classic premorbid symptoms of schizophrenia. (2) (MH; AS; PS; SD)

1 These symptoms are usually not associated with schizophrenia.

2 These symptoms are not associated with any particular type of disorder.

4 Same as answer 1.

218. 1 The presence of ego strengths is demonstrated by some level of adjustment before the occurrence of the precipitating event; these ego strengths can be used to help the client reorganize the personality. (1) (MH; AS; PS; SD)

2 This would tend to contribute to a poor prognosis.

3 Same as answer 2.

4 Same as answer 2.

219. 2 The usual age of onset of schizophrenia is adolescence or early adulthood. (2) (MH; AS; PS; SD)

1 Symptoms usually do not appear this early.

3 Same as answer 1.

4 Same as answer 1.

220. 4 By observing the client the nurse is able to adjust care and communications to reflect assessment of individual needs. (1) (MH; AS; TC; SD)

1 This is not vital to initially help the client; the nurse should meet the client where the client is now.

2 Specific clients differ; the nurse should meet the client where the client is now.

3 Same as answer 1.

221. 3 Most hallucinating clients hear voices without external stimuli. (1) (MH; AS; PS; SD)

1 Although hallucinating clients may see things without external stimuli, visual hallucinations are not as common as auditory hallucinations.

2 Tactile hallucinations are not very common.

4 Olfactory hallucinations are not very common.

222. 3 Neologisms are words that are invented and therefore understood only by the person using them. (1) (MH; AS; PS; SD)
1 Echolalia is the verbal repeating of exactly what is heard.
2 Concretism is a pattern of speech characterized by the absence of abstractions or generalizations.
4 Paleologic thinking is a disturbed system of logic in which subjects are made identical if two variables about them are the same.

223. 1 An illusion is a misinterpretation of an actual sensory stimulus. (2) (MH; AN; PS; SD)
2 A delusion is a false fixed belief.
3 Confabulation is filling in blanks in memory.
4 An hallucination is a false sensory perception without a stimulus being present.

224. 4 A somatic delusion is a fixed false belief pertaining to part of the body. (2) (MH; AN; PS; SD)
1 An illusion is a misinterpretation of an actual sensory stimulus.
2 Hallucinations are false sensory perceptions without stimuli being present.
3 Depersonalization is a feeling of unreality concerning the self.

225. 2 Ambivalence describes the existence of two conflicting emotions, impulses, or desires. (2) (MH; AN; PS; SD)
1 Double bind is two conflicting messages, not emotions, in a single communication.
3 Loose associations are not two conflicting emotions but the loosening of connections between thoughts.
4 Inappropriate affect is not two conflicting emotions but the inappropriate expression of emotions.

226. 2 Failure to accept the client and the client's fears establishes a barrier to effective communication. (1) (MH; AN; TC; SD)
1 Today, mental health therapy is directed toward returning the client to the community as rapidly as possible.

3 Electroconvulsive therapy (ECT) is not effective in clients with schizophrenia; in fact, it makes them more confused.
4 Family cooperation is helpful but not an absolute necessity; the client can get well in spite of the family.

227. 2 Depersonalization is a feeling of change or unreality about the self or the environment caused by a loss of ego boundaries and a loss of reality testing. (3) (MH; AN; PS; SD)
1 Paranoid ideations are beliefs that the individual is being singled out for unfair treatment.
3 Loose associations are verbalizations that are difficult to understand because the links between thoughts are not apparent.
4 Ideas of reference are false beliefs that the words and actions of others are concerned with or are directed toward the individual.

228. 1 The client cannot reach out to others because of lack of trust; withdrawal is used to defend against interpersonal threats and results in isolation. (2) (MH; AN; PS; SD)
2 Sleep disturbances are not common because clients tend to use sleep to withdraw from reality.
3 Most clients with schizophrenic disorders are not violent.
4 This is usually not associated with this disorder.

229. 4 Any other approach would be threatening, increase anxiety, and probably result in a physical confrontation. (3) (MH; PL; TC; SD)
1 This would increase anxiety, not foster decision making.
2 This would increase the client's anxiety and probably result in a physical confrontation.
3 This would increase anxiety, not increase self-esteem.

230. 4 The nurse must deal with these feelings and establish basic trust to promote a therapeutic milieu. (2) (MH; PL; PS; SD)
1 Continuous pacing is not really a problem because the nurse can walk back and forth with the client.

2 This may be of long-range importance but has little influence on the nurse's response to the client.

3 Same as answer 2.

231. 3 Helping the client to develop feelings of self-worth would reduce the client's need to use pathologic defenses. (2) (MH; PL; PS; SD)

1 Faith or the lack of faith is not the basic underlying problem but merely a symptom of it.

2 Self-control or the lack of self-control is not the basic underlying problem but merely a symptom of it.

4 Insight can only develop when the need to use the defense is reduced.

232. 2 This response accepts the client at the client's present level and, in addition, allows the client to set the pace of the relationship. (3) (MH; PL; TC; SD)

1 This approach to any client can be misinterpreted and may precipitate an aggressive response.

3 This response asks the client to reach out to the nurse; in the therapeutic relationship the nurse must reach out to the client.

4 Even if the client is too regressed to respond, the nurse's physical presence can be reassuring.

233. 3 Participating with one trusted individual gradually diminishes the need for withdrawal. (2) (MH; PL; TC; SD)

1 This activity fosters competition, which would not be helpful at this time.

2 This would not increase socialization but rather would promote withdrawal.

4 Same as answer 2.

234. 4 This is very helpful in decreasing hallucinations because it provides another stimulus to compete for the client's attention. (2) (MH; PL; TC; SD)

1 This would foster and support the hallucinations.

2 Same as answer 1.

3 Connections should be made to decrease the use of hallucinations.

235. 1 This would facilitate a one-to-one interaction and the development of a trusting relationship. (3) (MH; PL; TC; SD)

2 This activity would allow the client to withdraw.

3 This activity would foster competition and could increase anxiety.

4 Same as answer 2.

236. 2 The delusional system contains grandiose ideation that allows the client to feel important rather than inferior. (2) (MH; PL; PS; SD)

1 Although these individuals often feel guilty, feelings of inferiority, not guilt, precipitate delusions.

3 These individuals are usually able to express aggressive feelings without difficulty.

4 Delusions of persecution are not usually present in clients with undifferentiated schizophrenia.

237. 4 The client truly believes the voices are real because the voices reflect the client's thoughts; the voices are usually accusatory and derogatory and therefore very frightening. (2) (MH; IM; PS; SD)

1 Soft music played either before hallucinations begin or after they have started will not be strong enough to compete for the client's attention.

2 This would be too late; competing stimuli must be present to block the occurrence.

3 This is incorrect; the client cannot be talked out of a hallucination.

238. 4 This helps the client explore underlying feelings and allows the client to see the message the verbalizations are communicating. (3) (MH; IM; PS; SD)

1 This denies the client's feelings rather than accepting and working with them.

2 Attempting to divert the client denies feelings rather than accepting and working with them.

3 This focuses on the delusion itself rather than the feeling causing the delusion.

239. 1 This response accepts the client's behavior (desires) but lets the client know the nurse is not going to give up attempts to establish a relationship. (2) (MH; IM; PS; SD)

2 This response requests insight that the client does not have at this point.

3 This does not respect the client's wish for space at the present time.

4 This statement on an initial encounter does not show respect for the client's space and is inappropriately interpretive.

240. 3 Attempting to approach the client in a nonthreatening manner and using a calm, consistent, nonviolent approach often helps the agitated client to gain more self-control. (2) (MH; IM; PS; SD)

1 This action would increase, not decrease, agitation.

2 Action should not be postponed; escalation must be prevented.

4 This is premature; medication should not be used before trying to verbally calm the client down.

241. 3 Because making decisions is frequently difficult, the nurse can best help the client by limiting the number and scope of choices. (2) (MH; IM; PS; SD)

1 This is an unstructured question leaving too many choices; it would create great anxiety in the client.

2 Same as answer 1.

4 Same as answer 1.

242. 1 This response reflects the client's feelings and avoids focusing on the delusion. (2) (MH; IM; PS; SD)

2 This will not change the client's feelings because the belief is real to the client.

3 This will not change the client's feelings because the other pitcher could also be perceived as poisoned.

4 This will not change the client's feelings; the client would believe that the nurse was not really drinking the juice.

243. 1 This is all the staff can do until trust is established and the client is able to give up some of these defenses; forcing the client to attend will disrupt the group. (2) (MH; IM; PS; SD)

2 This will serve only to create a confrontation between clients.

3 This will serve little purpose and will result in a confrontation; behavior cannot be altered by arguing.

4 Same as answer 3.

244. 4 This approach gives the client and family an opportunity to discuss their feelings together and clarifies their expectations. (2) (MH; IM; PS; SD)

1 This is the nurse's responsibility and should not be passed to someone else.

2 This is not the nurse's role; the family may never be reassured.

3 This would do little to reassure the family.

245. 1 The fetal position represents regressed behavior; regression is a way of responding to overwhelming anxiety. (1) (MH; EV; PS; SD)

2 Making this interpretation assumes that the nurse controls the client's behavior; the client is not responding to the nurse any differently than to anyone else who tries to establish reality contact.

3 There are no data to substantiate this; further assessment is necessary to make this interpretation.

4 Same as answer 3.

246. 2 This allows the client to work off energy without upsetting other clients. (1) (MH; IM; PS; SD)

1 This causes isolation and should only be used as a last resort if the client presents an actual danger to himself or others.

3 The client's present emotional state would limit concentration and prevent interaction with others.

4 Same as answer 3.

247. 3 Regression is the defense mechanism commonly used by clients with schizophrenia to reduce anxiety by returning to earlier behavior. (2) (MH; AN; PS; SD)

1 This organized defense is used by clients with schizophrenia, paranoid type, in which the delusional system is well systemized.

2 This unconscious forgetting is not a major defense used by clients with schizophrenia; if it were they would not need to break with reality.

4 Rationalization, in which the individual blames others for problems and attempts to justify actions, is seldom used by clients with schizophrenia.

248. 3 This provides a stimulus that competes with and reduces hallucinations. (2) (MH; IM; PS; SD)

1 This is a direct question that the client probably could not answer; it would also increase anxiety.

2 If the nurse waits for the client to stop hallucinating, there may be no chance for contact with this client.

4 In addition to setting unrealistic standards, this response fails to recognize that the client believes the hallucinations are real.

249. 4 This statement points out reality, prevents the nurse from getting caught up in the client's illness, and recognizes feelings. (2) (MH; IM; PS; SD)

1 This is nontherapeutic; it supports and focuses on the hallucination.

2 This is an attempt to argue the client out of feelings by denying they exist.

3 Same as answer 1.

250. 3 The state in which the client feels unreal or believes that parts of the body are distorted is known as depersonalization or loss of personal identity. (1) (MH; AN; PS; SD)

1 This is not an example of an hallucination; an hallucination is a sensory experience for which there is no external stimulus.

2 The client's statement does not indicate any feelings that others are out to do harm, are responsible for what is happening, or are in control of the situation.

4 The statement is not an example of autistic verbalization.

251. 1 Clients with paranoid type schizophrenia usually become very anxious in social situations; the other client's closeness may have triggered latent homosexual feelings that are thought to play a part in these client's delusions. (2) (MH; AS; PS; SD)

2 This is an invalid interpretation given the data presented.

3 Same as answer 2.

4 Same as answer 2.

252. 3 The client's physical appearance and presentation, as well as the feelings of paranoia, are indicative of this diagnosis. (1) (MH; AN; PS; SD)

1 There is no evidence in the history to demonstrate that the client's feelings are shared by anyone else.

2 The individual with a paranoid disorder usually remains organized in the other areas of functioning; the paranoia is usually isolated to only one area.

4 The individual usually has generalized feelings of suspiciousness and awareness of imagined wrongs, but delusions and disintegration are rarely present.

253. 4 The client's statement depicts the cognitive disturbance called a delusion, which is a fixed false belief that cannot be corrected by reason. (2) (MH; AS; PS; SD)

1 An illusion is a perceptual disturbance; a misperception of an actual environmental stimulus.

2 Hallucinations are sensory experiences without external stimuli.

3 Neologisms are made-up words understood only by the maker.

254. 3 The client is fearful and suspicious; feeling in a powerful position helps the client deal with anxiety. (2) (MH; AN; PS; SD)

1 The client is not out of touch with his real identity; he has given his real identity an important role.

2 This is incorrect; the client is compensating for feelings of inadequacy.

4 Same as answer 2.

255. 1 Clients use a structured delusional system to justify and compensate for their feelings of worthlessness and low self-esteem. (2) (MH; AN; PS; SD)

2 Clients experiencing delusions of a paranoid nature are isolated and need contact with people to increase their contact with reality.

3 This is not the purpose of the delusional system.

4 There is nothing in the situation to indicate this client is not accepted by others.

256. 1 The client has low self-esteem, which forms the basis for the delusion that others do not see the client as worthy; a delusion is a fixed, false belief. (1) (MH; AN; PS; SD)

2 The client is not coining words with unusual meanings.

3 The client is not experiencing hallucinations, which are false sensory perceptions without external stimuli.

4 The client is not exhibiting ideas of reference, which are feelings that everything that is happening or is being said refers to to the client.

257. 4 This will help the client develop self-esteem and reduce the use of paranoid ideation. (2) (MH; AN; TC; SD)

1 It is impossible to remove all stress in any situation.

2 Because people must function in a social environment, it is almost impossible to avoid placing some demands on others.

3 This will only succeed in supporting the client's ideas of persecution and will lower the client's self-esteem.

258. 3 The client's verbalization reflects feelings that others are blaming the client for negative actions. (1) (MH; AN; PS; SD)

1 The data does not demonstrate feelings of greatness or power.

2 The data does not demonstrate that the client is experiencing confusing misinterpretations of stimuli.

4 The data does not demonstrate that the client is hearing voices at this time.

259. 3 The recommended approach for working with suspicious clients is to allow them to set the pace for the relationship. (3) (MH; PL; TC; SD)

1 This would be threatening and add to feelings of paranoia.

2 Same as answer 1.

4 Same as answer 1.

260. 3 This response demonstrates that the nurse understands the client's feelings; reflection opens channels of communication. (2) (MH; IM; PS; SD)

1 The client cannot be talked out of delusions by pointing out reality.

2 Focusing on delusional content only reinforces false beliefs.

4 This does not reflect the content of the client's statement.

261. 4 Clients with paranoia often feel safer selecting foods from a cafeteria-type display that is prepared for the general population rather than eating from a tray specifically prepared for them. (3) (MH; IM; PS; SD)

1 This would not provide security because part of the food could still be poisoned.

2 Same as answer 1.

3 Same as answer 1.

262. 2 This statement demonstrates recognition and acceptance of the client's feelings and also points out reality. (2) (MH; IM; PS; SD)

1 This provides false reassurance; the client has no reason to trust that the nurse can provide protection.

3 This is nontherapeutic; it denies the client's feelings and would increase anxiety.

4 Encouraging the client to focus on hallucinations tends to strengthen and confirm them.

263. 4 This response recognizes the client's feelings and points out reality. (3) (MH; IM; PS; SD)

1 This statement is inappropriate because it reinforces the client's delusional system.

2 Although this is an empathic response, it does not point out reality; the word "trick" does not have the same connotation as "out to get me."

3 This statement does not recognize the client's feelings and would place the client on the defensive.

264. 2 Suspicious individuals do not do well in groups because they are unable to tolerate the "give and take" that is necessary for successful group functioning. (3) (MH; AN; PS; SD)

1 Suspicious individuals do not trust others enough to do well in group therapy.

3 This is not always true for acutely ill psychiatric clients who may not be ready to accept reality.

4 This is not true; this is the purpose of remotivation, not a therapy group.

DELIRIUM, DEMENTIA, AND OTHER COGNITIVE DISORDERS

265. 2 Confabulation or the filling in of memory gaps with imaginary facts is a defense mechanism used by people experiencing memory deficits. (1) (MH; AS; PS; DD)

1 Concretism is demonstrated by speech where the major or salient point being made by the speaker is lost because it is buried in excessive verbal detail.

3 Flight of ideas is demonstrated by speech that jumps from one topic to another with no obvious connection for either the speaker or the listener.

4 Associative looseness is demonstrated by speech that is difficult to follow because the connections between the speaker's statements or train of thoughts are so loose they are not obvious to the listener.

266. 4 Moderate dementia is characterized by increasing dependence on environmental and social structure and by increasing psychological rigidity with accentuated previous traits and behaviors. (3) (MH; AS; PS; DD)

1 Although paranoid attitudes may be exhibited, the decrease in cognitive functioning, disorientation, and loss of memory usually do not lead to hypervigilance.

2 With the decrease in impulse control that is associated with dementia, decreased, not increased, inhibition would be present.

3 An enhancement of intelligence would not occur in dementia; initially intellectual deterioration is subtle.

267. 2 Routines and familiarity with activities or the environment provide for a sense of security. (2) (MH; PL; TC; DD)

1 Change is poorly tolerated; frustration and the inability to accomplish tasks lead to lowered self-esteem.

3 Challenging activities can be frustrating and can lead to hostility or withdrawal.

4 Decreased physical capacity and attention span limit active participation; frustration can result.

268. 3 Clients with dementia have the greatest loss in the area of recent memory. (2) (MH; PL; PA; DD)

1 Memory of remote events usually remains fairly intact.

2 Same as answer 1.

4 Same as answer 1.

269. 2 When the client is unable to perform a task, frustration occurs and results in more disorganized behavior. (3) (MH; PL; TC; DD)

1 The client's disorientation is documented and will not change although some day-to-day variations may occur; most important is the assessment of the client's ability to function.

3 There is no documentation of disruptive behavior; frustration must be avoided.

4 The client will probably never adjust any further.

270. 2 This client needs toileting every 2 hours to prevent soiling; physically seating the client on the toilet often prevents accidents and negates the use of diapers. (3) (MH; IM; TC; DD)
  1 The client needs to be physically placed on the toilet; confusion limits effectiveness of other actions.
  3 Same as answer 1.
  4 Same as answer 1.

271. 1 "Where are you?" is the best question to elicit information about the client's orientation to place because it encourages a response that can be assessed. (3) (MH; AS; PS; DD)
  2 This question focuses on recent memory; it does not assess orientation to place.
  3 This question would probably be answered by a yes or a no; this could not objectively determine the client's orientation.
  4 This question focuses on orientation to time, not place.

272. 2 Confabulation is used as a defense mechanism against embarrassment caused by lapse of memory; the client fills in the blanks in memory by making up details. (2) (MH; AN; PS; DD)
  1 Regression is a defense mechanism in which the individual moves back to earlier developmental defenses.
  3 Although the elderly fear being forgotten or losing others' affection, this is not the main reason for confabulation.
  4 Confabulation is not used to reminisce about past achievement.

273. 4 This action maintains, for as long as possible, the client's remaining intellectual functions by providing an opportunity to use them. (3) (MH; PL; PS; DD)
  1 All clients need adequate nutrition; this is not a particular priority of care for these clients.
  2 The main priority should be directed toward maintaining intellectual functioning; remotivation is not always possible with extensive organic damage.
  3 There are no data to indicate the client needs custodial care at this time.

274. 2 This client would require a structured environment, regardless of the cause of the behavior; this would help provide a safe environment. (2) (MH; PL; PS; DD)
  1 This is important, but is secondary to promotion of an environment conducive to safety and security.
  3 Same as answer 1.
  4 A battery of screening tests will probably be used in an attempt to determine the etiology of the dementia; however, provision for safety is necessary first.

275. 2 This allows the client to exercise the right to decide which articles to keep and provides for safety and cleanliness. (2) (MH; PL; TC; DD)
  1 This deceives the client, limits judgment, and creates mistrust toward the staff.
  3 Explanations alone will not provide for safety or meet this client's needs because of a decreased attention span and memory.
  4 This does not help because all of the objects the client is hoarding are not harmful.

276. 4 Cell damage seems to interfere with registering input stimuli which affects the ability to register and recall recent events; vascular dementia is related to multiple vascular lesions of the cerebral cortex and subcortical structures. (3) (MH; AN; PA; DD)
  1 The remote memory is usually not impaired to any great degree.
  2 The loss of abstract thinking is related to cell damage, not the emotional state.
  3 The inability to concentrate is related to cell damage, not decreased stimuli.

277. 2 The client needs constant reassurance because forgetfulness blocks previous explanations; frequent presence of staff serves as a continual reminder. (2) (MH; PL; TC; DD)
  1 The client needs continual reassurance and would not remember times for planned interactions or activities.
  3 This client would be unable to explain the reasons for concern.
  4 This client will not remember the explanation from one moment to the next.

278. 2   These clients require external controls to minimize danger of injury and to preserve human dignity. (2) (MH; PL; TC; DD)

    1   The client will not have excessive energy.

    3   The staff cannot prevent all gross motor activity; the client needs to use muscles or atrophy will occur.

    4   Further deterioration usually cannot be prevented in this disorder.

279. 2   This encourages verbalization, gives the client a feeling of security, and decreases the sense of isolation. (1) (MH; IM; PS; DD)

    1   This action discourages verbalization between the client and nurse; the client may be unable to function in a small group because of increased anxiety.

    3   This discourages verbalization of feelings and will lead to feelings of being unwanted.

    4   Same as answer 1.

280. 2   This assists the client in decision making; new situations may be stressful and lead to ambivalent feelings. (2) (MH; IM; PS; DD)

    1   This would make the client feel guilty and add to anxiety.

    3   This is not sharing decision making; hurrying the client will lead to feelings of frustration and resentment.

    4   The client may perceive this action as punishment.

DRUG-RELATED RESPONSES

281. 4   Psychoactive drugs have been shown to be capable of interrupting the acute psychiatric process, making the client more amenable to other therapies. (1) (MH; AN; PA; DR)

    1   This is untrue; ECT is more effective in treating depressed clients.

    2   Family therapy is effective but is a long-term, costly therapy; symptoms must be reduced before the client can participate.

    3   Clients with schizophrenia usually have little insight into their problems; confronting the client through insight therapy will increase anxiety.

282. 1   The user has an emotional and physiologic dependence on the drug, and the phenomenon of tolerance (more drug needed to achieve the same effect) occurs. (2) (MH; AN; PA; DR)

    2   Tolerance, even to levels that would be lethal in the nonaddicted individual, occurs.

    3   There is an emotional dependence.

    4   There is a physiologic dependence.

283. 2   A hypotensive reaction is a common adverse effect of chlorpromazine. (2) (MH; AS; PA; DR)

    1   Restraints of any type may increase the client's anxiety and result in struggling and increased agitation.

    3   Photosensitivity occurs most frequently when clients are taking large doses and are spending time outdoors in the sun.

    4   Tardive dyskinesia and akathisia usually result from prolonged large doses of phenothiazines in susceptible clients.

284. 4   Chlorpromazine suppresses central sympathetic activity, which reduces the discomfort of withdrawal and the risk of seizures. (3) (MH; AN; PA; DR)

    1   This drug helps to reduce the risk of convulsions but does not prevent physical injury during a convulsion.

    2   Although these benefits may occur, they are not the primary objectives for using the drug.

    3   The ability of the client to accept treatment depends on readiness to accept the reality of the problem.

285. 4   The lithium concentration is most stable at this time; absorption and excretion occur 8 to 12 hours after the last dose. (2) (MH; AN; TC; DR)

    1   Absorption and excretion rates vary; concentrations may be falsely higher at this time affecting the reliability of readings.

    2   Same as answer 1.

    3   Same as answer 1.

286. 2 Benztropine mesylate (Cogentin), an anticholinergic, helps balance neurotransmitter activity in the CNS and helps control extrapyramidal tract symptoms. (2) (MH; AN; TC; DR)
1 Hydroxyzine (Atarax) is a sedative that depresses activity in the subcortical areas in the CNS; it is used to reduce anxiety.
3 Sodium amobarbital (Sodium Amytal), a barbiturate, interferes with transmission of impulses to the cerebral cortex; it is used for the treatment of insomnia.
4 Acetaminophen chlorzoxazone (Parafon Forte), a skeletal muscle relaxant, depresses nerve transmission through polysynaptic pathways; it is used for the treatment of muscle spasms.

287. 2 Haloperidol (Haldol) reduces emotional tensions, excessive psychomotor activity, panic, and fear. (2) (MH; AN; PA; DR)
1 Clients exhibiting manic behaviors do not respond well to Haldol, and it can exacerbate their underlying feelings of depression.
3 Clients exhibiting excited-depressed behavior do not respond well to Haldol because it tends to increase the depression.
4 Haldol appears to have few stimulating effects and, in fact, increases feelings of lassitude and fatigue.

288. 4 Lithium's therapeutic window is very narrow and toxic levels could occur without routine monitoring of the blood's drug level. (2) (MH; PL; TC; DR)
1 A low sodium diet can lead to hyponatremia, which must be avoided because it limits the excretion of lithium and can result in toxicity.
2 Diuretics reduce serum sodium levels and lithium is not excreted when sodium levels are decreased; the retention of lithium can result in toxic levels.
3 This may or may not be true.

289. 2 The drug physostigmine (Antilirium) is essential to manage an overdose of a tricyclic antidepressant; it increases acetylcholine at cholinergic nerve terminals and reverses central and peripherial anticholinergic effects. (3) (MH; PL; PA; DR)
1 Dialysis or forced diuresis is an ineffective treatment for an overdose of a tricyclic antidepressant; immediate administration of physostigmine to counteract the effects of the tricyclic antidepressant is necessary.
3 Acetylcholine is already depressed from the tricyclic antidepressant; anticholinergics are most effective in managing the side effects of antipsychotic/neuroleptic drugs.
4 Prevention of suicidal behavior is always advantageous; however, in this case, immediate emergency intervention is necessary.

290. 3 Extreme photosensitivity is a common side effect of Prolixin. (3) (MH; PL; ED; DR)
1 Once the client's medication is adjusted and CNS response is noted, driving may be permitted; drowsiness usually subsides after the first few weeks.
2 This is untrue; energy is usually decreased.
4 Although this drug can cause hypotension, it does not consistently lower blood pressure; a sudden drop can be dangerous to a client with hypertension.

291. 1 This drug is a narcotic antagonist that displaces narcotics from receptors in the brain, reversing respiratory depression. (2) (MH; PL; PA; DR)
2 This is a synthetic opiate that causes CNS depression; it would add to the problem of overdose.
3 This drug would have no effect on respiratory depression related to the presence of an overdose of a narcotic.
4 Same as answer 3.

292. 3 Monoamine oxidase uptake is inhibited by the medication, increasing concentrations of endogenous epinephrine, norepinephrine, serotonin, and dopamine in CNS storage sites; high levels of these transmitters in the presence of tyramine can cause hypertensive crisis. (2) (MH; PL; ED; DR)

1 This may be an adverse reaction to the drug but is not related to drug-food interaction.

2 Same as answer 1.

4 This is not related to drug-food interaction.

293. 1 These products often contain an alcohol base and can cause a severe reaction in the presence of Antabuse. (2) (MH; IM; ED; DR)

2 These do not contain alcohol and need not be avoided.

3 Only wine vinegar should be avoided.

4 Same as answer 2.

294. 4 Blood levels must be checked monthly or bimonthly when the client is on maintenance therapy because there is only a small range between therapeutic and toxic levels. (1) (MH; IM; ED; DR)

1 The client receiving lithium is encouraged to maintain a normal diet.

2 There is no need to take lithium with milk because it does not normally cause gastrointestinal problems.

3 Lithium does not cause changes in the blood cells.

295. 3 Phenothiazine potentiates the action of alcohol and can cause death if the drug and alcohol are taken together. (1) (MH; IM; ED; DR)

1 This medication should be taken consistently to prevent recurrence of symptoms and maintain blood drug levels.

2 Same as answer 2.

4 Medication should be taken as ordered; taking it all at one time can interrupt the maintenance of a constant therapeutic blood level.

296. 3 This is too short a period of time; clients usually begin to feel a lightening of depression in approximately 14 to 20 days, with the full antidepressant effects being felt between 3 and 4 weeks. (1) (MH; EV; ED; DR)

1 Drowsiness usually occurs early in treatment but passes with time.

2 It usually takes this long before the full effects of the antidepressant are experienced.

4 Clients usually remain on these medications for a few months.

297. 4 The Parkinsonian symptoms are related to extrapyramidal tract effects and agranulocytosis is related to bone marrow depression. (2) (MH; EV; TC; DR)

1 Jaundice is an adverse reaction; vomiting is not.

2 Tardive dyskinesia is an adverse reaction; nausea is not.

3 Postural hypotension is an adverse reaction; hiccups are not.

298. 2 Tardive dyskinesia, an extrapyramidal response characterized by vermicular movements and protrusion of the tongue, chewing and puckering movements of the mouth, and a puffing of the cheeks, is often irreversible even when the antipsychotic medication is withdrawn. (1) (MH; EV; TC; DR)

1 This can usually be treated with antiparkinsonian or anticholinergic drugs while the antipsychotic medication is continued.

3 Same as answer 1.

4 Same as answer 1.

299. 2   Diarrhea is an early sign of lithium toxicity and the resulting loss of sodium tends to increase the lithium level even further. (2) (MH; EV; TC; DR)

1   Tinnitus can occur early in treatment, but, unless other progressive neurological symptoms develop, it is not considered a symptom of toxicity.

3   Akathisia is a symptom associated with the side effects of the antipsychotic drugs.

4   Torticollis is a symptom associated with the side effects of antipsychotic drugs.

300. 1   Hypotension is a major side effect of Valium that occurs early in therapy. (2) (MH; EV; PA; DR)

2   An alteration in urinary output is not a common side effect, but it may occur after prolonged use.

3   This is not a common side effect, but distention from constipation may occur after prolonged use.

4   CNS depression is not a common side effect, but it may occur after prolonged use.

301. 4   Anticonvulsants and Haldol exert a synergistic CNS depressant effect. (2) (MH; EV; TC; DR)

1   This is untrue; the effect is potentiated.

2   Anticonvulsants do not affect absorption or metabolism of Haldol.

3   Same as answer 2.

302. 2   This drug creates a general sense of well-being, increases appetite, and helps lift depression. (2) (MH; EV; ED; DR)

1   The client might not know the reason for the depression, and the drug does not cause amnesia.

3   Symptomatic relief usually begins after 2 to 4 weeks of therapy.

4   Concomitant use of monoamine oxidase inhibitors and tricyclic antidepressants is usually contraindicated.

303. 1   Medication should be discontinued immediately if these symptoms of lithium toxicity occur. (1) (MH; EV; TC; DR)

2   These are symptoms of toxicity, and a stimulant will not alter them; the medication must be stopped

3   There is no special diet required; these are symptoms of toxicity and the medication must be stopped.

4   The client maintains a normal salt and fluid intake; these are symptoms of toxicity and the medication must be stopped.

304. 2   As with other tricyclics, optimal therapeutic effects take 2 to 3 weeks to occur. (2) (MH; EV; PA; DR)

1   This is untrue; the maximum therapeutic effect of tricyclics takes up to 3 weeks to occur.

3   Same as answer 1.

4   Same as answer 1.

305. 4   A hypertensive crisis would not be associated with extrapyramidal tract symptoms. (2) (MH; EV; TC; DR)

1   Akathisia, characterized by restlessness and twitching or crawling sensations in muscles, is an extrapyramidal side effect.

2   Opisthotonos, characterized by hyperextension and arching of the back, is an extrapyramidal side effect.

3   Oculogyric crisis, characterized by the uncontrolled upward movement of the eyes, is an extrapyramidal side effect.

306. 1   The medication should be stopped immediately because the jaundice indicates possible liver damage which would prolong elimination of the drug and may result in toxic accumulation. (1) (MH; EV; TC; DR)

2   Milk does not change the effect of the drug.

3   The drug must be stopped, not reduced.

4   The drug is only available in an oral form; in addition, the route of administration would not influence the occurrence of toxic accumulation.

307. 3   Infection can indicate agranulocytosis, a serious side effect that can occur with therapy and can cause death. (3) (MH; EV; PA; DR)

1   This would be unsafe because the client may be developing agranulocytosis, a potentially life-threatening side effect that needs immediate treatment.

2 Same as answer 1.
4 Same as answer 1.

308. 2 For clients with bipolar disorders, it has been shown that long-term lithium therapy flattens the highs of the euphoric phase and the lows of the depressed phase. (1) (MH; EV; ED; DR)
1 This is untrue; the physician should be notified before medication is stopped.
3 This is untrue; clients should never adjust their own dosage of medication.
4 This is not true; the therapeutic level and the toxic level are very close, and serious side effects do occur.

309. 2 These are common side effects of lithium. (2) (MH; EV; ED; DR)
1 This is a side effect of the phenothiazine group of medications.
3 Neither problem is associated with lithium intake.
4 Lithium can cause polyuria and incontinence, not retention.

310. 2 Foods such as chocolate, aged cheese, pickled herring, and those containing excessive caffeine contain high levels of tyramine and cause dangerous hypertension in clients taking MAO inhibitors. (2) (MH; EV; ED; DR)
1 There is no need to limit intake of this food while taking MAO inhibitors.
3 Same as answer 1.
4 Same as answer 1.

311. 4 This acute dystonic reaction is a severe side effect of Haldol and requires intramuscular or intravenous administration of antiparkinsonian medication. (2) (MH; EV; TC; DR)
1 The medication would not be increased but discontinued, and antiparkinsonian medication would be administered.
2 At this point symptoms are so severe that this medication must be discontinued.
3 These symptoms are more severe than pseudoparkinsonism and require more than an adjustment in this medication.

THERAPEUTIC RELATIONSHIPS

312. 3 The answer to this question will provide the nurse with an idea of the client's hopes and frustrations without being threatening or probing. (3) (MH; AS; PS; TR)
1 This question is probing, disregards the client's statement, and provides little information for the nurse to use in planning care.
2 Same as answer 1.
4 Same as answer 1.

313. 2 Before deciding how to decrease the client's fears of addiction, the nurse must explore the full extent of the client's knowledge and feelings about taking the drug. (1) (MH; AS; PS; TR)
1 Information may or may not be helpful; the client's feelings are what must be addressed.
3 It is too early; exploration to find the basis of the fear is necessary first.
4 Same as answer 3.

314. 3 All behavior has meaning; the nurse must try to understand what the behavior means to the client. (3) (MH; AS; TC; TR)
1 The isolation of a client may increase anxiety and precipitate more acting-out behavior.
2 Ignoring behavior does little to alter it and it may even cause further acting out.
4 The nurse cannot explain the meaning of the client's behavior, only the client can.

315. 1 The client has the right to expect that all records of care will remain confidential; permission must be sought for use. (1) (MH; AN; TC; TR)
2 This right was not violated; this applies to the concept of holding clients against their will.
3 This right was not violated; this applies to the humane aspect of care.
4 This right was not violated; this applies to procedures and treatments to be performed on the client.

316. 3 This is a technique that avoids misunderstanding so that both the client and the nurse can work toward a common goal in the therapeutic relationship. (2) (MH; AN; PS; TR)
1 This would not provide for clarification or understanding.
2 Same as answer 1.
4 Same as answer 1.

317. 2 Evaluation includes assessing the client's response to care, judging the effectiveness of the nursing care plan, and changing the plan as necessary. (1) (MH; EV; PS; TR)
1 Planning includes the development of a plan that focuses on specific goals and actions unique to the client's needs.
3 Assessing entails collecting and reviewing objective and subjective data about the client's health status.
4 Implementation includes performing specific actions designed to achieve the stated goals.

318. 2 The psychoanalytic model studies the unconscious and uses the strategies of hypnosis, dream interpretation, and free association as a means of releasing repressed feelings. (1) (MH; AN; PS; TR)
1 The behaviorist model subscribes to the belief that the self and mental symptoms are viewed as learned behaviors that persist because they are consciously rewarding to the individual; this model deals with behaviors on a conscious level of awareness.
3 The psychobiologic model views emotional and behavioral disturbances as stemming from a physical disease; abnormal behavior is directly attributed to a disease process; this model deals with behaviors on a conscious level of awareness.
4 The social-interpersonal model affirms that crucial social processes are involved in the development and resolution of disturbed behavior; this model deals with behavior on a conscious level of awareness.

319. 2 During the working stage goals are met, problems are resolved, and changes in behavior occur. (1) (MH; AN; TC; TR)
1 During the initial stage trust is the primary focus, goals and contracts are set, and problems are identified.
3 There is no such stage in the nurse-client relationship; this is a step in the nursing process.
4 The evaluation/termination stage focuses on accomplishments, reinforces new behaviors, and closes the relationship.

320. 4 The preinteraction phase is the period before the nurse begins the interaction; it is the preparatory phase of a planned therapeutic relationship. (2) (MH; AN; TC; TR)
1 The working phase is the period in a relationship when the individuals are occupied with achieving goals and sharing facts and feelings.
2 The orientation phase is the initial period of the actual interaction; it is the introductory or exploratory phase.
3 The termination phase is the period in a relationship when the individuals are beginning to separate and move toward independent paths.

321. 2 This is a correct description of the working phase of a relationship; trust has been established and a relationship has been developed based on mutual respect. (2) (MH; AN; TC; TR)
1 This behavior would occur during the orientation phase before trust is established.
3 Same as answer 1.
4 Same as answer 1.

322. 2 The client's inability to recall is an example of repression, which is the unconscious and involuntary forgetting of painful events, ideas, and conflicts. (2) (MH; AN; PS; TR)
1 There is nothing to demonstrate that denial, an unconscious refusal to admit an unacceptable behavior or idea, has occurred.

3 There is nothing to demonstrate that regression, a return to an earlier, more comfortable developmental level, has occurred.

4 There is nothing to demonstrate that dissociation, the separation and detachment of emotional affect and significance from a particular idea, situation, or incident, has occurred.

323. 3 Realistic limits and controls provide a degree of security that adds to emotional safety by limiting choices, reducing the need for self-regulation, and decreasing decision making. (2) (MH; AN; PS; TR)

1 Passive acceptance is not conducive to psychologic safety and often signifies a degree of resignation.

2 It is impossible to meet all of a client's needs in any situation.

4 An orderly physical environment has little relationship to psychologic safety.

324. 3 This goal is related to the nursing diagnosis and is appropriate and measurable. (1) (MH; AN; PS; TR)

1 This is not related to the nursing diagnosis; this is true for everyone but the priority for this client is to facilitate interaction with others.

2 This is not related to the nursing diagnosis; acting-out behavior is not inherent in the situation.

4 This is not related to the nursing diagnosis and is not appropriate.

325. 1 Without an awareness of personal beliefs the nurse may unconsciously stop listening if the client expresses deviant beliefs. (1) (MH; AN; PS; TR)

2 Although this may create some anxiety, it usually does not interfere with accurate listening.

3 Same as answer 2.

4 Same as answer 2.

326. 4 This ethically sound response clearly defines who is involved in decision making and allows for parental expression of ideas and thoughts. (2) (MH; AN; PS; TR)

1 Discussion of the implication of a DNR order should not take place until after the family has spoken with the physician.

2 Although the answer promotes the physician-client relationship, it stops the nurse-client interaction.

3 This answer could be interpreted as negative; it also abdicates nursing responsibility.

327. 4 If nurses are unaware of their biases about rape, they will be unprepared to evaluate objectively and meet the client's needs. (1) (MH; AN; PS; TR)

1 This would interrupt communication; information can be solicited later.

2 The nurse should be able to deal with this client without assistance.

3 It is not necessary to know these to effectively respond to the client in a therapeutic manner.

328. 1 Value clarification is a technique that uncovers individuals' values so that the individuals can be more aware of them and their effect on others. (2) (MH; AN; TC; TR)

2 This is untrue; it merely helps individuals become aware of values and their effect on others.

3 Same as answer 2.

4 Same as answer 2.

329. 2 The ability to discuss feelings about others and life situations is necessary for positive mental health. (2) (MH; AN; TC; TR)

1 This is a long-term, not a short-term, goal.

3 Same as answer 1.

4 Same as answer 1.

330. 3 Past experiences are important and must be recognized because they set the parameters for the individual's values throughout life. (1) (MH; AN; TC; TR)

1 This is untrue; past experiences would not affect inherited traits.

2 This is untrue; past experiences play an important role in an individual's life.

4 Nothing establishes how an individual responds forever; new experiences continue to influence future responses.

331. 3 This is true; the client's goal is meaningful, and the nurse should do everything possible to help the client achieve it. (2) (MH; AN; PS; TR)

1 No evidence demonstrates the client is using denial.

2 There is no reason to attempt to move the client away from this meaningful goal.

4 If the client wants to work toward a goal, the energy expenditure is justified.

332. 3 An individual must feel a sense of control over self and the environment to feel secure, reduce anxiety, and function at an optimal level. (3) (MH; AN; PS; TR)

1 This is untrue; most emotionally ill people are too introspective to empathize with others.

2 No one functions optimally in all settings; the healthy individual can accept and handle temporary periods of confusion and loss of control.

4 This is not true; many individuals with mental illness do not demonstrate observable signs or socially inappropriate behavior.

333. 3 The greatest fear of an inexperienced nurse is of saying the wrong thing and doing harm to a client; it is important to recognize that it can actually become a therapeutic encounter whereby both the client and the nurse can learn from the situation. (3) (MH; AN; TC; TR)

1 Although this client presents a low risk of having the emotional or physical energy to hurt a caregiver, fear of injury is not as high as fear of saying the wrong thing.

2 Being rejected can occur with any client; fear of rejection usually is not an overwhelming concern of nurses.

4 This usually is not an overwhelming concern of nurses.

334. 4 Early notification provides an opportunity to prepare for change. (3) (MH; PL; TC; TR)

1 This may be a secondary gain but not the primary purpose.

2 Same as answer 1.

3 Same as answer 1.

335. 2 The client cannot be expected to accept or even respond to a plan that would be incompatible with the family's life style. (1) (MH; PL; TC; TR)

1 The family should not have to adjust to the nurse's biases; the nurse must deal with biases before they interfere with care.

3 All individuals respond differently to situations.

4 There is no documentation that misconceptions are present.

336. 3 Clients usually respond with better motivation for self-care if they feel someone is depending on them and they are needed. (2) (MH; PL; PS; TR)

1 Clients need to feel needed, not just to establish new social contacts.

2 This is untrue; emotionally healthy individuals do not feel better simply because others have more problems.

4 Same as answer 1.

337. 2 When planning a group the nurse must ensure that clients have similar needs to foster relationships and interactions; diverse needs do not foster group process. (2) (MH; PL; TC; TR)

1 Although important, this is not a primary consideration.

3 Behavior and needs, rather than diagnosis, are of primary importance.

4 This has little effect on group process.

338. 2 Members must feel comfortable to discuss things in the group; there must be an awareness that what is discussed in the group will remain in the group. (2) (MH; PL; PS; TR)

1 This will not establish trust and will increase anxiety because the members will feel their turn for exposure will come whether they want it or not.

3 Same as answer 1.

4 Talking about trust does little to foster it.

339. 1 To achieve the greatest therapeutic value from a group session, the members must be involved in deciding what will be discussed. (3) (MH; PL; PS; TR)

2 By this response the nurse leader abdicates the leadership role and places the entire responsibility for the success of the group on its members.

3 This response presents an extremely structured view of the purpose of a therapy group; the members must be involved in the selection of the topics to be discussed.

4 Same as answer 3.

340. 4 This action by the leader would be most therapeutic because it sets both the parameters of discussion and limits on behavior. (2) (MH; PL; PS; TR)

1 This would not be therapeutic for a group of clients with the diagnosis of schizophrenia; because of the disruption of cognitive processes these clients would be unable to make this contribution.

2 Same as answer 1.

3 Same as answer 1.

341. 2 The nurse must accept the client's statement and beliefs as real to the client to develop trust and move into a therapeutic relationship. (2) (MH; PL; PS; TR)

1 Clients cannot be argued out of any delusions.

3 These feelings and thoughts are constant; this would result in an overdose.

4 Redirecting the client's conversation whenever negative topics are brought up adds to the client's feelings that negative thoughts are correct.

342. 1 The client has been able to function well up to this time, and the client's usual behavior and routines should be supported. (2) (MH; PL; TC; TR)

2 At this time the data presented do not identify this as a need.

3 Same as answer 2.

4 Same as answer 2.

343. 2 Family therapy tries to view the whole (Gestalt) within the context in which the emotional problems are occurring. (3) (MH; PL; TC; TR)

1 Time efficiency is not an adequate rationale for choosing a therapeutic approach.

3 This may or may not be true; an astute nurse can control manipulation and alliance in any situation.

4 Promotion of truthfulness is a secondary gain achieved through this mode.

344. 3 This is the client's desire, and the nurse should do everything possible to assist the client to achieve it. (2) (MH; PL; PS; TR)

1 The client should be encouraged, not discouraged; mental activity should not be too taxing and it is not unrealistic if the client wishes to do it.

2 This would not be therapeutic; the client has an unmet need, and the nurse should not try to refocus the client away from the objective.

4 No data support the conclusion that the client needs to work through anger.

345. 4 If religion is a family concern, then the nurse should allow discussion of the family's thoughts and feelings on the subject. (2) (MH; PL; PS; TR)

1 If religion is a family concern, its discussion should be encouraged, not limited.

2 The minister is not part of the family unit; the minister would be invited only if requested by the family.

3 The role of the nurse is to facilitate and listen, not to have a mutual discussion.

346. 1 In behavior modification, positive behavior is reinforced and negative behavior is punished or not reinforced. (2) (MH; PL; TC; TR)

2 This may be a part of the program, but it is not a major component.

3 Same as answer 2.

4 Same as answer 2.

347. 1 Before therapy can begin, a trusting relationship must develop. (2) (MH; PL; TC; TR)

2 A client with major depression would not have the impetus or energy to investigate new leisure activities.

3 This is not appropriate initially; a trusting one-to-one relationship must be developed first.

4 This would not be successful unless the client had developed a trusting, comfortable relationship with the nurse.

348. 4 The client and the family should be included in discussion so that concerns can be addressed openly; this increases trust and fosters relationships. (2) (MH; PL; TC; TR)

1 This may be helpful, but the client should be made aware of the family's present feelings and concerns.

2 This provides false reassurance; the client has had periods where the behavior was acceptable, only to once again become disturbed.

3 This may be useful for the family later, but it would not help the immediate problem.

349. 4 Evaluation and termination are the foci of a discharge planning conference; it is important for the nurse to assist the family in viewing the hospitalization as a learning experience. (3) (MH; PL; PS; TR)

1 This should have been discussed prior to the discharge conference, where evaluation and future planning are the foci.

2 Same as answer 1.

3 Same as answer 1.

350. 1 The use of self is often the only tool available to the nurse to help a client cope; the nurse must be present, actively listening, and attentive to be therapeutic. (1) (MH; IM; TC; TR)

2 The environment is important, but it is not the most basic tool.

3 The client's intellect is not necessarily a therapeutic tool used by the nurse.

4 The nurse must first use self before the helping process can begin.

351. 1 Empathy is the projection of self into another's emotions to share the emotions and the other's state of mind; this technique helps the nurse understand the meaning and significance of the experience to the client. (1) (MH; IM; TC; TR)

2 Sympathy is a shared expression of sorrow over a real or imagined loss.

3 Projection is an unconscious defense, not a therapeutic technique.

4 This approach does not require the nurse to project the self into the client's emotions, but rather just to accept the client and the emotions.

352. 3 Focusing is indicated when communication is vague; the nurse attempts to concentrate or focus the client's communication on one specific aspect. (2) (MH; IM; TC; TR)

1 Touch would invade the client's space and would do nothing to help focus the client's communication.

2 Silence would only prolong the rambling communication; client needs to be focused.

4 Until the concern is identified and explored, summarizing would be impossible.

353. 1 This demonstrates that the staff believes that what the client has to say is important; this also encourages verbalization. (2) (MH; IM; TC; TR)

2 This would only increase feelings of worthlessness and persecution and would cut off communication.

3 This would accomplish little if anything; individuals cannot be talked out of feelings.

4 Feelings cannot always be explained; this also forces the client to further develop the delusional system.

354. 2 Silence is a tool employed during therapeutic communication that indicates the nurse is listening and receptive; it allows the client time to collect thoughts, gain control of emotions, or speak without hurrying. (2) (MH; IM; TC; TR)

1 Silence should be comfortable and should not create a feeling of pressure to break it by talking.

3 The nurse's facial expression should be projected outward, not inward.

4 This is incorrect; this would close communication.

355. 4 This verifies family and physician agreement and uses institutional policy developed by the ethics committee. (2) (MH; IM; PA; TR)
  1 The nurse should not accept this inappropriate burden.
  2 Same as answer 1.
  3 The order must be part of the written record.

356. 4 This lets the client know the nurse is trying to understand; it increases the client's feeling of self-esteem and points out reality. (3) (MH; IM; PS; TR)
  1 Clients with schizophrenia have problems with associative links, and these same problems will occur regardless of the topic.
  2 This statement cuts off communication and tells the client that the nurse will only speak if the client's communication makes sense.
  3 Same as answer 2.

357. 4 Depersonalization is the result of high anxiety levels; projecting empathy to the client will facilitate exploration of concerns. (2) (MH; IM; TC; TR)
  1 This response points out reality to the client from the nurse's perception, but does not acknowledge the frightening experience for the client.
  2 This is irrelevant; the nurse must deal with what the client is experiencing now.
  3 This response belittles the client's feelings and will make establishment of a therapeutic relationship difficult.

358. 1 This is the best response that reflects back the feelings being expressed at this time. (2) (MH; IM; PS; TR)
  2 This does not address the real concern; the mother's argument may have been justified and the daughter's behavior should not be rewarded.
  3 This avoids the issue; the fear may be that next time control may be lost and abuse may occur.
  4 False reassurance avoids the real issue.

359. 1 Recognizing the family's feelings and giving simple factual information helps to allay anxiety. (2) (MH; IM; ED; TR)
  2 This discourages further verbalization of concerns and promotes feelings of isolation and helplessness.
  3 This is an inappropriate statement, especially during this time of stress; it also gives little assurance to the family.
  4 This is false reassurance and does not allow the family to verbalize their anxieties or fears.

360. 1 Unless staff can share both positive and negative feelings, resentment, anger, and frustration will develop. (3) (MH; IM; ED; TR)
  2 This response does little to foster communication and relationships among staff members.
  3 This response attacks the speaker and cuts off communication in the group.
  4 Same as answer 3.

361. 4 Establishment of a therapeutic relationship begins with introductions. (2) (MH; IM; PS; TR)
  1 This provides no information except the speaker's name.
  2 This does not provide the client with any information about who the speaker is; use of the client's first name demonstrates lack of respect.
  3 In addition to not providing any information and using the client's first name, this greeting is probing and would place the client on the defensive.

362. 3 This response addresses the reality that the client is on the mental health unit and offers assistance. (2) (MH; IM; PS; TR)
  1 On the basis of the information available, it would be too early to make this decision.
  2 This is a rather hostile response that assumes the client is unable to follow conversation.
  4 This response assumes the client is disoriented as to place; it sounds like the beginning of a lecture.

363. 4 This response addresses the client's misconceptions about mental health services and specific fear of being crazy. (2) (MH; IM; PS; TR)
   1 This response ignores the feeling tones behind the client's statement and focuses on facts.
   2 Same as answer 1.
   3 Same as answer 1.

364. 4 This response is optimistic and supportive and clarifies the purpose of the relationship. (2) (MH; IM; PS; TR)
   1 This statement diminishes the client's response and sets up a challenge; it does not foster a therapeutic relationship.
   2 Same as answer 1.
   3 Same as answer 1.

365. 2 Unless the nurse answers the question, the client will continue to focus on the nurse rather than on the self; the nurse can best redirect after a brief answer. (2) (MH; IM; TC; TR)
   1 This moves the focus to the nurse's opinions rather than the client's feelings.
   3 Same as answer 1.
   4 This is not therapeutic; the client is being asked to share, and the nurse should also be willing.

366. 1 This response recognizes problems of the caregiver without a hint of blame for admission; it opens the channel of communication. (2) (MH; IM; TC; TR)
   2 This is a somewhat hostile response that would place the caregiver on the defensive.
   3 Same as answer 2.
   4 Same as answer 2.

367. 1 This response identifies the child's feelings and lets the child know the nurse can understand them. (3) (MH; IM; TC; TR)
   2 This denies the child's feelings and really does not offer support.
   3 This is an unrealistic response; the child would probably be unable to express his feelings to peers.
   4 This is an unrealistic response; the nurse cannot be sure that weight loss will improve the child's ability in gym.

368. 4 This response does not attack the client for behavior but places responsibility for allowing behavior to continue on the group; the client will recognize the message without feeling increased anxiety. (3) (MH; IM; TC; TR)
   1 This is not a confronting approach but an attack.
   2 This is not therapeutic; it allows behavior to continue without limits being set.
   3 This would increase anxiety by placing demands on other members; it does not deal with the identified problem.

369. 3 This response focuses the client on the behavior and what the client is trying to achieve by such behavior; it also helps the client to see how such behavior affects others. (3) (MH; IM; TC; TR)
   1 The group would not know what the client was trying to tell the nurse; only the client would know and should be asked directly.
   2 This response uses a nondirect approach to attack the client.
   4 This is an attacking, defensive response made without really knowing what the client was attempting to accomplish.

370. 2 The leader should not intervene at this point; the client addressed the statement to the group, and the group response should be fostered. (2) (MH; IM; TC; TR)
   1 This response would be viewed as an attack and would make other members fearful of contributing because they may be attacked.
   3 This denies the client's response.
   4 Same as answer 1.

371. 3 This is an open-ended, nonjudgmental response that points out incongruity between the client's verbal and nonverbal communication. (2) (MH; IM; PS; TR)
   1 This would not help the client recognize the incongruity.
   2 Same as answer 1.
   4 Same as answer 1.

372. 2 This response uses paraphrasing to restate the content of the client's statement; it encourages further communication. (1) (MH; IM; PS; TR)

  1 Feelings are personal and can really not be understood by others; this is an ineffective attempt to empathize and refocuses the attention on the nurse.

  3 This response negates the client's feelings and changes the subject; the client needs to talk and this response cuts off communication.

  4 This response negates the client's feelings, makes the feelings impossible to share, may make the client feel guilty for the feelings, and tells the client how to behave and feel.

373. 4 Helping the client to understand the meaning of the family member's behavior reduces the family member's emotional control over the client. (2) (MH; IM; PS; TR)

  1 This ignores the necessity of clarifying the family member's behavior.

  2 Distraction is not a therapeutic way to deal with realistic feelings.

  3 This is only a temporary measure and does not reduce the emotional conflict with the family member.

374. 3 These client behaviors indicate increased trust and comfort in the nurse-client relationship. (1) (MH; EV; TC; TR)

  1 This tells nothing about the client's behavior in the therapeutic nurse-client relationship.

  2 Same as answer 1.

  4 In a therapeutic relationship, the client is prepared in advance for the nurse's absence; the client may act out on these days but it cannot be attributed solely to the nurse's absence.

375. 2 This behavior is typical of the working stage of the group; trust has been established and a willingness to discuss any problems or needs is present. (2) (MH; EV; PS; TR)

  1 This can occur at any stage; it occurs in social, as well as therapeutic, relationships.

  3 This would occur in the early phase of the group before trust is established and when everyone is trying to fit in.

  4 Same as answer 3.

Mental Health Nursing Quiz

1. A client, who is admitted to the hospital for an elective prostatectomy, is extremely anxious and has hand tremors. The client's wife informs the nurse that the client has been drinking heavily for the last 5 years. While the client is unpacking his suitcase, the nurse notices him hiding a bottle of whiskey in the rear of the drawer. The nurse's responsibility in relation to the alcohol includes:
   1. Trying to catch the client drinking the alcohol
   2. Asking the client how much alcohol he really drinks
   3. Confiscating the alcohol when the client is not looking
   4. Waiting for the client to bring up the subject of drinking

2. When a female client who has pressured speech mumbles incoherently, the most appropriate intervention would be for the nurse to:
   1. Set limits on the client's behavior by refusing to talk with her unless she speaks clearly
   2. Consistently ask the client to repeat what she said, so she will learn to recognize she is mumbling
   3. Ignore the client's mumbling since she is using this pathological manner of speech to get attention
   4. Indicate to the client that she needs to slow down because what she says is important and cannot be understood

3. A 16-year-old arrested for assault and robbery has a history of truancy and prostitution. The client demonstrates little emotion and is unconcerned that this behavior has caused emotional distress to others. The diagnosis of antisocial personality disorder is made. The client's lack of remorse and repetitive behavior is probably related to an underdeveloped:
   1. Id
   2. Ego
   3. Superego
   4. Limbic system

4. The nurse can be most therapeutic in approaching a withdrawn toddler who is sitting in a corner rocking and spinning a top by:
   1. Gently stroking the toddler's arm to gain the child's attention
   2. Bending down and staring at the spinning top with the toddler
   3. Holding the toddler to provide a sense of support and security
   4. Waiting for the toddler to make the initial contact before moving close

5. The nurse evaluates that a client has understood the teaching about the side effects and precautions associated with the neuroleptic drug, haloperidol (Haldol), when the client states:
   1. "I will immediately report any diarrhea or vomiting to my doctor."
   2. "I will not eat any tyramine-containing foods while I'm taking Haldol."
   3. "I'll maintain an adequate fluid intake, since I may urinate more than usual."
   4. "I'll avoid direct sunlight and use sunburn preventatives when I go outdoors."

6. When caring for a middle-aged female client who has lost about 20 pounds over the last two months, cries easily, sleeps poorly, and refuses to participate in any family or social activities that she previously enjoyed, it is very important for the nurse to:
   1. Provide the client with a high-caloric, high-protein diet
   2. Set firm consistent limits to reduce the client's crying episodes
   3. Assure the client that she will regain her usual function in a short time
   4. Allow the client to externalize her feelings, especially anger, in a safe manner

7. A recently admitted client with the diagnosis of schizophrenia, paranoid type says to the nurse, "I know they're spying on me in here too. I'm not safe anywhere!" The most therapeutic response by the nurse would be:
   1. "Nobody's spying on you in here."
   2. "Why do you feel they'd want to follow you here?"
   3. "You don't feel safe anywhere, not even in the hospital."
   4. "You are safe in the hospital; nothing can happen to you here."

8. To foster a therapeutic relationship with a deeply depressed, unresponsive client who stares into space, remains curled up in bed, and refuses to talk, the nurse must first break through the client's withdrawal. Initially, this can best be achieved by:
   1. Sitting quietly next to the client for set periods of time each hour
   2. Urging the client to participate in simple games with other clients
   3. Gently touching the client on the arm when the opportunity arises
   4. Informing the client that dressing and going to the dayroom is required

9. An adolescent is arrested for shoplifting and is brought to the psychiatric unit. Although describing her child as intelligent, witty, entertaining, and friendly, the mother states, "My child is somewhat unreliable, untruthful, and insincere." The client is diagnosed as having a personality disorder. The most accurate nursing diagnosis for the client would be:
   1. Ineffective individual coping
   2. Antisocial personality disorder
   3. Potential for introverted and mature behavior
   4. Impairment of common sense, feelings of guilt and remorse

10. An elderly client, accompanied by family members, is admitted with the diagnosis of dementia. During the admission procedures the initial approach by the nurse that would be most helpful to this client would be:
    1. "You are somewhat disoriented now, but do not worry. You will be all right in a few days."
    2. "Do not be frightened. I am the nurse, and everyone here in the hospital will help you get well."
    3. "I am the nurse on duty today. You are at the hospital. Your family can stay with you for a while."
    4. "Let me introduce you to the staff here before you get acquainted with our ward policy and routine."

11. In her 8th month of pregnancy, a 24-year-old client is brought to the hospital by the police who were called when she barricaded herself in a ladies room of a restaurant. During the admission, the client shouts, "Don't come near me. My stomach is filled with bombs and I'll blow up this place if anyone comes near me." This is an example of:
    1. Ideas of reference
    2. Delusional thinking
    3. Loose associations
    4. Tactile hallucinations

12. The nurse is aware that a 6-year-old with normal psychosocial development would have achieved Erikson's developmental tasks of trust, autonomy, and:
    1. Identity
    2. Initiative
    3. Intimacy
    4. Belonging

13. A client who appears dejected, barely responds to questions, and walks very slowly about the mental health unit tells the nurse in a barely audible voice that life is no longer worth living. The nurse's most therapeutic response to this statement would be:
    1. "Have you been thinking about suicide?"
    2. "What could be so bad to make you feel that way?"
    3. "We'll talk about your feelings after you have rested."
    4. "Let's talk about something pleasant, and you'll feel better."

14. A client with a diagnosis of mood disorder, manic episode, is started on a regimen of chlorpromazine and lithium carbonate. The nurse is aware that the rationale behind this regimen is that the chlorpromazine:
    1. Potentiates the action of lithium for more effective results
    2. Acts with the lithium to prevent progression to the depressive phase
    3. Acts to quiet the client while allowing time for the lithium to take effect
    4. Helps decrease the incidence of lithium toxicity in the first week of therapy

15. The day care treatment team decides it would be therapeutic for a client with an obsessive compulsive personality disorder to get a part-time job. On the day of the job interview, the client comes to the center very anxious and displays an increase in compulsive behaviors. The nurse could best respond to these behavioral changes by stating:
    1. "I know you're anxious, but make yourself go and try to conquer your fear."
    2. "It must be that you really don't want that job after all. I think you should think more about it."
    3. "If going to an interview makes you this anxious, it seems to me that you're not ready to work."
    4. "Going for your interview triggered some feelings in you. Describe what you're feeling at this time."

16. After detoxification, a client with a long history of alcohol abuse has agreed to attend Alcoholics Anonymous meetings at the hospital. On the day of the second meeting the client states, "I cannot attend the AA meeting today because I am expecting an important phone call." The nurse's most therapeutic response would be:
    1. "You are expected to go to the meeting."
    2. "Is your phone call really that important?"
    3. "You can go to the meeting after the call."
    4. "You can wait for the call and skip the meeting."

17. When a client is receiving lithium, the nurse should assess the client's:
    1. Weight
    2. Visual acuity
    3. Bowel sounds
    4. Potassium level

18. When caring for a client with a somatoform disorder, conversion type paralysis, the nurse should:
    1. Avoid discussing the paralysis
    2. Explain the reason for the paralysis
    3. Ask how the client feels about being paralyzed
    4. Encourage the client to get up, pointing out that walking is possible

19. A client with bulimia nervosa eats two sandwiches, two salads, and four desserts for lunch. After the meal the nurse would expect to observe the client:
    1. Performing excessive exercises
    2. Hoarding more food for a later binge
    3. Withdrawing from the group to the bathroom
    4. Actively socializing with small groups of clients

20. A client who has been raped, aware of the possible legal implications, decides to prosecute the rapist. The nurse carefully listens and documents all observations. This is done because with a charge of rape the burden of proof:
    1. Rests with the rape victim
    2. Rests with the health team
    3. Is on the defendant to prove innocence
    4. Must be established before the case will be heard

21. When talking with the nurse a client with a mood disorder states, "I feel rotten and useless. I cannot think straight. I feel overwhelmed by everything. I don't know if I can go on." When recording this encounter in the client's record, the most objective description of the client's mood would be:
1. Client appeared to be very depressed for most of the morning. Little interest in self or environment
2. Client is not able to cope with her problems and this hospitalization; states, "I cannot think straight."
3. Client stated, "I feel rotten and useless. I feel overwhelmed by everything. I don't know if I can go on."
4. Client expressed suicidal thoughts about not being able to go on and has decreased ability to think clearly

22. A client has been experiencing delusions. The nurse understands that delusions are:
1. A defense against anxiety
2. Precipitated by external stimuli
3. The result of paleological thinking
4. Subconscious expressions of anger

23. A nurse on the psychiatric unit is assigned to work with a client who appears seclusive and mistrustful of everyone. The nurse can help the client to develop trust by:
1. Attempting to be prompt for their scheduled meetings
2. Stating simply and sincerely that the nurse cares about the client's feelings
3. Handing the client medication and not watching to see whether it is swallowed
4. Listening attentively to the client's positive feelings and ignoring negative feelings

24. A female client in the terminal stage of cancer is admitted to the hospital in severe pain. The client refuses medication for the pain because it puts her to sleep and she wants to be awake. One day, despite the client's objection, a nurse administers the pain medication saying, "You know that this will make you more comfortable." The nurse in this situation could be charged with:

1. Battery
2. Assault
3. Invasion of privacy
4. Lack of informed consent

25. After lunch one afternoon the nurse notes that a client with the diagnosis of dementia of the Alzheimer type is alone in the dayroom away from other clients. When the nurse approaches, the client says, "I am all alone. No one has any use for me." The response by the nurse that would be most appropriate at this time would be:
1. "You seem upset. Would you like to tell me what is bothering you?"
2. "We need to be alone sometimes. It helps us get to know ourselves better."
3. "You should focus on ways to change this. Let's play some games to improve your morale."
4. "Have you done anything to avoid feeling lonely? I think you should socialize more with others."

26. A 16-year-old female client is admitted to the adolescent psychiatric unit with a diagnosis of anorexia nervosa. The adolescent has lost 40 pounds during the last 6 months and her current weight is 75 pounds. When approaching this client, the nurse should initially:
1. Point out how bad she looks
2. Refrain from discussing her appearance
3. Recognize that she is deliberately trying to kill herself
4. State the rules about eating in a matter-of-fact manner

27. A 5-year-old with an attention-deficit hyperactivity disorder exhibits a short attention span and demonstrates intermittent head banging, hair pulling, and excessive motor activity. The most important nursing diagnosis for this child at this time would be:
1. Anxiety related to shortened attention span
2. Sleep pattern disturbance related to hyperactivity
3. Body image disturbance related to acting out behavior
4. High risk for violence: self-directed, related to self-destructive behavior

28. An elderly male is widowed suddenly when his wife is killed in an automobile accident. The first action by the nurse in the emergency room to best help the client at this time would be:
1. Asking the clergyman of his faith to visit him
2. Having the physician order a tranquilizer for him
3. Referring him to a support group that meets near his home
4. Assuring him that everything possible was done for his wife

29. A forgetful, elderly client suspected of having Alzheimer's disease becomes progressively confused and tries to climb out of bed. The physician orders that the client be restrained at night while in bed. The nurse should apply:
1. Mitt restraints secured under the bed
2. Leg restraints secured to the footboard
3. Arm restraints secured to the headboard
4. A jacket restraint secured to the under-bed frame

30. During the admission interview of a client with a diagnosis of mood disorder, manic episode, the nurse would expect the client to demonstrate:
1. Flight of ideas
2. Ritualistic behaviors
3. Associative looseness
4. Delusions of persecution

31. To therapeutically relate to parents who are known to have abused their children, the nurse must first:
1. Recognize the emotional needs of the parent
2. Identify personal feelings about child abusers
3. Call authorities to report the suspected incident
4. Gather information about child's home environment

32. A young woman who has just lost her first job comes to the Mental Health Clinic very upset and states, "Without warning, I just start crying without any reason." The nurse's initial response should be:

1. "Do you know what makes you cry?"
2. "Most of us need to cry from time to time."
3. "Crying unexpectedly must be very upsetting."
4. "Are you having any other problems at this time?"

33. A client with schizophrenia is started on an antipsychotic/neuroleptic medication. The nurse is aware that these drugs are used primarily to:
1. Keep the client quiet and relaxed
2. Reduce the need for physical restraints
3. Control the client's behavior and reduce stress
4. Make the client more receptive to psychotherapy

34. The nurse is aware that the major defense mechanism used by an individual with a phobic disorder is:
1. Projection
2. Avoidance
3. Regression
4. Repression

35. A young adult client is admitted with a diagnosis of schizophrenia, paranoid type. The client's family is concerned with the client's safety and well-being because the client has been stating, "The voices are telling me to kill myself." The nursing diagnosis that should have first priority for this client is:
1. Disturbed self-esteem
2. Impaired verbal communication
3. High risk for self-directed violence
4. Sensory-perceptual alterations (auditory)

36. When caring for individuals with a history of abuse of multiple drugs, the nurse is aware that the most serious life-threatening symptoms during withdrawal usually result from:
1. Heroin
2. Methadone
3. Barbiturates
4. Amphetamines

37. The nurse notices that each time the physician or head nurse visits a disturbed female client she becomes extremely anxious. Today after visiting with the physician the client sits wringing her hands. The best initial response by the nurse would be:
    1. "How do you handle your anxiety?"
    2. "I notice that you are wringing your hands."
    3. "Tell me why you are afraid of authority figures."
    4. "Do you realize why you are wringing your hands?"

38. The nurse should be aware that the statement by a client that would indicate an irreversible adverse response to long-term therapy with the antipsychotic medication thioridazine hydrochloride (Mellaril) would be:
    1. "My mouth is always dry."
    2. "I'm not eating like I should."
    3. "I can't seem to sleep at night."
    4. "My tongue and lips move themselves."

39. The staff of the psychiatric unit conducts a biweekly orientation meeting for newly admitted clients. When planning for this meeting the nurse recognizes that the beginning of the meeting should be directed toward defining the:
    1. Rules for client behavior
    2. Purpose of the group meeting
    3. Clients' role and the leader's expectations
    4. Development of trust between staff and clients

40. A female client is admitted to the psychiatric unit with the diagnosis of obsessive compulsive disorder demonstrated by an increasing, consuming obsession with dirt. The client feels her hands are dirty and has a need to wash them about 70 to 80 times a day. The client's hands are red and raw with some bleeding. An immediate nursing goal for this client would be to get the client to:
    1. Understand that her hands are not dirty
    2. Develop insight into her emotional problems
    3. Stop washing her hands so the skin will heal
    4. Limit the number of times she washes her hands

41. A client comes to the mental health clinic complaining about feelings of extreme terror when attempting to ride in an elevator and feeling very uneasy in large crowds. The client feels uncomfortable about these fears and is beginning to experience difficulty concentrating at work. When assessing the situation, the nurse should understand that the client's symptoms are probably associated with:
    1. The development of an obsession as a result of conflicts with society
    2. Depression about life events which frequently leads to unreasonable fears
    3. A terrifying incident in an elevator in the past that has been repressed but unresolved
    4. Generalized anxiety about conflicts which has been displaced into specific unreasonable fears

42. A husband and wife are admitted to the trauma unit with gunshot wounds sustained in a robbery. Shortly following admission, the husband succumbs to his wounds. A potential nursing diagnosis for the wife related to the death of the husband would be:
    1. Defensive coping
    2. Altered family processes
    3. Ineffective individual coping
    4. Personal identity disturbance

43. A 30-year-old high school dropout who is employed as a dishwasher and his 37-year-old wife of 9 years have five children between the ages of 2 months and 8 years. He drinks heavily, especially on weekends and it takes little or no provocation to send him into a rage, yelling obscenities, throwing and breaking furniture, and occasionally hitting his wife and the older children. The nurse recognizes that this abusive behavior is probably related to the client's:
    1. Feeling trapped in a marriage
    2. Living in the culture of poverty
    3. Low socioeconomic background
    4. Long-standing problem with alcohol

44. A client with a diagnosis of mood disorder, manic episode, has pressured speech punctuated with profanity. It would be most therapeutic for the nurse to deal with this client's behavior by:

1. Thoroughly explaining the type of behavior allowed in the facility
2. Quietly stating that the use of profanity is unbecoming and will not be tolerated
3. Encouraging an interaction with another client who is exhibiting similar behavior
4. Allowing for the expression of hostility in a safe manner without being judgmental

45. A 3-year-old child is admitted to a children's mental health unit with a diagnosis of infantile autism. The major goal of therapy for a child with this pervasive developmental disorder would be, The child will:
1. Develop language skills
2. Limit the use of regressive behavior
3. Be mainstreamed into a regular preschool group
4. Recognize the self as an independent person of worth

Mental Health Nursing Quiz Rationales

1. 2 This assesses the client's level of alcohol abuse by direct questioning. (2) (MH; AS; TC; SA)

    1 This is judgmental; it is not straightforward; catching the client would decrease the client's self-esteem.

    3 This is not straightforward and will decrease trust.

    4 The client probably would not bring up the subject, because denial is often used to cope with alcohol abuse.

2. 4 This response provides feedback, which helps communication stay on track and demonstrates the nurse's interest in the client as a person. (2) (MH; IM; PS; MO)

    1 This response would not set limits but would create feelings of rejection.

    2 This response would only increase the client's anxiety and anger; it may precipitate acting-out behavior.

    3 Ignoring a client does not help the situation, nor does it demonstrate the nurse's interest or concern.

3. 3 Lack of remorse indicates weak superego, the aspect of personality concerned with prohibitions. (2) (MH; AN; PS; PR)

    1 This aspect of personality is not underdeveloped in this person; the id acts to achieve self-gratification.

    2 The ego is not related to acting-out behavior.

    4 This is not underdeveloped; it is related to achieving pleasure.

4. 2 Autistic children relate best with objects, which can be used as a bridge in interpersonal relationships; this begins at the child's level. (2) (MH; IM; PS; BA)

    1 Autistic children usually have difficulty tolerating being touched.

    3 Autistic children often become agitated when movement is restricted and personal space is invaded.

    4 Autistic children will not initiate contact or interactions.

5. 4 Photosensitivity is a side effect of many antipsychotic medications. (3) (MH; EV; TC; DR)

    1 These symptoms are side effects of lithium, not of Haldol.

    2 Avoiding tyramine-containing foods is a precaution associated with MAO inhibitors, not with Haldol.

    3 This is a precaution associated with lithium, not with Haldol.

6. 4 The greatest danger associated with depression is self-inflicted injury when feelings, especially anger, are internalized. (2) (MH; PL; PS; MO)

    1 A low-calorie diet would be more appropriate because of the client's decreased physical activity.

    2 The client is unable to control or regulate behavior at this time.

    3 This is false reassurance; this is not supportive of the client's feelings at this time.

7. 3 Rephrasing allows for further communication, expresses understanding, and does not belittle the client's feelings. (3) (MH; IM; PS; SD)

    1 Presenting reality to the client at this time only raises anxiety and leads the client to defend the delusion.

    2 "Why" questions make a client defensive, and the wording implies the client's delusion could be true.

    4 This is false reassurance; in any event, a suspicious client would not believe the nurse.

8. 1 Sitting quietly with a severely withdrawn client can provide an opportunity for nonthreatening interaction. (2) (MH; PL; PS; MO)
2 The client is unable to deal with even a one-to-one relationship at this time.
3 Entering a withdrawn client's body space is intrusive and stressful; it often precipitates a need for further withdrawal.
4 Placing demands on the withdrawn client causes a sense of threat, increased anxiety, and a need for additional withdrawal.

9. 1 History demonstrates that the client has had a difficult time controlling impulsive behavior and has consistently exhibited poor judgment; this indicates ineffective coping. (1) (MH; AN; PS; PR)
2 This is a psychiatric diagnosis, not a nursing diagnosis.
3 This is not an accepted nursing diagnosis.
4 Same as answer 3.

10. 3 Familiarity with the environment and orientation to the staff may help promote security and feelings of trust. (2) (MH; IM; PS; DD)
1 This denies the client's feelings and provides false reassurance.
2 This statement denies feelings and is false reassurance because all personnel are not involved with the client.
4 A person under stress cannot assimilate much information; verbiage can only lead to more confusion and anger.

11. 2 Delusions are false, fixed beliefs that have a minimal reality base. (1) (MH; AN; PS; SD)
1 Ideas of reference are false beliefs that every statement or action of others relates to the individual.
3 Loose associations are verbalizations that sound disjointed to the listener.
4 Tactile hallucinations are false sensory perceptions of touch without external stimuli.

12. 2 A 6-year-old should have resolved the developmental task of initiative vs guilt. (1) (MH; AN; ED; PD)
1 Resolution of identity vs role diffusion occurs at adolescence.

3 Resolution of intimacy vs isolation occurs at adulthood.
4 This is part of Maslow's hierarchy of needs; the need for love and belonging arises once physical and safety needs are met.

13. 1 It is important to determine if the client is thinking about suicide; the direct approach is most appropriate. (1) (MH; AS; PS; MO)
2 This approach not only denies feelings but also tells the client it is not right to feel that way.
3 This approach tells the client that feelings do not have top priority.
4 This approach denies the client's feelings and may be false reassurance.

14. 3 Antipsychotics are usually prescribed to calm the agitated client during the period of time it takes for the lithium to become effective. (3) (MH; AN; TC; DR)
1 Chlorpromazine is a major tranquilizer that has a different, not a potentiating, mechanism of action.
2 The drugs are used to control symptoms of mania; most clients do not progress to depression from the manic phase.
4 Chlorpromazine is a major tranquilizer that has no effect on lithium toxicity.

15. 4 These symptoms are a defense against anxiety resulting from decision making, which triggers old fears; the client needs support. (2) (MH; EV; PS; PR)
1 This denies the client's overwhelming anxiety and lacks realistic support.
2 This is judgmental; an increase in anxiety does not necessarily mean the client does not want to attain the goal.
3 This is judgmental; the client should be encouraged to work through the symptoms, not to avoid risk.

16. 1 This helps the client recognize and adhere to established limits and goals. (2) (MH; IM; PS; SA)
2 This response can be degrading and reinforces the client's manipulative behavior.
3 This reinforces the client's pattern of manipulation.
4 Same as answer 3

17. 1 Weight gain may be indicative of fluid retention; renal problems have been reported with lithium therapy. (3) (MH; EV; TC; DR)

2 This has no relationship to the administration of lithium.

3 Same as answer 2.

4 Same as answer 2.

18. 1 Discussion should not be initiated by the nurse; symptoms should be accepted but should not be the focus of discussion. (3) (MH; PL; TC; AX)

2 This response would increase anxiety and take away the client's unconscious defense.

3 This response would increase anxiety because it focuses on unconscious feelings about the paralysis.

4 This response would increase anxiety and deny the client's symptoms; in reality this client cannot make the legs move to walk.

19. 3 Bulimia is characterized by the binge-purge cycle; most clients withdraw from others and vomit after an eating binge. (2) (MH; AS; TC; EA)

1 Although some individuals with bulimia may perform excessive exercises, this is a more common finding with the diagnosis of anorexia nervosa.

2 Although individuals with bulimia may hoard food, this behavior frequently occurs later, when limits are put on their intake.

4 Most individuals with bulimia do not seek support or socialization after a binge, although they may socialize at other times.

20. 1 When the rape victim chooses to prosecute the rapist, the victim must prove that rape occurred; the accused is innocent until proven guilty. (1) (MH; AN; TC; CS)

2 The medical team may be asked to provide evidence at the trial, but the victim must prove that the rapist is guilty.

3 The perpetrator tries to establish innocence in a rape case; the victim must prove that the rapist is guilty.

4 Guilt or innocence will be established by a jury, with the burden of proof placed on the victim.

21. 3 This is a direct quotation of the client's statement with no added value judgments. (2) (MH; AS; PS; MO)

1 This is a subjective judgment and an interpretation of what the client actually said.

2 Same as answer 1.

4 Same as answer 1.

22. 1 Delusions are a way the unconscious defends the individual from real or imagined threats. (2) (MH; AN; PS; SD)

2 Illusions are false interpretations of actual external stimuli.

3 This is logical thinking that is formulated from an illogical base

4 Delusions are precipitated by feelings of anxiety, not anger.

23. 1 This helps the client to feel important enough for the nurse to remember their meeting and be on time. (2) (MH; IM; PS; TR)

2 The client is mistrustful of others and will probably not believe the nurse; caring is best demonstrated through behavior.

3 This would not only be unsafe but may make the client feel that the nurse does not care enough to stay.

4 Feelings should never be ignored but should be accepted as important to the client.

24. 1 This is the intentional touching of one person by another without permission of the person touched. (2) (MH; EV; TC; CS)

2 This is an intentional act, without touching, that makes a person fearful or produces reasonable apprehension of bodily harm.

3 This refers to the right of clients to have their private affairs protected.

4 This applies to written permission for procedures and treatments to be performed.

25. 1 This is a therapeutic approach that indicates awareness of the client's feelings and encourages verbalizations. (1) (MH; IM; PS; TR)

2 Moralizing is a roadblock to effective communication.

3 This is diverting the client's attention to something else and ignoring the client's attempt to verbalize.

4 This conveys a judgmental or critical attitude toward the client's actions.

26. 2 Initially the nurse should not discuss the client's appearance because this focuses on a symptom rather than feelings. (2) (MH; IM; PS; EA)

1 This focuses on a symptom rather than feelings; in addition, the client does not believe she looks bad.

3 The client's objective is not suicide; the client has an unconscious desire to remain childlike.

4 Stating the rules would not accomplish anything and will not convince the client to eat.

27. 4 Excessive motor activity with intermittent head banging and hair pulling is self-destructive behavior that can result in injury; prevention of self-injury has the highest priority. (1) (MH; AN; TC; BA)

1 This is not the most important nursing diagnosis according to the data presented; prevention of self-injury is primary.

2 Same as answer 1.

3 Same as answer 1.

28. 4 This helps allay guilt, reduces anxiety, and assists with coping. (3) (MH; IM; PS; CS)

1 The client should be consulted before a clergyman is called.

2 This is a last resort because this delays the grieving process.

3 It is too soon for this intervention.

29. 4 This provides for turning in bed; putting siderails up and down will not interfere with the restraint, which can be easily removed in an emergency. (1) (MH; IM; TC; DD)

1 This is contraindicated; it would restrict shoulder, elbow, wrist, and upper trunk movement.

2 This is unsafe; it would restrict leg movement and turning; the client could be injured by partially falling from the bed.

3 Same as answer 1.

30. 1 This is a fragmented, pressured, nonsequential pattern of speech typically used during a manic episode. (1) (MH; AS; PS; MO)

2 These are repetitive, purposeful, and intentional behaviors that are carried out in a stereotyped fashion; they are typically found in clients with obsessive-compulsive disorders.

3 This is the pattern of speech found in clients with schizophrenia; usual connections between words and phrases are lost to the listener and meaningful only to the speaker.

4 These are fixed false beliefs that others are plotting to do harm; they are typically found in clients with paranoid schizophrenia.

31. 2 Self-awareness is an essential element in providing support, understanding, and empathy to others. (1) (MH; AS; PS; CS)

1 Meeting emotional needs cannot be accomplished until an interpersonal relationship is established.

3 Although essential, this may in reality be a deterrent to the interpersonal relationship.

4 Although important, these data do not take priority at this time.

32. 3 This identifies the client's feelings. (1) (MH; IM; PS; AX)

1 This is an unrealistic question; the cause of anxiety is on an unconscious level.

2 This response moves the focus away from the client.

4 This disregards the client's comment and avoids feelings.

33. 4 Antipsychotic/neuroleptic medications help control anxiety and acting-out behavior, making the client more approachable. (3) (MH; AN; TC; DR)

1 Although the medication may produce this effect, it is not the primary purpose of administration.

2 Same as answer 1.

3 Same as answer 1.

34. 2 The person transfers anxieties to objects, usually inanimate objects, which are then avoided to decrease anxiety. (1) (MH; AN; PA; AX)

1 Projection, the attributing of undesirable traits or unacceptable feelings or motivations to others, is not the main defense mechanism used by someone with a phobia.

3 Regression, the return to an earlier more comfortable level of development, is not the main defense mechanism used by someone with a phobia.

4 Repression, the pushing of unacceptable impulses or ideas into the unconscious, is not the main defense mechanism used by someone with a phobia.

35. 3 Client safety always has the highest priority over any other client needs. (1) (MH; PL; TC; SD)

1 This is a later priority.

2 Same as answer 1.

4 Same as answer 1.

36. 3 Anxiety, shakiness, and insomnia occur early; within 24 hours convulsions, delirium, tachycardia, and death can occur. (2) (MH; AN; PA; SA)

1 Withdrawal is rarely life threatening but does cause severe discomfort such as abdominal cramping and diarrhea.

2 Same as answer 1.

4 Withdrawal does not cause life-threatening symptoms but does result in severe exhaustion and depression.

37. 2 The nurse is making an observation; bringing it to the attention of the client is an initial step in understanding that behavior. (1) (MH; IM; PS; TR)

1 This is premature because the client may not even be aware of anxiety.

3 This is premature and does not allow for self-recognition of feelings.

4 This is requesting an explanation from the client that the client probably is incapable of making.

38. 4 This is characteristic of tardive dyskinesia, an irreversible, antipsychotic, drug-induced, neurologic disorder. (2) (MH; EV; PS; DR)

1 This is an anticholinergic-like side effect that is not considered serious.

2 This is unrelated to antipsychotic medications.

3 This drug would cause sedation, not insomnia.

39. 2 Clients should know why they are there, what to expect, and what is to be accomplished. (1) (MH; PL; PS; TR)

1 This would come after the explanation of the purpose of the group.

3 Same as answer 1.

4 This is not necessary to define; this is a long-term goal.

40. 4 This action still permits the client to deal with feelings of anxiety in an acceptable way. (2) (MH; AN; TC; PR)

1 The client is aware that her hands are not dirty; the anxiety is too great for the client to stop.

2 Recognition must precede the development of insight; neither can be done until the level of anxiety is reduced.

3 This will not allow the client any outlet for dealing with extreme anxiety, which is a priority need at this time.

41. 4 Phobias are specific fears that serve as a means of coping with generalized anxiety. (2) (MH; AN; PS; AX)

1 Anxiety, not obsession, is related to phobias.

2 Anxiety, not depression, is related to phobias; finding a direct connection to life events is often difficult.

3 A direct connection to life events is often difficult to find.

42. 3 Because of the shock and trauma it is expected that the client will have an alteration in normal coping mechanisms. (2) (MH; AN; PS; CS)

1 The client will probably not project falsely positive self-opinions to enhance self-regard; it is more likely that the problems will be meeting life's demands and handling stress.

2 No family is mentioned in the situation.

4 No information is presented to indicate that the client cannot distinguish between the self and the non-self.

43. 4 Alcohol frequently reduces inhibitions and is one of the leading causes of violent behavior. (1) (MH; AS; PA; SA)

1 This factor alone rarely precipitates abusive behavior.

2 Same as answer 1.

3 Same as answer 1.

44. 4 This shows acceptance and protects the client and others from possible aggressive behavior. (2) (MH; PL; PS; MO)

1 Explanations are not helpful because the client's easy distractibility interferes with understanding.

2 This is a threatening approach that increases feelings of inadequacy.

3 Both clients would be very responsive to external stimuli; therefore this action could lead to loss of control for both.

45. 4 In a pervasive developmental disorder the child does not have a self-concept or view the self as separate; until this goal is attained other therapies will produce little or no positive outcomes. (2) (MH; AN; ED; BA)

1 The child with autism may have language skills but usually does not use them; nonverbal behavior is most generally associated with autism.

2 Regressive behavior should be anticipated as the child undergoes therapy, especially when working through earlier phases of development.

3 To be mainstreamed, the child must first have a developing independence.

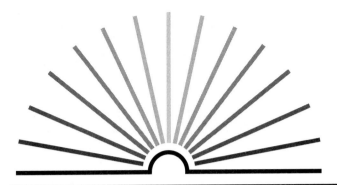

CHAPTER 6

Comprehensive Examination 1

Part A

1. The hypertonicity of the muscles in an infant with cerebral palsy causes scissoring of the legs. The nurse should suggest to the infant's mother that the best way to carry the baby is in a sitting position:
   1. Astride one of her hips
   2. Strapped in an infant seat
   3. Wrapped tightly in a blanket
   4. Under the arm using a football hold

2. A client with portal hypertension and ascites is given 2 units of salt-poor albumin IV. The purpose of salt-poor albumin is to:
   1. Provide parenteral nutrients
   2. Increase the client's protein stores
   3. Increase the client's circulating blood volume
   4. Temporarily divert blood flow away from the liver

3. A client, 36 weeks gestation, with moderate pregnancy-induced hypertension is admitted to the high-risk labor unit and placed on a fetal monitor as well as a blood pressure monitor. The continuous monitoring of the blood pressure is essential to reduce the potential for:
   1. Fetal death
   2. Convulsions
   3. Hemorrhage
   4. Premature delivery

4. The most important aspect of a therapeutic contract is:
   1. Discussing and defining the client's goals for treatment
   2. Determining the time and place of meetings with the client
   3. Understanding the professional responsibilities of the nurse
   4. Planning the frequency and duration of meetings with the client

5. After a mastectomy, a client returns from surgery with a portable suction unit in place and a dry sterile dressing covering the site of the incision. When observing this client for signs of bleeding, the nurse should:
   1. Empty and measure the output in the portable suction unit hourly
   2. Inspect the bedclothes under the axillary area for signs of drainage
   3. Turn the client on the affected side to inspect for blood that may flow backward
   4. Reinforce the operative site with a pressure dressing if any drainage appears on the dressing

6. The nurse empties a portable wound suction device when it is only half full because:
   1. It is easier and safer to empty the unit when it is only half full
   2. This facilitates a more accurate measurement of drainage output
   3. The negative pressure in the unit lessens as fluid accumulates in it, interfering with further drainage
   4. As fluid collects in the unit it exerts positive pressure, forcing drainage back up the tubing and into the wound

7. Before discharge after a myocardial infarction, a male client asks the nurse how long he should wait before having sexual relations with his wife. The nurse's best reply would be:
1. "It depends on how you are feeling."
2. "Two weeks is the usual waiting time."
3. "Have you discussed this with your physician?"
4. "You should wait until your heart feels stronger."

8. A female client and the nurse are standing next to each other in the mental health clinic when the client gets down on her hands and knees and says, "I am a table." It would be most effective for the nurse to:
1. State, "You were never a table before and you are not a table now."
2. State, "You are safe here in the clinic. You do not need to be a table."
3. Touch her arm while saying, "You must be very frightened to feel this way."
4. Offer a hand to help her up while saying, "You are not a table, you are a person."

9. To best help manage pain during burn dressing changes, the nurse can teach the client:
1. Deep breathing exercises
2. The importance of wound care
3. Active range of motion exercises
4. To alternately contract and relax muscles

10. A postpartum client who has insulin-dependent diabetes states that she does not want another baby for at least 3 years. The nurse provides family planning instructions and is satisfied that the teaching has been understood when the client states, "Because of my diabetes, the best type of contraception is:
1. An oral contraceptive."
2. The intrauterine device."
3. A diaphragm with foam."
4. Tying the fallopian tubes."

11. After the administration of epinephrine to a child with asthma, the nurse would carefully monitor for the common side effect of:
1. Flushing
2. Dyspnea
3. Tachycardia
4. Hypotension

12. A client is admitted to the psychiatric unit with a history of abuse of multiple drugs. In planning care after the withdrawal period the nurse should take into consideration that the client is probably:
1. Unable to give up drugs
2. Unconcerned with reality
3. Unable to delay gratification
4. Unaware of the dangers of drug addiction

13. A factor, learned during the nursing history, that probably predisposed a client to diabetes mellitus is:
1. Having diabetes insipidus
2. Eating low cholesterol foods
3. Being 20 pounds overweight
4. Drinking a daily alcoholic drink

14. After a pneumonectomy a client is receiving an intravenous infusion. In light of this particular surgery, the client is most vulnerable to the complication of:
1. Phlebitis
2. Infiltration
3. Air embolism
4. Pulmonary edema

15. The nurse tells a laboring client that she must avoid lying on her back during labor. The nurse bases this instruction on the knowledge that the supine position can:
1. Unduly prolong labor
2. Cause decreased placental perfusion
3. Interfere with free movement of the coccyx
4. Lead to transient episodes of hypertension

16. When planning care for a child with leukemia, the nurse must keep in mind that the prognosis of a child with acute lymphocytic leukemia who is receiving therapy is:
1. Very poor, but the therapy keeps them pain free
2. Limited to a few months in 70% of the children affected
3. Extended to at least 5 years in 60% of the children treated
4. Very positive, with a probable cure in 90% of the children affected

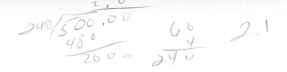

17. Methotrexate is to be administered IV to a 14-year-old. The appropriate amount has been added to 500 ml of D5W. The physician has ordered the 500 ml to be absorbed in 4 hours. The nurse should set the infusion device at:
    1. 50 ml/hr
    2. 75 ml/hr
    3. 100 ml/hr
    4. 125 ml/hr

18. A subclavian catheter is inserted and the client is started on total parenteral nutrition (TPN). To prevent the most common complication of TPN the nurse should plan to teach the client to:
    1. Avoid touching the dressing as much as possible
    2. Keep the head as still as possible whenever moving
    3. Weigh daily at the same time, wearing the same clothing
    4. Regulate the flow rate on the infusion pump as necessary

19. Care in a day treatment center is often indicated early in the treatment program for clients with incapacitating symptoms resulting from obsessive compulsive personality disorders because it:
    1. Limits the client's time to carry out the symptomatic rituals
    2. Allows the therapeutic staff to exert control over the client's activities
    3. Provides a neutral environment in which the client can work through conflicts
    4. Resolves client's anxiety, since opportunities requiring decision-making are reduced

20. To relieve the symptoms of Parkinson's disease the nurse should expect the physician to order:
    1. Levodopa
    2. Dopamine
    3. Vitamin B_6
    4. Isocarboxazid

21. After a transurethral prostatectomy, a client returns to the recovery room with a three-way Foley catheter with continuous bladder irrigation (CBI). An initial nursing priority in the client's care plan would be to:
    1. Observe for signs of confusion and agitation
    2. Maintain the client in a semi-Fowler's position
    3. Observe the suprapubic dressing for drainage
    4. Force fluids by mouth as soon as the gag reflex returns

22. A client has had a cesarean delivery because of fetal distress. When doing postoperative coughing and deep breathing she complains of localized pain in the incision which subsides in a few moments. The nurse should:
    1. Place her in the supine position and inspect the wound site
    2. Instruct her to splint the wound with a pillow when coughing
    3. Assess the intensity of the pain and give her the ordered analgesic
    4. Call her physician immediately and then check for wound dehiscence

23. While doing a newborn assessment, the nurse suspects that the infant has a talipes equinovarus when the infant's toes are:
    1. Lower than the heel with the foot pointing inward
    2. Higher than the heel with the foot pointing inward
    3. Lower than the heel with the foot pointing outward
    4. Higher than the heel with the foot pointing outward

24. Dehiscence is a complication with gastrointestinal surgery. A factor that would further predispose an obese 55-year-old client who had an abdominal cholecystectomy to wound dehiscence would be:
    1. The age of the client
    2. Presence of a T-tube
    3. The presence of excessive flatus
    4. Weight 25% over recommended level

25. A female client with chronic obstructive pulmonary disease (COPD) tells the nurse that although she smokes she limits it to a cigarette or two a day. She also tells the nurse that she has been lax in doing the prescribed pulmonary physiotherapy exercises because they are too tiring. The nurse should respond:
    1. "Tell me more about your typical day before you changed your routine."
    2. "Your being so sick is probably because of your smoking and not exercising."
    3. "Smoking is probably a primary cause of the increased severity of your disease."
    4. "I can't make you stop doing what you are doing. It's your choice to be sick or well."

26. A client with a diagnosis of bipolar disorder, manic episode is receiving lithium. During the third week of therapy with lithium, the nurse would be aware that the drug was effective when the client is:
    1. More high-spirited
    2. Able to laugh off criticism
    3. More appropriately groomed
    4. Able to spend the morning alone

27. The nurse is aware that an early sign of chronic lead poisoning (plumbism) in children is:
    1. Anemia
    2. Oliguria
    3. Convulsions
    4. Mental retardation

28. A neonate develops hyperbilirubinemia, and phototherapy is begun. The nursing care plan for an infant during phototherapy should include:
    1. Taking vital signs q1h
    2. Giving additional fluids q2h
    3. Drawing blood for a Guthrie test qd
    4. Dressing the neonate in a light shirt and diaper

29. The nurse assesses a client for increasing intracranial pressure by monitoring the pulse pressure. The nurse understands that a client's pulse pressure is actually the:
    1. Force exerted against an arterial wall
    2. Difference between the apical and radial rates
    3. Difference between systolic and diastolic readings
    4. Degree of ventricular contraction in relation to output

30. At night an elderly client with dementia becomes more disoriented and sleeps very little. Confusion caused by sleep deprivation can often be decreased by:
    1. Applying restraints so the client will remain in bed
    2. Giving the client a back rub and shutting the door tightly
    3. Administering the client's prescribed sedative medications
    4. Leaving a subdued light on in the client's room all night long

31. A pediatric client is receiving chloramphenicol. The child's blood work should be monitored for side effects which include:
    1. Polycythemia
    2. Hyperuricemia
    3. Aplastic anemia
    4. Hypoalbuminemia

32. The physician prescribes a low-fat, 2 gram sodium diet for a client with hypertension. The nurse understands that a low-sodium diet will:
    1. Chemically stimulate the loop of Henle
    2. Diminish the thirst response of the client
    3. Prevent reabsorption of water in the distal tubules
    4. Cause fluid to move toward the interstitial compartment

33. An open reduction and internal fixation is performed on a client with a fractured left hip sustained in a fall. The nurse plans postoperative care knowing that the client:
    1. Will not be permitted to lie on the affected side
    2. Should be positioned with the legs in adduction
    3. Cannot bear weight on the affected leg for three months
    4. Can be ambulated for short distances 1 to 2 days after surgery

34. A women with 5 children comes to the emergency room with multiple facial injuries. The client states her husband, who is an alcoholic, beat her up. Because the client appears to be a victim of abuse, it would be most therapeutic for the nurse to:
1. Discuss birth control with her
2. Report her experiences to the police
3. Let her talk about her family problems
4. Discuss the possibility of her leaving him

35. On the fourth postpartum day the client's vaginal discharge is pinkish in color and does not contain clots. This discharge is called:
1. Lochia alba
2. Lochia rubra
3. Lochia serosa
4. Lochia pinkosa

36. After an infant has the cast used to correct a talipes equinovarus (club foot) removed, the nurse teaches the mother how to exercise the baby's foot. The nurse would know that the mother understood the instructions when she says that she will exercise the foot:
1. With each diaper change
2. Every four hours without fail
3. Twice a day, in the AM and PM
4. Once a day, after the baby naps

37. A child is receiving chelation therapy for lead poisoning. The nurse should be aware that a condition that can be attributed both to lead toxicity and to the side effects of the chelating agent, Ca EDTA, is:
1. Hypocalcemia
2. Nephrotoxicity
3. Bone marrow depression
4. Increased intracranial pressure

38. Following a myocardial infarction a client begins a supervised progressive jogging regimen and asks the nurse how to tell if it is helping. The nurse should reply:
1. "Your intermittent claudication will be reduced."
2. "Your breathing will become regular and shallow."
3. "You will be able to run progressively longer distances before tiring."
4. "You will perspire less when you run, because you'll be using less energy."

39. A client returns from the operating room following a total laryngectomy with a laryngectomy tube in the permanent stoma. To facilitate respirations and promote comfort, the client should be placed in the:
1. Side-lying position
2. Orthopneic position
3. High-Fowler's position
4. Semi-Fowler's position

40. A neuromuscular blocking agent is administered to a client before ECT therapy. The nurse should observe the client for:
1. Convulsions
2. Loss of memory
3. Nausea and vomiting
4. Respiratory difficulties

41. An infant born with a cleft lip is to have a surgical repair of the lip at about 2½ months of age. In preparation for the postoperative period the nurse should instruct the infant's mother to:
1. Teach the infant to drink from a cup
2. Keep the infant's arms in restraints at all times
3. Burp the infant as little as possible after feeding
4. Place the infant in the supine position for extended periods

42. A couple interested in delaying the start of a family discuss the various methods of family planning. Together, they decide to use the basal body temperature method. Before they begin using this method they should understand that the fertility period surrounding ovulation usually extends from:
1. 12 hours before to 24 hours after ovulation
2. 72 hours before to 24 hours after ovulation
3. 24 to 48 hours before to 48 hours after ovulation
4. 72 to 80 hours before to 72 hours after ovulation

43. A long-term goal for a male client experiencing dysfunctional grieving after the death of his wife would be that the client will be able to:
1. Resume previously enjoyed activities
2. Eat at least two meals a day with another person
3. Decrease negativistic thinking about self and others
4. Relocate to a state in which other family members reside

44. During a routine examination an enlarged thyroid gland is discovered in a middle-aged female and hyperthyroidism is suspected. On assessment the nurse would expect this client to have:
1. Thickened and coarse skin
2. Tachycardia and palpitations
3. Apathetic attitude and masklike facies
4. Menstrual disturbances and loss of libido

45. A client with a history of chronic obstructive pulmonary disease develops a pneumothorax and a chest tube is inserted. The primary purpose of the chest tube is to:
1. Lessen the client's chest pain and discomfort
2. Drain accumulated fluid from the pleural cavity
3. Restore negative pressure in the pleural space
4. Prevent subcutaneous emphysema in the chest wall

46. When assessing a young infant, inspection, palpation, percussion, and auscultation are used. The technique the nurse should perform last is:
1. Percussion of the infant's lung fields
2. Palpation of the infant's abdominal organs
3. Inspection of the infant's general condition
4. Auscultation of the infant's heart and breath sounds

47. Following gastrointestinal surgery a client's condition improves and a regular diet is ordered. The food that will most likely be tolerated with little discomfort is:

1. Fresh fruit
2. Baked fish
3. Whole milk
4. Bran cereal

48. A pregnant client's last menstrual period was on February 11. By July 18, a physical assessment of the client should indicate that the top of the fundus is:
1. Even with the umbilicus
2. Just above the symphysis pubis
3. Two fingerbreadths above the umbilicus
4. Half way between the symphysis and umbilicus

49. A two-year-old requires close supervision to protect against potential accidents because at this age the child's learning occurs primarily from:
1. Playmates
2. The parents
3. Older siblings
4. Trial and error

50. The most important nursing objective when planning care for a young, hyperactive child with an attention-deficit disorder who engages in self-destructive behavior would be to:
1. Prevent the child from inflicting any self-injury
2. Help the child to develop the ability to test reality
3. Assist the child to formulate realistic ego boundaries
4. Provide the child with opportunities to discharge energy

51. A laboring client with a breech presentation is scheduled for a cesarean delivery. An important nursing intervention during labor to prevent postoperative complications would include:
1. Providing scrupulous skin care
2. Maintaining adequate hydration
3. Notifying the neonatal intensive care unit
4. Monitoring the maternal vital signs frequently

52. A client is to have a craniotomy for removal of a brain tumor. The client's preoperative preparation should include:
1. Forcing nutrient fluids
2. Gently shampooing the hair
3. Administering morphine sulfate
4. Administering cleansing enemas

53. Two days following a myocardial infarction a client has a temperature of 100.2°F. The nurse should:
1. Auscultate the chest for diminished breath sounds
2. Notify the physician immediately about the temperature
3. Encourage deep breathing and coughing every 2 hours
4. Record the temperature and monitor vital signs at routine intervals

54. A client with newly diagnosed hyperthyroidism is treated with propylthiouracil, an antithyroid drug, along with potassium iodide. The nurse teaches the client about these medications with the knowledge that:
1. Iodide solutions such as these must be taken on an empty stomach and diluted in water
2. The client should carefully observe for signs of infection or bleeding while on this therapy
3. Use of these drugs prior to thryroidectomy will increase the risk of postoperative hemorrhage
4. The drugs will be discontinued as soon as the client's temperature and pulse rate return to normal

55. During a well-baby visit the nurse recognizes that an 18-month-old's growth and development is within the normal range when the child:
1. Climbs up the stairs
2. Pedals a tricycle easily
3. Says 150 different words
4. Builds a tower of 8 blocks

56. A client with phobias about elevators and large crowds comes to the clinic for help because of feelings of depression related to these fears. An appropriate short-term goal would be that the client will:

1. Ride an elevator without anxiety when accompanied by the nurse
2. Describe the thoughts and feelings experienced in terrifying situations
3. Experience relief from feelings of depression and an elevation of mood
4. Identify the early childhood conflicts leading to the development of the fears

57. A client is admitted for a contraction stress test in the 42nd week of gestation. The nurse is aware that this test is being done because a prolonged pregnancy can:
1. Result in a baby that is LGA
2. Lead to placental insufficiency
3. Indicate subclinical gestational diabetes
4. Predispose the mother to postpartal infection

58. A client develops a small decubitus ulcer on the sacral area. The nurse should plan to deal with this problem by:
1. Keeping the area dry
2. Applying moist dressings
3. Providing a low-calorie diet
4. Keeping the client on the right side

59. When implementing a screening program for scoliosis, the most appropriate site would be in a:
1. Middle school
2. Well-baby clinic
3. Senior high school
4. Preschool day care center

60. The clinic nurse observes a 2-year-old girl sitting alone rocking and staring at a small shiny top she is spinning. Later, the mother relates to the nurse her concerns, stating, "She pushes me away. She does not speak and only shows feelings when I take her top away. Is it something I've done?" It would be most therapeutic for the nurse to respond by:
1. Asking the mother about her relationship with her husband
2. Asking the mother how she held the child when she was an infant
3. Telling the mother that it's nothing she has done and sharing observations of the child
4. Telling the mother not to be concerned, that the child will outgrow this phase of development

61. The nurse assesses a client with the diagnosis of bulimia nervosa for the psychological characterstics commonly associated with this disorder which include:
    1. A flattened affect
    2. Unmet dependency needs
    3. Rigidity of character and inflexibility
    4. An unwillingness to discuss problems

62. The physician prescribes propranolol (Inderal) 20 mg po qid for a client after double coronary artery bypass surgery. The discharge teaching plan should include telling the client to:
    1. Avoid abruptly discontinuing the medication
    2. Increase the medication if chest pain occurs
    3. Only drink alcoholic beverages in moderation
    4. Report a pulse rate below 70 beats per minute

63. A nurse is called upon to assist with an emergency home delivery. To facilitate the expulsion of the placenta after the baby is born, the nurse should:
    1. Push down vigorously on the fundus
    2. Have the mother breastfeed the baby
    3. Place gentle continuous tension on the cord
    4. Encourage the mother to vigorously bear down

64. As part of a high school sex education program the school nurse discusses herpes genitalis. The nurse should tell the students that:
    1. Herpes genitalis is curable with penicillin
    2. The disease generally is painless in women
    3. Herpes genitalis causes both local and systemic reactions
    4. The disease is not transmitted via fomites such as toilet seats

65. A client with a history of benign prostatic hypertrophy mentions that he has heard cranberry juice prevents bladder infection. The nurse replies that cranberry juice may be helpful because it:

1. Increases the acidity of the urine
2. Soothes the irritated bladder walls
3. Improves the glomerular filtration rate
4. Destroys microorganisms in the urinary tract

66. When a client is actively hallucinating, it would be most therapeutic for the nurse to:
    1. Ask to whom the client is speaking
    2. Request that the client speak softly
    3. Involve the client in a simple game of cards
    4. Allow the client to continue without interruption

67. When caring for a child with cystic fibrosis, the nurse plans to include times for postural drainage in the child's nursing care plan. This therapy should be scheduled:
    1. Once a day, after breakfast
    2. Three times a day, before meals
    3. Three times a day, halfway between meals
    4. Two times a day, on awakening and at bedtime

68. When giving discharge instructions to the parents of a child with cystic fibrosis, the nurse realizes that further explanation about the problems caused by cystic fibrosis is needed when the parents state, "We will:
    1. Keep our child in an air-conditioned room."
    2. Give our child the pancreatic enzymes with meals."
    3. Provide our child skin care after each bowel movement."
    4. Take our child to Florida this summer to visit both grandparents."

69. The nurse is aware that one reason the dialysate used in peritoneal dialysis is warmed to body temperature before its instillation into the peritoneal cavity is to:
    1. Force potassium back into the cells, thereby decreasing serum levels
    2. Encourage removal of serum urea by dilating the peritoneal blood vessels
    3. Add extra warmth to the body because metabolic processes are disturbed
    4. Help prevent cardiac dysrhythmias by speeding removal of excess serum potassium

70. After exposure to a nephrotoxic substance a client is hospitalized in the oliguric phase of acute renal failure. The client's estimated urine output for the last 24 hours is about 1 pint. The BUN level is 96 mg/dl. The physician orders 900 ml of water by mouth during the next 24 hours. In carrying out this order, the nurse realizes that the rationale for the order is that 900 ml of fluid will:
1. Equal the expected urinary output for the next 24 hours
2. Prevent the development of complicating hypostatic pneumonia
3. Compensate for both insensible and measured fluid losses over the next 24 hours
4. Prevent hyperkalemia, which could result in the client having serious cardiac dysrhythmias

71. A client, 38 weeks gestation, is experiencing painless bleeding, and has been diagnosed as having placenta previa. The client is concerned that she may have done something to cause the bleeding. Recognizing that the client appears worried, it would be most therapeutic for the nurse to say:
1. "You probably have a weak uterus."
2. "It's not your fault; these things happen."
3. "Don't worry; it's just a sign of beginning labor."
4. "The placenta is lying low and separates when you dilate."

72. When formulating a plan of care for a "paralyzed" client with a somatoform disorder, conversion type, the nurse must realize that:

1. The illness is very real to the client and the client needs good nursing care
2. Although the client believes there is an illness, there is no cause to be concerned
3. Good nursing care is needed even though the nurse recognizes the client is not ill
4. There is no physiological basis for the illness; therefore only emotional care is needed

73. A client with diabetes mellitus develops ketoacidosis. The laboratory value that would support a diagnosis of diabetic ketoacidosis would be:
1. A normal BUN
2. Elevated serum lipids
3. A decreased hematocrit
4. Low serum calcium levels

74. A client has a below-the-knee amputation of the right leg. The nurse should understand that after this type of surgery:
1. Strict bed rest is usually maintained for at least several days
2. The stump dressing is usually changed daily by the physician
3. Hemorrhage rarely occurs during the early postoperative period
4. The client is usually positioned with the stump elevated for the first 24 hours

75. After a gastric resection the nurse should expect to observe:
1. Vomiting
2. Gastric distention
3. Intermittent periods of diarrhea
4. Bloody drainage for the first 12 hours

Part B

76. Long-term plans for parents of children with sickle cell anemia includes periodic conferences with groups of parents whose children have sickle cell disease to:
   1. Find special schooling facilities for the child
   2. Make plans for moving to a more therapeutic climate
   3. Choose a means of birth control to avoid future pregnancies
   4. Air their feelings regarding the transmission of the disease to the child

77. The nurse would expect a client with a somatoform disorder, conversion type, to display an affect that is:
   1. Happy and cheerful
   2. Sad and depressed
   3. Frightened and upset
   4. Calm and matter-of-fact

78. A client, 36 weeks gestation, is admitted to the labor and delivery unit because she is having painless periods of bright red bleeding. A tentative diagnosis of placenta previa is made. The nurse is aware that the diagnosis of placenta previa is usually confirmed by:
   1. Amnioscopy
   2. Laparoscopy
   3. Amniocentesis
   4. Ultrasonography

79. One morning a female client with the diagnosis of schizophrenia tells the nurse that she is Joan of Arc and is going to be burned at the stake. The most therapeutic response by the nurse would be:
   1. "Tell me more about being Joan of Arc."
   2. "You and I both know you are not Joan of Arc."
   3. "You are safe here, we won't let you be burned."
   4. "It seems like the world is a pretty scary place for you."

80. When a student in a sex education class in high school asks if recurrent infection is possible with herpes genitalis, the nurse should reply that:
   1. Once herpes genitalis has been adequately treated, recurrence is rare
   2. The only sure way to prevent recurrent attacks is to abstain from sexual activity
   3. Unfortunately, recurrent attacks do occur but they are not as severe as the initial infection
   4. Good health practices such as getting adequate rest and maintaining good nutrition will prevent recurrences

81. The nurse prepares a client who has had coronary bypass surgery for discharge by teaching that there will be:
   1. No further drainage from the incisions after hospitalization
   2. A mild fever and extreme fatigue for several weeks after surgery
   3. Little incisional pain and tenderness after 3 to 4 weeks after surgery
   4. Increased edema in the leg used for the donor graft with progressive activity

82. The nurse should observe a client with the diagnosis of bulimia nervosa for symptoms of:
   1. Weight gain
   2. Dehydration
   3. Hyperactivity
   4. Hyperglycemia

83. When discussing the frequency of tub baths with an elderly client, the prime factor that the nurse should consider is the:
   1. Condition of the client's skin
   2. Client's ability to provide self-care
   3. Client's history of allergic reactions
   4. Degree of the client's orientation to the environment

84. The nurse teaches a new mother how to clean and disinfect the base of her infant's umbilical cord. The nurse explains to the mother that the cord stump is a potential source of infection because:

1. Wharton's jelly is no longer present.
2. It contains necrotic tissue and blood.
3. It is touched by blankets and clothing.
4. Newborns have no resistance to infection.

85. The behavior that would indicate that nursing interventions have been effective for a six-year-old male, hyperactive child with an attention-deficit disorder would be that the child:
    1. Is not inhibited by rules or routines
    2. Enjoys playing with his cars by himself
    3. Is no longer enuretic during the nighttime
    4. Has an increased attention span in a special school

86. The nurse knows that the most important aspect of the preoperative care of a child with Wilms' tumor is:
    1. Checking the size of the child's liver
    2. Monitoring the child's blood pressure
    3. Maintaining the child in a prone position
    4. Collecting the child's urine for culture and sensitivity

87. A client is scheduled for a hemicolectomy. The nurse's primary role in informed consent for surgery is one of client advocate. The nurse should recognize that in regard to informed consent:
    1. As a witness, the nurse must be present to see the client actually sign the form
    2. A consent is only valid for 7 days; if a longer time passes a new form must be signed
    3. Clients need to know about the procedure; they need not be frightened with information about potential risks
    4. Either a nurse or a physician can give the client the necessary information to obtain informed consent for surgery

88. When caring for a client with a chest tube in place, the nurse should plan to:
    1. Administer cough suppressants at appropriate intervals as ordered
    2. Empty and measure the drainage in the collection chamber each shift
    3. Apply clamps below the insertion site whenever getting the client out of bed
    4. Encourage coughing, deep breathing, and ROM to the arm on the affected side

89. Eight months following the traumatic death of a spouse, a client comes to the mental health clinic complaining of continuing depression. The client states, "I have not been seeing any of my friends or attending any of the activities I previously enjoyed. My married children live in another state and I rarely have any contact with them." The most accurate nursing diagnosis for this client would be:
    1. Impaired verbal communication related to social isolation
    2. Ineffective family coping related to separation from children
    3. Ineffective individual coping related to low motivation to resume activities of daily living
    4. Dysfunctional grieving related to difficulty reestablishing a lifestyle following the death of a spouse

90. The nurse in a family planning center knows that a client understands the discussion about the use of a diaphragm when the client states, "After intercourse, a diaphragm must be left in place for:
    1. 1 to 2 hours."
    2. 6 to 8 hours."
    3. 10 to 12 hours."
    4. 16 to 20 hours."

91. A client with a severe depression that has not responded to any of the antidepressant medications is to start electroconvulsive therapy (ECT) and asks how the treatment will help. The nurse should reply:
    1. "The important thing is it will help you."
    2. "It changes your usual behavior patterns."
    3. "Why don't you ask your physician to explain it better."
    4. "It works on chemical substances in the brain, and it does help."

92. When talking with a depressed client, the statement that would give the nurse a clue that the client may be going to attempt suicide would be:
    1. "I don't feel too good today."
    2. "I feel much better; today is a lovely day."
    3. "I'm very tired today, and I'd like to be alone."
    4. "I feel a little better, but it probably will not last."

93. A client's angina is usually very intense. To hasten the absorption of the nitroglycerin tablet, the nurse should instruct the client to:
1. Take the tablet with a glass of warm water
2. Move the tablet around with the tip of the tongue
3. Break up the tablet before placing it under the tongue
4. Swallow saliva before placing the tablet under the tongue

94. Focusing attention on individuals who may be at high risk for child abuse is an example of:
1. Legal prevention
2. Tertiary prevention
3. Primary prevention
4. Secondary prevention

95. To answer client questions about fluid and electrolyte imbalances, the nurse must understand that in the human body, where a semipermeable membrane divides two solutions, the solution with the greatest number of particles:
1. Draws water in its direction
2. Draws particles in its direction
3. Does not contribute particles to the other side
4. Gives up water to the side with fewer particles

96. A client with severe hypertension and dependent edema is admitted to the hospital. The physician orders furosemide (Lasix) 20 mg IV push. When administering the Lasix, the nurse should explain that the client:
1. May have problems with hearing
2. Will need to void in 5 to 10 minutes
3. Will feel some burning at the IV site
4. Should drink 240 ml of orange juice

97. If all of the following beds are available on a pediatric unit, a nurse should plan to place a child admitted with meningitis in:
1. A semiprivate room in the middle of the unit
2. A corner of a four-bed room next to the nurses' station
3. A private room two doors away from the nurses' station
4. An isolation room away from activity at the far end of the unit

98. When a client is receiving dexamethasone (Decadron), the nurse should plan nursing care considering the client's predisposition to:
1. Infection
2. Weight gain
3. Hypotension
4. Urinary stasis

99. A preterm newborn in the neonatal intensive care unit experiences occasional periods of apnea and is placed on an apnea monitor. If the apnea monitor sounds, the nurse's initial action should be to:
1. Provide oxygen by hood
2. Suction the nasopharynx
3. Provide light tactile stimulation
4. Institute resuscitative measures

100. The supervised activity that would be most therapeutic for a client during the early phase of hospitalization for a manic episode of a bipolar disorder would be:
1. Joining a brief swimming competition
2. Writing letters and doing needlepoint
3. Playing a board game with another client
4. Walking around the hospital grounds with one of the nurses

101. A 3-year-old is admitted to the hospital for chelation therapy for lead poisoning. The child's mother asks the nurse how the child got lead poisoning. The nurse bases the response on the knowledge that this problem in children is:
1. Clearly related to the child's ingestion of nonfood substances
2. Attributed to an indigent and passive mother who fails to supervise them
3. Considered to be an environment with lead available for oral exploration by unsupervised children
4. Unknown, but high-risk groups include those with pica and those exposed to environmental hazards

102. An intravenous solution of lactated Ringer's is ordered to replace the T-tube output of a client who has had a choledochostomy. To evaluate whether the solution was therapeutically effective, the nurse should observe the client for symptoms associated with:

1. Urinary stasis
2. A paralytic ileus
3. Metabolic acidosis
4. An increased potassium level

103. A mother whose child is born with a talipes equinovarus (club foot) tells the nurse that she would be afraid to have more children because they might have the same problem. The best intervention by the nurse would be to:
    1. Discuss the certainty of the defect occurring in later children
    2. Explore with her the environmental and hereditary factors involved
    3. Reassure her that this is unlikely to happen again in the same family
    4. Explain that future children will have a 1 in 4 chance of having the deformity

104. A 65-year-old retiree with prostatic carcinoma is scheduled for a transurethral prostatectomy. As he is being admitted to the surgical unit, he tells the nurse he is concerned that his operation will result in impotence. The nurse's best reply would be:
    1. "I can understand why you are worried; it is a very real possibility."
    2. "I can understand your concern, but this operation rarely causes impotence."
    3. "Most men worry about their ability to function. Why don't you speak with your physician?"
    4. "You may be impotent for a while, but normal functioning will probably return within 5 months."

105. When developing a plan of care for a female client with an obsessive compulsive personality disorder, the nurse should be aware that the client's anxiety level would be increased if the staff:
    1. Helped her to understand the nature of her anxiety
    2. Provided a nonjudgmental and accepting environment
    3. Involved her in establishing and implementing the therapeutic plan
    4. Permitted her ritualistic behaviors to be carried out at three set times during the day

106. After surgery for a brain tumor, the client is receiving intravenous mannitol (Osmitrol). During and after its administration the nurse should assess the client for:
    1. Respiratory failure
    2. Cardiac dysrhythmias
    3. A decrease in the heart rate
    4. A rebound increase in intracranial pressure

107. After the insertion of an intestinal tube, nursing care should include:
    1. Keeping the client on absolute bedrest
    2. Allowing the client frequent sips of water
    3. Securing the tube by taping it to the nose
    4. Confirming the tube's position by testing the pH of drainage

108. A client and her 2-week-old newborn are being seen by the visiting nurse at home. When the nurse arrives the client appears exhausted and the baby is crying. A most appropriate question by the nurse would be:
    1. "Oh, you're having a terrible day."
    2. "Tell me a little about your daily routine."
    3. "Is everything OK? You look exhausted."
    4. "When did the baby have the last feeding?"

109. A client with insulin-dependent diabetes mellitus is found unconscious having Kussmaul respirations; an acetone odor to the breath; and dry, hot, flushed skin. The nurse suspects that the client is experiencing:
    1. Diabetic ketoacidosis
    2. A hypoglycemic reaction
    3. The Somogyi phenomena
    4. Hyperosmolar, non-ketotic coma

110. A client is diagnosed as having diabetes mellitus. The nurse should expect the client's fasting blood glucose to be:
    1. 30 mg/100 ml
    2. 60 mg/100 ml
    3. 110 mg/100 ml
    4. 160 mg/100 ml

111. A young adult client who has a history of psychiatric problems and has been diagnosed as having an antisocial personality disorder is admitted to the hospital. The nurse should recognize that this client has probably had a long history of:
1. Sexual aberrations
2. Interpersonal difficulties
3. Stringent parental discipline
4. Diminished contact with reality

112. After delivery a neonate is given an injection of vitamin K. The nurse knows that this is done to:
1. Improve the absorption of biliary salts
2. Promote liver formation of clotting factors
3. Prolong the prothrombin time of the infant
4. Replace necessary bacteria in the intestine

113. A client with 36% of the body surface burned is receiving hydrotherapy. The best approach to wound care is to:
1. Use a consistent approach to care and encourage the client's participation
2. Prepare equipment while doing the procedure and explain interventions to the client
3. Change staff every 4 to 5 days and have the client select the time for the procedure to be done
4. Heat the water to 102°F to prevent loss of body temperature and prepare the equipment before starting

114. On admission to the mental health unit, a client with the diagnosis of schizophrenia, paranoid type says, "They all are trying to kill me. They all are." The nurse's best response would be:
1. "No one wants to hurt you."
2. "We are here to protect you."
3. "You are having very frightening thoughts."
4. "Tell me more about their wanting to kill you."

115. A nurse performs Leopold's maneuvers on a client who has been admitted in active labor. The examination reveals a soft rounded mass at the fundus, smooth irregular curvature on the right side of the abdomen, and bumpy projections on the left side. The fetal position is:
1. LSP
2. LOP
3. ROA
4. RScA

116. During the termination phase of a therapeutic relationship the client misses a series of appointments without any explanation. The nurse should:
1. Terminate the relationship immediately
2. Explore personal feelings with the supervisor
3. Contact the client to encourage another session
4. Attend the remaining designated meetings and wait

117. A major complication of hypertensive disease associated with pregnancy that the nurse should anticipate is:
1. Placenta previa
2. Isoimmunization
3. Oligohydramnios
4. Abruptio placentae

118. A 2-year-old child with cerebral palsy is admitted to the hospital for orthopedic surgery. During the admission interview the nurse should:
1. Tell the mother that her child will be put in a private room
2. Let the mother know at what hours she will be permitted to visit
3. Explain to the mother that the hospital will provide a pureed diet
4. Ask the mother about the therapy program used by the family at home

119. The nurse can determine that peristalsis has returned in a client who has had a gastrectomy when:

1. Borborygmi are auscultated
2. The feeling of nausea passes
3. The client has a bowel movement
4. The abdomen is no longer rigid and tender

120. An 8-year-old is being discharged after recovery from a sickle cell crisis. The nurse teaches the parents all the "dos and don'ts" concerning the child's care. The nurse is satisfied that the parents understand the principles of care when they state that they are:
1. Not allowing the child to play with other children
2. Keeping the child's fluid intake restricted at night
3. Getting the child a private tutor to help with school work
4. Not permitting the child to play soccer or go backpacking with the Scouts

121. Sterile warm saline soaks tid are ordered for a client with cellulitis from a puncture wound. A staff nurse has placed a clean basin, wash cloth, and protective pad at the bedside in preparation for the soak but is unable to continue the procedure. The nurse assigned to complete the soak should:
1. Continue the procedure as started
2. Collect new supplies before starting
3. Report the first nurse to the supervisor
4. Discuss the type of soak with the physician

122. A client was hospitalized because of an inability to walk. After a physiological basis for the problem was ruled out, a diagnosis of somatoform disorder, conversion type was made. The nurse realizes that the client's paralysis is a:
1. Nondisabling illness
2. Way of getting attention
3. Loss of contact with reality
4. Result of intrapsychic conflict

123. The diagnosis of placenta previa indicates to the nurse that the placenta is:

1. Infarcted
2. Low-lying
3. Immaturely developed
4. Separating prematurely

124. A client is scheduled for peritoneal dialysis. When explaining this procedure to the client, the nurse should review that its purpose is to:
1. Help do some of the work usually done by the kidneys
2. Prevent the development of complicating heart problems
3. Remove bad chemicals from the body so the condition will not worsen
4. Speed recovery because the kidneys are not responding to other therapy

125. An early symptom that the nurse commonly observes in newborns who are later diagnosed as having cystic fibrosis is:
1. Meconium ileus
2. Imperforate anus
3. Rapid respiratory rate
4. Elevated bilirubin level

126. The verbalizations of a client with schizophrenia contain many words that sound like the client is speaking a different language. The nurse recognizes that this communication is an example of:
1. Clanging
2. Echolalia
3. Neologisms
4. Echophrasia

127. The physician prescribes sulfamethoxazole and trimethoprim (Septra) for a sexually active female who has been experiencing frequency and burning on urination for 24 hours. The nurse knows the teaching about this medication was understood when the client says she will:
1. Strain all urine for calculi
2. Drink 6 glasses of water daily
3. Replace oral contraceptives with other methods
4. Notify the physician if the urine becomes orange

128. During an emergency delivery the nurse remembers that the most common complication associated with a too rapid expulsion of the fetus in a precipitate labor is:
 1. Pitting edema of the fetal scalp
 2. Prolonged retention of the placenta
 3. Dural or subdural tears in fetal brain tissue
 4. Premature separation of the placenta during the delivery

129. In the immediate postoperative period after coronary bypass surgery, the nurse should be particularly alert for the common complications of:
 1. Graft closure with recurrence of angina-like chest pain
 2. Supraventricular dysrhythmias, especially atrial fibrillation
 3. Postpericardotomy syndrome with fever and audible friction rub
 4. Elevation of hemoglobin and hematocrit levels with risk of embolization

130. A primary component of the nursing care plan for a client with bulimia nervosa would be:
 1. Intake and output
 2. Daily weighing before eating
 3. Careful observation after meals
 4. Daily room search for hoarded food

131. A client with a history of binge eating and purging is admitted to the eating disorder unit with a diagnosis of bulimia nervosa. The nurse is aware that bulimia nervosa can best be defined as the:
 1. Uncontrollable pilfering and hoarding of food for later consumption
 2. Refusal to eat in public and engaging in private excessive overeating
 3. Mood swings, ranging from euphoria to depression, associated with food
 4. Uncontrollable ingestion of large quantities of food in a short period of time

132. A child, who is newly diagnosed with idiopathic scoliosis, has a mild structural curve. The child's mother asks if the problem can be corrected with exercise and is told by the nurse that an exercise program will be:

 1. Used in conjunction with a Milwaukee brace
 2. Employed if the child appears highly motivated
 3. Avoided because it can exaggerate the curvature
 4. The only intervention needed to correct the curvature

133. A client with an acute exacerbation of rheumatoid arthritis is in severe pain and tells the nurse, "The only time I am pain-free is when I lie perfectly still." The nurse should explain that the client needs to exercise every day to prevent:
 1. Paresthesias of the feet
 2. Osteoblastic development
 3. Shortening of the muscles
 4. Loss of muscular coordination

134. By the third day of life an infant weighs 5% less than at birth. The nurse is aware that the weight loss most likely results from:
 1. The development of sepsis
 2. An obstructive gastrointestinal anomaly
 3. Generalized muscle response to stimuation
 4. An imbalance between nutrient intake and elimination

135. An obese client becomes pregnant and continues to gain excessive weight during pregnancy. The nurse understands that treating a client's obesity during pregnancy is not advisable because:
 1. Weight loss can best be achieved after pregnancy
 2. Additional calories are needed for her increased activity
 3. Calcium utilization varies proportionately with calorie intake
 4. Protein is utilized for energy when carbohydrates are decreased

136. A primigravida is admitted in active labor. The fetus is in a breech position. During this client's labor the nurse may note:
 1. Heavy bleeding from the vagina
 2. Irregularities of the fetal heart rate
 3. Meconium staining of the amniotic fluid
 4. Decelerations at the end of contractions

137. The nurse begins planning for the discharge of a client who had a cerebral vascular accident with residual hemiparesis and a hemianopia. Information which the nurse should include in the education program is the:
1. Importance of bedrest at home
2. Use of oxygen therapy at home
3. Importance of a safe environment
4. Need to decrease protein in the diet

138. The nurse is aware that a preschool child views death:
1. As permanent and irreversible
2. In a frightening and horrible way
3. As a departure from which the person returns
4. Without comprehending its meaning in any way

139. A 4-year-old is admitted with the diagnosis of Wilms' tumor. The nurse should place a sign on the child's bed that states:
1. Strain all urine
2. No IV medications
3. Do not use diapers
4. Do not palpate abdomen

140. A malnourished client with a history of cirrhosis is admitted with nausea, ascites, and gastrointestinal bleeding. The nurse recognizes that the ascites is primarily due to the client's malnourished state, especially the lack of adequate:
1. Iron to prevent proper hemoglobin synthesis
2. Vitamins to maintain cell coenzyme functions
3. Sodium to maintain its proper concentration in tissue fluid
4. Plasma protein to maintain proper capillary-tissue circulation

141. One morning during the working phase of a therapeutic relationship, the client suddenly becomes very hostile. The most appropriate interpretation of this behavior is that:

1. The client is exercising assertiveness, which implies improvement
2. Hostility is being used as a defense because the nurse has come too close
3. Flare-ups often occur when the nurse and client have a good working relationship
4. This behavior is a form of regression and implies deterioration in the client's condition

142. A 5-month-old is brought to the pediatric clinic because of probable exposure to an adolescent sibling with measles. The infant's mother anxiously asks the clinic nurse if the baby can be vaccinated against measles at this age. The nurse's reply should take into consideration the history of:
1. Immunization of this baby
2. Previous viral illnesses of this baby
3. Preexisting tuberculosis of the mother
4. Maternal diseases and immunizations

143. After attaching a cardiac monitor to a newly admitted client, the nurse notes six premature ventricular beats (PVBs) per minute. The nurse, following established protocols, should first:
1. Administer a bolus of cardiac Xylocaine
2. Obtain an orthostatic blood pressure reading
3. Encourage the client to cough and deep breathe
4. Initiate cardiopulmonary resuscitation on the client

144. Nursing care for a child admitted with acute glomerulonephritis should be directed toward:
1. Forcing fluids
2. Promoting diuresis
3. Enforcing strict bedrest
4. Eliminating sodium from the diet

145. A client who is an insulin dependent diabetic in her 34th week of pregnancy has been told by her physician that she may have to be delivered at about 38 weeks gestation instead of the usual 40 weeks. The client asks the nurse why an early delivery may be necessary. The best initial reply by the nurse would be:
    1. "Early delivery will reduce the chance of your infant developing hyperglycemia."
    2. "You need to be delivered early before the fetus gets too big to fit through the birth canal."
    3. "After 36 weeks the placenta may not be as efficient in providing for your fetus' needs."
    4. "You need to be delivered early so that you do not develop pregnancy-induced hypertension."

146. A 23-year-old male is admitted to the surgical unit with superficial wounds of both wrists as the result of an abortive suicide attempt. When the nurse enters the client's room, he states, "I suppose you're going to ask me about my suicide attempt!" The nurse's best response would be:
    1. "Do you want to talk about it?"
    2. "Tell me how you feel about it."
    3. "It's best not to dwell on it right now."
    4. "Why do you think I'd ask you about it?"

147. A 22-year-old client with an antisocial personality disorder is being discharged after an abortive suicide attempt and is to continue psychotherapy on an outpatient basis. When evaluating chances for improvement, the nurse recognizes that:
    1. The client's prognosis for adjusting to a limited lifestyle is excellent
    2. The client will not change unless the client's parents are willing to set and keep firm limits
    3. The client requires intensive psychotherapy combined with tranquilizers to produce a remission
    4. The client will not change unless there is a readiness to accept the pain associated with change

148. A client is placed on a 1500 calorie diet. The client should be taught that 1 gram of carbohydrate contains:

    1. 2 calories
    2. 4 calories
    3. 9 calories
    4. 12 calories

149. After a normal vaginal delivery, the nurse should plan the postpartum care of a Class 1 cardiac client based on the knowledge that:
    1. The client should increase her fluid intake, particularly if she is breastfeeding
    2. The client is out of immediate danger because the stress of pregnancy is over
    3. Clients with cardiac problems should be kept on bedrest for a minimum of 7 days
    4. The first 48 hours postpartum are the most stressful on the cardiopulmonary system

150. A child with leukemia is receiving vincristine. Nursing care for this child includes checking and recording bowel sounds bid. This action is necessary because a side effect of this drug is:
    1. Decreased innervation of the GI tract
    2. Hyperactivity of the bowel from diarrhea
    3. Nausea that decreases fluid intake and produces constipation
    4. Increased antigen/antibody reactions which cause edematous bowels

151. A client with lymphosarcoma is receiving allopurinol (Zyloprim) and methotrexate. The nurse can help the client prevent complications related to uric acid nephropathy by administering the:
    1. Allopurinol and promoting urine acidity
    2. Methotrexate after providing an antacid
    3. Allopurinol and encouraging the intake of fluid
    4. Methotrexate and restricting the intake of fluid

152. A client who had an above-the-knee amputation has an elastic bandage around the stump. The physician's orders include bathing the stump daily and rewrapping the elastic bandage prn. The nurse should:
    1. Reapply it only if the bandage slips off
    2. Apply it tightly so that it does not slip off
    3. Apply it smoothly without wrinkles or creases
    4. Reapply it while the stump is in the dependent position

153. A client receiving levodopa experiences orthostatic hypotension, a side effect of drug therapy. To help limit this adaptation the nurse should:
1. Initiate gait training
2. Apply elastic stockings
3. Withhold the next dose
4. Increase the fluid intake

154. A client, with a history of placenta previa in a previous pregnancy, is scheduled for an ultrasound. When preparing the client for the sonography the nurse should tell her to:
1. Empty her bladder before the ultrasound
2. Avoid eating for eight hours before the test
3. Take a laxative the night before the sonogram
4. Force fluids for one hour before the ultrasound

155. Before irrigating a client's nasogastric tube, the nurse must first:
1. Assess breath sounds
2. Instill 15 ml of normal saline
3. Auscultate for bowel sounds
4. Check the tube for placement

156. When helping to break the vicious cycle of fear, dyspnea, and avoidance of activities commonly found in clients with chronic obstructive pulmonary disease (COPD), the nurse should place primary emphasis in the teaching program on:
1. Learning to control or prevent respiratory infections
2. Education about the disease and breathing exercises
3. Teaching about priorities in carrying out daily activities
4. Judicious use of aerosol therapy, especially nebulizers

157. While caring for a client during a manic episode of a bipolar disorder the initial priority in planning care would be:

1. Arranging for the client to participate in a daily discussion group
2. Encouraging frequent close contact with the staff and a few selected clients
3. Reducing the number of people interacting with the client during any given day
4. Varying the staff assigned to care for the client to reduce the opportunity for manipulation

158. One evening, an elderly client with the diagnosis of dementia chokes on a piece of food and becomes panicky and cyanotic. The nurse performs the abdominal thrust maneuver and a wad of food pops out of the client's mouth. After several deep respirations the client's cyanosis passes. It would be most appropriate at this time for the nurse to:
1. Inform the client that everything is fine
2. Stand the client up and check the pulse
3. Provide psychological support to the client
4. Teach the client how to prevent future problems

159. A couple bring their 5-year-old daughter to the emergency room with a broken arm and contusions. It is decided that the child is a victim of abuse. Through conversation with the parents and the child, the nurse is unsure who is responsible for the abuse. The nurse suspects it may be the mother because of her:
1. Assertive and dominating personality
2. Effective use of defense mechanisms
3. Isolation and lack of emotional support
4. Lack of knowledge about child development

160. When assessing the rate of involution of a client's uterus on the second postpartum day, the nurse palpating the fundus would expect it to be:
1. At the level of the umbilicus
2. One fingerbreadth above the umbilicus
3. One to two fingerbreadths below the umbilicus
4. Three to four fingerbreadths below the umbilicus

161. Several days after a client has had a total laryngectomy, the physician orders a progressive diet as tolerated. The nurse should:
1. Keep a suction apparatus readily available in case aspiration occurs
2. Administer the diet through a nasogastric tube until the suture line heals
3. Encourage intake of pureed foods because they promote the swallowing reflex
4. Administer pain medication as ordered 30 minutes before meals to limit discomfort

162. For a few days following the repair of a cleft lip, an infant should be fed by:
1. Nasogastric tube
2. Intravenous infusion
3. A rubber-tipped syringe
4. A bottle with a preemie nipple

163. Nursing care for a client following surgery for a ruptured tubal pregnancy should include:
1. Assuring her that she is still capable of becoming pregnant
2. Administering Rho (D) immune globulin (RhoGAM) to prevent isoimmunization
3. Counseling for an intrauterine device (IUD) to prevent another tubal pregnancy
4. Telling her not to douche after intercourse because this may dislodge a fertilized egg

164. A nurse assesses a client who is experiencing a crisis and formulates a nursing diagnosis. The nursing diagnosis that is made could be defined as a statement:
1. To explain the client's present needs
2. That describes the client's health status and related factors
3. Of the client's responses that are within the scope of nursing
4. That rewords the client's medical diagnosis in nursing terminology

165. Gamma globulin and aspirin are ordered for a 3-year-old with Kawasaki disease. When administering the aspirin to the child the nurse should:

1. Disguise the medication in the child's favorite food
2. Let the child decide how the medication will be taken
3. Offer the child a reward for taking the prescribed medication
4. Not respond to questions about the taste of the drug to avoid lying

166. A client is in labor. When her cervix is 3 to 4 cm dilated and 60% effaced and the vertex is at −1 station, the client has a sudden spurt of dark blood from the vagina. The uterus is irritable on palpation and does not relax well between contractions. The nurse should immediately:
1. Transport her to the delivery room without delay
2. Perform a vaginal examination to determine dilation
3. Check her BP and FHR and monitor her uterine activity
4. Change the client's underpad and position her on her back

167. A 50-year-old male client has difficulty communicating because of expressive aphasia following a cerebral vascular accident. When the nurse asks the client how he is feeling, his wife answers for him. The nurse should:
1. Ask the wife how she knows how the client feels
2. Instruct the wife to let the client answer for himself
3. Acknowledge the wife but look at the client for a response
4. Return later to speak to the client after the wife has gone home

168. The physician orders dexamethasone (Decadron) for a client following a craniotomy for a brain tumor. The nurse recognizes that the expected response to this drug should be:
1. Reduced cerebral edema
2. Reduced cell proliferation
3. Increased renal reabsorption
4. Increased response to sedation

169. The physician orders aspirin therapy to be continued at home for a client with severe arthritis. When teaching regarding aspirin intake, the nurse should emphasize that the client should:
1. Switch to Tylenol if tinnitus occurs
2. See the dentist if bleeding gums develop
3. Avoid spicy foods while taking the medication
4. Take the medicine on a full stomach or with meals

170. A child who has head lice tells the school nurse, "My mother said I got lice because I don't keep myself clean." The nurse's best reply to this statement would be:
1. "You feel that your mother is putting you down?"
2. "You have problems getting along with your mother?"
3. "There is no relationship between cleanliness and lice."
4. "Lice are more common if you have poor personal hygiene."

171. Prior to obtaining informed consent for cardiac bypass surgery from a client the nurse should:
1. Explain to the client the risks involved in the surgery
2. Explain to the client that obtaining the signature is routine for surgery
3. Evaluate whether the client's knowledge level is sufficient to give consent
4. Witness the client's signature, since this is what the nurse's signature documents

172. One of the adaptations associated with toxoplasmosis that the nurse might observe when assessing an infant affected with this disease is:
1. Small size for the gestational age
2. Pigmentation spots on the buttocks
3. A head circumference of 34 cm (13.5 inches)
4. Irregular respirations when the infant is awake

173. A client who has repeated episodes of cystitis is scheduled for a cystoscopy to determine the possibility of urinary abnormalities. In answer to the client's questions the nurse describes the procedure as:
1. A computerized scan that clearly outlines the bladder and surrounding tissue
2. An x-ray film of the abdomen, kidneys, ureters, and bladder after administration of dye
3. The visualization of the urinary tract through ureteral catheterization using a radiopaque material
4. The visualization of the inside of the bladder with an instrument connected to a source of illumination

174. The nurse is aware that the most appropriate toy for a 2½-year-old would be a:
1. Plastic mirror
2. Set of nesting blocks
3. Colorful hanging mobile
4. Wooden puzzle with large pieces

175. After her 6-week-old baby's surgery for pyloric stenosis, the mother is reluctant to resume feeding the baby but readily in favor of assisting with all other aspects of infant care. The care plan for this infant specifically states that the mother should be encouraged to participate in the oral feedings. The rationale for the focus of nursing care is that the mother is:
1. Unaware that family involvement in care is permitted
2. Uncertain of how the thickened oral feedings are administered
3. Reluctant to feed the baby because of the present need to use a special nipple
4. Probably afraid to resume feedings because of the frequent vomiting before surgery

176. A client with cirrhosis of the liver and ascites fails to respond to chlorothiazide, and spironolactone (Aldactone) is prescribed in addition to the chlorothiazide. The advantage of Aldactone is that it:
    1. Stimulates H_2O excretion
    2. Stimulates sodium excretion
    3. Helps prevent potassium loss
    4. Reduces arterial blood pressure

177. The nurse can best initially prepare a client for the termination of their relationship by:
    1. Periodically summarizing the client's progress during the working phase
    2. Stating that, if the client feels it is necessary, their meetings could be extended
    3. Telling the client how long they will be working together during their first meeting
    4. Waiting until the termination phase, then reminding the client periodically of the duration of their meetings

178. The nurse would know that a client who had a mastectomy understands the discharge teaching when she states she will report to the physician any:
    1. Persistent itching around the incision
    2. Swelling and erythema around the incision
    3. Slightly irregular appearing skin around the incision
    4. Decreased sensations in the area around the incision

179. A client is brought to the emergency room with chest pain. The doctor orders an electrocardiogram (ECG). The client asks the nurse, "What is the purpose of this test?" The nurse replies, "This test will:
    1. Enable us to detect heart sounds."
    2. Enable us to detect heart damage."
    3. Help us to change your heart rhythm."
    4. Tell us how much stress your heart can endure."

180. When obtaining a health history of a 7-year-old admitted with acute glomerulonephritis, the nurse would expect the child's mother to report that:

    1. The child had a sore throat 3 weeks ago
    2. The child had just gotten over the measles
    3. The child's father has a history of urinary infections
    4. The child's immunizations for camp were completed last week

181. A 24-year-old client who has had insulin dependent diabetes for the past 6 years is concerned about how her pregnancy will affect her diabetes, especially her diet and insulin needs. The nurse should inform the client that pregnancy:
    1. Decreases the need for insulin because the excess glucose will be used by the fetus for growth
    2. Is a normal state, and that a revised diet and her usual insulin regimen will meet her and the fetus' needs
    3. Increases the need for protein, and adjustments have to be made to meet the need for increasing doses of insulin
    4. Will vary her diet and insulin needs, and she will have to monitor her blood glucose more often to make appropriate adjustments

182. A child with asthma is being discharged from the hospital on oral theophylline. The nurse recognizes that the parents understand the discharge teaching when they tell the nurse that they will monitor the child for the side effect of:
    1. Apneic episodes
    2. Frequent urination
    3. Nausea and vomiting
    4. Spasmodic hiccoughs

183. The primary difficulty in establishing long-range goals for clients with an antisocial personality disorder is related to the fact that such clients are usually:
    1. Reluctant to change their lifestyle
    2. Unwilling to accept their need for help
    3. Unable to deal with their feelings of guilt
    4. Resistant to any demonstration of feeling

184. A client with insulin dependent diabetes mellitus is taught the symptoms associated with hypoglycemia. The nurse would know

that the teaching was understood when the client states, "I will know I am having an insulin reaction when I experience:
1. Confusion, vomiting, and rapid deep breathing
2. Thirst and excessive urination and have blurred vision
3. Generalized nervousness, headache, and perspiration
4. Abdominal pain and nausea and have a fruity odor to my breath."

185. A 32-year-old client who had rheumatic fever as a child is now pregnant. She is classified as having Class 1 heart disease. Although this client will experience some symptoms during her pregnancy that are related to her cardiac pathology, she will also probably experience some normal symptoms of pregnancy such as:
1. Tachycardia
2. Dyspnea at rest
3. Progressive dependent edema
4. Shortness of breath on exertion

186. A 5-year-old boy with suspected leukemia is to have a bone marrow aspiration. Before the procedure the child should be told that:
1. He will be put to sleep and will not feel anything
2. After the test is over he will have to stay in bed until supper
3. He will feel a little pressure and when it's over a Bandaid will be applied
4. He will have a few stitches at the site, but he can get up and go to the playroom

187. A client is scheduled for an ileostomy. Preoperative teaching should include a statement that:
1. Skin irritation at the stoma site will occur easily
2. Fecal matter from the stoma can be controlled by daily irrigation
3. Regular bowel habits can be established within a few weeks postoperatively
4. Effluent discharge from the stoma will be formed fecal matter if diet is regulated

188. The physician orders Dextrose 5% in Water with 20 mEq of KCl per liter to infuse at 75 ml/hour. The client has a 250 ml bag of Dextrose 5% in Water infusing with 150 ml left in the bag. To deliver the ordered amount of potassium chloride without hanging a new bag of solution, the nurse should add to the remaining IV fluid:
1. 3 mEq KCl
2. 5 mEq KCl
3. 10 mEq KCl
4. 20 mEq KCl

189. Following a resection of the colon, a client returns from the operating room with a nasogastric tube in place. The nurse understands that the purpose of this tube is to:
1. Monitor the acidity of the gastric secretions
2. Provide a route for liquid tube feeding when possible
3. Permit continuous decompression of the large intestine
4. Remove fluids and gas from the upper gastrointestinal tract

190. While undergoing chemotherapy with doxorubicin (Adriamycin) for Hodgkin's disease, it is most essential for the client to immediately report to the nurse the presence of:
1. Nausea
2. A sore throat
3. A loss of hair
4. Constipation

191. A client with a chest tube is to be transported via a stretcher. When transporting the client, the nurse should keep the:
1. Collection device attached to mechanical suction
2. Collection device below the level of the client's chest
3. End of the chest tube covered with sterile 4x4s securely taped
4. Chest tube clamped between the water seal chamber and the client

192. If antithyroid medication is not effective in decreasing the symptoms associated with hyperthyroidism, an additional health problem may develop as a result of continued tachycardia. The nurse should tell the client taking an antithyroid medication to immediately report the development of:
    1. Nervousness and irritability
    2. Weight gain or pedal edema
    3. Flushed skin and diaphoresis
    4. Changes in appetite or bowel habits

193. Studies have shown that the grieving process may last longer for people who have:
    1. Feelings of guilt
    2. Failed to remarry within three years
    3. Ambivalent feelings about the death
    4. Had a close relationship with their family

194. A client with a ruptured tubal pregnancy is experiencing sharp shooting pains in the right lower quadrant of the abdomen. There is also vaginal spotting present. In view of the symptoms, the nurse should expect to prepare the client for a:
    1. Myomectomy
    2. Hysterectomy
    3. Salpingectomy
    4. Dilation and curettage

195. A couple interested in family planning asks the nurse about the cervical mucus method of family planning. The nurse explains that with this method the couple must avoid intercourse when the cervical mucus is:
    1. Clear and thick
    2. Yellow and thin
    3. Cloudy and viscid
    4. Clear and stretchable

196. Following an ECT treatment, a client complains of loss of memory. The nurse should reply:
    1. "I will help you try to remember when the treatments are over."
    2. "It is better if you forget what happened before you became ill."
    3. "The fact that you are getting well is the most important thing for you right now."
    4. "This is only temporary; your memory will return after the therapy is completed."

197. When caring for clients who are at risk for suicide, the nurse should be aware that:
    1. A client who fails in a suicide attempt will probably not try again
    2. It is best not to talk to clients about suicide because it may give them the idea
    3. The more formalized the plan, the greater the possibility that the client will attempt suicide
    4. Clients who talk about suicide never commit suicide; they just use the threat to gain attention

198. A wife, after visiting her husband who has been hospitalized with chest pain, says to the nurse, "He looks so pale." The nurse should reply:
    1. "Paleness is expected with heart problems."
    2. "You both must be terribly frightened by this."
    3. "I can understand why you are worried, but he will be all right."
    4. "Other clients get pale and recover without any complications."

199. A client with Parkinson's disease begins carbidopa-levodopa (Sinemet). A nursing priority should be to:
    1. Observe sleeping patterns weekly
    2. Assess the vital signs every 4 hours
    3. Perform a physical assessment daily
    4. Monitor the intake and output every 8 hours

200. A client, pregnant for the first time, questions the nurse about all the changes in her body. The nurse, when explaining these changes, is aware that the most profound change of all during pregnancy occurs in the:
    1. Urinary system
    2. Endocrine system
    3. Cardiovascular system
    4. Gastrointestinal system

201. The total bile drainage from a T-tube 24 hours after gallbladder surgery is 150 ml. The nurse should:

1. Clamp the T-tube and drain small amounts of bile every 4 hours
2. Empty the drainage bag and record amount on the I and O record
3. Check the tube for kinks because the drainage is less than expected
4. Notify the physician immediately of the excessive amount of bile drainage

202. A client with asthma is receiving intravenous aminophylline. The adverse reaction for which the nurse should observe is:
   1. Oliguria
   2. Bradycardia
   3. Hypotension
   4. Hypoventilation

203. Chelation therapy injections cause local discomfort. To relieve some of this discomfort the nurse should:
   1. Apply warm soaks to the affected area
   2. Give the child a cool tub bath after each injection
   3. Assist the child to ambulate immediately after each injection
   4. Vigorously massage the affected injection site with an alcohol swab

204. A nurse observes a new mother timidly approach her preterm son for the first time in the neonatal intensive care nursery. To aid the mother in the bonding process, the nurse should say to the mother:
   1. "He'll gain weight gradually and look better."
   2. "I will give you instructions on how to care for him."
   3. "It must be hard to let yourself love a baby when you're not sure he'll make it."
   4. "Many mothers are shocked when they first see their babies; you'll see him grow."

205. When working with clients who are spontaneously aborting a pregnancy, it is important for nurses to first deal with their own feelings about abortion, death, and loss so that they can:
   1. Share personal grief with the clients
   2. Allow the clients to express grief fully
   3. Maintain complete control of the situation
   4. Teach the clients to cope more effectively

206. The nurse assists a client, who has had a cerebral vascular accident, with lunch. The nurse suspects left hemianopia when the client:
   1. Asks to have all food moved to the left side of the tray
   2. Drops the coffee cup when trying to use the right hand
   3. Ignores the food on the left side of the tray when eating
   4. Complains about not being able to use the left arm to help eat

207. Before discharging a 4-year-old girl after a right nephrectomy for Wilms' tumor, the nurse teaches the parents that precautions will have to be taken to preserve the remaining kidney. The nurse is aware that the parents understand the teaching when they say, "We will:
   1. Limit our daughter's fluid intake to 3 glasses daily."
   2. Allow our daughter to participate in sports when she is older."
   3. Keep our daughter away from those individuals with infections."
   4. Teach our daughter to wipe from front to back after going to the bathroom."

208. A client delivers an infant by cesarean delivery. It is suspected that the infant has Down syndrome when the initial assessment reveals:
   1. Low-set ears, micrognathia, and rocker bottom feet
   2. High-pitched catlike cry, microcephaly, and low set ears
   3. Hypotonia, low-set ears, simian crease, and epicanthal folds
   4. Lymphedema of dorsum of hands and feet, webbed neck, and widely spaced nipples

209. A client is pregnant with her first child. About the eighth or ninth week of gestation, an assessment of the client's adaptations to pregnancy would reveal:
   1. Lightening
   2. Quickening
   3. Goodell's sign
   4. Braxton-Hicks' contractions

...

210. A client who has an adenocarcinoma of the descending colon with a partial obstruction is receiving doxorubicin (Adriamycin) IV to reduce the tumor mass. The nurse should assess for signs of toxicity which include:
1. A minor skin rash
2. A blue tinge to the urine
3. An alteration in cardiac rhythm
4. An increased feeling of nervousness

211. The first child of adolescent parents is brought to the pediatric unit with a diagnosis of nonorganic failure to thrive (NFTT). In light of this diagnosis and the family structure the priority nursing diagnosis for this family would be:
1. Altered parenting related to knowledge deficit
2. High risk for injury related to mothering failure
3. Altered nutrition: less than body requirements related to child abuse
4. Sensory-perceptual alterations (gustatory) related to infant deprivation

212. A client with an enlarged thyroid gland is referred to the laboratory for a radioactive iodine (RAI) uptake test. When teaching about this test, the nurse should explain that:
1. The urine will not contain any radioactive particles
2. Test results will not be influenced by any medications
3. This test is one of several needed for an accurate diagnosis
4. An accurate measure of thyroid hormone levels will be obtained

213. Formulating a nursing diagnosis for all clients, including clients experiencing a crisis, occurs during the stage of the nursing process known as:
1. Analysis
2. Planning
3. Evaluation
4. Assessment

214. A client with an abdominal aortic aneurysm, being prepared for surgery, complains of feeling light-headed. The client is pale and has a very rapid pulse. The nurse assesses that the client may be:

1. Hyperventilating
2. Going into shock
3. Extremely anxious
4. Developing an infection

215. Following a cleft lip repair, the nurse places elbow restraints on a 10-week-old infant boy. The mother questions the nurse about the reason for the restraints. The nurse's best response would be:
1. "They are used routinely on all children with lip surgery."
2. "The surgeon insists that all postoperative infants have them on."
3. "By keeping the arms straight, it is difficult for the hands to touch the mouth."
4. "We can't be with your child all the time to watch that the hands do not touch the mouth."

216. The mother of a ten-week-old infant demonstrates good understanding of the infant's postoperative needs following a cleft lip repair when she:
1. Cleanses the suture line after each feeding
2. Allows the infant to cry for short periods of time
3. Offers a pacifier when the infant becomes restless
4. Gives the feeding while the infant is in a side-lying position

217. A client who has had a total laryngectomy is using a pad and pencil to communicate. The client becomes very frustrated and writes, "When can I learn how to speak again?" The nurse's best response would be:
1. "Every client is different. It's difficult to say just how long it will be."
2. "It must be difficult for you, but be patient. These things take time."
3. "You have to give the incision time to heal before going to speech therapy."
4. "Perhaps I can arrange for a member of the Laryngectomy Club to speak with you."

218. A client is placed on a low-sodium, weight-reducing diet following a myocardial infarction. The nurse knows that the dietary teaching was effective when the client chooses:

1. Lean steak and carrots
2. Tuna fish salad with celery sticks
3. Baked chicken and mashed potatoes
4. Stir-fried Chinese vegetables and rice

219. On the day after delivery a client mentions that her nipples are becoming sore from breastfeeding. The nurse should:
1. Instruct her to apply warm compresses before she begins to breastfeed
2. Provide a breast shield for her to keep the infant's mouth off the nipples
3. Assess her breastfeeding and hygiene techniques to identify possible causes
4. Instruct her to limit breastfeeding to 5 minutes per side until the soreness subsides

220. While caring for a client who had an open reduction and internal fixation of the hip, the nurse encourages active leg and foot exercises of the unaffected leg every 2 hours. This activity will specifically help to:
1. Reduce leg discomfort
2. Maintain muscle strength
3. Prevent formation of clots
4. Limit venous inflammation

221. When providing teaching about a 2-gram sodium diet, the nurse should instruct the client to:
1. Use lemon juice to season meat
2. Refrain from eating canned fruits
3. Restrict the intake of green vegetables
4. Drink carbonated beverages instead of decaffeinated coffee

222. A child is receiving an IV of 500 ml of D5 $\frac{1}{2}$NS at 55 ml/hour via a microdrip set. The flow rate should be regulated at:
1. 55 gtt/minute
2. 60 gtt/minute
3. 9 to 10 gtt/minute
4. 13 to 14 gtt/minute

223. When planning care for an 85-year-old newly admitted client with the diagnosis of dementia of the Alzheimer type, the nurse should remember that confusion in the elderly:

1. Follows transfer to new surroundings
2. Is always progressive and will get worse
3. Is a common finding and is to be expected with aging
4. Results from brain pathology and cannot be cured or stopped

224. The mother of a young man suspected of having Cushing's syndrome expresses anxiety about her son's condition. To help the mother better understand the illness, the nurse should inform her that:
1. He will need to take exogenous steroids for several months
2. His condition is improving as demonstrated by his weight gain
3. His physical changes are permanent but will improve with time
4. He may have mood swings or depression as a result of his disease

225. At 5 AM, two hours after a vaginal delivery, a client is transferred to the postpartum unit. When planning morning care for this client, the nurse's highest priority would be:
1. Arranging an individual session in which the client can learn all that is necessary about successful breastfeeding
2. Preparing for the probability of hemorrhage and assessing the client's uterus every 15 minutes for firmness and position
3. Anticipating possible safety needs and instructing the client to remain in bed and call for assistance before attempting to ambulate
4. Planning activities so that the client has time to rest and offering mild analgesics as ordered and other comfort measures to facilitate this rest

226. X-rays reveal that a client has sustained an intracapsular fracture of the left hip during a fall. The client is temporarily placed in Buck's traction. When providing care the nurse should:
1. Turn the client from side to side every 2 hours
2. Monitor the client for tenderness in the left calf
3. Put each extremity through passive range of motion
4. Raise the head of the bed to a semi-Fowler's position

227. When making rounds a nurse finds a client having a seizure. The nurse should:
1. Hyperextend the client's neck
2. Move obstacles away from the client
3. Restrain the client's head and limb movements
4. Attempt to place an airway in the client's mouth

228. A child with meningitis suddenly assumes an opisthotonic position. The nurse should place the child in a:
1. Side-lying position
2. Knee-chest position
3. High-Fowler's position
4. Trendelenburg position

229. When caring for a client after an ileostomy, the nurse should expect drainage from the ileostomy in the first 24 to 48 postoperative hours to be:
1. Fecal with flatus
2. Bloody with clots
3. Clear with mucoid shreds
4. Mucoid and serosanguinous

230. A client with sprue develops signs of tetany. The nurse is aware that this is caused by inadequate absorption of:
1. Sodium
2. Calcium
3. Potassium
4. Phosphorus

231. The ritual of a female client with an obsessive compulsive personality disorder focuses on checking her pocketbook for her keys and other belongings every four minutes. If prevented from doing this, she gets quite upset. The nurse should:
1. Allow her to continue to check her pocketbook for as long as she wants and wait for her to get tired
2. Keep her actively involved in projects to distract her so she will forget about checking her pocketbook
3. Lock her pocketbook in a safe place in the morning, thereby relieving her of the necessity to check it
4. Allow the behavior, but with the client's agreement, set limits on the amount of time and the frequency of the checks

232. The physician has ordered alternate liters of D5W and D5RL at the rate of 175 ml/hour. The drop factor of the IV set is 15 gtt/ml. The nurse should adjust the flow to provide:
1. 40 gtt/min
2. 42 gtt/min
3. 44 gtt/min
4. 46 gtt/min

233. A client returns from surgery after an abdominal cholecystectomy for a gangrenous gallbladder. The location of the surgical site high in the abdominal cavity places the client at high risk for the postoperative complication of:
1. Atelectasis
2. Hemorrhage
3. Paralytic ileus
4. Wound infection

234. A client with chronic obstructive pulmonary disease (COPD) continues to smoke and does not perform the prescribed chest physiotherapy exercises because they cause fatigue. The nursing diagnosis that is most indicated for this client is:
1. Self-care deficit related to fatigue
2. Altered thought processes related to cerebral hypoxia
3. Noncompliance with therapeutic regimen related to nonacceptance
4. Knowledge deficit related to causal relationship of smoking to lung disease

235. Chelation therapy with Ca EDTA is started on a child with chronic lead poisoning. The nurse can evaluate the success of this therapy by monitoring for:
1. Elevated blood lead levels
2. Increased fecal excretion of lead
3. Increased urinary excretion of lead
4. Decreased deposition of lead in the bones

236. While observing a mother visiting her preterm infant son in the neonatal intensive care nursery, the nurse recognizes that the mother has still not begun the normal bonding process when the mother says:
1. "It looks like such a tiny baby."
2. "Do you think he will make it?"
3. "He looks so much like my husband."
4. "Why does he need to be in an incubator?"

237. Clinical manifestations of Cushing's syndrome that the nurse might observe in a client who is suspected of having a pituitary tumor include:
1. Retention of sodium and water
2. Hypotension and a rapid, thready pulse
3. Increased fatty deposition in the extremities
4. Hypoglycemic episodes in the early morning

238. An elderly client, whose conformance to social norms, hygiene, and dress requirements has deteriorated over the last three months is admitted to the psychiatric unit. The nurse notes the client seems quite anxious, frequently paces about, has a short attention span, and is very forgetful. The nurse can best cope with the behaviors associated with dementia by:
1. Providing a restrictive environment, including restraints, to prevent self-injury
2. Ignoring instances when denial is used as well as the client's memory lapses
3. Consistently having all staff members reinforce reality with each client contact
4. Focusing on the client's coping skills to avoid precipitating feelings of inadequacy

239. A 4-year-old is admitted to the hospital to rule out a leukemic process. On admission the most important nursing assessment is to determine:
1. The parents' ability to cope in stressful situations
2. What the child has been told about the diagnosis
3. The child's growth percentile and developmental abilities
4. The child's previous experience with illness and hospitalization

240. A client who has had a tremendous weight loss is told by the physician that more protein foods must be eaten to provide the needed essential amino acids. The client asks the nurse why these substances in protein foods are "essential." The nurse should respond:
1. "They will give you the added energy you need."
2. "They are essential for rebuilding your body tissue protein."
3. "They contain the necessary nitrogen you need for healing."
4. "Your body can't make them so you must get them in your food."

241. The physician prescribes regular insulin each morning for a client with diabetes mellitus. After administering the insulin at 8:00 AM, the nurse should observe the client for a potential insulin reaction:
1. At breakfast
2. Before lunch
3. Before dinner
4. In the early afternoon

242. A male client with a history of an antisocial personality disorder is admitted to a medical unit. The client threatens the staff and other clients. He refuses to turn off his television set at bedtime and is often found in other clients' rooms. One client on the unit states that a watch is missing, and another has lost a wallet. The nurse's best response to this situation would be to:
1. Call the hospital security and tell them the client is stealing
2. Have the client transferred to the psychiatric unit or discharged
3. Tell the client that the staff knows he took the articles in question
4. Search the client's belongings for the missing articles without telling him

243. An 8-year-old with a history of severe asthma is admitted to the hospital after an asthma attack at home. The child is extremely short of breath. To facilitate breathing and to promote respiratory drainage, the nurse should place the child in a:
1. Supine position
2. Left-lateral position
3. High-Fowler's position
4. Trendelenburg position

244. A client who has been severely burned receives an autograft. One week after the graft the client, who has been taught to do dressing changes, notices the edges of the graft curling up and asks the nurse about it. The nurse's best response would be:
1. "May I take a look at it?"
2. "It's time for another graft."
3. "Let me see if it is infected."
4. "Is there any sign of redness?"

245. A male client with the diagnosis of schizophrenia, paranoid type appears very suspicious of the nurse. The most effective approach to this problem would be for the nurse to:
1. Assign various caregivers to the client
2. Make brief, frequent contacts with the client
3. Engage the client in a discussion about his thoughts
4. Allow the client to stay in his room without interruption

246. The coach of a primigravida in active labor for about 6 hours asks the nurse, "How much longer will this take? She is having a lot of back pain and is so uncomfortable." The nurse could best respond:
1. "It shouldn't be much longer now."
2. "I think you should take a break for awhile."
3. "Everything is progressing nicely as expected."
4. "Let me show you how to provide back pressure."

247. On the first postoperative day after a mastectomy, the nurse encourages the client to perform exercises such as flexion and extension of fingers and pronation and supination of the forearm. These interventions are done primarily to:
1. Preserve muscle tone
2. Prevent joint contractures
3. Assess extent of lymphedema
4. Stimulate peripheral circulation

248. A client with a history of a ruptured nucleus pulposus is scheduled for a total hip replacement. To prevent the most common complication associated with total hip replacement surgery, the nurse should teach the client to perform:
1. Straight leg raises
2. Burger-Allen exercises
3. Deep-breathing and coughing
4. Plantar- and dorsiflexion exercises

249. A client with a chronic progressive disease repeatedly expresses the fear of becoming a burden and states, "I want to die." The client asks the nurse for help. Before responding, the nurse recognizes that a nurse actively or passively aiding a client with euthanasia is:
1. Liable to be tried for a crime
2. Acting within the law in most states
3. Practicing medicine without a license
4. Negligent in performing nursing duties

250. On the third postpartum day a client tells the nurse that her breasts feel warm, firm, and tender. The skin appears shiny and taut. The nurse suspects that the cause of the client's breast discomfort is:
1. Overdistention of the acini with milk
2. Stasis of milk in the mammary ducts
3. Inadequate emptying of the breast during each feeding
4. Increased lymphatic and venous circulation in the breasts

251. An elderly client with a chronic degenerative disease progresses to the stage where self care is no longer possible, and admission to a nursing home becomes necessary. According to Erikson the major developmental conflict for this client would be:
1. Intimacy vs isolation
2. Identity vs role diffusion
3. Ego integrity vs despair
4. Generativity vs stagnation

252. A thirteen-year-old with newly diagnosed idiopathic scoliosis is very upset about the treatment regimen and is worried about being different from friends. To help the child develop a positive self-image during treatment the nurse should:
1. Refer the child for psychologic counseling until the treatment program is over
2. Remind the child how crooked the back would be if treatment were not started
3. Exaggerate the child's positive attributes and avoid focusing on negative attributes
4. Assist the mother to help the child select appropriate clothing to minimize the condition

253. While walking to the examination room with the nurse, a toddler with autism suddenly runs over and begins head-banging on the wall. The nurse's initial action should be to:
1. Allow the toddler to act out feelings
2. Ask the toddler to stop this behavior
3. Restrain the toddler to prevent head injury
4. Tell the toddler that the behavior is unacceptable

254. After a cardiac catheterization, a client is discharged and is scheduled to return for coronary bypass surgery. The client asks, "When I get chest pain at home, how will I know if I should call the doctor?" The nurse should teach the client to call the physician if the pain:
1. Radiates to the arms, neck, or jaw
2. Is accompanied by mild diaphoresis
3. Repeatedly occurs after mild exercise
4. Is not relieved by rest or by nitroglycerin

255. Before a client's scheduled open heart surgery, the nurse should plan to include in the teaching plan a:
1. Thorough discussion of discharge plans
2. Detailed description of the surgical procedure
3. Visit by a postanesthesia-unit nursing staff member
4. Discussion of the specific areas of the body that will be shaved

256. Immediately after assisting with an emergency delivery, the nurse should be especially concerned with:
1. Expelling the placenta
2. Keeping the infant warm
3. Cutting the umbilical cord
4. Controlling maternal bleeding

257. The nurse should expect the physician's orders for a client with moderate pregnancy-induced hypertension to include:
1. Bedrest, intake and output, diuretics
2. Diuretics, low-salt diet, intake and output
3. Daily weights, glucose monitoring, bedrest
4. Intake and output, daily weights, high-protein diet

258. A mother, whose infant was diagnosed with cerebral palsy at 6 months of age, asks why she was not told that her baby had cerebral palsy when the infant was born. The nurse should reply:
1. "The joint deformities of cerebral palsy appear only after 6 months of age."
2. "The health care personnel in the clinic did not want to alarm you until it was necessary."
3. "The neurologic lesions responsible for the child's condition may have changed as the child matured."
4. "Early diagnosis of cerebral palsy is difficult in infants until they develop control of voluntary movements."

259. The nurse is aware that the genotypic make-up of the parents of a child with sickle cell anemia is:
1. Father–normal   Mother–heterozygous
   homozygous
        ↓   ↓
   (no sickle trait)   *(sickle trait)*
2. Father–heterozygous   Mother–homozygous
        ↓   ↓
   (sickle trait)   *(no sickle trait)*
3. Mother–homozygous   Father–homozygous
        ↓   ↓
   (has sickle cell disease)   *(normal)*
4. Mother–heterozygous   Father–heterozygous
        ↓   ↓
   (sickle trait)   *(sickle trait)*

260. A client with non-insulin dependent diabetes mellitus (NIDDM) is admitted for elective surgery. The client is now being given regular insulin even though oral hypoglycemics were adequate prior to hospitalization. The nurse recognizes that regular insulin is now needed because:
1. The client will need a higher serum glucose level while on bedrest
2. The possibility of acidosis is greater when a client is on oral hypoglycemics
3. The dosage can be adjusted to changing needs during recovery from surgery
4. Regular insulin is readily available in the event of any complications after surgery

261. A client with an antisocial personality disorder continually uses manipulative behavior. The nurse is aware that this behavior can best be controlled by having the staff:
1. Avoid focusing on this aspect of the client's behavior
2. Develop and use a unified approach in response to this behavior
3. Assign members who are not easily manipulated to care for the client
4. Designate one staff member to approach the client about this behavior

262. A client in acute renal failure says to the nurse, "My doctor said I am going to be given some insulin. Do I also have diabetes?" The response by the nurse that best demonstrates an understanding of the use of insulin in acute renal failure would be:
1. "No, the insulin will help your body handle a chemical called potassium."
2. "Why don't you ask that question when your physician comes to see you today?"
3. "You probably had an elevated blood glucose level and your physician is cautious."
4. "No, but insulin will reduce the toxins in your blood by lowering your metabolic rate."

263. In view of the adaptations of cystic fibrosis, the diet the nurse should provide for a child affected with this disease should be:
1. Low in fat and low in salt
2. High in fat and high in protein
3. Low in fat and high in carbohydrate
4. Low in salt and high in carbohydrate

264. A 19-year-old college sophomore is admitted to the hospital with schizophrenia, undifferentiated type. The client sits in a corner for long periods of time rocking and responds to voices using words that the staff cannot understand. When developing the plan of care for this client, the nurse should:
1. Plan to spend short periods of time with the client
2. Include the client in a discussion group on the unit
3. Encourage the client to talk to other clients during the day
4. Allow the client to be alone, but maintain observation from a distance

265. After treatment for a bladder infection, a female client asks if there is anything she can do to prevent cystitis in the future. The nurse tells her to plan to:
1. Avoid the regular use of tampons
2. Void immediately after intercourse
3. Increase her intake of orange juice
4. Cleanse from vaginal orifice to urethra

Answers and Rationales for Comprehensive Examination 1

Part A

1. 1 Straddling the hip would prevent scissoring by keeping the infant's legs abducted. (2) (PE; IM; PA; NM)
2 An infant seat would not prevent scissoring.
3 Tight wrapping would maintain the infant's legs in a scissored position.
4 When the football hold is used the infant is carried in a supine position with the legs adducted, which promotes scissoring.

2. 3 This increases oncotic pressure, which pulls interstitial fluid into the blood vessels, restoring blood volume. (3) (ME; AN; PA; FE)
1 Nutrients are provided by total parenteral nutrition, not salt-poor albumin.
2 Salt-poor albumin is not given to increase protein stores.
4 Salt-poor albumin has no effect on diverting blood flow away from the liver.

3. 2 Rising blood pressure with a widening pulse pressure indicates cerebral edema, which can cause convulsions. (1) (CW; EV; TC; HP)
1 Cessation of fetal heart beat would indicate fetal death rather than a change in maternal blood pressure.
3 Bleeding is not associated with pregnancy-induced hypertension unless abruptio placentae occurs.
4 This generally does not occur unless the sedated client is not carefully observed; premature delivery is not indicated by blood pressure changes.

4. 1 This gives direction to the relationship and provides a blueprint for future evaluation of progress. (2) (MH; AN; TC; TR)
2 This is an aspect of the therapeutic relationship but is not the most important; what the client wants to achieve takes priority.

3 Same as answer 2.
4 Same as answer 2.

5. 2 Drainage will flow with the force of gravity; therefore the dependent area should be checked for the presence of blood. (2) (CW; EV; TC; WH)
1 The drainage is assessed for amount and characteristics; it is not emptied hourly, only once per shift or when necessary.
3 Turning the client on the affected side is usually painful and should be avoided; the client should turn to the unaffected side.
4 Pressure dressings are rarely used when a portable suction device is employed; if the drainage on the dressing is excessive, the physician should be notified.

6. 3 As drainage collects and occupies space, the original level of negative pressure decreases; the less negative pressure, the less effective the drainage. (1) (SU; AN; TC; IT)
1 It is easy and safe to empty regardless of the amount of drainage in the unit.
2 Drainage can be accurately measured by the calibrations on the unit or in a calibrated container after emptying.
4 A one-way valve between the tubing and the collection chamber prevents drainage from entering the tubing and causing trauma to the wound.

7. 3 The physician must be consulted because the decision depends on the amount of damage and extent of healing. (3) (ME; IM; TC; EH)
1 This is a medical decision that depends on the amount of damage, not how the client feels.
2 It would be false reassurance to determine an exact time and date; this would be too early.
4 Same as answer 1.

8. 4 This simply states reality without attempting to argue the client out of the delusion; actual physical contact should be initiated by the client. (3) (MH; IM; PS; SD)

1 This denies the client's feelings and directly attacks the delusional system forcing the client to defend it.

2 This is false reassurance; the client does not feel safe and the nurse's saying it does not make it so.

3 Touching the client's arm can be frightening and overwhelming.

9. 1 Deep breathing provides an active role in controlling pain; this is a positive coping skill. (3) (SU; PL; ED; NM)

2 Understanding the importance of wound care will not reduce severe pain; health teaching should be initiated before, not during, a procedure.

3 This could increase pain.

4 Distraction techniques are usually ineffectual in the presence of severe pain; contraction may increase the pain.

10. 3 The properly fitted diaphragm, when used correctly with spermicidal gel, is 98 to 99% effective and has low risk for complications. (2) (CW; EV; ED; RC)

1 Oral contraceptives are not recommended for women with diabetes mellitus because of their effect on carbohydrate metabolism and the risk of major cardiovascular complications.

2 The intrauterine device carries a risk of infection which is already increased in women with diabetes mellitus.

4 Sterilization is recommended only if there is severe renal disease or proliferative retinopathy associated with diabetes mellitus.

11. 3 Epinephrine produces sympathetic nervous system side effects such as tachycardia and hypertension. (2) (PE; EV; TC; DR)

1 Pallor, not flushing, is a common side effect.

2 This is not a common side effect; this medication is given to decrease respiratory difficulty.

4 Hypertension, not hypotension, is a common side effect.

12. 3 The person addicted to drugs is unable to adequately deal with reality; drugs help blur reality and reduce frustrations. (3) (MH; PL; PS; SA)

1 It is possible, although not easy, but it does require a change in attitude and a deconditioning process.

2 People who abuse drugs are concerned with reality; drug use is often an attempt to blur the pains of reality.

4 Education of the public has been extensive but the individual who experiments with drugs does not believe addiction will develop.

13. 3 Obesity is a known predisposing factor to diabetes mellitus; the exact relationship is unknown. (2) (ME; AS; PA; EN)

1 Diabetes insipidus is a disease caused by too little ADH and has no relationship to diabetes mellitus.

2 High-cholesterol diets and atherosclerotic heart disease are associated with diabetes mellitus.

4 Alcohol intake is not known to predispose to diabetes mellitus, and alcohol lowers the blood glucose.

14. 4 A lung is a highly vascular area that accommodates a large portion of intravascular volume; once a portion is removed the remaining lung tissue is at risk for pulmonary congestion. (3) (SU; AN; PA; RE)

1 When an intravenous solution is administed correctly, this should not occur.

2 Same as answer 1.

3 Same as answer 1.

15. 2 In this position the gravid uterus impedes venous return; this causes decreased cardiac output and results in reduced placental circulation. (1) (CW; AN; TC; HC)

1 This may be partially true, but more significantly, it is the least comfortable position and may cause hypotension and reduced placental perfusion.

3 Even if true, this is not significant as a factor of labor.

4 This is false; it can lead to supine hypotension.

16. 3 Today, 5-year survival rates for children with acute lymphocytic leukemia exceed 60% in most treatment centers. (3) (PE; AN; PA; BI)

1 This projected prognosis is too fatalistic; 5-year survival occurs in about 60% of children treated.

2 Same as answer 1.

4 This projected prognosis is too favorable; 5-year survival occurs in about 60% of children treated.

17. 4 500 ml divided by 4 hours equals 125 ml per hour. (2) (PE; AN; TC; FE)

1 This rate would deliver less than the prescribed amount in the prescribed time.

2 Same as answer 1.

3 Same as answer 1.

18. 1 Infection is the most common complication; sterile technique at the catheter insertion site must be maintained. (2) (SU; PL; TC; GI)

2 This is not necessary; the catheter is sutured in place, and reasonable movement is permitted.

3 Excessive weight gain or loss is not a complication of total parenteral nutrition.

4 The client should be taught to leave the infusion pump as set and to call the nurse if the alarm rings.

19. 3 These clients can better work through their underlying problems when the environment is controlled, demands are reduced, and the routine is simple. (2) (MH; AN; PS; PR)

1 Preventing these clients from carrying out rituals can precipitate panic reactions.

2 The intent of therapy should be to help the client gain control, not to enable others to do the controlling.

4 Because anxiety stems from unconscious conflicts, the environment alone is not enough to effect resolution.

20. 1 Levodopa can cross the blood-brain barrier and be converted to dopamine, a substance depleted in Parkinson's disease. (2) (ME; PL; TC; DR)

2 Dopamine is not given because it does not cross the blood-brain barrier.

3 Vitamin B_6 can reverse the effects of some anti-Parkinson's disease medications and is contraindicated.

4 Isocarboxazid is an MAO inhibitor used for the treatment of severe depression, not symptoms of parkinsonism.

21. 1 Clients may develop cerebral edema caused by excessive absorption of irrigating solution by the venous sinusoids during surgery. (3) (SU; EV; TC; RG)

2 The procedure is usually performed under spinal anesthesia; the supine position is maintained for 8 to 12 hours.

3 The surgery is performed through the urinary meatus and urethra; there is no suprapubic incision.

4 The client is initially npo and then advanced to a regular diet as tolerated; continuous irrigation supplies enough fluid to flush the bladder.

22. 2 This relieves some of the pain because it provides support to the incised abdominal wall. (1) (CW; IM; TC; HP)

1 The symptoms do not indicate a need for this action.

3 Analgesics will not relieve the discomfort associated with coughing unless stress placed on the incision by coughing is relieved.

4 Same as answer 1.

23. 1 This is a correct description of talipes equinovarus. (2) (PE; AS; PA; SK)

2 This describes talipes calcaneovarus.

3 This describes talipes equinovalgus, also known as rocker-bottom foot.

4 Same as answer 2.

24. 4 Being overweight is a predisposing factor to wound dehiscence because of decreased vascularity and fragility of adipose tissue. (2) (SU; AS; PA; GI)

1 Age does not really contribute to dehiscence.

2 This does not contribute to dehiscence; a T-tube helps remove bile from the common bile duct.

3 This causes discomfort, not dehiscence.

25. 1 More data is needed about activities of daily living to evaluate noncompliance before revising the care plan. (2) (ME; AS; TC; RE)
    2 This is nonproductive because it places blame for the illness on the client.
    3 Same as answer 2.
    4 Same as answer 2.

26. 3 The client will be able to attend to grooming because lithium effectively controls and reduces grandiosity, poor judgment, and psychomotor hyperactivity. (2) (MH; EV; TC; DR)
    1 This would not reflect an effective response to lithium.
    2 Same as answer 1.
    4 Same as answer 1.

27. 1 Bone marrow is most susceptible to lead toxicity; interference with hemoglobin biosynthesis leads to early signs of anemia. (3) (PE; AS; PA; BI)
    2 This is a late response indicating kidney shut-down; loss of protein and other substances occurs first.
    3 This is a serious, life-threatening, late response.
    4 This is a late response indicating central nervous system involvement.

28. 2 Insensible and intestinal fluid losses are increased during phototherapy; extra fluid prevents dehydration. (3) (CW; PL; TC; HN)
    1 This is unnecessary unless changes from the baseline occur.
    3 A Guthrie test is done for PKU screening.
    4 The total body needs to be exposed to light.

29. 3 The pulse pressure is obtained by subtracting the diastolic from the systolic blood pressure reading; pulse pressure widens as intracranial pressure increases. (1) (SU; AN; PA; NM)
    1 This is reflected in the actual blood pressure readings and indicates cardiovascular function.
    2 This is the definition of a pulse deficit.
    4 This is determined by various diagnostic techniques used in cardiology; this is the role of the physician, not the nurse.

30. 4 A small light in the room may prevent misinterpretation of shadows, which can heighten fear and alter the perception of the environment. (2) (MH; IM; TC; DD)
    1 Less restrictive intervention should be used first; restraints may not be necessary.
    2 This is unsafe; a disoriented and confused client should not be isolated but closely observed.
    3 This is unnecessary; sedatives should be used sparingly in the aged because they may further confuse and agitate the aged client.

31. 3 A serious side effect of chloramphenicol (Chloromycetin) is aplastic anemia, a common reaction to the drug; blood studies would monitor RBCs. (3) (PE; EV; TC; DR)
    1 A decrease, not an increase, in RBCs occurs.
    2 This is unrelated to chloramphenicol.
    4 Same as answer 2.

32. 3 Sodium absorbs water in the kidney's renal tubules; when dietary intake is decreased, water is not reabsorbed and edema is reduced. (2) (ME; AN; PA; FE)
    1 This is untrue; a decrease in sodium will prevent the reabsorption of water; furosemide stimulates the loop of Henle.
    2 Adequate hydration is the major factor that diminishes the thirst response.
    4 This will not be caused by a low-sodium diet; a low-sodium diet will cause fluid to enter the intravascular compartment.

33. 1 Lying on the affected side causes adduction, which may result in dislocation of the femoral head. (3) (SU; PL; PA; SK)
    2 This is contraindicated; it would put too much pressure on the operative site; the leg on the operative side should be kept in abduction.
    3 This is too long a period of time; partial weight bearing will be permitted sooner, depending on the extent of surgery and the progression of healing.
    4 Partial weight bearing on the affected leg is generally contraindicated for at least 2 to 3 weeks.

34. 3 Encouraging conversation allows the abused individual an opportunity to verbalize feelings and may ultimately lead to the development of possible coping strategies. (2) (MH; IM; PS; CS)

1 This focuses on a topic that may not be the client's concern; the client should be permitted to direct the topic of conversation.

2 This is not the legal responsibility of the nurse at this time.

4 Same as answer 1.

35. 3 Lochia serosa is similar in appearance to serosanguinous drainage and generally appears on the third or fourth postpartum day. (1) (CW; AS; PA; HC)

1 Lochia alba consists of leukocytes, decidua, epithelial cells, mucus, and serum; this appears 10 days postpartum and lasts 2 to 6 weeks.

2 Lochia rubra is initially bright red, changing to dark red or reddish brown; it consists mainly of blood, decidua, and trophoblastic debris; it occurs immediately after delivery, lasting for 2 to 3 days.

4 There is no such term.

36. 1 Exercising should be done often; association with a specific activity makes it easier to incorporate it into the lifestyle, leading to increased compliance. (2) (PE; EV; ED; SK)

2 Although this is frequent enough, such a rigid schedule is difficult to follow with an infant, and compliance becomes more difficult.

3 This is not frequent enough.

4 Same as answer 3.

37. 2 Lead toxicity and Ca EDTA both damage the proximal renal tubules, resulting in the abnormal excretion of protein and other substances. (3) (PE; EV; TC; RG)

1 This does not occur with lead toxicity, nor is it likely to occur with the Ca EDTA preparation, which replaces calcium.

3 Bone marrow damage is caused by lead toxicity only.

4 Lead encephalopathy causes serious elevation of intracranial pressure; this is not related to Ca EDTA.

38. 3 The ability to endure progressive activity indicates that collateral circulation has improved cardiopulmonary functioning. (3) (ME; IM; ED; CV)

1 Intermittent claudication is related to peripheral arterial occlusive disease, not cardiopulmonary function.

2 Breathing when jogging should be regular and deep to meet the oxygen demands of the body during exercise.

4 Perspiration is an expected and desired adaptation to promote heat loss through evaporation.

39. 4 The semi-Fowler's position helps to maintain the head in proper body alignment and facilitates respiration. (2) (SU; PL; PA; RE)

1 The side-lying position inhibits respiratory excursion.

2 This position may cause flexion of the neck, which would inhibit respiration and place pressure on the suture line.

3 Same as answer 2.

40. 4 Neuromuscular blockers, such as Anectine or Pavulon produce respiratory depression because they inhibit contractions of respiratory muscles. (1) (MH; EV; TC; DR)

1 As a muscle relaxant, the neuromuscular blocking agent prevents convulsions.

2 The loss of memory results from the ECT treatment, not from the neuromuscular blocking agent.

3 Because the client is not permitted anything by mouth for 8 to 10 hours before the treatment, this is not a major problem.

41. 4 Because the infant will be kept supine after surgery to prevent irritation to the lips, using this position early prepares the infant for its use later. (2) (PE; IM; ED; GI)

1 The infant is too young and will miss out on some oral gratification with this method.

2 Constant restraint of the arms would be injurious to arm growth, as well as to the infant's need to move about.

3 Infants with a cleft lip need increased burping time because they tend to swallow large amounts of air during feeding.

42. 3 The ovum is fertilizable for 12 to 24 hours, and sperm remain motile for about 72 hours. (1) (CW; PL; PA; RC)
1 The fertility period is longer than this.
2 This time period is too long before ovulation and too short after ovulation.
4 The period of fertility is shorter than this.

43. 1 This is realistic, specific, and measurable; it relates to the client's stated nursing diagnosis. (1) (MH; PL; PS; CS)
2 This is an unrealistic goal.
3 There are no data to indicate the client is thinking negatively about himself or others.
4 This may be unrealistic and cannot be made without involvement of the family.

44. 2 Hyperthyroidism raises the metabolic rate and need for oxygen; this results in increased heart rate and myocardial irritability. (2) (ME; AS; PA; EN)
1 These are signs associated with myxedema and hypothyroidism.
3 Same as answer 1.
4 Same as answer 1.

45. 3 Negative pressure is exerted by gravity drainage or by suction through the closed system. (1) (SU; AN; PA; RE)
1 Though the discomfort may be lessened, this is not the primary purpose.
2 In a pneumothorax associated with COPD there is an accumulation of air, not fluid.
4 Subcutaneous emphysema in the chest wall is most frequently associated with clients receiving air under pressure, such as received on a ventilator.

46. 2 Palpation is the most invasive technique of the assessment skills; infants do not tolerate invasive procedures as well as they do less threatening maneuvers. (2) (PE; AS; TC; GD)
1 Percussion of the lung fields can be frightening to an infant but is generally tolerated better than palpation; it should be done toward the end of the assessment but before palpation.

3 Inspection is the least invasive procedure and should be done first.
4 Auscultation is less invasive than palpation; the accuracy of auscultation may be affected if it is done after a more invasive technique that produces crying, thus making auscultation more difficult.

47. 2 Baked fish is a low-residue, low-fat, high-protein, and non-gas-producing food that is usually well tolerated. (2) (SU; EV; PA; GI)
1 This has fiber and irritates the gastrointestinal tract.
3 This irritates the gastrointestinal tract and stimulates mucus production.
4 Same as answer 1.

48. 1 At about the twentieth to twenty-second week of gestation, the top of the fundus is at the level of the umbilicus. (3) (CW; AS; PA; HC)
2 In a normal pregnancy this would be too low for a pregnancy between the fifth and sixth month.
3 In a normal pregnancy, this would be too high for 20 to 22 weeks of gestation.
4 Same as answer 2.

49. 4 The child is developing autonomy, is curious, and learns from own experience. (1) (PE; AN; PA; GD)
1 The toddler is still learning from own experiences not from others; this is the level of parallel, not interactive, play.
2 The toddler is still attempting to distinguish self as separate from the parents; the struggle for autonomy limits learning from parents.
3 The struggle for autonomy at this age limits learning from older siblings, even though the toddler attempts to copy their behaviors; older siblings often are not good role models because they tend to be careless.

50. 1 All nursing care should be directed toward preventing injury, particularly with a self-destructive client. (2) (MH; PL; TC; BA)
2 Although this is important, prevention of injury is the priority.

3   Same as answer 2.
4   Same as answer 2.

51.   2   Because of increased blood loss associated with cesarean delivery, the client should be well hydrated before surgery to maintain adequate blood volume. (3) (CW; PL; PA; HP)
1   This is not relevant; just before surgery is done, the skin will be cleansed.
3   Unless the fetus is extremely premature or in distress, there is no reason for admission to the neonatal intensive care unit.
4   Only routine monitoring of vital signs is necessary unless there has been some indication of infection or pregnancy-induced hypertension.

52.   2   Shampooing is done carefully to avoid scratching the scalp, which would provide a portal of entry for microorganisms. (2) (SU; PL; TC; IT)
1   Fluids are withheld preoperatively; they may also be restricted because of cerebral edema.
3   Narcotics are not used because of possible central nervous system depression.
4   Enemas are contraindicated; the client should avoid straining because it increases intracranial pressure.

53.   4   Myocardial necrosis causes a rise in body temperature within the first 24 to 48 hours, which gradually returns to normal within a week. (2) (ME; PL; PA; CV)
1   This temperature did not result from a respiratory complication.
2   This is unnecessary; this is an expected response and not an emergency.
3   Coughing necessitates the use of the Valsalva maneuver, which is contraindicated because it can precipitate dysrhythmias.

54.   2   Propylthiouracil can cause a depression of leukocytes and platelets. (3) (ME; EV; TC; DR)
1   They are given with milk, juice, or food to prevent gastric irritation.

3   Drug therapy decreases the risk of postoperative hemorrhage because it decreases the size and vascularity of the thyroid gland.
4   Therapy will be continued for at least 6 to 8 weeks, even if the client's temperature and pulse return to normal.

55.   1   This is normal developmental behavior for 18-month-olds; however, they may have trouble coming down the stairs. (2) (PE; EV; PA; GD)
2   This is above the level of an 18-month-old child.
3   Same as answer 2.
4   Same as answer 2.

56.   2   This is a realistic essential first step; the problem and related feelings must be thoroughly explored before solutions can be developed. (1) (MH; AN; PS; AX)
1   This would be a long-term goal.
3   Same as answer 1.
4   This is an inappropriate goal; a direct connection to life events is often difficult to find.

57.   2   The placenta begins to age after term, and the fetus may be deprived of oxygen and nutrients. (3) (CW; AN; PA; HP)
1   Usually these infants lose weight because of placental deprivation.
3   This is unrelated; maternal diabetes usually results in early delivery.
4   Infection may be caused by premature rupture of membranes or a lack of sterile technique, not postmaturity.

58.   1   This encourages tissue regeneration and prevents creation of a moist area conducive to infection. (1) (ME; PL; TC; IT)
2   This creates a warm, moist, protein-containing medium that is ideal for growing pathogens.
3   A high-caloric diet is appropriate to provide energy for tissue repair.
4   Placing the client in one position will promote development of additional decubitus ulcers.

59. 1 Preadolescents and young adolescents are most at risk and can be most successfully treated. (1) (PE; PL; TC; SK)

2 Scoliosis would not be identifiable in children of this age.

3 Some students with scoliosis might be identified, but it may be too late for adequate treatment.

4 80% of clients with idiopathic scoliosis are preadolescents and young adolescents, not preschoolers.

60. 3 The nurse provides support in a nonjudgmental way by sharing information and observations about the child. (3) (MH; IM; PS; BA)

1 This indirectly indicates that the parent may be at fault; it negates the mother's need for support and increases her sense of guilt.

2 Same as answer 1.

4 This is false reassurance that does not provide support; the mother recognizes something is wrong.

61. 2 Individuals with bulimia have many unmet dependency needs that they attempt to meet by the use of food. (3) (MH; AS; PS; EA)

1 Individuals with bulimia tend to be extroverted rather than demonstrating a flattened affect.

3 Individuals with bulimia tend to be unable to make decisions; although they may appear obstinate at times, there is no rigidity of character.

4 Individuals with bulimia talk freely about their problems, although the discussion is usually on a superficial level.

62. 1 Abrupt discontinuation of Inderal may cause an acute myocardial infarction. (2) (SU; IM; ED; DR)

2 Clients should never increase medications without a physician's direction.

3 Alcohol is contraindicated for clients taking Inderal.

4 The pulse rate can go much lower as long as the client feels well and is not dizzy.

63. 2 Suckling will induce neural stimulation of the posterior pituitary gland, which in turn will release oxytocin and cause uterine contractions. (2) (CW; IM; PA; HC)

1 This will not help if the uterus is not contracting.

3 If the placenta is still attached to the uterine wall, this may disconnect the cord from the placenta.

4 This could cause a uterine prolapse.

64. 3 Fever, malaise, and headache may accompany local reactions. (2) (CW; AS; ED; WH)

1 Herpes is of viral origin; there is no cure, and antibiotics are ineffective.

2 Vesicles on genitalia rupture, causing painful ulcerations.

4 Although uncommon, a virus can survive for short periods of time on fomites.

65. 1 An acid-ash diet, including cranberries, lowers the pH of the urine and discourages pathogenic growth. (1) (ME; AN; ED; RG)

2 Acid urine does not soothe bladder walls.

3 The glomerular filtration rate is not affected.

4 An acid medium will discourage further growth but will not kill existing organisms.

66. 3 The nursing goal is to promote orientation by involving the client in activities with others; even though the client probably could not follow any game rules, the activity provides involvement with the nurse. (3) (MH; IM; TC; SD)

1 This is not therapeutic and implies that the client is actually talking to someone.

2 This would have no effect on the client's behavior.

4 This is not therapeutic; it allows for further withdrawal rather than orienting the client to reality.

67. 3 Treatment is done several hours after meals to avoid regurgitation and several hours before meals so that unpleasant odor and taste do not affect eating. (2) (PE; PL; PA; RE)

1 Treatment is done more frequently than this.

2 Postural drainage should not be done before meals because the unpleasant odor and taste will interfere with eating.
4 Same as answer 1.

68. 4 Hot climates are contraindicated for children with cystic fibrosis because sweating brings about excessive loss of sodium chloride. (3) (PE; EV; ED; EN)
1 This is advisable because it will keep the child from sweating.
2 Pancreatic enzymes are essential to help digest the nutrients so that they can be absorbed by the intestinal mucosa.
3 After passage of the feces associated with this disorder, the rectum may become inflamed if not properly cleaned.

69. 2 Heat promotes vasodilation, which aids the shift of urea, a large molecular substance, from blood vessels into the dialyzing solution. (3) (SU; AN; PA; RG)
1 Heat does not affect the shift of potassium into the cells.
3 The ability to remove metabolic wastes is affected in renal failure; the metabolic processes themselves are not disturbed.
4 Excess serum potassium is removed by dialyzing with a potassium-free solution, not by heat.

70. 3 The client's measured output is about 500 ml in 24 hours based on the available history; insensible losses are 400 to 500 ml in 24 hours. (3) (ME; AN; PA; FE)
1 Based on the history, the client's expected urinary output should be about 400 ml in the next 24 hours; this is far less than 900 ml.
2 This is insufficient fluid to help prevent hypostatic pneumonia; fluid intake is only one of many factors involved.
4 Hyperkalemia in acute renal failure is caused by inadequate glomerular filtration and is not related to fluid intake.

71. 4 This response presents facts that help to reduce guilt. (2) (CW; IM; PS; EC)
1 This is very unreassuring, as well as incorrect, because placenta previa can occur in a woman with a normal uterus.

2 This is an inadequate explanation and gives the client no idea of what is happening.
3 This is untrue, and labor may not be beginning at this time.

72. 1 Individuals who have somatoform disorders are really ill; they need care and a nonthreatening environment. (3) (MH; PL; TC; AX)
2 The client requires physiologic and emotional care; without movement, venous stasis and atrophy of the "paralyzed" limbs can occur.
3 The client is ill and requires good physical and emotional care.
4 Same as answer 2.

73. 2 With diabetic ketoacidosis, serum lipid levels can go so high that the serum appears opalescent and creamy. (3) (ME; AS; PA; EN)
1 With diabetic ketoacidosis the BUN is generally elevated because of dehydration.
3 With diabetic ketoacidosis the hematocrit is generally elevated because of dehydration.
4 This is unrelated to diabetic ketoacidosis.

74. 4 Elevation in the first 24 hours helps prevent edema; continued elevation may lead to hip contractures. (1) (SU; PL; PA; SK)
1 The client is usually out of bed on the second postoperative day.
2 The stump dressing is usually a pressure dressing and it is not changed daily.
3 Hemorrhage and infection are the two most common complications.

75. 4 Drainage is bright red initially and gradually becomes darker red during the first 24 hours. (2) (SU; EV; PA; GI)
1 If the nasogastric tube is functioning correctly, secretions will be removed and vomiting will not occur.
2 If the nasogastric tube is functioning correctly, gastric distention will not occur.
3 Because the bowel was emptied before surgery and the client is now npo, there would be no expected intestinal activity.

How to Use Worksheet 1: Errors In Processing Information

Common errors in processing information are listed in the left-hand column of this worksheet. At the top of the worksheet is a row of blank spaces for inserting the number of the question missed. Directly below each number, check any errors you made in answering that question. You may have made more than one type of error in an answer.

Worksheet 1: Errors in Processing Information

Question number																									
Did not read situation/ question carefully																									
Missed important details																									
Confused major and minor points																									
Defined problem incorrectly																									
Could not remember terms/ facts/concepts/principles																									
Defined terms incorrectly																									
Focused on incomplete/incorrect data in assessing situation																									
Interpreted data incorrectly																									
Applied wrong concepts/ principles in situations																									
Drew incorrect conclusions																									
Identified wrong goals																									
Identified priorities incorrectly																									
Carried out plan incorrectly/ incompletely																									
Was unclear about criteria for evaluating success in achieving goals																									

How to Use Worksheet 2: Knowledge Gaps

Types of common knowledge gaps are listed along the top of this worksheet. Write a brief description of topics you want to review in the spaces provided. For example, if you missed a question on administration of a particular drug, write the drug name and problem (e.g., dosage) in the appropriate space under the column labeled *Pharmacology*.

Worksheet 2: Knowledge Gaps

Basic science	Skills/ procedures	Basic human needs	Growth and develop- ment	Normal nutrition	Psycho- social factors	Clinical area/ topic	Stressors/ coping mechanisms	Patho- physiology	Pharma- cology	Therapeutic nutrition	Legal implications	Other

Part B

76. 4 Discussion with parents who have children with similar problems helps to reduce some of their discomfort and guilt. (2) (PE; PL; PS; EH)

1 When not in crisis, the child should be allowed to attend school and should not be developmentally damaged by social isolation.

2 There is no recommended therapeutic climate for these children, and moving may not be beneficial to the child or the family.

3 Some parents do not choose to avoid future pregnancies and should not be forced to do so.

77. 4 The symptoms prevent the individual from being forced to move in either direction on the conflict; symptoms thus reduce anxiety and remove the conflict. (2) (MH; AS; PS; AX)

1 The individual is not happy and cheerful but is relieved by the reduction in anxiety.

2 The individual is not sad and depressed but is relieved by the reduction in anxiety.

3 The individual is not frightened or upset because the symptoms relieve the anxiety.

78. 4 This is a noninvasive, relatively harmless way to visualize the location of the placenta. (2) (CW; AN; PA; HP)

1 This is a visualization of the amniotic fluid via vaginal examination; it is contraindicated because it may detach the placenta.

2 This is an invasive surgical procedure used for diagnostic purposes other than the location of the placenta.

3 This is used for removing amniotic fluid for diagnosis and fetal evaluation, not for diagnosing placenta previa.

79. 4 This statement attempts to understand the symbolism, reflects and acknowledges the client's feelings, and helps to preserve ego integrity. (3) (MH; IM; PS; SD)

1 This validates the client's delusion and does not test reality.

2 This rejects the client's feelings and does not address the client's fears of being harmed; clients cannot be argued out of delusions.

3 This is false reassurance; the nurse cannot fully understand the symbolism and therefore cannot make this promise.

80. 3 The initial attack is both local and systemic; recurrent attacks are milder and localized. (1) (CW; IM; ED; WH)

1 There is recurrence in 50% of clients.

2 Recurrent attacks are precipitated by physical and emotional stress, not by sexual activity.

4 Although optimal health habits may limit recurrence, they will not totally prevent it.

81. 4 Because the client is up more at home, edema usually increases. (3) (SU; IM; ED; CV)

1 Serosanguinous drainage will persist after discharge.

2 These should not be expected and are in fact signs of postpericardotomy syndrome.

3 These symptoms will persist longer, because it takes 6 to 12 weeks for the sternum to heal.

82. 2 The nurse should be alert for dehydration caused by fluid loss through vomiting in the binge-purge cycle. (2) (MH; AS; TC; EA)

1 Weight gain would not be expected because of the purging that usually follows a binge.

3 Hyperactivity would not be expected because most individuals with bulimia withdraw and vomit after a binge.

4 Hyperglycemia would not be expected because of the vomiting that follows a binge.

83. 1 Aging causes reduction in skin lubrication that results in dry skin. (1) (ME; PL; PA; IT)

2 This influences how much assistance is necessary, not the frequency of bathing.

3 This influences what bath products may be used, not the frequency of bathing.

4 This influences safety factors applicable during the bath, not the frequency of bathing.

84. 2 Necrotic tissue and blood in an area that is moist, warm, and dark make an excellent culture medium. (2) (CW; AN; ED; NN)

1 This is untrue; Wharton's jelly is present and provides a protective barrier.

3 The diaper is kept below the level of the umbilicus; although the site may be touched by clothing, the clothing should be 100% cotton to allow for drying of the cord.

4 This is untrue; newborns carry antibodies from the mother.

85. 4 An increased attention span in school indicates that the child has improved. (2) (MH; EV; PS; BA)

1 This would indicate that the child has not made sufficient progress.

2 This would indicate that the child has not made progress because children should enjoy playing with peers at this age.

3 A child of age six is not usually enuretic at night even without hyperactivity; there is no data to indicate enuresis in this situation.

86. 2 Because the tumor is of renal origin, the renin-angiotensin mechanism can be involved and blood pressure monitoring is very important. (3) (PE; PL; TC; RG)

1 This could put pressure on the involved area, causing rupture of the tumor and seeding of cancer cells.

3 Same as answer 1.

4 This is unnecessary; no infection is present.

87. 1 At the very minimum, the role of a witness is to attest to the validity of the signature. (1) (SU; AN; TC; EH)

2 A consent is valid for the length of the hospital stay.

3 Clients also need to know about the outcomes and risks of surgery.

4 This is the responsibility of the physician.

88. 4 All these interventions promote aeration of the reexpanding lung and maintenance of function in the arm and shoulder on the affected side. (3) (SU; PL; PA; RE)

1 Cough suppressants would not be indicated, because coughing and deep breathing are to be encouraged.

2 Drainage is marked with time tapes on the side of the device; the closed system is not entered for emptying; when full, the entire device is replaced.

3 Clamps are not necessary and should be avoided in almost all instances because of the danger of tension pneumothorax.

89. 4 The client's grieving process is severe and extended, indicating dysfunction. (2) (MH; AN; PS; CS)

1 The data does not support this; the client is communicating effectively with the nurse.

2 There is not enough data to support this conclusion.

3 This is not as specific as identifying grieving; also, low motivation is not the reason for the client's inability to cope.

90. 2 The diaphragm is used in conjunction with spermicidal jelly or cream, which remains active for only 6 to 8 hours. (1) (CW; EV; ED; RC)

1 Removal this soon would allow motile sperm to pass through the cervical os.

3 The diaphragm may be left in place as a mechanical barrier but the spermicidal jelly or cream becomes inactive after 6 to 8 hours.

4 The diaphragm may be left in place for this period of time but may cause an unpleasant odor.

91. 4 This is a true statement that assures the client that it is effective. (2) (MH; IM; PS; MO)

1 This response does not answer the client's question.

2 ECT does not change usual patterns of behavior although it does interrupt disturbed or disturbing acting-out behavior.

3 This response puts off answering the client's question by referring it to the physician.

92. 2 A rapid mood upswing and psychomotor change frequently signals that the client has made a decision and has developed a plan for suicide. (2) (MH; EV; PS; MO)

1 This statement is typical in the depressed client and does not really signal a change in mood.

3 Same as answer 1.

4 Same as answer 1.

93. 3 Breaking up the tablet increases the surface area of the tablet, which permits it to dissolve faster. (2) (ME; IM; ED; DR)

1 If taken with water, the tablet is held away from the site of absorption or may even be swallowed.

2 This does not hasten absorption and may even impair the tablet's ability to dissolve.

4 This would slow absorption because saliva helps to dissolve the tablet.

94. 3 Identifying potential health problems and planning and implementing programs aimed at these problems is primary prevention. (2) (MH; AN; TC; CS)

1 There is no such term; legal intervention would be a form of secondary prevention.

2 These are interventions such as long-term or permanent removal of the child from the home.

4 These are interventions such as legal orders of protection or temporary removal of the child from the situation.

95. 1 The solution with the greatest number of particles is hyperosmolar and exerts an osmotic force, pulling fluid in its direction. (2) (ME; AN; ED; FE)

2 This is untrue; fluids are pulled in.

3 Some particles can move.

4 On the contrary; water moves to the side with the greater number of particles.

96. 2 Furosemide (Lasix) is a diuretic with a rapid onset of action, particularly when given intravenously. (1) (ME; IM; ED; DR)

1 Hearing loss is associated only with high doses; 20 mg is a small dose.

3 Burning is not associated with IV administration of furosemide.

4 This is contraindicated; at this time, the client has a fluid volume excess; potassium needs will be addressed later.

97. 3 This private room will provide isolation; also, being close to nurses' station will facilitate frequent neurologic monitoring. (2) (PE; PL; TC; NM)

1 This is unsafe; it would permit cross-infection; a private room is necessary to prevent transmission of airborne droplets.

2 Same as answer 1.

4 This is unsafe; it interferes with frequent monitoring of the client.

98. 1 Corticosteroids inhibit the inflammatory response and increase an individual's susceptibility to infection. (3) (SU; EV; TC; DR)

2 With therapy, a slight weight gain may occur.

3 The client will be hypertensive, not hypotensive, until stabilized.

4 Urinary stasis is unrelated to Decadron; Decadron will promote cerebral diuresis.

99. 3 Immature neurologic and chemical respiratory mechanisms cause apnea in preterm infants; tactile stimulation will start breathing. (2) (CW; IM; PA; HN)

1 This is not done unless the infant is cyanotic or the blood PO_2 is low.

2 This is not done unless the infant shows signs of an obstructed airway.

4 This is done only if the infant does not respond to tactile stimulation.

100. 4 This involves no element of competition and still allows for channeling of excessive energy. (2) (MH; PL; TC; MO)

1 The sense of competition and increased stimulation may raise the client's anxiety.

2 This requires fine motor skill from a client who is hyperactive and whose attention span is limited.

3 The client is too hyperactive to complete this task and may respond with distractibility or aggressiveness toward others.

101. 4 The exact reason is unknown, but three factors appear related: lead in the environment; toxins in the environment; and characteristics of the child and the parents. (3) (PE; IM; ED; NM)

1 This is only one of the three etiologic factors.

2 Same as answer 1.

3 Same as answer 1.

102. 3 Lactated Ringer's is an alkaline solution that replaces bicarbonate ions lost from T-tube bile drainage, thus preventing or treating acidosis. (3) (SU; EV; TC; FE)

1 This is unrelated to the effectiveness of this IV solution.

2 Same as answer 1.

4 Same as answer 1.

103. 2 Exploration allows the nurse to assess the client's knowledge and fears. (2) (PE; IM; ED; EH)

1 This is not true; this would imply a dominant mode of transmission.

3 This is false reassurance; it may occur again.

4 This is not true; this would imply an autosomal recessive mode of transmission.

104. 2 This response recognizes the concern and provides accurate information that may reduce anxiety. (2) (SU; IM; ED; EH)

1 This is inaccurate information; impotence usually does not result; it is possible after perineal prostatectomy.

3 This reply closes off communication and transfers responsibility to the physician.

4 This does not recognize feelings and provides inaccurate information; impotence rarely if ever occurs with this operation.

105. 4 This sets an unrealistic limit that would increase anxiety by removing a defense the client needs at this time; rituals cannot be this controlled until other defenses are developed to replace them. (2) (MH; EV; PS; PR)

1 This is done in therapy as the client's condition improves; insight must be developed slowly to minimize anxiety.

2 This would reduce, not increase, anxiety because the client would feel free to express feelings.

3 This would increase self-esteem and self-control, not increase anxiety.

106. 4 This is an adverse reaction that may occur about 8 to 12 hours after diuresis occurs. (3) (SU; EV; PA; DR)

1 Although mannitol may cause respiratory congestion, it does not cause respiratory failure.

2 This is not an expected response; mannitol does not directly affect the heart, but injudicious use can cause electrolyte imbalances which can eventually cause dysrhythmias.

3 Tachycardia, not bradycardia, is an adverse reaction related to mannitol.

107. 4 An acid pH means the tube is still in the stomach; a pH greater than 7 indicates the tube has reached the small intestine. (3) (SU; IM; TC; GI)

1 The client does not need to remain in bed.

2 A client with a nasogastric or intestinal tube is kept npo.

3 This tube must advance to the intestine; securing it would inhibit this movement.

108. 2 This provides for collection of more data. (1) (CW; AS; ED; EC)

1 This is a negative comment that closes communication.

3 This implies that things are not well, and the mother may be to blame.

4 This could make the mother feel guilty about not meeting her baby's needs.

109. 1 Ketoacidosis occurs when insulin is lacking and carbohydrates cannot be used for energy; this increases the breakdown of protein and fat causing Kussmaul respirations, decreased alertness, decreased circulatory volume, metabolic acidosis, and an acetone breath. (1) (ME; EV; PA; EN)

2 Hypoglycemia is manifested by cool moist skin, not hot dry skin or Kussmaul respirations.

3 The Somogyi phenomenon is a rebound hyperglycemia induced by severe hypoglycemia; there is not enough data to determine if this occurred.

4 Hyperosmolar non-ketotic coma usually occurs in non-insulin dependent diabetes because available insulin prevents the breakdown of fat.

110. 4 160 mg/100 ml is above the normal fasting blood glucose level which is between 60 to 110 mg/100 ml; this is indicative of diabetes mellitus. (2) (ME; AS; PA; EN)

1 This would indicate hypoglycemia, not hyperglycemia.

2 Same as answer 1.

3 This is an expected blood glucose level in the nondiabetic individual.

111. 2 There is usually a history of interpersonal difficulties; clients are unable to engage in the give and take a relationship requires. (2) (MH; AN; PS; PR)

1 There is no direct relationship between antisocial personality disorders and sexual aberrations.

3 The parents of these individuals rarely impose any discipline or limits at all.

4 There is no diminished contact with reality; these clients are in contact with reality; they just do not care about it.

112. 2 Because the newborn's GI tract is sterile, the infant does not have the bacteria that are necessary to synthesize vitamin K; it is vitamin K that functions to stimulate the liver's production of clotting factors. (1) (CW; AN; PA; DR)

1 Vitamin K has no relation to the absorption of biliary salts.

3 A prolonged prothrombin time indicates potential clotting problems for the newborn and would not be deliberately produced.

4 The vitamin K does not replace the necessary bacteria; the bacteria will develop once oral feedings are established.

113. 1 Client participation provides for a sense of control, and a consistent approach provides a routine with no surprises; these approaches may limit pain and promote compliance with the regimen. (2) (SU; PL; TC; IT)

2 Preparation of the equipment and explanation of the procedure should be performed before the procedure; when performed during the procedure it wastes time, which can prolong pain.

3 Changing staff disrupts the client's routine and sense of trust.

4 This is too hot; the water should be approximately 100°F.

114. 3 This statement leaves communication lines open. (3) (MH; IM; PS; SD)

1 This response discounts the client's thoughts and may increase agitation.

2 This provides false reassurance; it does not provide security because the client may believe the nurse is one of those involved in the plot to kill.

4 This supports the client's delusional system.

115. 3 Right occiput anterior is a vertex presentation; the fundus has a soft rounded mass, which is the buttock and therefore this is a cephalic presentation; the irregular curvature on the right indicates the fetal spine, and the bumpy projections on left indicate the extremities. (2) (CW; AS; PA; HC)

1 Left sacrum posterior is a breech presentation; the fetal part in the fundus would be firm.

2 The fetal spine would be on the left side in left occiput posterior position.

4 This is a transverse lie with right scapula (shoulder) presenting anteriorly.

116. 3 An additional meeting is important to deal with the problem of termination with the client. (2) (MH; IM; PS; TR)

1 This would not be a therapeutic termination because the issues would not be resolved for the client.

2 The nurse may want to do this; however, the focus should be on the needs of the client.

4 The client is avoiding the nurse, and the nurse must reach out to help the client with the termination process.

117. 4 Vasospasms of placental vessels occur because of elevated blood pressure, and the placenta may separate prematurely (abruptio placentae). (2) (CW; PL; TC; HP)

1 Placenta previa is an abnormal placental implantation and is not related to hypertension.

2 Isoimmunization in pregnancy is associated with Rh problems, not hypertension.

3 This is scant amniotic fluid and is usually not associated with hypertensive disorders of pregnancy.

118. 4 The therapy program in use in the home should be incorporated into the nursing care plan to maintain continuity. (1) (PE; PL; TC; SK)

1 The child has social needs, and interaction should be promoted; there is no need for a private room.

2 The parents should be encouraged to stay with the child and actively participate in care.

3 The child should have a regular diet appropriate for the developmental age.

119. 1 The nurse should auscultate the abdomen and listen for bowel sounds, which signify the passage of flatus. (1) (SU; IM; PA; GI)

2 Nausea may be present even though peristalsis has begun.

3 The first bowel movement occurs after peristalsis returns and usually after food is eaten.

4 Peristalsis should return before the tenderness of the abdomen subsides.

120. 4 Strenuous exercise leads to increased cellular metabolism, causing tissue hypoxia, which can precipitate sickling. (2) (PE; EV; ED; BI)

1 This is unnecessary unless the other children have an infectious disease; peer relationships should be encouraged.

2 Fluid should never be restricted; keeping the child well hydrated helps to prevent sickling.

3 This is detrimental to the child's developmental needs and may result in social isolation.

121. 2 An open wound needs sterile technique; the supplies at the bedside are not sterile and the physician ordered sterile soaks. (2) (SU; IM; TC; IT)

1 This is unsafe; a clean basin and washcloth are not sterile.

3 Client safety is the priority.

4 This is unnecessary; the physician has already indicated the type of soak desired.

122. 4 When action on either side of a conflict creates anxiety, a physical reason for not acting at all may unconsciously be used. (3) (MH; AN; PS; AX)

1 These disorders are disabling; the client truly believes the symptoms are real.

2 These individuals do not enjoy their illness; their anxiety is relieved by it.

3 These individuals are in contact with reality.

123. 2 Because normal implantation occurs in the upper third of the uterus, a low-lying placenta would be an abnormal implantation. (2) (CW; EV; PA; HP)

1 Infarctions may appear on a placenta because of some interference with the blood supply; this is not related to position.

3 Placenta previa usually occurs with a fully developed, normal placenta that is abnormally located.

4 Abruptio placentae is the premature separation of a normally implanted placenta.

124. 1   Dialysis removes chemicals, wastes, and fluids usually removed from the body by the kidneys. (1) (SU; IM; PA; RG)
2   The mention of heart problems is a threatening response and may cause increased fear or anxiety.
3   This is a threatening response and can cause an increase in the client's level of anxiety.
4   Dialysis does not speed recovery; it helps maintain fluid and electrolyte balance.

125. 1   The intestine is obstructed by thick, tenacious, pasty meconium. (2) (PE; AS; PA; EN)
2   Imperforate anus is a congenital malformation in which the anal opening is obliterated; it is not associated with cystic fibrosis.
3   A rapid respiratory rate is normal in infants; respirations accelerate with movement and crying.
4   This is common in most newborns because of destruction of immature erythrocytes; it may be physiologic or pathologic.

126. 3   Neologisms are newly coined words with personal meanings to the client with schizrenia. (2) (MH; AN; PS; SD)
1   Clanging is the association of words by sound rather than meaning.
2   Echolalia is parrot-like echoing of spoken words or sounds.
4   Echophrasia (echolalia) is parrot-like echoing of spoken words or sounds.

127. 3   This medication decreases the effectiveness of oral contaceptives and alternate contraceptive measures will have to be used. (2) (CW; EV; ED; WH)
1   Although the urine should be observed for crystals, straining is not necessary.
2   This is a sulfa based medication; this fluid intake is inadequate and would not prevent crystal formation.
4   The urine will not turn orange with this medication; if bloody or smoky urine were present prior to treatment, it would become a normal color once treatment was initiated.

128. 3   The sudden change of pressure tends to tear away the dural linings. (3) (CW; AN; PA; HP)
1   This occurs normally during labor as the baby's head descends into the birth canal.
2   Although this could occur, the placenta usually is expelled shortly after the fetus.
4   This occurs before delivery and is unrelated to precipitate labor; this may occur in placenta previa or abruptio placentae.

129. 2   These dysrhythmias may result from postoperative inflammation around the SA node. (3) (SU; EV; TC; CV)
1   This syndrome occurs later, not immediately.
3   Same as answer 1.
4   Hemoglobin and hematocrit levels usually fall; anemia can be a problem.

130. 3   This is the only way the nurse can be certain of the amount of food and fluid vomited. (3) (MH; PL; TC; EA)
1   An accurate intake and output is difficult to maintain unless the individual is closely observed.
2   Weighing daily would not help to assess the individual's electrolyte or nutritional status.
4   Searching for hoarded food establishes a negative relationship and documents lack of trust.

131. 4   This is the most complete definition of bulimia. (2) (MH; AN; PS; EA)
1   This may occur with bulimia, but it is not the definition.
2   Although clients with bulimia do consume large amounts of food in private, they do eat in public.
3   Same as answer 1.

132. 1   An exercise program and the Milwaukee brace are the treatments of choice for mild structural scoliosis. (2) (PE; IM; ED; SK)
2   Although compliance will affect the ultimate outcome of treatment, exercises alone are not helpful in this type of scoliosis.

3   Exercises are to be encouraged regardless of the type or extent of scoliosis.

4   Exercises alone are used only with scoliosis that is related to posture, not structure.

133. 3   Flexion and extension prevents tightening of muscles and tendons. (2) (ME; PL; ED; SK)

1   This is an abnormal sensation and is related to neurologic, not musculoskeletal, alterations.

2   Weightbearing, not exercise, would promote the development of osteoblasts.

4   This is the result of cerebellar changes; it is not related to immobility.

134. 4   The newborn's intake of milk is gradual and small and at the same time the bowel is emptying of meconium; thus a weight loss occurs. (2) (CW; AN; PA; NN)

1   This is untrue; slight weight loss after delivery is a normal physiologic response.

2   Same as answer 1.

3   Same as answer 1.

135. 4   If carbohydrate intake is reduced, protein is utilized for energy, thereby lowering the recommended elevated protein requirements for pregnancy. (2) (CW; AN; PA; HP)

1   This is not the reason for avoiding dieting during pregnancy.

2   Additional calories are needed to spare protein.

3   This is untrue.

136. 3   This is not uncommon in breech presentation because the contracting uterus exerts pressure on the lower colon, forcing out the meconium. (3) (CW; AS; PA; HC)

1   Mild vaginal show is expected; a heavier flow might indicate placenta previa or severe abruptio placentae.

2   This is not observable during usual external monitoring; the fetus would have to be attached to a special ECG apparatus.

4   This would not only be unusual with a breech position but also ominous, because it may be an indication of fetal distress.

137. 3   Safety becomes a priority when the client has hemiparesis and hemianopsia. (2) (ME; PL; ED; NM)

1   Although a balance between activity and rest is important, the client does not have to maintain bedrest.

2   Oxygen is generally not necessary.

4   All the basic nutrients should be included in the diet; there is no need to reduce protein intake.

138. 3   Between the ages of 3 and 5 years, death is viewed as a departure or sleep, which is reversible. (3) (PE; AN; PS; GD)

1   This is the concept of death held by children 9 or 10 years of age; death is viewed as reversible by the preschooler.

2   The early school-age child of 6 or 7 years personifies death and sees it as horrible and frightening; this is consistent with the concrete thinking present at this age.

4   Children of all ages have some concept of death.

139. 4   Palpation would create a risk of rupturing the tumor mass. (2) (PE; IM; TC; RG)

1   This is unnecessary; no calculi are present.

2   There is no related contraindication for IV medication.

3   Diapers can be worn as long as there is no palpation.

140. 4   Malnutrition and liver damage lead to a reduced serum albumin level and failure of the capillary fluid shift mechanism, resulting in ascites. (2) (ME; AN; PA; FE)

1   Iron promotes hemoglobin synthesis; this is unrelated to cirrhosis.

2   Vitamins are unrelated to ascites.

3   The sodium level is usually excessive with cirrhosis.

141. 2 Closeness increases anxiety, which cannot be tolerated; hostility is used to keep people away. (2) (MH; EV; PS; TR)

1 Hostility is more extreme than assertiveness and is not an indication of improvement.

3 This is true, but the expression of hostility is not really a flare-up in this situation.

4 Regressive behavior is the resumption of behavior characteristic of an earlier stage of development; hostility does not fit this definition.

142. 4 This is important in determining whether the baby has maternally transmitted antibodies against measles. (2) (PE; AS; PA; BI)

1 This baby has no vaccination against measles because this is not done until the baby is older than 1 year of age.

2 This has no relationship to the present exposure to measles.

3 Same as answer 2.

143. 1 Xylocaine usually reduces the irritability of the heart. (3) (ME; IM; TC; CV)

2 Treating the PVBs is the first priority.

3 Stimulating the cough reflex will not affect an irritable heart muscle.

4 At present, manually stimulating the heart is not needed.

144. 2 With the reduction of edema the child's health improves, the appetite increases, and the blood pressure normalizes. (2) (PE; PL; TC; RG)

1 Fluids should not be forced because the kidneys are inflamed and cannot tolerate large amounts.

3 Ambulation does not have an adverse effect on the disease; most children voluntarily restrict their activities during the acute phase.

4 Sodium is lowered not eliminated; sodium restriction is not tolerated well by children and may further restrict their appetite.

145. 3 This is giving correct information in a non-threatening manner; fetal-placental status may deteriorate because of falling estriol levels, which occur in a mother with diabetes mellitus. (3) (CW; IM; ED; HP)

1 Neonates generally develop hypoglycemia shortly after birth; however, early delivery has no effect on this development.

2 Fetal viability as determined by lung maturity, not size, would influence the time of delivery; the route would be determined by fetal and maternal status, not just size.

4 This client does not show any signs of pregnancy-induced hypertension; in addition, delivering early does not prevent development of pregnancy-induced hypertension; however, the client with severe preeclampsia may be delivered early to prevent eclampsia.

146. 2 This moves the emphasis from facts to feelings; it focuses on the client without setting the direction for communication. (3) (MH; IM; PS; MO)

1 This elicits a 'yes' or 'no' response; the client has already brought up the topic.

3 This denies the client's feelings and cuts off further communication.

4 This asks a direct question that the client will probably be unable to answer.

147. 4 Change is always accompanied by some anxiety and pain; without motivation, change will not occur. (2) (MH; EV; PS; PR)

1 The lifestyle of these individuals is rarely limited because they tend to be rather gregarious and outgoing; in reality, they attempt to live by their guile.

2 The reactions of the client's parents would be of little influence at this age.

3 These usually do not work unless the individual is motivated to change.

148. 2 This is an accurate statement; each gram of carbohydrate contains 4 calories per gram. (1) (ME; PL; ED; GI)

1 This provides too few calories; carbohydrates contain 4 calories per gram.

3   This provides too many calories; fat contain 9 calories per gram.

4   This provides too many calories; no nutrient contains this many calories per gram.

149. 4   In the first 48 hours there is a rapid fluid shift, which causes an increase in cardiac output and blood volume; this taxes an already compromised heart. (2) (CW; PL; PA; HP)

1   This is not recommended because this will further increase circulating blood volume and necessitate an increase in cardiac workload.

2   This is false; the first 48 hours are crucial because of the rapid fluid shift and the stress of increased cardiac output on a compromised heart.

3   Progressive ambulation starting 48 hours after delivery is recommended.

150. 1   Constipation and paralytic ileus are frequent problems because of decreased nerve innervation of the GI tract; they are symptomatic of neurotoxicity. (2) (PE; EV; TC; DR)

2   This is not a toxic effect; it is not necessary to check bowel sounds if diarrhea is present.

3   This is not a factor in the development of constipation; fluid can be given intravenously if nausea is present.

4   Vincristine causes leukopenia, which increases susceptibility to infection; it does not cause antigen/antibody reactions.

151. 3   Allopurinol decreases serum uric acid levels before and during chemotherapy; increased fluid intake aids in the increased excretion of uric acid; allopurinol and increased fluids help prevent renal tubular impairment and kidney failure because of hyperuricemia. (3) (ME; PL; PA; DR)

1   The client should be encouraged to follow a diet that promotes urine alkalinity.

2   If the oral route is used, this will limit gastric irritation not uric acid nephropathy.

4   Fluid intake should be increased to 2 to 3 liters per day to prevent urate deposits and calculi formation.

152. 3   The elastic bandage must be applied smoothly without wrinkles, folds, or creases because these can cause excessive pressure or irritation. (2) (SU; PL; TC; SK)

1   The bandage should be reapplied whenever necessary; this may be necessary if it slips off, if it is too tight or too loose, or if it has wrinkles or creases.

2   This would be unsafe because it could impede circulation; the bandage should be snug, not tight.

4   This would be unsafe because the dependent position allows the blood vessels to become engorged; the bandage should be applied with the leg level with the heart.

153. 2   Elastic stockings help decrease venous pooling of blood and help maintain systemic blood pressure when the client stands up. (2) (ME; IM; PA; CV)

1   Orthostatic hypotension occurs on rising to an upright position; gait training will not affect this.

3   An alteration in dosage may be ordered by the physician, but sudden withdrawal is dangerous and unwarranted.

4   This may increase the intravascular fluid volume temporarily but will not affect reflexes involved in orthostatic hypotension.

154. 4   Forcing fluids fills the bladder, which is necessary to push the uterus up for optimal ultrasound viewing. (2) (CW; IM; TC; HC)

1   The bladder must be full, not empty, for better visualization of the uterus.

2   This has no relation to ultrasound preparation; fasting places the fetus in jeopardy.

3   The gastrointestinal tract is not involved.

155. 4   This reduces the risk of introducing the irrigant into the lungs. (1) (SU; AS; TC; GI)

1   This is irrelevant to nasogastric tube irrigation.

2   This increases the risk of introducing irrigant into the lungs if tube placement is not checked first.

3   Same as answer 1.

156. 2 Clients need to understand the cycle as a physiologic event that can be dealt with, not as a life-threatening crisis. (2) (ME; PL; ED; RE)
1 This is insufficient to break the cycle.
3 Same as answer 1.
4 Though helpful, this is not primary in helping to break the cycle of fear, dyspnea, and inactivity.

157. 3 This will help decrease irritability and impulsiveness caused by the client's increased responsiveness to changing stimuli. (2) (MH; PL; PS; MO)
1 This is not helpful because of the client's easy distractibility and minimal attention span.
2 At this time, the client may misidentify this approach as threatening and may retaliate by aggression.
4 A strange environment and new staff tend to increase the anxiety level, not reduce manipulation.

158. 3 The client will need reassurance and support after this frightening experience. (1) (MH; IM; PS; CS)
1 This provides false reassurance.
2 This is inappropriate; the priority is to allay anxiety; also, there is no need to stand the client up to take the pulse.
4 This is inappropriate; the client has dementia and will have limited recall of recent teaching.

159. 3 Parental role support and contact with other adults is very important in parenting. (2) (MH; AS; PS; CS)
1 No personality type is specifically associated with abusive behavior.
2 This is untrue; present defenses are ineffective when an adult engages in child abuse.
4 Although lack of knowledge may lead to unrealistic expectations of the child, this factor alone does not significantly contribute to abusive behavior.

160. 3 The fundus tends to stay at or slightly above the umbilicus for about 24 hours, then decreases in size about one finger-breadth per day. (1) (CW; AS; PA; HC)
1 This would be the position in the first 24 hours postpartum.
2 Same as answer 1.
4 This would be the position on the fourth or fifth day.

161. 1 Initial attempts at oral feeding may cause a choking feeling that may produce severe coughing and raise secretions. (3) (SU; IM; PA; RE)
2 Swallowing does not have an adverse effect on the suture line; a nasogastric tube would not be used because it could traumatize the suture line.
3 A progressive diet is started with liquids, not pureed foods.
4 The pain medication may cause a decrease in the client's respiratory effort and may also depress the cough reflex.

162. 3 This would minimize the sucking and yet not be irritating to the suture line. (2) (PE; PL; TC; GI)
1 This is not used because it would be irritating to the nostrils.
2 Intravenous infusions do not supply the necessary caloric intake.
4 No nipple should be used because the baby should not suck.

163. 1 Removing a tube does not impair the ovary on the unaffected side from releasing an egg, which may be fertilized in the remaining tube. (1) (CW; PL; ED; RP)
2 There is no information given that states the client is Rh negative.
3 There is no absolute way of knowing whether or not another tubal pregnancy will ensue.
4 This is unrelated to tubal pregnancy, as well as incorrect information, because douching cannot reach a fertilized egg.

164. 2 The nursing diagnosis consists of two parts: the statement of the client's health status (health problem) and the related factors (probable causes). (3) (MH; AN; TC; CS)
1 The nursing diagnosis includes a statement of the problem; the client's needs are addressed in the plan of care.
3 Although the client's responses may reflect health status, this is only one part of the diagnosis.
4 A medical diagnosis describes a disease process; a nursing diagnosis describes a person's response to a disease process, condition, or situation.

165. 2 When children are allowed to have some control in their care, their cooperation and willingness to tolerate procedures and medications are enhanced. (2) (PE; PL; PS; EH)
1 A child's favorite food should never be used to disguise medication because it will likely cause an aversion to that food and can affect the child nutritionally.
3 Bribing sets up a nontherapeutic relationship between the child and the nurse and should not be used.
4 The nurse should be truthful about the taste of medication so that the child can have an opportunity to suggest ways to deal with the taste.

166. 3 The client should be assessed further for signs of abruptio placentae by looking for cessation of uterine activity, fetal heart deceleration, and falling blood pressure. (2) (CW; IM; TC; HP)
1 This is unsafe; the status of the fetus and mother must be assessed immediately.
2 This is not the priority; the status of the fetus is paramount.
4 This is unsafe; the status of the fetus is primary; in a partial abruptio placentae, placing the client in a supine position would further compromise blood flow to the fetus.

167. 3 The opportunity must be provided for the client to practice language skills; family participation must be accepted and recognized. (1) (ME; IM; PS; NM)
1 This demeans the spouse and cuts off communication.
2 Same as answer 1.
4 The spouse should be included and involved in the client's care.

168. 1 Decadron is a corticosteroid with antiinflammatory effects. (1) (SU; EV; TC; DR)
2 Decadron will not keep the tumor from growing; it will only reduce fluid content and therefore cell size, not the number of cells.
3 Decadron does not promote fluid reabsorption, which is undesirable because it increases fluid retention and therefore cerebral edema.
4 Decadron does not promote sedation; sedation is not desired because it could mask symptoms.

169. 4 ASA is irritating to the stomach lining and can cause ulceration; the presence of food, fluid, or antacids decreases this response. (1) (ME; IM; ED; DR)
1 Tylenol does not contain the antiinflammatory properties present in aspirin; tinnitus should be reported to the physician.
2 This should be reported to the physician, not the dentist.
3 This is unnecessary as long as aspirin is taken with food.

170. 1 This statement focuses on the client's perceptions and promotes further communication. (3) (PE; IM; PS; EH)
2 This reads too much into the client's statement and may be too emotionally charged.
3 This is untrue; there is a higher incidence of lice in people with inadequate personal hygiene.
4 This statement is valid but accusatory; it discourages further communication.

171. 3   Informed consent means the client must comprehend the surgery, the alternatives, and the consequences. (2) (SU; IM; TC; CV)

1   This explanation is not within nursing's domain.

2   This is true, but it does not determine the client's ability to give informed consent.

4   The nurse's signature documents that the client has given informed consent; however, this follows after the nurse determines the client's comprehension.

172. 1   Growth retardation is evident and common in infants with toxoplasmosis. (3) (CW; AS; PA; HN)

2   This is a normal characteristic in the dark-pigmented neonate.

3   This is a normal assessment in a healthy neonate.

4   Same as answer 3.

173. 4   This answers the client's question and provides an accurate description of a cystoscopy. (1) (SU; AN; ED; RG)

1   This is not a computerized examination.

2   This procedure does not involve x-ray films or dye.

3   Radiopaque material is not used and the catheter is inserted via the urethra, not the ureters.

174. 4   A 2½-year-old is capable of fitting large wooden pieces into the puzzle; this activity challenges the child's ability to recognize shapes. (2) (PE; PL; ED; GD)

1   This is a toy suitable for the young infant.

2   This is more appropriate for the child of 12 months who is becoming adept at motor skills.

3   Same as answer 1.

175. 4   Previous experiences with projectile vomiting are frightening; an explanation that surgery has eliminated this, as well as support and encouragement of the parents as they resume care of their infant, are necessary. (1) (PE; EV; PS; EH)

1   This is untrue; the data indicate the mother is eager to assist with other aspects of care.

2   These are not used initially; oral feedings are reinstituted with clear liquids and electrolytes and progress to formula as tolerated.

3   No special nipple is required; these are used for infants with cleft lip and/or palate.

176. 3   Aldactone is a potassium-sparing diuretic often used in conjunction with thiazide diuretics. (1) (ME; AN; PA; DR)

1   Both diuretics do this, so it is not a particular advantage of Aldactone.

2   Same as answer 1.

4   Same as answer 1.

177. 3   A first step in any therapeutic relationship should include setting parameters of meetings such as time and frequency. (3) (MH; PL; PS; TR)

1   This is part of the working phase of a therapeutic relationship and, therefore, not an initial intervention.

2   The nurse should not deviate from the original contract.

4   There is no need to carry this out during the termination phase because it is part of the initial ground rules.

178. 2   These would be signs of infection and should be reported to the physician. (1) (CW; EV; ED; WH)

1   This is a sign of healing that is expected and normal.

3   There is little subcutaneous fat in the thoracic area, and the skin may be taut at the operative site, appearing irregular; this commonly occurs.

4   This results from severance of nerves and formation of scar tissue, which are expected and normal.

179. 2   Various waveforms can indicate damage to different areas of the heart. (1) (ME; IM; ED; CV)

1   Auscultation can detect various heart sounds.

3   Cardioversion, not an ECG, is used to change heart rhythm.

4   An ECG taken during a stress test determines endurance of the heart.

180. 1 Glomerulonephritis is associated with a history of a prior streptococcal infection of the throat. (1) (PE; AS; PA; RG)
2 A streptococcus infection, not the measles virus, is associated with glomerulonephritis.
3 Glomerulonephritis is not an inherited disease; it usually follows a streptococcal infection.
4 There are no immunizations that would cause glomerulonephritis.

181. 4 Insulin needs may decrease in early pregnancy because of increased fetal needs for nutrients and the possibility of maternal nausea and vomiting; insulin needs increase in the second and third trimesters as a resistance to insulin develops; the blood glucose is monitored to prevent ketoacidosis and ensuing harm to the fetus. (1) (CW; IM; ED; HP)
1 This is true only during early pregnancy; during the second and third trimesters of pregnancy there is a resistance to insulin and more insulin is required.
2 This is untrue; even the nondiabetic woman makes a dietary adjustment to keep pace with the increased demands of pregnancy; in addition, insulin needs increase in the second and third trimesters.
3 Most nutrient requirements, not just protein, increase in pregnancy.

182. 3 This drug is a local irritant to the GI tract. (3) (PE; EV; ED; DR)
1 This is not a side effect; theophylline is given to ease respirations.
2 This is not considered a side effect; frequent urination is expected because this drug often produces diuresis.
4 This is not a side effect.

183. 2 Anxiety about the behavior is absent, as is motivation for change; these persons are unwilling to accept help. (2) (MH; AN; PS; PR)
1 More than lifestyle needs to change; the client's entire view of life and interpersonal response is involved.

3 These individuals do not experience feelings of guilt about their behavior.
4 It is not a resistance to demonstrating feelings but a total lack of feeling for others.

184. 3 These are early signs of hypoglycemia or too much insulin; the client should be taught to take additional food or an oral glucose solution. (3) (ME; EV; ED; EN)
1 These are symptoms of hyperglycemia.
2 Same as answer 1.
4 Same as answer 1.

185. 4 This is a normal cardiopulmonary symptom in pregnancy; it is caused by an increased ventricular rate and an elevated diaphragm. (2) (CW; AS; PA; HC)
1 This is pathologic, a sign of impending cardiac decompensation.
2 Same as answer 1.
3 Same as answer 1.

186. 3 The child needs to know that he will remain awake, and he should be prepared to experience the pressure of the aspiration or the biopsy needle entry, and he should know that he will not be incapacitated following the test. (2) (PE; IM; ED; BI)
1 This is a false statement; false statements must be avoided or the child will not trust what is said in the future.
2 The child will be permitted to ambulate freely.
4 A bone marrow specimen is obtained through a puncture wound; sutures are not necessary.

187. 1 Drainage from the small intestine contains residual digestive enzymes that cause the skin to break down. (1) (SU; PL; PA; GI)
2 An ileostomy is not irrigated; the stool is liquid in quality and drains unassisted.
3 An ileostomy will continually drain liquid stool; control of fecal elimination is impossible.
4 An ileostomy will continually drain liquid stool; this is unrelated to diet; the stool is excreted before fluid can be reabsorbed in the large intestine.

188. 1 Using ratio and proportion:

$$20 \text{ mEq} : 1000 \text{ ml} = X \text{ mEq} : 150 \text{ ml}$$
$$1000 X = 20 \times 150$$
$$1000 X = 3000$$
$$X = 3000 \div 1000$$
$$X = 3 \text{ mEq} \ (2)$$

(ME; AN; TC; FE)

    2 This is too much; this should be added to 250 ml of fluid.

    3 This is too much; this should be added to 500 ml of fluid.

    4 This is too much; this should be added to 1000 ml of fluid.

189. 4 This procedure removes fluids and gas from the GI tract, which permits better healing of the surgical area and minimizes nausea. (1) (SU; AN; TC; GI)

    1 This is not the purpose in this situation; the tube is used to decompress the stomach.

    2 Tube feeding would be contraindicated after gastrointestinal surgery.

    3 The tube decompresses the stomach, not the large bowel.

190. 2 Respiratory tract infection may be the first clinical sign of bone marrow suppression. (2) (ME; EV; TC; DR)

    1 This is an expected, non-life-threatening side effect.

    3 Same as answer 1.

    4 This is not a side effect of doxorubicin.

191. 2 The collection device must be kept below the level of the chest to prevent backflow of fluid into the pleural space. (1) (SU; IM; TC; RE)

    1 For transport, suction should be turned off and the tubing disconnected distal to the water seal connection.

    3 There is no reason to disconnect the chest tube from the water seal system; this would allow atmospheric air to enter the pleural space.

    4 The chest tube should almost never be clamped; this may precipitate a tension pneumothorax.

192. 2 These are signs of congestive heart failure, which may develop with the persistent tachycardia that is present with hyperthyroidism. (3) (ME; EV; PA; EN)

    1 These are expected to occur with hyperthyroidism and need not be reported immediately.

    3 Same as answer 1.

    4 Same as answer 1.

193. 1 Guilt feelings can prolong the grieving process because the individual is overwhelmed by both the guilt and grief, and consequently the energy needed to cope with both is excessive. (3) (MH; AN; PS; CS)

    2 There are no research data to support this.

    3 Ambivalent feelings about the deceased, not the death itself, can prolong grief.

    4 Usually the opposite is true; the support provided would hasten resolution of grief.

194. 3 The ruptured tube usually will be removed; if the tube is repaired it may result in scarring, predisposing to another tubal pregnancy. (1) (CW; PL; TC; RP)

    1 This is a procedure for removing myomas (fibroids) from the uterus.

    2 The uterus is usually uninvolved in a tubal pregnancy, and this would make the woman incapable of future pregnancy.

    4 The D and C would be effective only in cleaning out the uterine cavity; no pregnancy contents are in the uterus with a tubal pregnancy.

195. 4 The cervical mucus is clear and stretchable (spinnbarkeit) at ovulation because of maximum estrogen stimulation. (3) (CW; IM; PA; RC)

    1 These characteristics do not normally occur at any point during the cycle.

    2 Same as answer 1.

    3 Same as answer 1.

196. 4 This is a true statement that addresses the client's concern. (2) (MH; IM; PE; MO)

    1 This approach denies the client's fears and feelings and really does not address the current concern.

2   This approach denies the client's fears and feelings and could be frightening and upsetting.

3   This approach denies the client's fears and feelings and may not be the most important thing to the client at this time.

197. 3   A formal plan demonstrates determination, concentration, and effort, with conclusions already thought out. (2) (MH; AS; PS; MO)

1   Failure to successfully complete the suicidal act can add to feelings of worthlessness and stimulate further acts.

2   Talking about suicide does not give clients the idea; verbalizing feelings may help reduce clients' need to act out.

4   Many clients verbalize their suicidal thoughts as they are working on their decision and plan of action; suicide is not always attempted for the attention it achieves.

198. 2   This response recognizes the client's and family's concerns and encourages further verbalization of feelings. (2) (ME; IM; PS; EH)

1   This response does not focus on the client's and family's underlying concerns and keeps the discussion on a physiologic level.

3   This provides false reassurance and cuts off further verbalization of feelings.

4   Same as answer 3.

199. 3   Because of the serious side effects of Sinemet, a thorough daily nursing assessment is a priority. (3) (ME; PL; TC; DR)

1   This is incomplete; it is only one part of a thorough nursing assessment.

2   This is an incomplete assessment; vital signs would be a priority if there were an additional abnormality or indication beyond the drug therapy.

4   This is an incomplete assessment; isolating this as a priority would be indicated if there were a fluid imbalance.

200. 3   Total blood volume increases 50%, which necessitates the heart pumping harder and working more to accommodate this increase. (2) (CW; AN; PA; HC)

1   Although the renal threshold is lowered, the major changes occur in the cardiovascular system.

2   Changes in hormonal levels occur but are not as profound as changes in the cardiovascular system.

4   There are no changes in this system, but pressure from the growing uterus can result in altered patterns of elimination.

201. 3   Bile drainage for the first 24 hours is usually 300 to 500 ml; kinks in the tubing hinder the flow. (3) (SU; IM; TC; GI)

1   Clamping the tube is contraindicated in the first 24 hours.

2   Further intervention is necessary because this amount of bile is less than normal.

4   Drainage of 150 ml is less than expected in the first 24 hours.

202. 3   Aminophylline acts as a vasodilator, and hypotension results when vessels are dilated. (3) (ME; EV; TC; DR)

1   Increased diuresis, not oliguria, is a common side effect.

2   Tachycardia, not bradycardia, is a common side effect.

4   Tachypnea, not hypoventilation, is a common side effect.

203. 1   Applying moist or dry heat relieves muscle pain through vasodilation, increases circulation to the area, and facilitates drug absorption. (2) (PE; PL; TC; NM)

2   This will prolong the discomfort by slowing the rate of absorption of the drug because of vasoconstriction.

3   Movement most likely will be difficult and cause more discomfort.

4   This will cause more discomfort because the injection site is tender.

204. 3 Focusing on the client's feelings permits her to work through her fears. (2) (CW; IM; PS; EC)
 1 This statement does not encourage the client to focus on her feelings.
 2 This closes off communication and does not allow the client to verbalize her feelings.
 4 Same as answer 1.

205. 2 The nurse can be more sensitive to the needs of the client by dealing with personal emotions first. (3) (CW; AS; PS; EC)
 1 The focus should be on the client's feelings, not the nurse's.
 3 Complete control is not, and should not, be the goal of the nurse.
 4 A time of crisis is not the time to teach; the client is not ready to learn.

206. 3 Clients with left hemianopia ignore whatever is in the left field of vision. (3) (ME; EV; PA; NM)
 1 This would occur if the client had right hemianopia and wished to see better when eating.
 2 This would occur with right hemiparesis, not with hemianopia.
 4 This indicates hemiplegia, not hemianopia.

207. 4 This moves from clean to dirty and keeps microorganisms away from the urinary meatus to prevent an ascending infection. (2) (PE; EV; ED; RG)
 1 Fluid should be encouraged to maintain urinary function and prevent urinary stasis.
 2 Contact sports should be avoided to prevent trauma to the remaining kidney.
 3 This is not necessary; the child's immune system is not depressed.

208. 3 These are characteristics associated with children who have Down syndrome; a slant of the eyes is also present. (1) (CW; AS; PA; HN)
 1 Only low-set ears occur with Down syndrome; all of these symptoms occur with Trisomy 18.

 2 Although low-set ears occur with Down syndrome, microencephaly and a high-pitched cry may indicate a variety of neurologic problems; the last two symptoms are part of a syndrome known as cri-du-chat.
 4 Webbed neck and widely spaced nipples are associated with Turner's syndrome.

209. 3 Goodell's sign, or softening of the cervix, occurs at 8 to 9 weeks gestation. (3) (CW; AS; PA; HC)
 1 Lightening or settling of the fetal presenting part into the pelvis usually occurs 2 weeks before the onset of labor in nulliparas.
 2 This refers to the fetal movements usually perceived by the mother between the sixteenth and twentieth weeks of gestation.
 4 Braxton-Hicks are intermittent, cramplike contractions that usually occur toward the end of pregnancy and may be mistaken by the mother for the onset of labor.

210. 3 Doxorubicin is cardiotoxic and causes dysrhythmias. (2) (ME; EV; TC; DR)
 1 Toxicity causes severe, not minor, dermatitis.
 2 This is a side effect of doxorubicin, not a toxic effect.
 4 Same as answer 2.

211. 1 This is the most appropriate family nursing diagnosis because it is the alteration in parenting that forms the basis for the other problems experienced by the child and family. (3) (PE; AN; ED; GD)
 2 High risk for injury is not an actual problem at this time because there is no history or evidence of physical abuse.
 3 Altered nutrition is a problem for the child but only indirectly for the family; the history does not support child abuse.
 4 Sensory-perceptual alteration is a diagnosis that is related most specifically to the infant; the problem can be resolved by addressing the parenting problems.

212. 3 Additional studies such as T_3 and T_4 will be necessary to confirm hyperthyroidism; it is not reliable to base the diagnosis on RAI alone. (3) (ME; IM; ED; EN)

1 This test uses ^{131}I, which emits radioactive particles for at least 24 hours; these are excreted in the urine.

2 Test results are affected by many medications, especially those containing iodine.

4 This test measures uptake of ^{131}I by the thyroid gland; it does not measure levels of thyroid hormones.

213. 1 During this stage the nurse comes to a conclusion about the collected data and makes a diagnosis. (3) (MH; AN; TC; CS)

2 During this stage, the nurse sets priorities, establishes goals, identifies outcome criteria, and develops a nursing care plan.

3 The client's response to nursing care is assessed in relation to the stated outcome criteria to determine if goals have been met.

4 The nurse gathers and clusters data during this stage of the nursing process.

214. 2 These are early signs of shock; shock ensues rapidly in a ruptured aortic aneurysm because of profound hemorrhage; this is a surgical emergency. (3) (SU; EV; PA; CV)

1 The nurse can observe hyperventilation by watching the client's breathing patterns; rapid respirations, rather than a rapid pulse, would be expected.

3 Extreme anxiety is not usually associated with lightheadedness unless there is hyperventilation.

4 The symptoms are not inclusive enough to indicate infection; there is no indication of fever or a rising white blood count.

215. 3 An explanation of how the restraints work and why may reassure the mother. (2) (PE; AN; TC; GI)

1 Using things routinely does not explain why they are being used now; this is an unsatisfactory response.

2 This implies strict adherence to the physician's wishes without any thinking or understanding by the nurse.

4 This is most unreassuring because it gives the mother the feeling that the baby is not being watched at all times.

216. 1 Cleansing after feeding keeps the suture line from becoming infected. (2) (PE; EV; ED; IT)

2 This exerts pressure on the suture line and may cause wound separation.

3 Same as answer 2.

4 The baby should be held and cuddled during feeding.

217. 4 This frustration reveals readiness to deal with the problem of speech that may be best demonstrated by a person with a laryngectomy. (3) (SU; PL; PS; EH)

1 This type of answer leaves the client in limbo and offers no plans for goal setting.

2 This closes off communication and the client's frustration reveals a need for positive action.

3 The healing of the incision is not a factor in the initial activities of learning a new way of speaking; initially, discussions, demonstrations, and breathing exercises are performed.

218. 3 These foods are low in sodium and calories. (1) (ME; EV; ED; CV)

1 Beef is high in calories, and carrots are high in sodium.

2 Canned tuna fish and celery are high in sodium.

4 Stir-fried Chinese vegetables are made with soy sauce, which is very high in sodium, and cornstarch, which is high in calories.

219. 3 Nipple soreness often occurs when there is incorrect positioning of the newborn's mouth on the breast; also, nipples still need to toughen in response to sucking. (2) (CW; AS; PA; HC)

1 This is premature; the cause of soreness must be determined first and will dictate what type of intervention is necessary.

2 Same as answer 1.

4 Same as answer 1.

220. 3 Active ROM increases venous return from the unaffected leg, preventing complications of immobility, including thrombophlebitis (2) (SU; AN; PA; CV)

1 These isotonic exercises are being performed on the unaffected extremity; there should be no discomfort.

2 Although isotonic exercises do promote muscle strength, that is not the purpose at this time; the priority is to prevent thrombi from developing.

4 These activities will prevent, not limit, venous inflammation.

221. 1 Lemon juice adds flavor and is low in sodium. (1) (ME; IM; ED; FE)

2 This is unnecessary; canned vegetables generally contain sodium.

3 This is unnecessary.

4 Carbonated beverages generally contain sodium; coffee, whether it is decaffeinated or not, does not contain sodium.

222. 1 With a microdrip set, the nurse should know that the number of ml/hr equals the number of micro gtts/min; thus 55 ml/hr = 55 micro gtts/min. (2) (PE; AN; TC; FE)

2 This rate is too high; it would deliver more than the required amount of solution.

3 This is too low; this rate would not deliver the required amount of solution.

4 Same as answer 3.

223. 1 A change in environment and introduction of unfamiliar stimuli precipitate confusion in the elderly client with dementia type disorders; with appropriate intervention, including frequent reorientation, confusion can be reduced. (2) (MH; AN; PA; DD)

2 This is untrue; reality orientation can reduce confusion.

3 This is untrue; this is a stereotype.

4 Same as answer 2.

224. 4 High levels of steroids result in emotional changes; the actual cause is unknown, but knowing the response may help the client to better cope with her son's behavior. (2) (ME; IM; ED; EN)

1 This is unnecessary; the problem has been excessive production of steroids.

2 Weight loss, not weight gain, would indicate an improving condition.

3 The changes are not permanent with adequate therapy.

225. 4 After laboring all night the client is tired. (3) (CW; PL; PA; HC)

1 This would be premature; the client is not ready to learn.

2 This assessment would be too frequent and would interfere with the client's rest.

3 This is necessary only the first time the client ambulates; otherwise the client can ambulate ad lib.

226. 2 Thrombophlebitis is a common complication of immobility in situations related to the application of traction. (2) (SU; AS; TC; SK)

1 This is contraindicated during use of Buck's traction; positioning with a pillow to relieve back pressure is permitted for short periods.

3 This is contraindicated in the affected extremity; this could cause further soft tissue injury and pain for the client.

4 This interferes with the pull of traction; it would cause further soft tissue injury and pain for the client.

227. 2 This prevents trauma from hitting obstacles during the tonic-clonic phase of the seizure. (1) (ME; IM; TC; NM)

1 This is contraindicated; it could injure the client.

3 Same as answer 1.

4 If done during the tonic-clonic phase of the seizure it could cause injury; if necessary, this is done immediately after the seizure to establish an airway.

228. 1 The position of maximal safety and comfort is side-lying because the client's neck and back are hyperextended. (2) (PE; IM; TC; NM)

2 This would be impossible because the child is in a rigid opisthotonic position; this could be injurious to the child.

3 Same as answer 2.

4 This is contraindicated; this would increase intracranial pressure.

229. 4   The stoma secretes mucus immediately following surgery and continues to secrete mucus mixed with serum and blood because of surgical trauma; fecal drainage begins in about 72 hours. (2) (SU; EV; PA; GI)

1   This would not occur until about 72 hours after surgery.

2   Drainage that is bloody with clots would indicate hemorrhage; the expected drainage is mucoid and serosanguinous.

3   Drainage will not be clear; it will be serosanguinous because of the trauma of surgery.

230. 2   The normal muscle contraction-relaxation cycle requires a normal serum calcium-phosphorus ratio; the reduction of the ionized serum calcium level associated with sprue causes tetany (spastic muscle spasms). (2) (ME; AN; PA; GI)

1   Sodium is the major extracellular cation; the major route of excretion is the kidneys under the control of aldosterone; although it plays a part in neuromuscular transmission, it is not related to the development of tetany.

3   Potassium is the major intracellular cation; it is part of the sodium/potassium pump and helps to balance the response of nerves to stimulation; it is not related to the development of tetany.

4   Although phosphorus is closely related to calcium because they exist in a definite ratio, phosphorus is not related to the development of tetany.

231. 4   It is important to set limits on behavior, but it is also important to involve the client in decision making. (2) (MH; IM; PS; PR)

1   This is a nontherapeutic approach; some limits must be set by the client and the nurse together.

2   This is a nontherapeutic approach; rarely can a client be distracted from a ritual.

3   This would increase anxiety, because the client uses the ritual as a defense against anxiety.

232. 3   This is the correct flow rate; multiply the amount of fluid to be infused (175 ml) by the drop factor (15) and divide this result by the amount of time in minutes (1 hr ×60 min). (2) (SU; AN; PA; FE)

1   This rate would deliver less than the prescribed amount of fluid.

2   Same as answer 1.

4   This rate would deliver more than the prescribed amount of fluid.

233. 1   Subcostal incisional pain causes the client to splint and avoid deep breathing, which impedes air exchange in the alveoli. (3) (SU; AN; PA; GI)

2   The location of the incision does not increase the risk of hemorrhage.

3   This can be a postoperative problem, but it is unrelated to the site of the incision.

4   The site is not specifically a vulnerable location for infection.

234. 3   The client's behaviors are contrary to the medical regimen and are not conducive to positive self interests. (2) (ME; AN; PS; RE)

1   The behavior does not indicate a self-care deficit.

2   The client's behavior does not indicate altered thought processes.

4   There are no data to support this conclusion.

235. 3   The desired outcome is the increased excretion of lead in the urine. (2) (PE; EV; TC; DR)

1   This is expected when lead initially equilibrates to the blood; until the lead is excreted in the urine, the treatment is not considered a success.

2   The elimination of lead via the GI tract is less than via the urinary tract and would be an unsatisfactory measure of the success of the chelation therapy.

4   This is a desirable effect, but it does not determine the success of therapy; also, the amount is difficult to determine.

236. 1 By failing to acknowledge the baby as a person, the client indicates that she has not released her fantasy baby and accepted the real one. (1) (CW; AN; PS; EC)

2 The mother has acknowledged the infant by using "he," and her question denotes a relationship.

3 The mother incorporated the infant into the family by this statement.

4 Same as answer 2.

237. 1 Increased levels of steroids and aldosterone cause sodium and water retention. (3) (ME; AS; PA; EN)

2 Hypertension, not hypotension, would be expected because of sodium and water retension.

3 The extremities would be thin; subcutaneous fat deposits occur in the upper trunk, especially the back between the scapula.

4 Hyperglycemia, not hypoglycemia, occurs because of increased secretion of glucocorticoids; hyperglycemia is sustained and not restricted to the morning hours.

238. 3 This will help to decrease the client's anxiety, provide a safe environment, and compensate for impaired cognition. (2) (MH; PL; PS; DD)

1 Restraints may increase confusion and agitation; they should be used only when absolutely unavoidable.

2 Reality orientation should be employed when necessary.

4 Focusing on coping skills would increase the client's feelings of inadequacy; coping skills are on the unconscious level.

239. 4 Positive and negative experiences connected with previous illness or hospitalization will influence the child's response and adaptation to this and subsequent hospitalization. (3) (PE; AS; PS; GD)

1 The priority care at this time should be directed to the child's coping abilities.

2 This will not be too meaningful because a 4-year-old may not have too great an understanding of the illness.

3 This is not a priority; the child's present acute illness must be attended to first.

240. 4 All amino acids are needed for the synthesis of various proteins, but the term essential refers to those amino acids the body cannot make which are thus essential in the diet. (2) (SU; IM; ED; GI)

1 All amino acids in a protein contribute the same number of calories for energy.

2 All amino acids, not just essential amino acids, are necessary for rebuilding body tissue.

3 All amino acids, not just essential amino acids, contain nitrogen.

241. 2 Regular insulin is short acting, and it peaks in 2 to 4 hours which is just at or before lunch. (1) (ME; PL; TC; DR)

1 This is too soon; regular insulin peaks in 2 to 4 hours.

3 This is too late; regular insulin peaks in 2 to 4 hours.

4 Same as answer 3.

242. 2 This client does not need to be on the medical unit; the client's problem is emotional; it is unfair to upset the other clients; the client should be removed from this unit. (3) (MH; EV; PS; PR)

1 An individual cannot be accused of stealing unless actual proof is obtained.

3 This would accomplish little because the client would deny taking them.

4 This action supports the client's feelings that any means can be used to justify a desired goal.

243. 3 This position allows the lungs more room to expand, thus affording more comfort; this enables the child to breathe better. (1) (PE; IM; PA; RE)

1 This position would increase difficulty in breathing; it does not allow for chest expansion.

2 Same as answer 1.

4 Same as answer 1.

244. 1 An autograft is a permanent graft that should not be rejected; the nurse needs to assess the site immediately. (1) (SU; EV; TC; IT)

2 An autograft is a permanent graft that should not need to be replaced.

3 This could raise the client's anxiety and draws a conclusion before assessment of the site; infection is usually associated with purulent drainage.

4 The nurse needs to assess the site; the responsibility of assessment should not be left up to the client.

245. 2 Brief, frequent contacts are less threatening and help to build trust. (2) (MH; PL; TC; SD)

1 This would increase suspiciousness; the client needs consistent caregivers to help increase the level of trust.

3 This supports the client's delusional system, thus increasing suspiciousness.

4 The client needs to be observed to prevent self-harm as a result of delusional thinking.

246. 4 Counterpressure against the sacrum during contractions affords some relief from the discomfort of back pain. (1) (CW; IM; PA; HC)

1 It is difficult to predict the length of labor for any client.

2 This does not respond to the situation; the coach should be included in providing comfort to the client.

3 Same as answer 2.

247. 4 These movements require muscle contraction, putting pressure on blood vessels, increasing tissue oxygen, and thus promoting circulation. (3) (CW; AN; PA; WH)

1 Muscle atrophy is not a common complication following a mastectomy.

2 Contractures are a rare complication following a mastectomy.

3 Lymphedema is assessed by measuring the circumference of the extremity, not by doing exercises.

248. 4 These exercises promote venous return which helps prevent venous thrombi formation. (2) (SU; IM; ED; SK)

1 This exercise would be contraindicated in a client who had a history of ruptured nucleus pulposus.

2 These exercises stimulate collateral circulation for clients with peripheral vascular disease; they are seldom used because walking is considered a more effective exercise.

3 Although these should be encouraged to prevent respiratory complications, thrombus formation is a more common complication than respiratory complications following a total hip replacement.

249. 1 Euthanasia is a crime and is against the law in every state. (1) (ME; AN; PS; EH)

2 Euthanasia is against the law in all states.

3 Neither physicians nor nurses have the legal authority to perform acts of euthanasia; it is a crime.

4 This is not negligence; it is a crime.

250. 4 This is breast engorgement, which immediately precedes milk production on the second to fourth day postpartum. (2) (CW; AN; PA; HC)

1 Acini cells do not become overdistended because of the supply-and-demand nature of milk production; in addition, milk production is not yet established; the client is engorged.

2 Milk production has not yet begun; this is engorgement, which precedes milk production.

3 This is impossible because the breasts have not filled with milk yet; engorgement is occurring.

251. 3 The need for acceptance of life as fulfilling and meaningful is the major task of the elderly. (2) (ME; AN; ED; GD)

1 This is the task of young adulthood (20 to 30 years); it involves establishment of an intimate relationship and occupation.

2 The task of the adolescent (13 to 19 years) is establishing identity through relationships, particularly with peers.

4 This is the task of adulthood (31 to 45 years); it involves establishment of a family and guiding of the next generation.

252. 4   Properly chosen clothes can minimize the appearance of the brace, especially if an effort is made to keep up with the current styles. (1) (PE; IM; PS; EH)
   1   There are no data to indicate that the child will not adjust to the treatment regimen.
   2   This has a negative connotation that emphasizes the client's problem.
   3   This may be misinterpreted as false praise, and a trusting nurse-client relationship may not develop.

253. 3   The autistic child needs protection from self-injury. (2) (MH; IM; TC; BA)
   1   This can only be permitted if it does not place the child in jeopardy.
   2   The autistic child has difficulty following directions, especially when out of control.
   4   The autistic child cannot separate the self from her behavior; a punitive approach will decrease the child's self-esteem further.

254. 4   When neither rest nor nitroglycerin relieves the pain, there may be an acute myocardial infarction. (1) (SU; IM: ED; CV)
   1   This is expected; anginal pain can, and often does, radiate.
   2   This is expected; acute myocardial infarction causes profuse, not mild, diaphoresis, which should be reported.
   3   This is expected; activity increases cardiac output, causing angina.

255. 3   Clients should be familiar with these people and hear from them what will be experienced. (2) (SU; PL; ED; CV)
   1   Although discharge plans should be mentioned, they are not the primary focus at this time.
   2   Most clients do not want or need a minutely detailed description.
   4   The client's whole body, not just the specific area, will be prepped and shaved.

256. 2   Immature thermoregulation necessitates keeping the infant warm to prevent acidosis. (3) (CW; IM; TC; NN)
   1   There is no hurry; the placenta may not separate for 30 minutes without danger.

   3   There is no hurry; as soon as the infant breathes, the umbilical cord no longer functions.
   4   It is too soon to evaluate the hemorrhagic condition of the mother; the placenta has not yet been delivered.

257. 4   Changes in weight and intake and output are indicators of an edematous state; the high-protein diet is essential for fetal growth. (2) (CW; PL; PA; HP)
   1   Diuretics are contraindicated in pregnancy because they decrease circulating fluids and may impair fluid supply to the placenta.
   2   Diuretics and low-salt diets will gradually decrease circulating fluid, creating hypovolemia, which decreases placental circulation.
   3   Elevated serum glucose levels are unrelated to pregnancy-induced hypertension.

258. 4   Cortical control of voluntary muscles occurs between 2 and 4 months. (3) (PE; IM; ED; NM)
   1   Cerebral palsy is not diagnosed by the presence of joint deformities; these may develop later because of spastic muscle imbalance.
   2   Parents have a right to be informed of their child's diagnosis as soon as possible.
   3   The neurological lesions are fixed and will neither progress nor regress.

259. 4   This is an autosomal-recessive disorder; each parent contributes one affected gene. (2) (PE; AN; PA; BI)
   1   There is only a 50% chance that a child will have the sickle cell trait, not sickle cell anemia.
   2   Same as answer 1.
   3   All of the children from these parents will have the sickle cell trait but not sickle cell anemia.

260. 3   There is better control with short-acting (regular) insulin, and emergencies can be handled more quickly. (3) (SU; AN; PA; EN)
   1   This is untrue; the level of glucose must be maintained as close to normal as possible.

2   This is untrue; the occurrence is greater when the client is receiving exogenous insulin.

4   This is not the reason for using regular insulin; both oral hypoglycemics and insulin are available.

261. 2   Limit setting must be consistent with a client who is using manipulative behavior; a unified approach is vital because the client will play the staff against each other. (1) (MH; IM; PS; PR)

1   Limit setting is required to control inappropriate behavior.

3   The most important concept is unity of approach, not the ability of a few to resist manipulation.

4   This must be a group decision, not the responsibility of one staff member alone; the client is unable to set self-limits.

262. 1   Insulin causes an increased rate of flow of potassium into the cells, which will then reduce the circulating blood levels of potassium. (3) (ME; AN; PA; FE)

2   This response halts communication and is nonsupportive.

3   Blood glucose levels are usually not elevated in clients with acute renal failure.

4   Insulin will not lower the metabolic rate.

263. 3   Impaired fat absorption necessitates lowering dietary fat; more calories are needed because of poor absorption of nutrients. (3) (PE; PL; PA; EN)

1   A low-fat diet is recommended, but these children need high-salt diets to replace the large amount of salt lost when sweating.

2   A high-protein diet is recommended, but fat must be avoided because fat absorption is impaired.

4   A high-carbohydrate diet is correct, but because salt depletion via sweating is a hazard, children are encouraged to use salt generously.

264. 1   Withdrawn clients can tolerate personal contact only for short periods of time. (2) (MH; PL; PS; SD)

2   The client could not function in this type of group.

3   The client has a problem with interpersonal relations, therefore this would not work.

4   Allowing the client to be alone would not relieve anxiety; it would foster withdrawal.

265. 2   Voiding flushes the lower portion of the urinary tract of microorganisms introduced during intercourse. (3) (CW; PL; ED; WH)

1   When used correctly, tampons do not increase the risk of cystitis.

3   Most citric juices will increase the alkalinity of the urine, promoting bacterial growth.

4   This promotes the transfer of microorganisms to the urethra, where they could ascend to the bladder.

How to Use Worksheet 1: Errors In Processing Information

Common errors in processing information are listed in the left-hand column of this worksheet. At the top of the worksheet is a row of blank spaces for inserting the number of the question missed. Directly below each number, check any errors you made in answering that question. You may have made more than one type of error in an answer.

Worksheet 1: Errors in Processing Information

Question number																						
Did not read situation/ question carefully																						
Missed important details																						
Confused major and minor points																						
Defined problem incorrectly																						
Could not remember terms/ facts/concepts/principles																						
Defined terms incorrectly																						
Focused on incomplete/incorrect data in assessing situation																						
Interpreted data incorrectly																						
Applied wrong concepts/ principles in situations																						
Drew incorrect conclusions																						
Identified wrong goals																						
Identified priorities incorrectly																						
Carried out plan incorrectly/ incompletely																						
Was unclear about criteria for evaluating success in achieving goals																						

How to Use Worksheet 2: Knowledge Gaps

Types of common knowledge gaps are listed along the top of this worksheet. Write a brief description of topics you want to review in the spaces provided. For example, if you missed a question on administration of a particular drug, write the drug name and problem (e.g., dosage) in the appropriate space under the column labeled *Pharmacology*.

Worksheet 2: Knowledge Gaps

Basic science	Skills/ procedures	Basic human needs	Growth and develop- ment	Normal nutrition	Psycho- social factors	Clinical area/ topic	Stressors/ coping mechanisms	Patho- physiology	Pharma- cology	Therapeutic nutrition	Legal implications	Other

CHAPTER 7

Comprehensive Examination 2

Part A

1. Two days after delivery, a neonate's head circumference is 16 inches (40.6 cm) and the chest circumference is 13 inches (33 cm). These measurements:
   1. Are both normal parameters at birth
   2. Suggest the presence of microcephaly
   3. Indicate that the baby's head is enlarged
   4. Demonstrate a smaller than normal chest

2. The nurse notes six premature ventricular beats (PVBs) in a row on the cardiac monitor of a client in the coronary care unit (CCU). Using the protocol generally established in most CCUs, the nurse should first:
   1. Encourage the client to cough and deep breathe
   2. Initiate cardiopulmonary resuscitation immediately
   3. Administer a 50 to 100 mg bolus of cardiac xylocaine
   4. Notify the client's physician of the findings immediately

3. A client paces back and forth across the floor, speaks incoherently, and spends a great deal of time talking and verbally fighting with persons who are not present. The initial therapeutic intervention by the nurse should be directed toward:
   1. Setting limits on the client's verbal aggression
   2. Isolating the client to decrease the aggressive behavior
   3. Engaging the client in a structured, reality-oriented activity
   4. Establishing a relationship to reduce the client's loneliness

4. The laboratory calls to state that a client's lithium level is 1.9 mEq/liter after 10 days of lithium therapy. The nurse should:
   1. Immediately report the finding to the physician since the level is dangerously high
   2. Monitor the client closely because the level of lithium in the blood is slightly elevated
   3. Continue to administer the medication as ordered because the level is within the therapeutic range
   4. Report the findings to the physician so the dosage can be increased because the level is below the therapeutic range

5. To check for wound hemorrhage after a client has a thyroidectomy the nurse should:
   1. Loosen an edge of the dressing and lift it to visualize the wound
   2. Observe the dressing at the back of the neck for the presence of blood
   3. Outline the blood as it appears on the dressing to observe any progression
   4. Press gently around the incision to express accumulated blood from the wound

6. A 16-year-old primigravida comes to the labor suite. She is in her 38th week of gestation and states that she is in labor. To verify that the client is in true labor the nurse should:
   1. Obtain slides for a fern test
   2. Time any uterine contractions
   3. Prepare her for a pelvic examination
   4. Place nitrazine paper at the cervical mouth

7. As part of a diagnostic work-up for pulmonic stenosis, a child has a cardiac catheterization. The nurse is aware that children with pulmonic stenosis have increased pressure:
   1. In the pulmonary vein
   2. In the pulmonary artery
   3. On the left side of the heart
   4. On the right side of the heart

8. A client with cholecystitis is placed on a low-fat, high-protein diet. The nurse should teach the client that this diet can include:
   1. Boiled beef
   2. Skimmed milk
   3. Poached eggs
   4. Steamed broccoli

9. As a very anxious female client is talking to the nurse, she starts crying. She appears to be upset that she cannot control her crying. The most appropriate response by the nurse would be:
   1. "Is talking about your problem upsetting you?"
   2. "It is OK to cry, we can talk when you're ready."
   3. "Sometimes it helps to get it out of your system."
   4. "You look upset, let's talk about why you are crying."

10. As a postpartum client is being prepared for discharge, she says to the nurse, "I don't think I'll be able to take care of the baby when I go home." The nurse's best response would be:
    1. "What is it that makes you think that?"
    2. "It will come naturally. Give yourself time."
    3. "Is there anything specific that concerns you?"
    4. "I know it can be frightening, but you'll do just fine."

11. The nurse initiates preparation of a 9-year-old girl for an infratentorial craniotomy. The nurse plans to:
    1. Encourage doll play with blunt tools and dressings
    2. Schedule role playing with others having similar surgery
    3. Have the child draw her concept of the brain and briefly clarify any misconceptions
    4. Provide a minutely detailed explanation of anatomy and the surgery to be performed

12. MOPP therapy for a client with Hodgkin's disease has been ineffective and an ABVD combination chemotherapeutic treatment regimen is begun. This protocol includes doxorubicin HCl (Adriamycin), bleomycin sulfate (Blenoxane), vinblastine (Velban), and dacarbazine (DTIC). Because Adriamycin is part of this therapy, the nurse should teach the client to:
    1. Cease taking any medication that contains vitamin D
    2. Keep the Adriamycin in a dark area, protected from light
    3. Expect urine to turn red for 1 to 2 days after taking this drug
    4. Take the Adriamycin on an empty stomach with plenty of fluids

13. After a muscle biopsy, the nurse should teach the client to:
    1. Change the dressing as needed
    2. Resume a usual diet as soon as desired
    3. Bathe or shower according to preference
    4. Expect a rise in body temperature for 48 hours

14. A client had an open reduction and internal fixation of the head of the femur. In the post-anesthesia unit the client's vital signs remained stable for an hour at BP 130/78, P 68, R 16. An hour after returning to the surgical unit the client's vital signs are BP 100/60, P 74, R 22, and the client is restless. The nurse should:
    1. Increase the IV flow rate
    2. Raise the head of the bed
    3. Check the client's dressing
    4. Continue to monitor the vital signs

15. A fetal monitor is attached to a client in active labor. When the client has a contraction the nurse notes a 15 beat per minute acceleration of the fetal heart rate above the baseline. The nurse should:
    1. Turn the client on her left side
    2. Call the physician immediately
    3. Prepare for immediate delivery
    4. Record this normal fetal response

16. A male client receiving prolonged steroid therapy complains of always being thirsty and urinating frequently. The best initial action by the nurse would be to:
    1. Perform a finger stick to test the client's blood glucose level
    2. Have the physician assess the client for an enlarged prostate
    3. Obtain a urine specimen from the client for screening purposes
    4. Assess the client's lower extremities for the presence of pitting edema

17. A client is placed on the "Prudent Diet" advocated by the American Heart Association and designed to control saturated fats and cholesterol. To best explain the dietary nature of these two food substances the nurse should teach the client that:
    1. Cholesterol is a necessary body constituent and cannot be eliminated
    2. Polyunsaturated fats come from animal foods such as meat and cheese
    3. Plant sources of cholesterol must also be controlled in the diet every day
    4. The more saturated fats come from plant foods such as seeds and grains

18. After 3 months of supplemental oral iron therapy there is no significant rise in a child's hemoglobin level. The physician orders iron dextran (Imferon). When administering this medication, the nurse should:
    1. Use the Z-track method
    2. Massage the injection site
    3. Use a 25 gauge 5/8 inch needle
    4. Avoid aspiration before injection

19. On admission to the neonatal intensive care nursery after delivery, priority care for the neonate of a diabetic mother would include:
    1. Doing a Dextrostix test on heel blood
    2. Double clamping the cord immediately
    3. Starting an IV with 10% glucose in water
    4. Instilling prophylactic ophthalmic medication

20. An emergency tracheotomy is performed on a toddler in acute respiratory distress from laryngotracheobronchitis (viral croup). In addition to routine suctioning of the tracheotomy, the nurse should also suction if the toddler:
    1. Becomes restless, diaphoretic, and cyanotic
    2. Has severe substernal retractions and stridor
    3. Verbalizes an increased difficulty in breathing
    4. Becomes restless, pale, or has an increased pulse rate

21. The nurse understands that ascites related to cirrhosis is most likely the result of:
    1. Impaired portal venous return
    2. Inadequate secretion of bile salts
    3. Excess production of serum albumin
    4. Decreased interstitial osmotic pressure

22. A client in the hospice homecare program is experiencing severe pain. The physician orders MS Contin (morphine) for pain management. The nurse should explain to the client that:
    1. It is given automatically at regular intervals around the clock
    2. A heparin lock will be inserted for intermittent IV administration
    3. The medication must be requested before the pain becomes severe
    4. The potential for dependency or addiction is decreased with this drug

23. Obvious right-sided paradoxical motion of a client's chest indicates multiple rib fractures, resulting in a flail chest. The complication the nurse should carefully observe for is:
    1. Mediastinal shift
    2. Tracheal laceration
    3. Open pneumothorax
    4. Pericardial tamponade

24. A client refuses to eat saying, "They want to kill me." The most therapeutic response by the nurse would be:
    1. "No one is trying to harm you."
    2. "You feel someone is attempting to poison your food."
    3. "That's not true. It's the same food everyone else is eating."
    4. "If you want, I'll taste your food before you do so you'll know it's okay."

25. When planning care for a client admitted with placenta previa, the nurse's primary goal is to:
    1. Provide a calm, quiet environment
    2. Prevent further episodes of bleeding
    3. Prepare for a possible cesarean delivery
    4. Arrange periods of diversional activity and rest

26. A mother, exceedingly upset about her child being diagnosed as having a pinworm infestation, is taught by the public health nurse how the pinworm infestation is transmitted. The nurse evaluates that the teaching was effective when the mother states:
    1. "I'll need to be sure the cat stays off my child's bed at night."
    2. "I'll have to reinforce my child's handwashing especially before eating or handling food."
    3. "I'll be sure to disinfect the toilet seat after my child's bowel movements for the next few days."
    4. "My child contracted this infestation from the dirty school toilets, and I'll report that to the school nurse."

27. When assessing the thorax of a client with chronic obstructive pulmonary disease, the nurse would expect to find:
    1. Decreased breath sounds
    2. Atrophic accessory muscles
    3. A shortened expiratory phase
    4. A decrease in the A-P diameter

28. A client has a chest tube inserted to treat a right hemopneumothorax. To facilitate chest drainage, the client should be encouraged to lie:

1. In the supine position
2. On the right (affected) side
3. On the left (unaffected) side
4. Immobilized as much as possible

29. An adolescent client with anorexia nervosa refuses to eat, stating, "I'll get too fat." The nurse can best respond to this behavior initially by:
    1. Not talking about the fact that the client is not eating
    2. Stopping all of the client's privileges until food is eaten
    3. Pointing out to the client that death can occur with malnutrition
    4. Telling the client that tube feedings will eventually be necessary

30. The nurse should plan to assist a client with an obsessive compulsive disorder to control the use of ritualistic behavior by:
    1. Providing repetitive activities that require little thought
    2. Attempting to reduce or limit situations that increase anxiety
    3. Getting the client involved with activities that will provide distraction
    4. Allowing the client to perform menial tasks to expiate feelings of guilt

31. Immediately after a child is admitted with acute bacterial meningitis, the nurse should plan to:
    1. Assess the child's vital signs every 4 hours
    2. Administer oral antibiotic medications as ordered
    3. Check the child's level of consciousness every hour
    4. Restrict parental visiting until isolation is discontinued

32. A client with the diagnosis of otosclerosis undergoes a stapedectomy with insertion of a middle ear prosthesis. A few days after the operation the client is discouraged because there is no improvement in hearing. The nurse should bear in mind that this is most likely due to:
    1. Swelling within the ear canal
    2. Damage to the organ of Corti
    3. Perforation of the tympanic membrane
    4. The graft having slipped out of position

33. After a transurethral resection of the prostate a client has a three-way Foley catheter with a continuous bladder irrigation. The client complains that he needs to void. The nurse should first:
    1. Obtain the client's vital signs and notify the physician
    2. Assess the client's total intake and output for the day
    3. Explain to the client that the balloon inflated in the bladder causes this feeling
    4. Check the tubing connected to the client's collection bag to see whether it is draining

34. A client with the diagnosis of multiple sclerosis develops hand tremors. When performing a physical assessment, the nurse should take into consideration that the tremors associated with multiple sclerosis usually occur when the client:
    1. Is asleep
    2. Is inactive
    3. Gets nervous or upset
    4. Attempts to do something

35. An elderly client is hospitalized with the diagnosis of dementia. Considering the client's diagnosis the behavior that the nurse would most likely observe is an:
    1. Increased attention span and perceptual disturbances
    2. Inability to learn new things and disturbance in thinking
    3. Acceptance of personality and social changes due to declining years
    4. Increased capacity for adaptation to environment based on past life experiences

36. After delivery, the nurse assesses a client who had an abruptio placentae and suspects that disseminated intravascular coagulopathy (DIC) is occurring when observations demonstrate:
    1. A boggy uterus
    2. Multiple vaginal clots
    3. Hypertension and tachycardia
    4. Bleeding from the venipuncture site

37. During a client's second stage of labor, the nurse should:

1. Watch for bulging of the client's perineum
2. Give the client pain medication as ordered
3. Teach the client how to pant with each contraction
4. Catheterize the client so that the head can be delivered

38. A client with diabetes mellitus receives 36 units of intermediate acting insulin before breakfast. The nurse should be alert to the symptoms of an insulin reaction, which include:
    1. Dry skin, drowsiness, and tachycardia
    2. Excessive thirst, anorexia, and malaise
    3. Headache, nervousness, and diaphoresis
    4. Ataxia, dilated pupils, and Kussmaul respirations

39. The most beneficial between-meal snack for a client who is recovering from full-thickness burns would be a:
    1. Cheeseburger and a malted
    2. Piece of blueberry pie and milk
    3. Bacon and tomato sandwich and tea
    4. Chicken salad sandwich and soft drink

40. A client with a fractured right head of the femur and osteoporosis is placed in Buck's traction before surgical repair. Until surgery is performed the nurse should plan to:
    1. Remove the weights from the traction every 2 hours to promote comfort
    2. Inspect the skin and circulation of the affected leg hourly to prevent trauma
    3. Turn the client from side to side every 4 hours to prevent pressure on the coccyx
    4. Raise and maintain the knee gatch on the bed to limit the shearing force of traction

41. A 16-month-old has had large, frothy, foul-smelling stools since the introduction of table food and cow's milk into the diet. The child's mother also noted that the child changed from pleasant and outgoing to irritable and apathetic. The child is diagnosed as having celiac disease and is placed on a gluten-free diet. When evaluating the child's response to the diet after 2 days, the nurse anticipates the first change will be:
    1. A return of appetite
    2. An increase in weight
    3. A cessation of diarrhea
    4. An improved personality

42. The nurse recognizes that failure of a newborn to make the appropriate adaptation to extrauterine life would be indicated by:
1. Cyanotic lips and face
2. A respiratory rate of 40
3. Cyanotic feet and hands
4. A liver 2 cm below right costal margin

43. A tricyclic antidepressant is prescribed for a depressed client. After 1 week, a member of the client's family comes to speak with the nurse and expresses concern that there does not seem to be much improvement after taking the medication. When responding to the family member the nurse explains that:
1. As the client's physical condition improves, the antidepressant medication will act more effectively
2. The client may require other drugs in addition to the antidepressants before behavioral changes are noted
3. In clients who have been depressed for a prolonged period the drug takes additional time to be effective
4. The tricyclics are slow-acting drugs and it may take 3 to 4 weeks until therapeutic effectiveness is achieved

44. A 2-year-old who is HIV positive from multiple blood transfusions is seen in the emergency room. Presently the child has been ill for a week with a temperature of 103°F. The child's mother states that the child is losing weight and has a whitish film on the gums. When doing the health history the nurse determines that the child is at high risk for developing AIDS because of:
1. A positive HIV antibody screening test
2. An immature reticuloendothelial system
3. The multiple blood transfusions received
4. The presence of an opportunistic infection

45. A client stops taking birth control pills because she and her husband want to start a family. After 18 months of unsuccessful attempts at conception the client is diagnosed as having primary infertility related to anovulatory cycles. Clomiphene citrate (Clomid) is prescribed for 6 months. The nurse knows that the teaching about the correct time to take the Clomid is understood when the client states, "I will begin to take the pills on the:

1. Fifth day of my cycle."
2. Last day of my period."
3. First day I start my period."
4. Fourteenth day of my cycle."

46. One day a young adult client's mother confides to the nurse that she is very troubled by her child's emotional illness. The nurse's most therapeutic initial response would be:
1. "It is very important that you become involved in volunteer work at this time."
2. "You must lessen your feelings of guilt and loneliness by seeing a psychiatrist."
3. "I recognize it's hard to deal with this. Try to remember that this too shall pass."
4. "Getting together with others who are coping with this problem can be quite helpful."

47. For a pregnant client whose blood pressure has been averaging 92/64 mmHg on her prenatal visits, pregnancy-induced hypertension should be suspected when the blood pressure first rises to:
1. 110/80 mmHg
2. 114/80 mmHg
3. 124/80 mmHg
4. 140/90 mmHg

48. While a client is on intravenous magnesium sulfate therapy for pregnancy-induced hypertension, it is essential for the nurse to monitor the client's deep tendon reflexes to:
1. Determine her level of consciousness
2. Evaluate the mobility of the extremities
3. Determine her response to painful stimuli
4. Avoid development of respiratory depression

49. The nurse makes notes on a female rape victim's record during the interview and physical examination, because the record may go to court as evidence. It is most important when charting that the nurse include:
1. The client's verbatim statements about the rape and the rapist
2. Observations about the client's reaction to male staff members
3. General statements about the client's previous knowledge of the rapist
4. A summarized statement about the client's description of the rape and the rapist

50. A preschooler is admitted with a diagnosis of acute glomerulonephritis. The child's history reveals a 5 pound weight gain in one week and periorbital edema. For the most accurate information on the status of the child's edema, nursing intervention should include:
    1. Obtaining the child's daily weight
    2. Doing a visual inspection of the child
    3. Measuring the child's intake and output
    4. Monitoring the child's electrolyte values

51. The physician orders the drug ranitidine (Zantac) to help treat a client's gastric ulcer. The nurse realizes the drug will help the client's condition by:
    1. Lowering the gastric pH
    2. Promoting the release of gastrin
    3. Regenerating the gastric mucosa
    4. Inhibiting the histamine H_2 receptors

52. The nurse teaches a 9-year-old and the child's parents about insulin-dependent diabetes and the occurrence of hyperglycemia. The nurse would be aware that they understand the teaching when they state that ketoacidosis is most often precipitated by:
    1. An infection
    2. An insulin overdose
    3. Decreased fluid intake
    4. Excessive physical exercise

53. An adolescent is admitted after having had a tonic-clonic seizure at college. The client has a 2-year history of a seizure disorder but the seizures have been well controlled by phenytoin (Dilantin) for the last 6 months. The client says to the nurse, "I am so upset. I didn't think I was going to have more seizures." The nurse's best response would be:
    1. "Did you forget to take your medication?"
    2. "You are worried about having more seizures?"
    3. "You must be under a lot of stress at school right now."
    4. "Don't be too concerned. Your medication needs to be increased."

54. Four hours after a liver biopsy the client complains of pain and the nurse notes that there is a leakage of a moderately large amount of bile on the dressing. Based on these findings the nurse should:

    1. Medicate the client for pain as ordered
    2. Tell the client to remain flat on the back
    3. Notify the client's physician immediately
    4. Monitor the client's vital signs q10 minutes

55. After surgery the physician orders gentamicin sulfate (Garamycin) 75 mg IVPB q6h and daily "peak" and "trough" levels. This is done primarily so that:
    1. A drop in the client's fever may be correlated with the "peak" level
    2. The blood culture can be obtained when gentamicin is at its lowest level
    3. Any allergy that the client might have to the drug would be detected early
    4. Presence of an adequate therapeutic level of the drug can be determined

56. On entering a depressed client's room one morning, the nurse finds the client still in bed. The client states, "I am unable to get dressed and go to breakfast." The nurse's best response would be:
    1. "You cannot just lie in bed. You must get up now and go to breakfast."
    2. "I'll get you dressed. I recognize that you have difficulty helping yourself."
    3. "Take your time. It is not necessary to hurry. I'll help you if you need me to."
    4. "You can lie there for awhile if you promise me you'll get dressed for lunch."

57. A four-year-old boy with acute lymphocytic leukemia is to have a bone marrow aspiration. While involving the child in therapeutic play prior to the procedure the nurse should help him understand that:
    1. He needs to have a positive attitude
    2. His parents are concerned about him
    3. He did nothing to cause his present illness
    4. His problem was caused by an environmental factor

58. The nurse recognizes that the most important factor in predicting a client's potential reaction to grief is the client's:
    1. Family interactions
    2. Emotional relationships
    3. Social support systems
    4. Earlier experiences with grief

59. The public health nurse presents a program on breast self-examination. The nurse realizes that certain aspects of the teaching program would have to be reviewed when, during the return demonstration, one of the women in the class:
1. Palpates her breasts while in the sitting position
2. Checks her nipples for alterations in size or shape
3. Palpates her breast with the palmar surface of her extended fingers
4. Observes her breasts for symmetry while holding her arms above her head

60. Based on the diagnosis of cancer of the pancreas, the nurse understands that a client's jaundice is caused by:
1. Necrosis of the parenchyma caused by the neoplasm
2. Excessive serum bilirubin caused by red cell destruction
3. Obstruction of the common bile duct by the pancreatic neoplasm
4. Impaired liver function resulting in incomplete bilirubin metabolism

61. Realizing that hypokalemia is a side effect of steroid therapy, the nurse should monitor a client taking steroid medication for:
1. Hyperactive reflexes
2. An increased pulse rate
3. Nausea, vomiting, and diarrhea
4. Leg weakness with muscle cramps

62. A woman with an active herpes infection can transmit the virus to her infant during a vaginal delivery. The nurse understands that the incidence of infection in the infant following a vaginal delivery is:
1. 15% to 20%
2. 20% to 35%
3. 40% to 60%
4. 75% to 90%

63. In addition to being non-constipating, the diet for a child who is in traction should be:
1. Low in calories and purine
2. High in calories and phosphorus
3. Moderate in calories and high in protein
4. Adequate in calories and high in calcium

64. The behavior that would indicate to the nurse that the mental status of a client with the diagnosis of schizophrenia, paranoid type was improving would be the client's:
1. Absence of or freedom from anxiety
2. Development of insight into the problem
3. Decreased need to use defense mechanisms
4. Ability to function effectively in activities of daily living

65. Because a severely depressed client has not responded to any of the antidepressant medications, the psychiatrist decides to try electroconvulsive therapy (ECT). Before the treatment the nurse should:
1. Have the client speak with other clients receiving ECT
2. Give the client a detailed explanation of the entire procedure
3. Limit the client's intake to a light breakfast on the days of the treatment
4. Provide a simple explanation of the procedure and continue to reassure the client

66. The nurse plans early postoperative ambulation for a client who has had a continent urostomy formed to prevent:
1. Wound infection
2. Urinary retention
3. Abdominal distention
4. Incisional evisceration

67. The day after a cesarean delivery, a client complains of abdominal pain and abdominal distention. The physician orders a Harris drip. After administering the Harris drip, the nurse can evaluate its effectiveness when:
1. The client has a bowel movement
2. The client's returns are finally clear
3. The client's abdomen is less distended
4. The client is able to retain 500 ml of fluid

68. A blonde-haired, blue-eyed farmer goes to the physician because he has a large, crusty patch of skin on his cheek. The client states that it bleeds easily and has not gotten better even after using different remedies. From the client's history, the nurse suspects skin cancer, because the major precipitating factor associated with skin cancer is:

1. Position of the lesion
2. Exposure to radiation
3. Self-treatment of lesions
4. Contact with soil contaminants

69. During a group therapy session, one of the clients asks a male client with the diagnosis of antisocial personality disorder why he is in the hospital. Considering this client's type of personality disorder, the nurse might expect him to respond:
1. "I need a lot of help with my troubles."
2. "Society makes people react in odd ways."
3. "I decided that it's time I own up to my problems."
4. "My life needs straightening out and this might help."

70. A child comes for a 6 weeks checkup following a tonsillectomy and adenoidectomy. In addition to assessing hearing, the nurse should include an assessment of the child's:
1. Smell and taste
2. Speech and taste
3. Swallowing and smell
4. Swallowing and speech

71. The nurse should plan to observe a client awaiting surgery for intestinal carcinoma for signs of:
1. Diarrhea
2. Dehydration
3. Intestinal obstruction
4. Abdominal peritonitis

72. A slow pulse rate during the early postoperative period following open heart surgery can be indicative of:

1. Shock
2. Hypoxia
3. Heart block
4. Congestive heart failure

73. When a 3-month-old baby is at the well baby clinic for a checkup, the parents express concern that their baby still has a soft spot on the top of the head. The nurse explains that normal closure time for the anterior fontanel is between the ages of:
1. 6 and 8 months
2. 9 and 12 months
3. 13 and 18 months
4. 19 and 24 months

74. In a childbirth preparation class, the instructor teaches the clients to control their urge to push until the cervix is fully dilated by:
1. Hyperventilating
2. Doing pelvic rocking exercises
3. Deep breathing between contractions
4. Panting or blowing breathing patterns

75. A client who had a CVA is discharged with a hemiparesis but is able to ambulate with assistance. Whenever the client gets up from a lying down position, a feeling of being light-headed and dizzy occurs. The nurse recognizes that this feeling is:
1. Relieved by resting before performing activities
2. Caused by blood pooling in the lower extremities
3. A temporary response that will go away with time
4. Precipitated by the medication which may have to be changed

Part B

76. A client who has had a continent urostomy created complains of postoperative pain. Initially the nurse should:
    1. Interview the client for more data
    2. Tell the client to take deep breaths
    3. Measure the client's current vital signs
    4. Administer the prescribed analgesic to the client

77. A client, who has been an insulin-dependent diabetic since childhood, is pregnant for the third time. Her first child is 4 years old and her second pregnancy resulted in a stillbirth. She is admitted for a contraction stress test (CST) at 33 weeks gestation. The nurse is aware that the client's history indicates she is a candidate for a CST primarily because:
    1. A CST is indicated for high-risk clients with possible placental insufficiency
    2. A CST measures plasma levels of maternal estriols, which indicate fetal distress
    3. The client's diabetes was probably the major causative factor in the previous stillbirth
    4. The client is past the 28th week of gestation and a CST has no clinical value before this time

78. A client is worried about what to expect after having a Whipple procedure for cancer of the pancreas. When assisting the client to plan, it would be most important for the nurse to know:
    1. Any history of alcohol or tobacco use
    2. The state and grade of the client's cancer
    3. Any previous exposure to known carcinogens
    4. The survival rate for individuals with pancreatic cancer

79. After a modified radical mastectomy, the nurse recognizes that a female client understands the schedule for self-examination of her remaining breast when she states she will carry out the procedure:

1. Several days before an expected menstrual period
2. Two to three days following the completion of each menstrual period
3. Halfway between menstrual periods, preferably after taking a shower
4. The same date every month, regardless of when menstruation occurs

80. The parents of a child, who has recently been diagnosed with leukemia, ask the nurse why the physician said that their child had too many white blood cells. The nurse's best response would be:
    1. "You seem to be focusing on your child's white blood cells."
    2. "Your doctor is the best one to answer that question for you."
    3. "It sounds like you really do not understand what occurs in leukemia."
    4. "The bone marrow isn't working properly and makes too many white cells."

81. An elderly couple, who live alone in their own home, both need help with dressing, bathing, and meal preparation. The condition that would rule out care in the home for this couple is:
    1. The home being located in a rural area
    2. The need for part-time multidisciplinary services
    3. The need for skilled nursing care on a 24-hour basis
    4. The need for part-time assistance for all personal care activities

82. Steroid therapy is ordered for a client with multiple sclerosis. The change that the nurse would expect to observe is decreased:
    1. Emotional lability
    2. Muscular contractions
    3. Pain in the extremities
    4. Episodes of vision loss

83. A client with the diagnosis of obsessive-compulsive disorder uses paper towels to open doors to avoid touching dirty doorknobs. The nurse's best response to this behavior would be to:

1. Point out that the towels may be dirty
2. Prevent the client from using the towels
3. Ignore the behavior for the present time
4. Quietly remove the paper towels from the area

84. After an automobile accident, a client who sustained multiple injuries is oriented as to person and place but is confused as to time. The client complains of a headache and drowsiness but assessment reveals that the pupils are equal and reactive. A significant nursing intervention would be to:
1. Keep the client alert and responsive
2. Prevent unnecessary movement by the client
3. Prepare the client for the administration of mannitol
4. Monitor the client for symptoms of increased intracranial pressure

85. In discussions with the nurse, a child newly diagnosed with insulin-dependent diabetes mellitus learns that insulin acts by:
1. Preventing the glucose from being stored in the liver
2. Helping to carry sugar into cells where it is burned for energy
3. Helping to break down protein and fat to provide needed glucose
4. Preventing the wasting of blood glucose by converting it to glycogen

86. After an uneventful pregnancy, a client delivers a baby who has a meningomyelocele. The baby has an Apgar score of 9/10. An immediate priority of nursing care for this newborn would be:
1. Administering O_2 by nasal catheter
2. Protecting the sac with sterile moist gauze
3. Transferring the infant to the intensive care nursery
4. Placing a name bracelet on the ankle and taking foot prints

87. A client becomes increasingly agitated and screams at, curses at, fights with, and bites other clients. The physician orders a stat injection of haloperidol decanoate (Haldol). The nurse should carry out the order to administer the Haldol:

1. Quickly with an attitude of concern
2. After the client agrees to take the injection
3. Before the client suspects what is happening
4. Quietly, without any explanation about the reason for it

88. The laboratory finding that reflects a major problem commonly found in pregnant adolescents is:
1. Urine glucose 2+
2. Hemoglobin 9.1 g
3. Platelets 75,000/mm^3
4. White blood cells 12,000/mm^3

89. A slightly overweight client is to be discharged from the hospital after a cholecystectomy. When teaching the client about nutrition the priority intervention should be:
1. Listing those fatty foods that may be included in the diet
2. Explaining that fatty foods may not be tolerated for several weeks
3. Teaching the importance of a low-calorie diet to promote weight reduction
4. Encouraging the client to join a weight reduction program in the local community

90. The nurse is aware that 60% of brain tumors in children result in symptoms of increased intracranial pressure and are most commonly found in the:
1. Cortex
2. Cerebellum
3. Temporal lobe
4. Subarachnoid space

91. When caring for a client during the period of acute alcohol withdrawal, the nurse should:
1. Apply restraints to provide security and keep the client calm
2. Encourage the client to relate hallucinations and delusions in detail
3. Continually reassure the client that the symptoms are part of the withdrawal syndrome
4. Keep the room dimly lit to counter the visual distortions the client probably will experience

92. In response to a client's question concerning the etiology of polyarteritis nodosa, the nurse should respond that:
    1. The disease affects both males and females in equal numbers
    2. With current therapy, clients with this disease have an excellent prognosis
    3. Arteriolar pathology of the disease affects only the kidneys and the retina of the eye
    4. The disease is considered one of hypersensitivity, but the exact cause is not known

93. A client has an open reduction and internal fixation of the hip. The client is to be transferred to a chair on the second postoperative day for a half hour. Before the transfer the nurse should:
    1. Assess the strength of the affected leg
    2. Explain how the transfer will be accomplished
    3. Instruct the client to bear weight evenly on both legs
    4. Encourage the client to keep the affected leg elevated

94. A class A pregnant diabetic client attends the high-risk clinic. When assessing a client with class A diabetes, the nurse would probably find that the client has:
    1. Vascular changes in the eyes
    2. No demonstrable vascular disease
    3. Retinal changes seen on eye examination
    4. A history of diabetes for at least 15 years

95. A client is admitted for acute gastritis and ascites secondary to alcoholism and cirrhosis. It is important for the nurse to routinely assess this client for:
    1. Obstipation
    2. Blood in the stool
    3. Any food intolerances
    4. Complaints of nausea

96. A client is at high risk for developing ascites. To assess for this condition the nurse should:
    1. Observe for signs of respiratory distress
    2. Percuss the abdomen, listening for dull sounds
    3. Palpate the lower extremities over the tibia and observe for edema
    4. Auscultate the abdomen, listening for decreased or absent bowel sounds

97. When the nurse approaches a delusional female client, the client yells, "You're the one that made my lover leave me." The nurse should recognize that the client:
    1. Is confused and disoriented
    2. Is actively hallucinating at this time
    3. Feels a great sense of vulnerability
    4. Needs to have limits set after quieting down

98. A pregnant client with a history of delusions, hallucinations, and suspiciousness tells the nurse she is fearful about her upcoming delivery and the health of her baby. The most supportive approach by the nurse would be to:
    1. Reassure the client that she will have plenty of help with the delivery
    2. Commend the client on her ability to express her fears and concerns
    3. Share with the client the staff's concerns about how she will handle the infant
    4. Provide the client with a detailed explanation of what occurs during labor and delivery

99. A 6-year-old female is being discharged after diagnostic studies and treatment for frequent urinary tract infections. The statement by the girl's mother that would indicate that further teaching is necessary would be:
    1. "I guess I should not use the bubble bath I got my daughter for her birthday."
    2. "When it doesn't hurt my daughter to urinate I can stop giving her these pills."
    3. "I hope my daughter can remember to always wipe from the front to the back."
    4. "I will tell my daughter's teacher to let her go to the toilet as soon as she needs to."

100. One day the mother of a 7-year-old previously hospitalized with nephrotic syndrome several months before, calls the clinic nurse. She reports that for the past week her child has had a muddy pale appearance, a poor appetite, and has been unusually tired after school. The nurse suspects that the child:
    1. Is not taking her medications
    2. Is developing a viral infection
    3. May be in impending renal failure
    4. May be overextending herself at school

101. A 5-month-old with tetralogy of Fallot is to be discharged with a prescription for digoxin (Lanoxin) and furosemide (Lasix). The nurse instructs the mother to notify the physician if:
1. The child's pulse rate goes above 100
2. Feeding difficulties and vomiting occur
3. Cyanosis occurs during periods of crying
4. The child requires several naps each day

102. The nurse recognizes that a client understands how to appropriately take the antacids prescribed by the physician when the client states, "I will take my antacids:
1. With the onset of pain."
2. 30 minutes after meals."
3. Every 4 hours around the clock."
4. Every time I have anything to eat."

103. The mother of a preschooler with acute glomerulonephritis asks the nurse if her child will have to stay in bed. The nurse should tell the mother that bedrest:
1. Is not part of the usual treatment unless the child is seriously ill
2. Will be necessary for 3 to 4 weeks regardless of the response to therapy
3. Is limited to 72 hours after the institution of antihypertensive drug therapy
4. Will be necessary until the child's blood pressure is normal and the urine clear

104. A client who has been on IV magnesium sulfate therapy for pregnancy-induced hypertension delivers an infant weighing 4 lbs in the thirty-seventh week of gestation. The nurse is aware that a finding in the newborn that may indicate magnesium sulfate toxicity is:
1. Pallor
2. Tremors
3. A pulse of 200
4. Respirations of 16

105. A teenager, hospitalized for pregnancy-induced hypertension, is anorexic and appears depressed. The nurse plans to further explore the client's emotional status when the client comments:
1. "I'm tired of feeling so clumsy."
2. "I'll be glad when I can sleep all night."
3. "I dreamed my baby had only one arm."
4. "I was really happy before I got pregnant."

106. A client, who has been diagnosed as having atherosclerosis and hypertension, has always been an active individual. The client is interested in measures that would help maintain health. The nurse explains that maintenance of vessel patency can be promoted by:
1. Practicing relaxation techniques
2. Decreasing the amount of exercise
3. Increasing saturated fats in the diet
4. Leading a more sedentary lifestyle

107. The nurse teaches a client with hypertension to reduce dietary sodium. The nurse should emphasize that:
1. The taste for salt is inherent but it can be overcome with practice
2. Salt-free natural seasonings can be used and taste the same as salt
3. The taste for table salt is learned and increases over time, but it is not a biologic necessity
4. Salt substitutes with potassium chloride bases can be used freely with foods to provide the same taste

108. The delivery room nurse does an Apgar on a newly delivered infant and knows that an Apgar value of 2 should be assigned to:
1. A strong, lusty cry
2. Body pink, extremities blue
3. Arms and legs slightly flexed
4. Heart rate of 90 beats per minute

109. When preparing a toddler with celiac disease for discharge, the nurse should caution the parents that the toddler characteristic that would make their child most susceptible to a celiac crisis is:
1. Invention
2. Autonomy
3. Narcissism
4. Negativism

110. When performing the initial assessment of a client in ketoacidosis the nurse notes:
1. Nervousness and cool pale skin
2. Erythema toxicum rash and pruritus
3. Diaphoresis and instability as with intoxication
4. Deep respirations and fruity odor to the breath

111. A client develops bronchopneumonia. To help determine the effectiveness of therapy, the nurse should refer to the results of the client's:
1. Lung scan
2. Bronchoscopy
3. Pulmonary function study
4. Culture and sensitivity of sputum

112. Cor pulmonale is a frequent complication of COPD. The sign that would lead the nurse to suspect that the client is developing cor pulmonale would be:
1. Peripheral edema
2. A productive cough
3. Twitching of the extremities
4. Lethargy progressing to coma

113. A client has chest tubes inserted to treat a hemopneumothorax resulting from a crushing chest injury. When connecting the two-chamber water-seal drainage system ordered, the nurse must understand that the chamber attached to the chest tube provides the:
1. Suction
2. Water seal
3. Seal and suction
4. Drainage receptacle

114. The nurse should plan to involve a client with anorexia nervosa in activities that will:
1. Save the client's depleted energy
2. Force the client into decision making
3. Focus the client on sexual attractiveness
4. Provide the client with peer group involvement

115. A client, with the diagnosis of obsessive compulsive disorder, who has a need to wash the hands about 50 to 60 times a day, tearfully tells the nurse, "I know my hands are not dirty, but I just can't stop washing them." The nurse's best response would be:
1. "Let's talk about why you feel you must wash your hands."
2. "I think you're getting better; you're beginning to understand your problem."
3. "Don't worry about it; these actions are part of your illness, and these feelings will pass."
4. "I understand that, but maybe we can work together to limit the number of times you wash them."

116. A child is admitted for surgical incision and drainage of a puncture wound and intravenous antibiotic therapy. The nurse administers tetanus toxoid immunization. The rationale for this is that the toxoid confers:
1. Life-long passive immunity
2. Longer-lasting active immunity
3. Life-long active natural immunity
4. Temporary passive natural immunity

117. A client with the diagnoses of multiple sclerosis had a sudden loss of vision and asks the nurse what caused it. The nurse explains that the temporary blindness was probably caused by:
1. Virus-induced iritis
2. Intracranial pressure
3. Closed angle glaucoma
4. Optic nerve inflammation

118. An elderly client is hospitalized with the diagnosis of dementia of the Alzheimer's type. Her daughter tearfully tells the nurse, "I should never have allowed my mother to live alone as she wanted to do. But she has not been this bad. I am to blame. She did not even recognize me immediately." The response by the nurse that would be the most helpful would be:
1. "I do not think that anybody could blame you. You did what she wanted. Your being here tells us that you care."
2. "I realize that you are upset now. You can visit again when she is more responsive. I am sure you'll see a change."
3. "Why do you think your mother's condition has deteriorated? Her forgetfulness is temporary. You'll help if you don't cry."
4. "This must be a difficult time for both of you. Would you like to share your other observations to help us plan for her care?"

119. A client in a birthing room is having contractions every 3 to 4 minutes which last about 35 seconds. A vaginal examination reveals that the cervix is 50% effaced and 6 cm dilated. From the results of the examination the nurse knows that the client is:
1. Early in the first stage of labor
2. In the transitional phase of labor
3. Beginning the second stage of labor
4. Midway through the first stage of labor

120. A public health nurse visits the home of a female client in the terminal stage of cancer 3 days a week to provide physical care and emotional support. The nurse observes that the client's adolescent children are having difficulty talking with their mother. The nurse suggests family meetings with the hospice nurse, knowing that:
1. It is important to solve family problems before death occurs
2. They will be unable to deal with their feelings until after their mother dies
3. A deeper level of understanding will help the children comprehend what their mother is going through
4. Opening communication systems reduces the intensity of a family's emotional reaction to terminal illness

121. After a modified radical mastectomy a female client tells the nurse, "This diagnosis is as good as a death sentence and I would rather go now than to suffer." At this time it would be most important for the nurse to:
1. Encourage her to admit herself to the psychiatric unit of the hospital
2. Determine whether she has experienced self-destructive or suicidal thoughts
3. Explore the possibility of a vacation after hospitalization to reduce her stress level
4. Encourage her to think positively and to try and focus on the good things in her life

122. A client with Crohn's disease is to have an upper gastrointestinal series. The nurse understands that an upper GI series with barium would be contraindicated if the client had:
1. Hemorrhoids
2. A perforation
3. Hyperkalemia
4. An inflamed colon

123. The teaching plan for a client with Crohn's disease should focus on:
1. Meeting nutritional needs
2. Anticipating sexual alteration
3. Controlling severe constipation
4. Preventing increased weakness

124. A client's contraction stress test (CST) is positive and indicates potential problems. The nurse understands that a positive test:
1. Indicates the need for induction of labor
2. Showed excessive late decelerations of the fetal heart rate
3. Showed a consistent fetal heart rate of 120 to 160 beats per minute
4. Indicates the need for a cesarean delivery in order to ensure viability of the fetus

125. A male client with the diagnosis of schizophrenia, paranoid type, frequently displays overt sexual behavior toward female clients and nurses. The nurses can best respond to the client's behavior by:
1. Refusing to speak with the client until he stops this behavior
2. Sending the client to his room when the behavior is observed
3. Matter-of-factly telling the client that his behavior is unacceptable
4. Ignoring this behavior until the client is more in control of his responses

126. Considering the anticholinergic-like side effects of many of the psychotropic drugs, the nurse should encourage clients taking these drugs to:
1. Suck on hard candy
2. Restrict their fluid intake
3. Eat a diet high in carbohydrates
4. Avoid products that contain aspirin

127. During the administration of an enema prior to gastrointestinal surgery, a client complains of cramps. The nurse should:
1. Discontinue the enema and try again at a later time
2. Close the lumen of the tubing until the client's cramps subside
3. Lower the container to the floor to decrease intestinal pressure
4. Administer the enema rapidly to permit a quicker evacuation of fluid

128. Nursing care for the child in the acute phase of nephrotic syndrome should include:
    1. Forcing fluids every hour
    2. Providing time for active play periods
    3. Encouraging frequent change of position
    4. Feeding low-protein, high-carbohydrate, and low-salt foods

129. The nurse teaches the mother of a child with a pinworm infestation how to collect a Scotch tape specimen. The nurse recommends that the specimen be collected:
    1. At night after the child has had a bath
    2. At night after the child has had a bowel movement
    3. In the late morning after the child has had a bowel movement
    4. In the morning before the child has had a bowel movement or a bath

130. A grand multigravida, 34 weeks gestation, is brought to the emergency room by her husband because she is experiencing vaginal bleeding. The nurse would suspect that the client has a placenta previa if the bleeding is:
    1. Painful vaginal bleeding in the first trimester
    2. Painful vaginal bleeding in the third trimester
    3. Painless vaginal bleeding in the first trimester
    4. Painless vaginal bleeding in the third trimester

131. A female client who has been delusional is found staring at the television set which is on. The client suddenly rises and shouts, "Stop saying that. Who do you think you are?" It would be most therapeutic for the nurse to:
    1. Attempt to distract the client by taking her for a walk
    2. Point out the inappropriateness of her behavior to her
    3. Take the client to her room so they can have a quiet place to talk
    4. Tell her that the voices she hears are coming from the television set

132. A female client is dying of cancer. Her family is concerned because she appears to be accepting less and less responsibility for her own care. To help the family plan for her care, the nurse should:
    1. Point out that denial is a normal response and will be temporary
    2. Assist them to identify methods for giving her more control over the situation
    3. Encourage them to accept her regression until she can cope more effectively
    4. Explain that her anger is normal and identify ways for the family to deal with it

133. A client has a paracentesis and the physician removes 1500 ml of fluid. It is most essential that the nurse observe the client for:
    1. A hypertensive crisis
    2. Abdominal distention
    3. An increased pulse rate
    4. Dry mucous membranes

134. A client is scheduled for an amniocentesis. Before the procedure the nurse should:
    1. Remind the client to empty her bladder
    2. Instruct the client to take nothing by mouth
    3. Give the client the ordered sedation to minimize fetal movement
    4. Administer a Fleet's enema to the client to prevent contamination

135. An episiotomy is performed to facilitate delivery and prevent tearing of maternal tissues. The physician orders sitz baths three times a day. The nurse should include in the teaching plan that sitz baths promote healing by:
    1. Promoting vasodilation
    2. Softening the incision site
    3. Cleansing the perineal area
    4. Tightening the rectal sphincter

136. A client with osteoporosis is encouraged to drink milk. The client refuses the milk explaining that it causes gasiness and bloating. A food rich in calcium which may be easily digested by those clients who do not tolerate milk is:

1. Eggs
2. Yogurt
3. Potatoes
4. Bananas

137. A client receiving steroid therapy states, "I have had difficulty controlling my temper, which is so unlike me, and I don't know why this is happening." The nurse's best response would be to:
1. Tell the client it is nothing to worry about
2. Encourage the client to talk further about these findings
3. Tell the client to attempt to avoid situations that cause irritation
4. Try to determine if the client has been experiencing mood swings

138. A client who is scheduled for a muscle biopsy tells the nurse, "They better give me a general anesthetic. I don't want to feel anything." The most therapeutic response by the nurse would be:
1. "You seem to be worried about the test."
2. "Try not to think about it, you won't feel a thing."
3. "This test is always done under local anesthesia."
4. "Tell them when you have pain, and they'll take care of it."

139. A client who is experiencing acute alcohol withdrawal appears frightened and points toward the bed and says, "Bugs are crawling all over my bed and on me." The most therapeutic response by the nurse would be:
1. "I do not see any bugs on your bed."
2. "The bugs will go away when you feel better."
3. "Do you want me to brush them away for you?"
4. "Those are not bugs; it is just the design on the bedspread."

140. A client is to receive nitrogen mustard as part of a drug protocol for Hodgkin's disease. The nurse should explain that the nitrogen mustard is believed to act by:

1. Interfering with cellular protein synthesis
2. Inhibiting the synthesis of purine and pyrimidine
3. Binding the DNA to interfere with RNA production
4. Binding the DNA strands and interfering with cell replication

141. A biopsy of a brain tumor removed from a child identifies the tumor as a cerebellar astrocytoma. The nurse is aware that this tumor is:
1. Fast growing and highly malignant
2. Benign and associated with a high rate of cure
3. A cause of pituitary malfunction as the child grows
4. Close to vital centers and only partial excision is possible

142. A 9-year-old is admitted with a diagnosis of possible infratentorial brain tumor. The nurse identifies the common presenting symptoms of this type of tumor when the child demonstrates:
1. Ataxia
2. Seizures
3. Papilledema
4. Cranial enlargement

143. One morning a male client, whose thought processes are marked by ideas of reference and persecutory ideation, appears very upset. The client tells the nurse that the reporter on television told everyone that he is "a queer." The most therapeutic response by the nurse would be:
1. "It sounds to me like you're having some frightening feelings."
2. "I will call the station and ask why the reporter said that about you."
3. "You seem upset by this. Why do you think the reporter said that about you?"
4. "Sometimes when we are unsure of ourselves we project our feelings on others."

144. The physician's order for a client in ketoacidosis states: add 500 units Humulin R insulin to 500 ml Ringer's lactate IV and run to administer 60 units of insulin in the next 30 minutes. To administer the correct amount of medication, the nurse should set the IV infusion device at:
1. 30 ml/hr
2. 60 ml/hr
3. 90 ml/hr
4. 120 ml/hr

145. When preparing a teaching plan for the parents of a child with celiac disease, the nurse recalls that the basic problem in celiac disease is the:
1. Presence of meconium stool
2. Clumping of the intestinal villi
3. Absence of the enzyme peptidase
4. Susceptibility to profound dehydration

146. The best nursing action to prevent heat loss in the neonate would be to:
1. Administer oxygen to prevent shivering
2. Dress the baby in a shirt and gown immediately
3. Bathe the baby in warm water as soon as possible after birth
4. Maintain skin-to-skin contact between mother and baby under a cover

147. A client thinks she is pregnant. The nurse is aware that a positive sign of pregnancy is:
1. Hegar's sign
2. Uterine enlargement
3. A positive pregnancy test
4. Fetal movements felt by the examiner

148. A young adult client with schizophrenia is started on haloperidol (Haldol). When the nurse gives the client the medication, the client asks, "What's this for?" The nurse could best respond, "This medication:
1. Will help you to relax and think more clearly."
2. Fights 'the blues' and keeps your thoughts together."
3. Will raise your seizure threshold letting you think more clearly."
4. Maintains an even mood while keeping your temper under control."

149. A young pregnant client, who has had inadequate prenatal care, is admitted to the hospital at 37 weeks gestation with pregnancy-induced hypertension (PIH). Assessment of the client reveals a nutritional deficit. A physical finding that would be related to inadequate protein intake is:
1. Petechiae
2. Bradycardia
3. Bleeding gums
4. Peripheral edema

150. An infant is admitted to the nursery and is classified as being small for gestational age (SGA). A priority intervention for this infant would be to:
1. Test the infant's stools for occult blood
2. Monitor the infant's blood glucose levels
3. Place the infant in the Trendelenburg position
4. Measure the infant's head circumference every shift

151. After several days on bedrest, a preschooler with the diagnosis of acute glomerulonephritis becomes demanding and will not listen to the nurses. The child was found in the playroom twice on the previous shift. To best meet the needs of this child the nurse should:
1. Ask the child not to get up again and explain the reason for bedrest
2. Place soft restraints on the child when family members cannot be present
3. Have a color television set moved into the child's room as soon as possible
4. Move the child into a room with another five-year-old who has a fractured femur

152. A client with laryngeal cancer has a partial laryngectomy and tracheostomy. To facilitate communication postoperatively, the nurse should:
1. Provide a pad and pencil for writing
2. Allow more time for the client to articulate
3. Face the client and speak slowly and distinctly
4. Use visual clues such as gestures and objects

153. When planning the development of a nurse-client relationship with a client, the nurse is aware that the most important aspect of this relationship during the early phase of its development is:
1. Trust
2. Empathy
3. Personal rapport
4. Open communication

154. A client with a peptic ulcer is scheduled for a subtotal gastrectomy. Nursing intervention directed toward minimizing the postoperative complication of dumping syndrome includes teaching the client to:
1. Ambulate after every meal
2. Remain on a diet low in fat
3. Eat in a semirecumbent position
4. Increase the fluid intake with meals

155. When teaching the parents of an 8-year-old who is a newly diagnosed insulin dependent diabetic, it is important to differentiate between insulin dependent and non-insulin dependent diabetes. The nurse should tell them that with insulin dependent diabetes it is more common to develop:
1. Obesity
2. Ketoacidosis
3. Resistance to treatment
4. Hypersensitivity to other drugs

156. An 11-year-old has just been diagnosed as an insulin dependent diabetic. The child, who likes sweets, asks about sugar and sugar substitutes in the diet. The nurse and the dietitian tell the child that:
1. Honey can be used as a natural sugar substitute
2. Simple sugars such as sucrose or fructose should be avoided
3. Sugar substitutes such as saccharin or aspartame can be used
4. The sweet taste habit can be broken by eliminating sweets altogether

157. Before a client's discharge after having a tonic-clonic seizure, the nurse should reinforce previous teaching related to the anticonvulsant phenytoin (Dilantin). The nurse should instruct the client to:

1. Report immediately any unsteadiness of gait
2. Expect transient joint discomfort on occasion
3. Avoid massaging the gums during oral hygiene
4. Immediately discontinue the drug if a skin rash appears

158. A full term neonate, born with a meningomyelocele, is scheduled for surgery. The priority preoperative nursing goal is to make certain that this baby:
1. Remains sedated
2. Continues infection free
3. Gains one ounce per day
4. Develops a strong sucking reflex

159. The physician prescribes the "Prudent Diet" advocated by the American Heart Association for a male client with angina. The client's wife says to the nurse, "I guess I'm going to have to cook two meals, one for my husband and one for my daughter and myself." The most appropriate response by the nurse would be:
1. "I wouldn't bother. This diet is really easy to follow; just cut down the salt you use and fry foods in peanut oil."
2. "You're right, and be careful not to cook his favorite meals because he will probably not want to adhere to the diet."
3. "The diet that has been prescribed for your husband is a healthy diet that is recommended for all of us to follow."
4. "This is a very difficult diet to follow. I would recommend that you shop daily for food so there are no temptations in the kitchen."

160. When administering hydroxyzine hydrochloride (Vistaril), the nurse should monitor the clients for the common side effects of this drug which include:
1. Ataxia and confusion
2. Drowsiness and dry mouth
3. Vertigo and impaired vision
4. Slurred speech and headache

161. After head and neck surgery hyperextension of the neck for the first few postoperative days may cause:
1. Cervical trauma
2. Laryngeal spasm
3. Laryngeal edema
4. Wound dehiscence

162. When checking the cervical dilation of a client in labor, the nurse notices that the umbilical cord has prolapsed. The nurse's first action should be to:
1. Take the fetal heart rate
2. Turn the client on her side
3. Cover the cord with sterile saline soaks
4. Put the client in a modified Trendelenburg position

163. After abdominal surgery a goal is to have the client achieve alveolar expansion. This goal would be most effectively achieved by:
1. Blow bottles
2. Postural drainage
3. Prolonged exhalation
4. Sustained inspirations

164. A young woman comes to the mental health clinic because she has lost her job and does not know what to do. The client lives alone and her family lives in another state. The client states she feels like a failure. An appropriate nursing diagnosis for this client would probably be:
1. Altered thought processes related to impaired judgment
2. High risk for violence self-directed related to panic state
3. Social isolation related to absence of satisfying personal relationships
4. Personal identity disturbance related to inability to distinguish self from nonself

165. A client with advanced cancer of the bladder is scheduled for a cystectomy and ileal conduit. Physical preparation for the surgery should include:
1. Insertion of a Foley catheter
2. Well-balanced diet with vitamins
3. Administration of neomycin sulfate
4. Administration of urinary antiseptics

166. The nurse should be aware that the most therapeutic activity for a depressed client would probably be:
1. Putting together a jigsaw puzzle
2. Stuffing envelopes for a local charity
3. Assembling and whip-stitching a wallet
4. Participating in an aerobic exercise group

167. A few days after an automobile accident in which a fractured femur was sustained, the laboratory reports of the child, who is now in Bryant's traction, indicate a slight decrease in hemoglobin and hematocrit. The most appropriate nursing action would be to:
1. Order a type and crossmatch
2. Notify the physician immediately
3. Provide additional meat for dinner
4. Assess the child's abdomen for internal bleeding

168. A client with active genital herpes had a cesarean delivery and is now in the recovery room. When providing care to this client, the nurse should:
1. Wear a gown and gloves
2. Use meticulous hand washing
3. Use bacteriostatic hand scrubs
4. Wear a gown, gloves, and a mask

169. The physician prescribes the drug cholestyramine, an anion exchange resin, to treat a client's persistent diarrhea. This drug reduces the absorption of fat which may produce a deficiency of:
1. Thiamine
2. Vitamin A
3. Riboflavin
4. Vitamin B_6

170. A client with colitis is started on steroid therapy. The nurse would know that teaching was effective when the client says, "When taking this medication I should:
1. Take the medicine at bedtime with a snack."
2. Take the drug 1 hour before or 2 hours after eating."
3. Divide the dose into equal parts and take with each meal."
4. Take the drug in the early morning with food or an antacid."

171. When reviewing the breast self-examination procedure with a client, the comment by the client that the nurse should consider significant is:
1. "My bra feels tight when I am menstruating."
2. "My breasts feel lumpy just before menstruation."
3. "My left breast was always slightly larger than my right."
4. "My right breast feels and looks thicker than my left breast."

172. A terminally ill client is furious with one of the staff nurses. Over the next several days the client refuses the nurse's care and insists on doing self care. A different nurse is assigned to care for the client. The nurse's initial step in revising the nursing care plan to meet the client's needs would be to:
1. Get a full report from the first nurse and adjust the plan accordingly
2. Ask the physician for a report on the client's condition and plan accordingly
3. Speak with the client about the change in staff responsibilities and assess the client's reaction
4. Assess the client's present status and capabilities and include the client in a discussion of revisions

173. The membranes of a laboring client rupture spontaneously. An observation by the nurse at this time that would necessitate immediate notification of the obstetrician would be:
1. Bloody show
2. Greenish fluid
3. Clear fluid with specks of mucus
4. Shortened intervals between contractions

174. The nursing care plan of a client who is being admitted with a diagnosis of abruptio placentae should include careful assessment for signs and symptoms of:
1. Jaundice
2. Hypertension
3. Hypovolemic shock
4. Impending convulsions

175. When developing a plan of care for an elderly client with the diagnosis of dementia the nurse should:
1. Be considerate of the client's various likes and dislikes
2. Be firm in dealing with the client's attitudes and behaviors
3. Explain to the client the details of the therapeutic regimen
4. Provide consistency in carrying out nursing activities for the client

176. After a suprapubic prostatectomy, a client returns from the operating room with a suprapubic tube and a three-way Foley catheter with a continuous drip of a GU irrigant. The nurse realizes that the purpose of this therapy is to:
1. Promote continuous formation of urine
2. Prevent the formation of clots in the bladder
3. Facilitate the measurement of urinary output
4. Provide continuous pressure on the prostatic fossa

177. A child with a puncture wound, whose history of immunizations is uncertain, is given tetanus immune globulin (Hyper-Tet). The nurse knows that the chief reason for using tetanus immune globulin instead of tetanus antitoxin is that it:
1. Is as effective as the antitoxin
2. Is more convenient to administer
3. Is not likely to cause anaphylaxis
4. Can be safely given to everyone who needs it

178. A 2½-year-old is admitted with a fever of 103°F, stiffness of the neck, and generalized malaise. The child is diagnosed as having acute bacterial meningitis. Priority nursing care for this child would include:
1. Hydrating the child
2. Administering oxygen
3. Placing the child in isolation
4. Giving the child a tepid sponge bath

179. A client with a fractured tibia and fibula is to be discharged with a right leg cast and crutches. In addition to teaching the technical aspects of crutch walking, the nurse plans to advise the client to:
    1. Avoid taking showers until the cast is removed
    2. Increase the intake of vitamin C to enhance healing
    3. Gradually increase weight bearing on the injured leg
    4. Remove loose rugs and rearrange furniture as necessary

180. X-ray films reveal that a client has closed fractures of the right femur and tibia. Multiple soft-tissue contusions are also present. An important short-term intervention is to:
    1. Prepare the client for application of skeletal traction
    2. Reassure the client that these injuries are not that serious
    3. Prepare the client for operative reduction of the injured extremity
    4. Assess the circulatory, motor, and sensory status of the client's injured extremity

181. The primary goal of therapy for a client with chronic obstructive pulmonary disease is to:
    1. Limit hydration
    2. Improve ventilation
    3. Increase oxygenation
    4. Correct the bicarbonate deficit

182. The adaptation in a child with nephrotic syndrome that would necessitate that the nurse check vital signs, especially pulse quality and rate and blood pressure is:
    1. Hypovolemia
    2. Hyperkalemia
    3. Pulmonary emboli
    4. Congestive heart failure

183. In a childbirth preparation class a client learned a number of exercises that could be performed on the first day after a cesarean delivery. The nurse on the postpartum floor recognizes that further teaching is necessary when the client states that one of the exercises learned was:
    1. Leg bends
    2. Foot circles
    3. Pelvic rocking
    4. Shoulder circles

184. A pregnant client comes to the emergency room because of vaginal bleeding. The nurse asks the client to approximate how much bleeding is occurring. The best gauge for the client to use is:
    1. Whether or not clots are present
    2. Any change in fetal activity with the bleeding
    3. The amount in relation to her usual menstrual flow
    4. How weak she has become since the bleeding began

185. After 3 weeks of mental health therapy a client tells the nurse, "I feel I am ready for discharge." The nurse can best evaluate the client's readiness for discharge by:
    1. Testing the client's level of trust of self and staff
    2. Exchanging views with the client about the prognosis
    3. Asking the client to explain any changes in behavior since admission
    4. Requiring the client to identify specific behaviors viewed as examples of wellness

186. The results of a biopsy indicate a client has a malignant sarcoma of the liver, and chemotherapy via regional perfusion is the treatment of choice. This method of drug administration probably was selected for this client because:
    1. The drug therapy can be continued at home with little difficulty
    2. Larger doses of drugs can be delivered to the actual site of the tumor
    3. The toxic effects of the chemotherapeutic drugs will be confined to the area of the tumor
    4. Combinations of drugs can be used to attack neoplastic cells at various stages of the cell cycle

187. When caring for a child in acute respiratory distress from laryngotracheobronchitis, who has a temperature of 103°F, the nurse should give priority to:
1. Delivering 40% humidified oxygen
2. Initiating measures to reduce fever
3. Constantly assessing the child's respiratory status
4. Providing support to reduce the child's apprehension

188. A client with diabetes mellitus develops persistent, alternating episodes of hyperglycemia and hypoglycemia despite increased amounts of insulin daily. The nurse recognizes that this effect is caused by:
1. Increased glycogen formation in the liver
2. Excessive insulin that causes glycogenolysis
3. Insufficient levels of insulin to lower blood glucose
4. Excessive glucose intake that causes gluconeogenesis

189. After an open reduction and internal fixation of a hip fracture in an elderly individual the assessment that would require immediate nursing intervention would be:
1. Complaints of pain in the chest 6 days postoperatively
2. An inability to cough productively 2 days postoperatively
3. A rectal temperature of 100.2°F three days postoperatively
4. Fatigue in the leg on the unaffected side 5 days postoperatively

190. When assessing the head of a 2-hour-old infant, the nurse would normally expect to find:
1. Closed suture lines
2. A sunken anterior fontanel
3. Open anterior and posterior fontanels
4. A soft fluctuant mass that outlines a bone

191. A 4-year-old with AIDS is placed on appropriate isolation precautions. These precautions include:

1. Gloves should be worn whenever approaching the bedside
2. Gloves should be worn when in contact with blood and body fluids
3. Limited physical contact should be made when care is administered
4. Gowns, masks, and gloves should be worn when providing direct care

192. The nurse is aware that the psychiatrist is concerned that one of the client's receiving haloperidol (Haldol) may be developing neuroleptic malignant syndrome. The nurse should carefully assess the client for symptoms that would include:
1. Jaundice, malaise, and pruritus
2. Sore throat, seizures, and tremors
3. Diaphoresis, muscle rigidity, and hyperpyrexia
4. Loss of visual acuity, dry skin, and hyperbilirubinemia

193. In the third trimester of pregnancy, a client develops extensive edema, hypertension, a low serum albumin level, and albuminuria. The nutritional therapy that requires primary emphasis is the:
1. Control of kilocalories to limit weight gain during this period
2. Elimination of all salt to reduce the edema and hypertension
3. Inclusion of protein to restore normal circulation of tissue fluids
4. Use of iron supplements to help restore circulating blood volume

194. An infant's discharge is being delayed because of a rising reticulocyte count. The infant's mother who is being discharged asks the nurse why the baby must stay. The nurse's response is based on an understanding that the infant needs to be observed for:
1. Significant jaundice
2. A bacterial infection
3. Bleeding tendencies
4. Adequate oxygenation

195. A young female client admitted to the trauma center after being raped continues to talk about the rape. The primary nursing intervention should be directed toward:
1. Getting her involved with a rape therapy group
2. Remaining available and supportive to limit destructive anger
3. Exploring her feelings about men to promote future relationships
4. Helping her restore emotional control to expiate feelings of shame

196. A client develops subcutaneous emphysema after a laryngectomy. This is most readily detected by:
1. Palpating the neck or face
2. Auscultating the lung fields
3. Evaluating the blood gases
4. Reviewing the chest x-ray film

197. A client who complains of memory loss, nervousness, insomnia, and fear of going out of the house is admitted after several days of increasing incapacitation. Initially, considering this client's history, the nurse should give priority to:
1. Evaluating the client's adjustment to the unit
2. Providing the client with a sense of security and safety
3. Exploring the client's memory loss and fear of going out
4. Assessing the precipitating factors for the client's hospitalization

198. After gastric surgery a client has a nasogastric tube in place. The nurse should plan to:
1. Change the tube at least once every 48 hours
2. Monitor the client for signs of electrolyte imbalance
3. Connect the nasogastric tube to high continuous suction
4. Assess placement by injecting 10 ml of water into the tube

199. A 9-year-old, recently diagnosed as having insulin dependent diabetes, attends the center for diabetic teaching with the parents. The nurse notes that the child's concerns about the illness center on:

1. How the parents will react to the diagnosis of the disease
2. How much school might have to be missed because of the disease
3. Whether or not the physician will be successful in controlling the diabetes
4. Whether having diabetes means it will be impossible to have children as an adult

200. A client comes to the clinic complaining of a productive cough with copious yellow sputum, fever, and chills for the past two days. The first thing the nurse should do when caring for this client is to:
1. Administer oxygen
2. Begin to push fluids
3. Collect a sputum specimen
4. Take the client's temperature

201. The nurse recognizes that the increased incidence of fractures with osteoporosis in the United States occurs because of the:
1. Dietary use of skim milk
2. Aging of the American population
3. Increased number of hysterectomies
4. Immobility associated with early retirement

202. A client's leg is placed in Buck's extension to reduce pain from muscle spasms until surgery can be performed. The nurse knows that Buck's traction is a type of:
1. Skin traction
2. Transfixation
3. Skeletal traction
4. Balanced suspension

203. When planning for a client's care during the detoxification phase of acute alcohol withdrawal, the nurse should anticipate the need to:
1. Supervise the client at all times
2. Keep the client's room lights dim
3. Speak to the client in a loud, clear voice
4. Restrain the client during periods of agitation

204. A client with Hodgkin's disease is to receive the cyclic antineoplastic vincristine (Oncovin) as part of a therapy protocol. The nurse explains that Oncovin helps destroy the malignant cells by:

1. Arresting mitosis in metaphase
2. Inhibiting the synthesis of pyrimidine
3. Alkylating nucleic acids needed for mitosis
4. Inactivating DNA and inhibiting RNA synthesis

205. During the postoperative period following a craniotomy for the removal of an astrocytoma, a child develops a sudden right pupillary dilation. The nurse recognizes this as a sign of:
1. Severe pain
2. Intense fear
3. Uncal herniation
4. Reduced intracranial pressure

206. When a client in active labor begins to experience contractions every 2 minutes that last 50 to 70 seconds, she complains of a severe backache and becomes very irritable. The nurse determines that the client is in the stage of labor known as:
1. Early first
2. Transition
3. Early third
4. Late second

207. A married, male client with three children has lost his job and feels useless. He is tearful, upset, and embarassed. A goal of care appropriate for this client would be:
1. Limiting tearfulness
2. Increasing self-esteem
3. Controlling feelings of sadness
4. Promoting acceptance by others

208. Following major surgery, a 4-year-old girl is in the intensive care unit and is told that she can have medication to keep her comfortable. The nurse should tell her that when she hurts:
1. She will be given a pill to make the hurt better
2. The nurses will give her an injection to take the hurt away
3. The nurses will put medicine in her IV to make the hurt go away
4. She will be given medicines that will make all the hurt go right away

209. To meet the needs of a client who has a seizure disorder and who has recently had a tonic-clonic seizure, the nurse should plan to:
1. Outline ways to prevent physical trauma from occurring during a seizure
2. Teach that anticonvulsant medications should be taken on an empty stomach
3. Explain that the client need not tell others of the illness because the medication will be increased
4. Teach the client that the symptoms and treatment of seizure disorders are similar, regardless of etiology

210. After surgery for a meningomyelocele, an infant is being fed by gavage feedings. When checking placement of the nasogastric tube, the nurse is unable to hear the air injected because of noisy breath sounds. The nurse should:
1. Notify the physician
2. Advance the tube 1 to 2 cm
3. Carefully insert 1 ml of formula
4. Attempt to aspirate the stomach contents

211. The physician orders 10 ml of a 10% solution of calcium gluconate for a client with a severely depressed serum calcium. The client also is receiving an IV solution of D5W and digoxin (Lanoxin) 0.25 mg daily. The nurse should be aware that calcium gluconate:
1. Is compatible with all IV solutions
2. Is nonirritating to surrounding tissues
3. Cannot be added to the IV of 1000 ml D5W
4. Potentiates the action of digitalis preparations

212. When lithium therapy is instituted the nurse should teach the client to maintain a normal daily intake of:
1. Iron
2. Sodium
3. Potassium
4. Magnesium

213. The nurse is aware that after a thyroidectomy the client should be observed carefully for symptoms indicating:
1. Perforation of the lung
2. Laceration of the esophagus
3. Fracture of the laryngeal cartilage
4. Accidental removal of the parathyroids

214. A 7 lb baby is delivered and admitted to the normal newborn nursery with an order for phytonadione (AquaMEPHYTON, vitamin K) 1 mg IM. The nurse is aware that this treatment is administered to:
1. Facilitate bilirubin excretion
2. Stimulate normal bowel flora
3. Increase liver glycogen stores
4. Promote normal blood clotting

215. After surgery to create an ileal conduit, a client awakens and asks for a sip of water. The nurse informs the client that water by mouth cannot be given until the:
1. Ileal loop begins to drain in 6 hours
2. Intestinal anastomosis heals in 10 days
3. Nasogastric suction is discontinued in 3 days
4. Client leaves the recovery room in a few hours

216. A severely depressed male client responds to therapy and with the help of the staff begins to set some immediate goals. The goal that would most indicate improvement would be the client's plan to:
1. Talk with at least one person on the unit daily
2. Stay clear of people who seem to make him anxious
3. Show the staff that he can do what they want him to do
4. Take at least 3 to 4 hours daily to sit alone and think about things

217. A young child is placed in Bryant traction for a fractured femur. The parents of the child ask the nurse about the traction. The nurse explains that with this system:

1. A Thomas splint, a sling, and pulleys keep the femur aligned
2. A system of pulleys keeps the affected leg elevated in a sling
3. Traction is placed on both legs, even though the left femur is fractured
4. Moleskin and weights are applied to the affected extremity to keep it extended

218. A client with active genital herpes has a cesarean delivery. The nurse teaches the mother how to limit transmission of the virus to her newborn. The nurse would evaluate that the instructions were understood when the mother states:
1. "I should avoid kissing my baby on the lips."
2. "I must wear gloves when I'm holding my baby."
3. "I have to wash my clothes and my baby's clothes separately."
4. "I should wash my hands thoroughly with soap and water before handling the baby."

219. A terminally ill client's oldest son is very concerned about his mother's condition. He asks the nurse, "Will she get better?" The nurse's most appropriate response would be:
1. "Her vital signs are stable, so she is holding her own."
2. "Of course she will. You can't give up. You must hope for the best."
3. "I don't know. You'll have to ask the doctor. I'll leave a note that you are here."
4. "Her condition is very serious. Would you like to discuss your concerns with me?"

220. The nurse encourages a terminally ill client to make decisions about daily activities and care. The nurse would know that the client, who had been extremely angry with everything and everybody, had resolved some of the anger when the client states:
1. "You've got a busy morning ahead of you! I'm really a mess."
2. "What are you going to let me do this morning? You know I can help."
3. "It's so hard to let someone do so much for me. It just doesn't seem right."
4. "I can do my face, hands, arms, and chest today but I think you'd better do the rest."

221. A male client, age 67, visits his physician complaining of frequency, dysuria, nocturia, and difficulty starting his urinary stream. A cystoscopy and biopsy of the prostate gland are done. The client is unable to void after the cystoscopy. The nurse should:
1. Limit oral fluids until he voids
2. Assure him that this is normal
3. Insert a urinary retention catheter
4. Palpate above the pubic symphysis

222. An IV of 800 ml/24 hours is ordered for a 2½-year-old. It is set up via a pediatric administration set (Buretrol). The solution should be set to infuse at:
1. 3 drops/minute
2. 6 drops/minute
3. 33 drops/minute
4. 60 drops/minute

223. A client is admitted to the emergency room with head and chest injuries received in an automobile accident. When evaluating the client's responses to the emergency room treatments, the assessments that indicate that the client can safely be transferred to a critical care unit are:
1. Alert but restless, stable vital signs, cyanosis
2. Stable vital signs, apprehension, complaints of pain
3. Drowsy but easily roused, improving tissue perfusion, fluctuating vital signs
4. Elevated temperature, slowing pulse and respiration, pain in the injured extremity

224. The nurse observes a client with acute bronchitis and chronic obstructive pulmonary disease sitting up in bed, appearing very anxious and dyspneic. The nurse should:
1. Provide oxygen at 2 L per minute
2. Administer the prescribed sedative
3. Have the client breathe into a paper bag
4. Encourage the client to cough and deep breathe

225. A primary nursing goal for a grand multipara in the event a cesarean delivery is performed is:
1. Prevention of hemorrhage
2. Prevention of perineal infection
3. Avoidance of wound dehiscence
4. Assistance with mother-infant bonding

226. Several hours after admission with laryngo-tracheobronchitis (viral croup), the nurse notes the child has developed tachypnea and tachycardia, accompanied by intercostal and substernal retractions and increased restlessness. The nurse should immediately:
1. Suction secretions from the child's trachea
2. Dislodge mucus by striking the child on the back
3. Report the child's respiratory status to the pediatrician
4. Increase the level of oxygen being delivered to the child

227. After surgery for a fractured hip a client is restless and appears anxious. When the nurse and nursing assistant enter the room to provide evening care the client becomes upset. The nurse should:
1. Explain that hip fractures are not life threatening
2. Reassure the client that they will be very careful
3. Describe the need for various personnel at this time
4. Suggest that the client can turn on the television for diversion

228. When a nurse suspects that a child has been abused, the nurse's primary responsibility must be to:
1. Treat the child's traumatic injuries
2. Confirm the suspected child abuse
3. Protect the child from any future abuse
4. Have the child examined by the physician

229. A 35-year-old male client is admitted to the hospital for confirmation of the diagnosis of Hodgkin's disease. The client and his wife are concerned that he may have cancer. The wife states, "Wouldn't it be unlikely for someone like my husband to have cancer?" Before responding to the emotional aspects of the question, the nurse should recall that:
1. It is impossible to predict who will develop cancer or when
2. Hodgkin's disease occurs most often in males aged 20 to 40
3. Hodgkin's disease is more common among women than men
4. Cancer is typically a disease of older rather than younger adults

230. The nurse avoids placing a client in the supine position during labor primarily because it can:
1. Lead to transient episodes of hypertension
2. Cause decreased perfusion of the placenta
3. Impede free movement of the symphysis pubis
4. Prolong labor because of the influence of gravity

231. A client who is bottle feeding her infant complains of discomfort from her engorged breasts. The measure most appropriate to relieve the engorgement would be:
1. Expression of breast milk to relieve pressure
2. Application of ice packs and a binder to her breasts
3. Use of hot moist towels as compresses on the breasts
4. Restriction of oral fluid intake to less than 1000 ml daily

232. The physician prescribes propylthiouracil for a client with hyperthyroidism. Two months after being started on the antithyroid medication the client calls the nurse and complains of feeling tired and looking pale. The nurse should:
1. Advise the client to get more rest
2. Schedule an appointment for the client
3. Instruct the client to skip one dose daily
4. Tell the client to increase the medication

233. A client, who is suspected of having had a silent myocardial infarction and is to have an electrocardiogram (ECG), asks the nurse, "Why are they doing this test?" To reply the nurse must understand that this test will:
1. Reflect heart sounds
2. Detect heart damage
3. Change the heart's rhythm
4. Assess the stress one can tolerate

234. Twelve hours after sustaining full-thickness burns to the chest and thighs, a client is complaining of severe thirst. The client's urinary output has been 60 ml/hr for the past 10 hours. No bowel sounds are heard. The nurse should:
1. Increase the client's IV flow rate
2. Give the client orange juice by mouth
3. Give the client 4 oz of water by mouth
4. Moisten the client's lips with wet gauze

235. The nursing diagnosis that takes priority when planning care for a client who has sustained partial- and full-thickness burns of the chest in a fire is:
1. High risk for infection related to burn trauma
2. Impaired physical mobility related to bedrest
3. Impaired gas exchange related to smoke inhalation
4. High risk for fluid volume deficit related to decreased intake

236. A depressed client frequently repeats doubts about going on and admits to thinking about suicide while denying a plan has been developed. During this period it is essential that the nurse:
1. Have a staff member stay with the client at all times
2. Plan to involve the client in activities that are interesting and absorbing
3. Explain in detail how the staff will protect the client against self-harm
4. Use frequent unobtrusive observations of the client's moods and activities

237. Eight days after starting antidepressant medication therapy, the nurse notices that a client who has been severely depressed is neatly dressed and well-groomed. The client smiles at the nurse and states, "Things sure look better today." Based on an awareness of depressed behavior the nurse should:
1. Begin preparing the client for discharge
2. Increase the client's privileges as a reward
3. Compliment both the client's appearance and smile
4. Assign a staff member to provide constant surveillance of the client

238. The nurse begins terminating the consistent one-to-one relationship with a client who is soon to be discharged. The nurse might expect the client to respond to termination by manifesting symptoms of:
1. Grief
2. Testing
3. Splitting
4. Manipulation

239. A young female client comes to the trauma center stating that she had been raped. She is disheveled, pale, and staring blankly. Taking what has occurred into consideration, the nurse asks the client to describe in detail what happened because:
1. It will help the nursing staff in giving legal advice and providing counseling
2. Talking about what led to the rape will help her see what may have precipitated it
3. It helps the victim put the event in better perspective and helps begin the resolution process
4. Discussing details will keep the victim from covering up the intimate happenings in the rape situation

240. A client's respiratory status may be affected after abdominal surgery. When planning care to provide for this need, the behavioral objective for this client should be:

1. Respirations will improve with coughing and deep breathing
2. Demonstrates the technique of coughing and deep breathing
3. Coughing and deep breathing will facilitate output of secretions
4. Will cough and deep breathe five or six times every hour while awake

241. After abdominal surgery a client develops hyperpyrexia, and peritonitis is suspected. When caring for this client the nurse should use:
1. Surgical asepsis
2. Protective isolation
3. Enteric precautions
4. Wound precautions

242. During the assessment of a pyrexic client who was admitted because of a productive cough, fever, and chills the nurse percusses an area of dullness over the right posterior lower lobe. Considering the presenting signs and symptoms, the nurse is aware that this finding may be indicative of:
1. Pleurisy
2. Bronchitis
3. Pneumonia
4. Emphysema

243. A male client with aortic stenosis is scheduled for a valve replacement in 2 days. He tells the nurse, "I told my wife all she needs to know if I don't make it." The response by the nurse that would be the most therapeutic would be:
1. "Men your age do very well."
2. "You are worried about dying."
3. "I'll get you a sleeping pill tonight, I know you will need it."
4. "I know you are concerned but your physician is excellent."

244. To decrease or control the sensory and cognitive disturbances that can occur after a client has open heart surgery, the nurse should:
1. Restrict all visitors
2. Withhold analgesic medications
3. Plan for maximum periods of rest
4. Keep the room light on most of the time

245. A client with cancer of the sigmoid colon is to have an abdominoperineal resection with a permanent colostomy. In preparation for surgery, the client is placed on a low-residue diet to:
1. Lower the bacteria in the intestine
2. Limit the amount of flatus produced
3. Reduce the amount of stool in the bowel
4. Prevent irritation of the intestinal mucosa

246. A 5-year-old girl is admitted for elective surgery. The nurse can best determine why the child thinks she is in the hospital by asking:
1. "Do you know what place this is?"
2. "Why did you come to the hospital?"
3. "Do you know what's going to happen to you?"
4. "You do know why you are in the hospital, don't you?"

247. A pregnant client is taught about warning signs that should be reported immediately to the obstetric care practitioner. The client indicates that she understands the information presented by stating that the sign that she would report immediately is:
1. Low back pain
2. White vaginal discharge
3. Braxton-Hicks contractions
4. Leakage of fluid from the vagina

248. A client with left ventricular failure is digitalized and placed on a maintenance dose of digoxin 0.25 mg qd. If a therapeutic effect is achieved the nurse would expect to observe:
1. Decreased pulse rate, diuresis, decreased edema
2. Decreased pulse pressure, increased blood pressure, weight loss
3. Increased pulse rate, stable fluid balance, decreased blood pressure
4. Decreased pulse rate, reduced heart murmur, increased blood pressure

249. A child with acute spasmodic bronchitis who is in a mist tent is taken out of the tent for morning care. During the bath, the nurse observes that the child has increased respiratory distress. The nurse should:
1. Do postural drainage and clap the child's chest
2. Suction the child's nasal passages to clear the airway
3. Discontinue the bath and place the child in the mist tent
4. Put the child in the orthopneic position and call the physician

250. Oral feedings for an infant with acute spasmodic bronchitis are stopped and intravenous fluids are ordered to:
1. Relieve laryngospasm
2. Lessen physical exertion
3. Decrease vagal stimulation
4. Meet the infant's caloric needs

251. A client has a permanent colostomy. During the first 24 hours there is no drainage from the colostomy. The nurse should realize that this is a result of the:
1. Edema following the surgery
2. Absence of intestinal peristalsis
3. Decrease in fluid intake prior to surgery
4. Proper functioning of the nasogastric tube

252. A client is admitted for surgery for a possible intestinal carcinoma. The client complains of malaise, constipation, and stomach rumbling. When obtaining a health history the nurse should expect the client to report changes in:

1. The shape of stools
2. The daily intake of fats
3. The amount of fluid intake
4. The use of spices in the diet

253. An infant who had been in a mist tent because of dyspnea caused by acute spasmodic laryngitis is being discharged. The parents ask the nurse about caring for their baby at home. The nurse's best response would be:
1. "Give 2 ounces of water after the feeding of formula."
2. "No one should be allowed to visit the baby for a while."
3. "All allergen producers such as animals should be avoided."
4. "No specific restrictions are necessary after your child goes home."

254. A child is receiving an infusion. The nurse notes some erythema at the infusion site. On palpation, the child cries and draws away. There is a blood return in the tubing when the solution container is held briefly below the insertion site. The nurse should:
1. Decrease the flow rate of the IV solution
2. Realize that additives may have this effect
3. Have the venipuncture site changed to a new area
4. Maintain the IV but continue to observe the insertion site

255. The nurse tells the parents of a child who is being discharged following a tonsillectomy and adenoidectomy that the child may have an objectionable mouth odor, slight ear pain, and a low-grade fever for the next few days. The nurse recommends that the parents:
1. Apply an ice collar for the pain
2. Give aspirin for pain as necessary
3. Let the child suck on peppermint candies
4. Encourage the child to gargle with warm salt solution

256. When caring for a client with an antisocial personality disorder, the staff should use a consistent approach that is:
1. Warm and firm without being punitive
2. Indifferent and detached but nonjudgmental
3. Conditionally acquiescent to client demands
4. Clearly communicative of personal resentment

257. The nurse is aware that group therapy with abusing parents should be designed to help these parents to:
1. Confront their own rage at being abused as children
2. Admit publicly and to themselves that they are child abusers
3. Recognize the long range psychologic effects of child abuse
4. Share information about their parenting techniques and skills

258. The day after having a cesarean delivery, a client is encouraged to ambulate. The client angrily asks the nurse, "Why am I being made to walk so soon after surgery?" The nurse's best reply would be:
1. "Early walking lowers the incidence of urinary infection."
2. "Walking about early will prevent your wound from opening."
3. "You can get to hold your baby more quickly if you walk around."
4. "Walking keeps the blood from pooling in your legs and prevents clots."

259. A male client with a cerebrovascular accident (CVA) frequently cries when his family visits. The family members are obviously upset by the crying. The nurse should explain to the family that the client is:
1. Mourning his obvious loss of function
2. Having difficulty controlling his emotions
3. Demonstrating his usual premorbid personality
4. Conveying his unhappiness about the situation

260. A client is admitted to the hospital with a diagnosis of left ventricular failure secondary to rheumatic heart disease. The nurse should be aware that the symptoms of heart failure occur because the:
1. Arterial system is less flexible due to hypertension or arteriosclerosis
2. Excessive blood volume increases the workload of the heart muscles
3. Heart can no longer pump blood adequately in relation to venous return
4. Heart valves have become stenotic or regurgitant and impede blood flow

261. After a basal cell carcinoma is removed by fulguration a client is given a topical steroid to apply to the surgical site. The nurse would recognize that the teaching regarding steroids and skin lesions was effective when the client states that the purpose of the medication is to:
1. Prevent infection of the wound
2. Decrease fluid loss from the skin
3. Reduce inflammation at the surgical site
4. Limit itching around the area of the lesion

262. Intestinal infestation with enterobius vermicularis (pinworm) is suspected in a 6-year-old. The nurse can assist in confirming the child's diagnosis by:
1. Asking the mother to collect stools for three consecutive days for culture
2. Instructing the mother to do an anal Scotch tape test early in the morning
3. Assisting the mother to schedule hypersensitivity tests of the child's blood serum
4. Having the mother bring in the child's stools for visual examination for three days

263. Considering the fact that a client with a right-sided cerebrovascular accident (CVA) is right handed, the task that will probably present the most difficulty is:
1. Eating meals
2. Writing letters
3. Combing the hair
4. Dressing every morning

264. The nurse would know that childbirth preparation classes were effective when during the transition phase a couple who attended the classes use the breathing pattern known as:
1. Pant-blow
2. Slow chest
3. Shallow chest
4. Accelerated-decelerated

265. The nipples of a client who is breastfeeding her baby become sore and cracked. The nurse should instruct the client to:
1. Apply continuous ice packs to her nipples
2. Take her analgesic medication as ordered
3. Remove the baby from the breast for a few days
4. Expose her nipples to the air several times a day

Answers and Rationales for Comprehensive Examination 2

Part A

1. 3 Normal head circumference is 13 to 14 inches (33 to 35.5 cm) and about 1 inch greater than the chest circumference. (2) (PE; AS; PA; NM)
   1 The head is too large.
   2 Same as answer 1.
   4 The chest circumference is within normal limits.

2. 3 Multiple premature ventricular beats (PVB) can eventually fall on a T wave, causing ventricular fibrillation; PVBs must be immediately interrupted with a drug that reduces cardiac irritability. (3) (ME; IM; TC; CV)
   1 This will not interrupt the dysrhythmia.
   2 This is unnecessary; a cardiac arrest has not occurred.
   4 This is unsafe; the dysrhythmia must be interrupted immediately; the physician can be notified later.

3. 3 Clients who have lost contact with reality can be assisted to reestablish contact by being provided structured activities. (2) (MH; PL; PS; SD)
   1 This client is responding to voices, not reality; limit setting is reality oriented and is usually ineffective unless it involves directing the client to dismiss the voices.
   2 The client represents no immediate threat to the self or others; isolating the client would decrease contact with reality and would most likely increase the hallucinations.
   4 Although this may decrease the hallucinations, it takes a long time to establish such a relationship and the client needs help now.

4. 1 Levels close to 2 mEq/liter are dangerously close to the toxic level; immediate action must be taken. (3) (MH; EV; TC; DR)
   2 The level is dangerously high; and the priority is the immediate notification of the physician rather than continued monitoring.
   3 Same as answer 2.
   4 The level is dangerously high; the therapeutic range for lithium is 0.6 to 1.2 mEq/liter.

5. 2 Drainage flows by gravity. (3) (SU; EV; TC; EN)
   1 This is unsafe; lifting and replacing a dressing would contaminate the surgical site.
   3 Although this might be done, it does not take into consideration that drainage flows by gravity.
   4 This is unsafe; this would interfere with the healing process.

6. 3 A pelvic examination would reveal dilation and effacement. (3) (CW; AS; PA; HC)
   1 This indicates only the presence of estrogen in cervical mucus; this determines ovulation, not true labor.
   2 Contractions are also present with Braxton-Hicks contractions, which are not true labor.
   4 This only differentiates between amniotic fluid and urine; rupture of the membranes can occur with or without the onset of true labor.

7. 4 Pulmonic stenosis increases resistance to blood flow, causing right ventricular hypertrophy; with right-ventricular heart failure there is an increase in pressure on the right side of the heart. (3) (PE; AN; PA; CV)

1 The pressure would be decreased in pulmonic stenosis.

2 Same as answer 1.

3 Same as answer 1.

8. 2 During acute cholecystitis, low-fat liquids are permitted; skim milk is low in fat and contains protein, which will eventually promote healing. (3) (SU; PL; ED; GI)

1 Beef, even if it is lean, contains fat and should be avoided.

3 Egg yolks contain fat and should be avoided.

4 Gas-forming vegetables should be avoided.

9. 2 This portrays a nonjudgmental attitude that recognizes the client's needs. (2) (MH; IM; PS; AX)

1 The client is upset that she cannot control her crying.

3 This is untrue; it implies that crying will make it all better.

4 This is unrealistic; the cause of the anxiety, and hence the crying, is on an unconscious level.

10. 3 This offers the mother the opportunity to identify what is bothering her about caring for her baby. (3) (CW; IM; PS; HC)

1 This response could put the client on the defensive.

2 This minimizes the client's feelings and offers false reassurance.

4 Same as answer 2.

11. 3 This indicates the child's level of understanding to the nurse, and the explanation can then proceed at this level. (3) (PE; PL; ED; GD)

1 Doll play is more appropriate for younger children; it is inappropriate in this instance.

2 Role playing is inappropriate and nontherapeutic at this time.

4 Although the school-age child appreciates some detail, extensive detail is inappropriate.

12. 3 This occurs with the administration of Adriamycin and may alarm the client. (3) (ME; EV; ED; DR)

1 This is true for mithramycin, not the drugs in this protocol.

2 This is unnecessary.

4 Adriamycin is not given orally, only via the IV route.

13. 2 As long as the client has no nausea or vomiting, there are no diet restrictions. (2) (SU; IM; ED; IT)

1 The client should not disturb the dressing; it should be changed by the physician on a follow-up visit.

3 The biopsy site will be sutured and should not get wet.

4 Temperature elevation is not a usual response and may indicate infection.

14. 3 The data indicate impending shock; the dressing should be assessed for signs of hemorrhage. (3) (SU; EV; TC; CV)

1 Although this may eventually be done, it is not the priority.

2 There are no signs of respiratory distress; if hemorrhage is confirmed, the supine position is preferable.

4 This is unsafe; the client may be hemorrhaging and needs immediate assessment.

15. 4 Stimulation of the autonomic nervous system is a normal response to cord compression during uterine contraction. (3) (CW; EV; PA; HC)

1 This is unnecessary; this is a normal response to cord compression during a contraction.

2 Same as answer 1.

3 Same as answer 1.

16. 1 The client has signs of diabetes, which may result from steroid therapy; testing the blood glucose level is a method of screening for diabetes mellitus, thus gathering more data. (2) (ME; AS; PA; EN)

2 The symptoms are not those of benign prostatic hypertrophy.

3 Assessing the urine for glucose and ketones is not as accurate as a blood glucose level.

4 The symptoms presented are not those of fluid retention, but of diabetes mellitus.

17. 1 Cholesterol is an essential precursor of body substances such as vitamin D and steroid hormones; although some is synthesized by the body, a small amount is needed in the diet. (3) (ME; IM; ED; CV)

2 Polyunsaturated fats come from vegetable sources; saturated fats come from animal sources, coconut oil, and palm oil.

3 The diet must contain some cholesterol, and this should come from plant sources.

4 Same as answer 2.

18. 1 This prevents seepage of Imferon up through the needle track, thereby limiting staining of the skin. (1) (PE; IM; TC; DR)

2 This is unsafe; massage would force Imferon into the subcutaneous tissue, causing irritation and staining.

3 This length needle is too short to get into a muscle; a 1½ to 2 inch needle is required; the gauge of the needle is too small for the viscosity of Imferon; a 19- to 22-gauge needle is required.

4 Aspiration would still be performed with the Z-track method.

19. 1 Hypoglycemia may be present because of sudden withdrawal of maternal glucose and increased insulin production by the infant. (3) (CW; AN; TC; HN)

2 The umbilical vein may be used for starting an IV; it should not be obliterated.

3 This is not the priority until the blood glucose level is determined.

4 This can be delayed for 2 hours; determination of the blood glucose level is the priority.

20. 4 These are some of the first signs of hypoxia; the airway must be kept patent to promote oxygenation. (2) (PE; AS; PA; RE)

1 These are late signs of hypoxia; suctioning should have been done well before this time.

2 These are late signs of respiratory difficulty; suctioning and other measures should have been done well before this time.

3 The client will not be able to communicate verbally after a tracheotomy.

21. 1 The congested liver impairs venous return, leading to increased portal vein hydrostatic pressure and fluid shift into the abdominal cavity. (3) (ME; AN; PA; GI)

2 Bile plays an important role in digestion of fats, but it is not a major factor in fluid balance.

3 Increased serum albumin causes hypervolemia, not ascites.

4 Ascites is not related to the interstitial fluid compartment.

22. 1 A continual level of this drug is maintained to keep the terminally ill client comfortable. (1) (ME; PL; PA; NM)

2 This medication is not administered intermittently; in addition, for clients' management at home it is usually prescribed in liquid form and is taken orally.

3 The client should not have to request this medication; it should be given routinely.

4 Addiction is not a major concern for the terminally ill client.

23. 1 Mediastinal structures move toward the uninjured lung, reducing oxygenation and venous return. (3) (SU; AS; PA; RE)

2 This is unusual with a crushing chest injury.

3 Flail chest is a closed chest injury; open pneumothorax results from a penetrating injury to the chest wall.

4 This is a result of cardiac contusion and usually occurs from sternal, not lateral, compression.

24. 2 This reflects the client's feelings and opens channels of communication. (3) (MH; IM; PS; SD)

1 This response denies the client's feelings; this will not foster development of trust.

3 This provides false reassurance; it is really not the same food, because it is on the client's plate.

4 This is false reassurance; the delusional client would believe the nurse knows what part to taste.

25. 3 If the bleeding continues, both mother and fetus are at risk and a cesarean delivery would be indicated. (1) (CW; PL; TC; HP)

1 This is desired in all situations, not just in placenta previa.

2 This may be a medical decision and would be difficult for the nurse to control.

4 It is best to deal with reality; diversion at this time is unrealistic.

26. 2 This infestation is transferred by the anal-oral route, and handwashing is the most effective method to prevent transmission. (1) (PE; EV; ED; GI)

1 Cats do not transmit this disease.

3 This is unnecessary; pinworms are found in the rectum or colon and travel to the perianal area only when the person sleeps.

4 This is not the usual mode of transmission.

27. 1 Decreased normal breath sounds result from reduced air flow, pleural effusion, and destruction of lung tissue. (3) (ME; AS; PA; RE)

2 There is enlargement of accessory muscles, which are used during the expiratory phase to help force air out.

3 There is an increased expiratory phase because of entrapment of air and collapse of airways.

4 There is an increased A-P diameter (barrel chest) because of air trapping and enlargement of the lungs with a loss of recoil ability.

28. 2 Lying on the affected side increases drainage and allows the unaffected lung to expand to the fullest extent. (3) (SU; IM; PA; RE)

1 This will not facilitate drainage and leads to pooling of drainage in the operative site.

3 Same as answer 1.

4 This is undesirable because this may not allow the unaffected lung to fully expand and provide maximum oxygenation.

29. 1 The client expects the nurse to focus on eating, but the emphasis should be placed on feelings rather than actions. (2) (MH; IM; PS; EA)

2 This is a threat that will not convince the client to eat; privileges are associated with a contracted weight gain.

3 This is a threat that will not convince the client to eat; the client is not concerned about the effects of malnutrition.

4 Threats will not convince the client to eat; this response sets up a challenge that the nurse will not win.

30. 2 Reducing anxiety limits the need for these obsessive-compulsive actions. (3) (MH; PL; TC; PR)

1 Simple repetitive activities are not therapeutic for this client and could increase anxiety.

3 This is a temporary action that does not deal with the feelings that cause anxiety.

4 Menial tasks may decrease feelings of self-worth; these individuals do not have a need to expiate guilt.

31. 3 This measure assesses for increasing intracranial pressure, which may occur if drainage channels are obstructed by the bacterial infection. (2) (PE; PL; TC; NM)

1 This is insufficient monitoring; many changes could occur in this time span.

2 Antibiotics are administered intravenously throughout the course of treatment.

4 Parents can visit if they are taught how to carry out the isolation procedures.

32. 1 Edema associated with the inflammatory reaction after surgery limits the conduction of sound. (3) (SU; AN; PA; NM)

2 This should not happen because the inner ear is not involved in this surgery.

3 This is extremely unlikely.

4 If the graft slips out, the hearing loss would be worse than before surgery.

33. 4 This action monitors the tube for patency; retained fluid raises intravesicular pressure, causing discomfort similar to the urge to void. (2) (SU; IM; TC; RG)

1 The need to take vital signs is not indicated by the client's complaint; the physician is not called unless a blocked tube cannot be corrected.

2 Total intake and output have no relationship to the client's present feeling that there is a need to void.

3 This is true; however, the integrity of the gravity system should be ascertained before this reason can be assumed.

34. 4 Muscle contractions cause neuronal stimulation; multiple foci of demyelination cause interruption or distortion of the impulse, resulting in intention tremors. (2) (ME; AN; PA; NM)
  1 There are no tremors when the person is asleep.
  2 There are no tremors when the client is inactive; this is a resting tremor that is usually associated with parkinsonism.
  3 Intention tremors are associated with muscle contraction, not feelings; stress can exacerbate the symptoms of MS.

35. 2 Destruction of brain cells decreases cognitive abilities, and learning and thinking are compromised. (2) (MH; AS; PA; DD)
  1 The attention span would be decreased.
  3 This is not specific to dementia or aging; it depends on the individual.
  4 Psychologic stress and changes caused by aging result in a decreased capability to adapt to the environment; familiar routines provide security.

36. 4 This indicates afibrinogenemia; massive clotting in the area of the separation has resulted in a lowered circulating fibrinogen level. (2) (CW; AS; PA; HP)
  1 A boggy uterus indicates a relaxed uterus with either placental membranes or clots present.
  2 Blood clots indicate normal fibrinogen levels; however, clots may indicate a failure of the uterus to contract and should be explored further.
  3 This is not indicative of shock, which would be a likely occurrence with the uncontrolled bleeding of DIC.

37. 1 Bulging of the perineum is caused by the presence of the fetal head and usually signifies imminent delivery. (2) (CW; IM; PA; HC)
  2 Pain medication at this time is harmful to the fetus; it crosses the placental barrier and causes respiratory distress.
  3 During the second stage of labor, the client is encouraged to push, not pant, with each contraction.

  4 Catheterization is indicated earlier in labor so that uterine contractions are not impeded; voiding will occur spontaneously with pushing.

38. 3 Hypoglycemia affects the central nervous system, causing headache and nervousness, and the sympathetic nervous system, causing diaphoresis. (2) (ME; EV; TC; EN)
  1 Dry skin and drowsiness are associated with ketoacidosis.
  2 These are not signs of an insulin reaction; excessive thirst and malaise are clinical symptoms of diabetes; hunger, not anorexia, is related to an insulin reaction.
  4 All of these signs are associated with ketoacidosis.

39. 1 Of the selections offered this is the highest in calories and protein, which are needed for the increased basal metabolic rate and for tissue repair. (3) (SU; PL; TC; IT)
  2 These foods do not provide as high an amount of calories and protein as the correct choice.
  3 Same as answer 2.
  4 Same as answer 2.

40. 2 Arterial perfusion and the presence of hemorrhage must be assessed hourly to prevent complications or identify problems early. (1) (SU; EV; TC; SK)
  1 This is unsafe; this will interfere with the pull of traction.
  3 Same as answer 1.
  4 Same as answer 1.

41. 4 Favorable personality change within 1 to 2 days attests to the effectiveness of the diet; other improvements take longer. (3) (PE; EV; PA; GI)
  1 Usually anorexia is not a problem; if it does occur, it does so during bouts of diarrhea.
  2 This occurs after the personality change.
  3 Same as answer 2.

42. 1 Central cyanosis (blue lips and face) indicates lowered oxygen of the blood caused by either decreased lung expansion or right-to-left shunting of blood. (2) (CW; AS; PA; HN)

2 This is normal in the newborn.

3 This is not an abnormal finding because peripheral circulation of the infant is unstable; blueness disappears when the baby is warm.

4 Same as answer 2.

43. 4 The effects of the tricyclic antidepressants are cumulative; it may be some time before improvement is noted. (2) (MH; IM; ED; DR)

1 This is false; antidepressants help relieve the physical and mental discomforts of the depressed client.

2 It is not a nursing function to prescribe drugs for the client.

3 Antidepressant drugs are effective in the treatment regardless of the length of the depression.

44. 1 A large percentage of HIV-positive individuals eventually develop AIDS. (2) (PE; AS; PA; BI)

2 An immature reticuloendothelial system does not indicate the potential development of AIDS.

3 Although blood transfusions can place someone at risk, a positive serologic status for HIV places a person at highest risk for AIDS.

4 The presence of an opportunistic infection alone is not an indication of AIDS.

45. 1 The objective is to stimulate ovulation near the fourteenth day of the menstrual cycle, which is achieved by taking the drug on the fifth through the ninth days; there is an increase in the pituitary gonadotrophins LH and FSH, with subsequent ovarian stimulation. (2) (CW; EV; ED; RP)

2 There are insufficient hormones for Clomid to be effective.

3 There is insufficient estrogen at this time for Clomid to be effective this early in the cycle.

4 This is too late in the cycle.

46. 4 Talking with others in similar circumstances provides support and allows for sharing of experiences. (1) (MH; IM; TC; TR)

1 This avoids the client's concerns and cuts off communication.

2 The feeling of guilt has not been expressed.

3 This is not therapeutic; it offers false reassurance.

47. 3 The client's systolic reading is 32 mmHg above the baseline reading and the diastolic reading is 15 mmHg above the baseline; a marked increase indicating a hypertensive disorder of pregnancy would be 30 mmHg for the systolic reading and 15 mmHg for the diastolic reading. (3) (CW; AS; TC; HP)

1 This is an insufficient rise to indicate a hypertensive disorder of pregnancy.

2 Same as answer 1.

4 Although this would indicate hypertension, it would be too far advanced for a person who normally exhibits a low blood pressure.

48. 4 Respiratory distress or arrest may occur when the serum level of magnesium sulfate reaches 12 to 15 mg/dl; deep tendon reflexes disappear when the serum level is 10 to 12 mg/dl; the drug is withheld in the absence of deep tendon reflexes. (3) (CW; EV; TC; DR)

1 This is an inappropriate assessment to determine client response to magnesium sulfate; deep tendon reflexes need to be assessed.

2 Same as answer 1.

3 Same as answer 1.

49. 1 This eliminates the nurse's subjectivity from the report. (1) (MH; IM; TC; CS)

2 This is unrelated to the rape itself; this would allow for subjectivity.

3 This is not part of the responsibility of the nurse.

4 This would allow for subjectivity.

50. 1 Weight monitoring is the most useful means of assessing fluid balance and changes in the edematous state; 1 liter of fluid weighs about 2.2 pounds. (2) (PE; PL; TC; FE)

2 This would be subjective and inaccurate.

3 This is not as accurate as daily weights; fluid can be trapped in the third space with no alteration in intake and output.

4 This is unreliable; these may or may not be altered with fluid shifts.

51. 4 Ranitidine inhibits histamine at H_2 receptor sites in parietal cells, which limits gastric secretion. (3) (ME; AN; PA; DR)

1 This is not the direct action of this drug; this is the action of antacids.

2 This would be undesirable; gastric hormones increase gastric acid secretion.

3 This drug does not regenerate the gastric mucosa; the drug prevents its erosion by gastric secretions.

52. 1 An infection will increase the metabolic rate, which eventually results in hyperglycemia. (3) (PE; EV; ED; EN)

2 This would cause hypoglycemia.

3 Same as answer 2.

4 Same as answer 2.

53. 2 This recognizes the client's feelings and encourages communication. (2) (ME; IM; PS; EH)

1 This question sounds accusatory; it ignores the client's feelings and discourages communication.

3 Although this may be true, it does not encourage further communication.

4 This statement negates the client's feelings and discourages communication.

54. 3 A small amount of bile-colored spotting is expected, a moderately large amount is abnormal; the physician should be notified. (2) (SU; IM; TC; GI)

1 The findings need further assessment; this intervention only treats one symptom and disregards the need for medical evaluation of the complication.

2 The client should be on the right side to compress the liver capsule against the chest wall.

4 Although this is important, the priority is to notify the physician.

55. 4 Drug dose and frequency are adjusted according to these results to enhance efficacy; therapeutic levels are maintained. (1) (SU; EV; TC; DR)

1 A sustained drop in fever is the desired outcome, not reduction just at peak serum levels of the drug.

2 Blood cultures are obtained when the client spikes a temperature; they are not related to "peak" and "trough" levels for gentamicin.

3 Peak and trough levels reveal nothing about allergic reactions.

56. 3 This response recognizes capability without adding stress or increasing dependency. (3) (MH; IM; PS; MO)

1 This does not address the client's needs and is punitive.

2 This increases dependency, which is not therapeutic.

4 This attempts to manipulate compliance; the client cannot accept responsibility for the future.

57. 3 This will help to elicit any fantasy the child may have; it helps the child understand that treatment is not a punishment. (3) (PE; IM; PS; EH)

1 This is inappropriate for a 4-year-old and does not elicit feelings.

2 This is inappropriate; it may be frightening.

4 This is not currently supported as a cause; this is an inappropriate discussion for a 4-year-old.

58. 4 How people handled grief in the past provides clues to their coping patterns when dealing with current grieving. (2) (MH; AN; PA; CS)

1 Although these are important, past experiences with grief are paramount.

2 Same as answer 1.

3 Same as answer 1.

59. 1 Breast palpation should be done in the supine position with a small towel roll under the shoulder of the palpated side. (1) (CW; EV; ED; WH)
    2 This is a correct procedure for breast self-examination.
    3 Same as answer 2.
    4 Same as answer 2.

60. 3 The common bile duct passes through the head of the pancreas; it is often constricted or obstructed by the neoplasm. (3) (ME; AN; PA; GI)
    1 This would not cause jaundice.
    2 This is the prehepatic cause of jaundice; it is not applicable in this situation.
    4 This is a hepatic cause of jaundice; it is not applicable in this situation.

61. 4 Impulse conduction of skeletal muscles is impaired with decreased K^+ levels; muscular weakness and cramps may occur with hypokalemia. (2) (ME; EV; PA; FE)
    1 Hyperactive reflexes indicate hyperkalemia, not hypokalemia.
    2 The pulse would be weak and irregular with hypokalemia because of an impaired conduction system in the cardiac muscle.
    3 Diarrhea is caused by hyperkalemia, not hypokalemia.

62. 3 Statistics show that 40% to 60% of the infants develop herpes. (2) (CW; AN; PA; HN)
    1 This is too low; 40% to 60% of the infants develop herpes.
    2 Same as answer 1.
    4 This is too high; 40% to 60% of the infants develop herpes.

63. 4 Calcium promotes osteoblastic activity, and calories support the growth and energy needs of the child. (1) (PE; PL; ED; SK)
    1 The level of purine does not affect bone repair; a decrease in calories would not support growth and development.
    2 Extra calories are converted to adipose tissue; if calcium needs are met, sufficient phosphorus will be ingested.
    3 Bone tissue responds to sufficient calcium in the diet; if injury had occurred to the soft tissues, a high-protein diet would be necessary.

64. 4 A person who can handle the activities of daily living and function in society is considered mentally healthy. (2) (MH; EV; PS; SD)
    1 Some anxiety is necessary; anxiety causes problems when it is overwhelming for an extended period of time.
    2 Insight into one's problems is of no use if one is unable to function in society.
    3 Everyone uses defense mechanisms; the degree to which they are used determines mental health.

65. 4 The nurse should offer support and use clear, simple terms to allay the client's anxiety. (1) (MH; IM; ED; MO)
    1 This may be too frightening or confusing to the client.
    2 When anxiety is high, the client cannot retain details, and details may lead to added fears.
    3 The client generally is kept npo before ECT to prevent aspiration during the treatment.

66. 3 Bedrest weakens the perineal and abdominal muscles used in defecating; ambulation promotes peristalsis and improves muscle tone, thereby facilitating expulsion of flatus and promoting defecation. (1) (SU; PL; PA; GI)
    1 Early ambulation will not prevent this complication.
    2 There will be no retention because the surgery involved removal of the bladder and the creation of a permanent urinary diversion.
    4 Same as answer 1.

67. 3 The Harris drip or flush removes accumulated gas in the intestine, which reduces distention of the abdomen. (2) (CW; EV; PA; HP)
    1 Stimulating evacuation is not the purpose of a Harris drip; a bowel movement would indicate the procedure was done improperly.
    2 The returns of a Harris drip usually contain small amounts of fecal material; it is not for cleansing the bowel.
    4 The fluid is not retained; small amounts are instilled slowly and then permitted to return, taking gas with them.

68. 2 The major cause of skin cancer is exposure to the sun's ultraviolet light, a form of radiation. (1) (ME; AN; PA; IT)
1 This is not a causative factor.
3 Same as answer 1.
4 Although environmental pollutants may have some bearing, they are not considered the major cause of skin cancer.

69. 2 The client is incapable of accepting responsibility for self-created problems and blames society for the behavior. (2) (MH; AS; PS; PR)
1 This response demonstrates insight, and these individuals rarely develop insight into their problems.
3 Same as answer 1.
4 Same as answer 1.

70. 1 Adenoids can obstruct nasal breathing, interfering with the senses of taste and smell. (2) (PE; EV; PA; RE)
2 Speech should not be affected because the vocal cords are not within the operative area.
3 The operative site should be healed and not cause discomfort when swallowing.
4 The vocal cords are outside the operative area; the site should be healed and not cause discomfort when swallowing.

71. 3 The intestinal lumen is narrowed by the large mass, and contraction of the proliferate fibrous tissue causes an obstruction. (2) (SU; AS; PA; GI)
1 Diarrhea may occur but usually alternates with constipation.
2 Dehydration usually does not occur unless there is severe vomiting and/or diarrhea.
4 This usually results from a perforation of the bowel that is caused by a buildup of pressure behind the obstruction.

72. 3 During open heart surgery the conductive system of the heart can be damaged because of the trauma of surgery. (3) (SU; EV; PA; CV)
1 Shock results in a weak, rapid pulse, not bradycardia.

2 Hypoxia causes tachycardia, not bradycardia.
4 Congestive heart failure causes a rapid pulse rate, not bradycardia.

73. 3 According to the standards of normal growth and development the anterior fontanel closes between 13 and 18 months of age. (3) (PE; IM; ED; GD)
1 This is too early; early closure may impede the growth of the infant's brain, impairing mental development.
2 Same as answer 1.
4 The closure should have occurred by 18 months; delayed closure may indicate neurologic difficulties.

74. 4 Panting or blowing breathing patterns make it impossible to push. (1) (CW; IM; ED; HC)
1 This causes respiratory alkalosis and fetal acidosis, which would be undesirable.
2 Pelvic rocking exercises are used to alleviate backache.
3 Deep-breathing exercises between contractions increase oxygenation and help maintain relaxation; this is unrelated to pushing.

75. 2 Dilation of blood vessels causes dependent pooling when the client moves to an upright position, resulting in cerebral hypoxia. (1) (ME; AN; PA; NM)
1 Resting will not help; the client can limit this response by moving gradually when changing positions.
3 This is false reassurance; the client needs teaching regarding changing positions gradually.
4 This is an expected response when moving from a horizontal to a vertical position; this single symptom is not enough reason for changing any medications the client may be taking.

How to Use Worksheet 1: Errors In Processing Information

Common errors in processing information are listed in the left-hand column of this worksheet. At the top of the worksheet is a row of blank spaces for inserting the number of the question missed. Directly below each number, check any errors you made in answering that question. You may have made more than one type of error in an answer.

Worksheet 1: Errors in Processing Information

Question number																								
Did not read situation/ question carefully																								
Missed important details																								
Confused major and minor points																								
Defined problem incorrectly																								
Could not remember terms/ facts/concepts/principles																								
Defined terms incorrectly																								
Focused on incomplete/incorrect data in assessing situation																								
Interpreted data incorrectly																								
Applied wrong concepts/ principles in situations																								
Drew incorrect conclusions																								
Identified wrong goals																								
Identified priorities incorrectly																								
Carried out plan incorrectly/ incompletely																								
Was unclear about criteria for evaluating success in achieving goals																								

How to Use Worksheet 2: Knowledge Gaps

Types of common knowledge gaps are listed along the top of this worksheet. Write a brief description of topics you want to review in the spaces provided. For example, if you missed a question on administration of a particular drug, write the drug name and problem (e.g., dosage) in the appropriate space under the column labeled *Pharmacology*.

Worksheet 2: Knowledge Gaps

Basic science	Skills/ procedures	Basic human needs	Growth and development	Normal nutrition	Psycho-social factors	Clinical area/ topic	Stressors/ coping mechanisms	Patho-physiology	Pharma-cology	Therapeutic nutrition	Legal implications	Other

Part B

76. 1 The nurse should determine the location, intensity, and other characteristics of the pain before initiating intervention. (1) (SU; EV; TC; NM)

2 Assessment should occur before nursing intervention.

3 This is an incomplete assessment.

4 Same as answer 2.

77. 1 Diabetic mothers have a tendency toward placental insufficiency, which can threaten fetal well-being during labor; a CST can determine if placental insufficiency is a problem with this client. (3) (CW; AN; TC; HP)

2 The CST does not measure any plasma levels.

3 This would be an assumption; the situation gives no reason to deduce this because the mother had a living child the first time.

4 This is true, but it is not the reason for doing the test.

78. 2 This individualized information would be the best basis for predicting the outcome of therapy. (2) (SU; PL; TC; EH)

1 This knowledge would not be helpful in understanding the likelihood of additional problems associated with the current cancer.

3 Same as answer 1.

4 This would be useful, but it is not specific for this client.

79. 2 At this time breast engorgement is minimal, and this provides a regular examination cycle. (1) (CW; EV; ED; WH)

1 Premenstrual breast engorgement may cause the breast to feel lumpy.

3 Ovulation is occurring, and hormones may influence breast consistency.

4 Breast consistency is altered by the menstrual cycle; the same date each month would fall in a different stage of the cycle.

80. 4 This accurately responds to the parents' question, reinforcing what the physician explained. (2) (PE; IM; ED; BI)

1 This is an insensitive response that places the parents in a defensive position.

2 This would abdicate teaching responsibilities.

3 This statement reinforces parental insecurity about the information they have recently received from the physician; this may increase anxiety.

81. 3 It is too costly and a poor delegation of manpower to use a professional nurse indefinitely in the home. (1) (ME; PL; TC; GD)

1 Clients prefer to stay in a familiar environment and will achieve their maximal potential regardless of the area.

2 Multidisciplinary services on a part-time basis in the home would be more therapeutic and cost effective than placement in a nursing home.

4 Part-time personal care assistance in the home would be more therapeutic and cost effective than placement in a nursing home.

82. 4 Steroids decrease the inflammatory process around the optic nerve, thus improving vision. (2) (ME; EV; PA; DR)

1 Steroids are usually associated with increased emotional lability.

2 Steroids are not effective in easing muscle contractions.

3 Pain in the extremities is not common unless spasms are present; steroids do not relieve spasms.

83. 3 A therapeutic relationship is easier to establish when anxiety is lowered; the use of paper towels may ultimately facilitate communication. (2) (MH; IM; PS; PR)

1 This is untrue and only reinforces the use of dirt as a defense against real feelings and increases anxiety.

2 This may increase anxiety further, thus hindering the development of a therapeutic relationship.

4 Same as answer 2.

84. 4 Limitation of increased intracranial pressure and resultant brain damage depends on frequent systematic observation. (3) (ME; AS; PA; NM)

1 This is unrealistic; the state of consciousness should be observed, but otherwise rest is not contraindicated.

2 There is no indication that hyperactivity is present.

3 Mannitol is administered to reduce cerebral edema; there is no indication as yet that this will be needed.

85. 2 Specialized insulin receptors on insulin-sensitive cells transport glucose through cell membranes, making it available for use. (1) (PE; AN; ED; DR)

1 This is not the action of insulin.

3 Same as answer 1.

4 Same as answer 1.

86. 2 Preventing infection and trauma are the priorities; rupture of the sac may lead to meningitis. (1) (CW; IM; TC; HN)

1 The Apgar is 9/10; there is no respiratory complication.

3 The sac must be protected before this is done.

4 This can be done before the infant leaves the delivery room; the priority is care of the sac.

87. 1 Quickness is used for safety; an attitude of concern may help to reduce client anxiety. (2) (MH; IM; TC; SD)

2 A client this upset would never agree; the client may harm self or others and must be sedated.

3 The client must be told why sedation is being used.

4 Same as answer 3.

88. 2 The iron needs of the adolescent are high because of growth requirements and often inadequate nutrition; the iron needs are increased by the demands of pregnancy. (2) (CW; AS; PA; HP)

1 This is not common in pregnant adolescents.

3 Same as answer 1.

4 Same as answer 1.

89. 2 Bile, which aids in fat digestion, is not as concentrated as before surgery; once the body adapts to the absence of the gall bladder, the client should be able to tolerate a regular diet that contains fat. (2) (SU; IM; ED; GI)

1 Initially the client should still avoid fatty foods unless the physician indicates otherwise.

3 This is an inappropriate priority at this time; a temporary avoidance of fatty foods with the gradual resumption of a regular diet is the priority.

4 Same as answer 3.

90. 2 The cerebellum is the most common area; symptoms of increased intracranial pressure result from obstruction of cerebrospinal fluid flow. (2) (PE; AN; PA; NM)

1 This is an uncommon site in children.

3 Same as answer 1.

4 Same as answer 1.

91. 3 This provides reality-based feedback for the client withdrawing from alcohol. (2) (MH; IM; PS; SA)

1 Physical restraints will increase agitation and should be applied only as a last resort.

2 This focuses on hallucinations and delusions rather than on reality.

4 Shadows will increase the chance of distortions and illusions.

92. 4 Autoimmune response plays a role in the development of polyarteritis, although drugs and infections may precipitate it. (3) (ME; IM; ED; CV)

1 Men are affected three times more frequently than women.

2 The disease is often fatal, usually as a result of congestive heart failure or renal failure.

3 Arteriolar pathology can affect any organ or system.

93. 2 The client needs to know details of transfer to assist appropriately and avoid injury. (1) (SU; IM; ED; SK)
1 This is not advisable because this could disrupt the repair of the affected hip.
3 More commonly, no weight bearing is permitted on the operative leg at first.
4 This is unnecessary; the client may touch the floor with the foot but may not bear weight on this extremity.

94. 2 Class A diabetes is gestational diabetes, and the woman demonstrates symptoms only when pregnant; this is the client's first pregnancy and her first sign of diabetes; it is too early for secondary complications. (1) (CW; AS; PA; HP)
1 Retinopathy is usually present in class D diabetes or higher.
3 Same as answer 2.
4 This is class C diabetes, which is more severe than class A.

95. 2 Erosion of blood vessels may lead to hemorrhage, a life-threatening situation further complicated by decreased prothrombin production. (3) (ME; AS; PA; GI)
1 Although increased intraabdominal pressure may cause this, there is no immediate threat to life; assessment for bleeding takes priority.
3 Although this may cause gastritis, there is no immediate threat to life; assessment for bleeding takes priority.
4 Same as answer 1.

96. 2 Percussing over fluid produces a dull sound, not the normal tympanic sound. (3) (ME; AS; PA; GI)
1 Respiratory distress occurs with ascites but is not an early sign.
3 This would assess for dependent edema, not ascites.
4 Bowel sounds do not indicate much about early ascites; when ascites is extensive, bowel sounds may diminish.

97. 3 The client's low self-esteem makes her doubt her lover; her statements reflect her feelings. (3) (MH; AS; PS; SD)
1 The client's statements do not reflect confusion or disorientation, but false beliefs.
2 The client's statements do not represent hallucinations because they are not false sensory perceptions.
4 Setting limits after the fact would not be effective in any situation; limits must be set when the situation occurs.

98. 2 Because suspicious clients lack trust and have difficulty sharing feelings, this healthy behavior should be recognized. (2) (MH; EV; PS; SD)
1 The client's feelings are rejected when blanket statements are given; this only responds to part of the client's concerns.
3 Focusing on the staff's concerns ignores the client's needs; the staff's attitude could decrease self-esteem.
4 A detailed description at this time may increase the client's fears.

99. 2 This would indicate a lack of understanding of the necessity of taking antibiotics for a full 10 to 14 days or until a follow-up urine culture is negative. (1) (PE; EV; ED; RG)
1 Bubble bath can be a source of irritation to the meatus, which can predispose to a urinary tract infection and thus should be avoided.
3 Wiping from front to back prevents contamination of the urinary meatus with feces.
4 Stasis is the primary predisposing factor to a urinary tract infection, thus voiding when feeling the urge is important; the bladder should be emptied every 3 to 4 hours.

100. 3 Poor appetite and decreased energy are associated with an accumulation of toxic waste; associated anemia accounts for the pallor. (3) (PE; AN; PA; RG)
1 Discontinuing the corticosteroids and diuretics if prescribed might result in recurrence of edema in steroid-dependent children; pallor would not occur.

2 An elevated temperature would be present with an infection; an infection would not cause muddy pallor.

4 Once remission has occurred, usual activities can be resumed with discretion.

101. 2 Vomiting and feeding difficulties are early signs of digoxin toxicity in infants. (2) (PE; IM; PA; DR)

1 The pulse rate of an infant receiving digoxin should remain above 100 beats per minute.

3 This is expected; tetralogy of Fallot causes cyanosis which will be pronounced when crying occurs.

4 Infants routinely require several naps, and an infant with heart disease requires additional rest periods daily.

102. 2 Antacids are most effective when taken after digestion has started but before the stomach begins to empty. (2) (ME; EV; ED; DR)

1 Antacids should be taken before the onset of pain; pain indicates that gastric irritation has begun, and the aim of treatment is to protect the GI mucosa.

3 The antacids would interfere with the absorption of nutrients.

4 Same as answer 3.

103. 4 Bedrest promotes decreased cardiac output; it also decreases tissue catabolism, which lowers the workload of the kidneys, eventually increasing filtration by the renal glomeruli; limiting activity also helps lower the blood pressure. (2) (PE; PL; ED; RG)

1 Bedrest is necessary during the acute phase of this illness.

2 The activity level depends on the response to therapy.

3 Same as answer 2.

104. 4 Respiratory depression occurs in magnesium sulfate toxicity because of CNS depression. (3) (CW; EV; TC; HN)

1 This is not a sign of magnesium sulfate toxicity.

2 Same as answer 1.

3 Same as answer 1.

105. 4 This indicates failure to resolve conflicting feelings about pregnancy that commonly occur in the first trimester. (3) (CW; PL; PS; EC)

1 This is a normal feeling in the third trimester.

2 Same as answer 1.

3 Concerns about the expected baby having physical abnormalities are common in the third trimester.

106. 1 Research has shown that decreasing stress will slow the rate of atherosclerotic development. (1) (ME; PL; ED; CV)

2 Exercise is thought to decrease atherosclerosis and the formation of lipid plaques.

3 Saturated fats in the diet increase atherosclerosis.

4 Same as answer 2.

107. 3 The taste for salt is learned from habitual use and can be unlearned or reduced with health improvement motivation and creative salt-free food preparation. (3) (ME; IM; ED; FE)

1 The taste for salt is learned.

2 This is untrue; substitutes often have a metallic taste.

4 This is unsafe; abnormally high potassium levels can result.

108. 1 A strong cry indicates effective respiratory function and is assigned a value of 2. (1) (CW; AS; PA; NN)

2 A value of 1 is assigned when the body is pink and the extremities are blue.

3 If the flexion of the arms and legs is only slight and movement is diminished, the value assigned is 1.

4 The heart rate should be over 100 per min and therefore is assigned a value of 1.

109. 2 Autonomy leads to exploring and self-feeding; the child may eat food not on the diet. (2) (PE; AS; ED; GD)

1 Although this is a common characteristic of a toddler, it would not lead to the child eating restricted foods.

3 Same as answer 1.

4 Same as answer 1.

110. 4 These are classic symptoms of ketoacidosis because of the respiratory system's attempt to compensate by blowing off excess carbon dioxide, a component of carbonic acid. (2) (ME; AS; PA; EN)
 1 This is indicative of an insulin reaction (diabetic hypoglycemia).
 2 This is a hypersensitivity reaction; it is unrelated to diabetes mellitus.
 3 Diaphoresis is associated with an insulin reaction, not diabetic ketoacidosis.

111. 4 The aim of therapy is to eliminate the causative agent, which can be determined from culture and sensitivity tests of sputum. (1) (ME; EV; TC; RE)
 1 A lung scan permits visualization of lung vasculature but does not provide data on the condition of the lung tissue itself.
 2 Bronchoscopy shows the appearance of the bronchi but does not indicate the presence or absence of microorganisms.
 3 Pulmonary function studies indicate air volume that may fall within the expected range despite the presence of bronchopneumonia.

112. 1 Cor pulmonale is right-ventricular heart failure caused by pulmonary congestion; edema results from increasing venous pressure. (3) (ME; AS; PA; CV)
 2 A productive cough is symptomatic of the original condition — COPD.
 3 This is caused by alterations in oxygen and hydrogen ion levels and their effects on the central nervous system.
 4 Same as answer 3.

113. 4 The chamber closest to the client collects drainage, and the second chamber acts as the water seal. (3) (SU; AN; TC; RE)
 1 Suction requires the addition of a third chamber or a modified system.
 2 The water seal in a two-chamber system is provided by the second chamber.
 3 In a one-chamber system the seal and drainage are combined and there is no suction chamber.

114. 4 These individuals need peer group relations to validate their feelings and to experience peer group pressures. (3) (MH; PL; PS; EA)
 1 These individuals have a remarkable store of energy that does not reflect their malnourished state.
 2 These individuals rarely have trouble making decisions, so they do not have to be forced into the role.
 3 These individuals totally relate their attractiveness to thinness; they have diminished libido and in addition women have amenorrhea.

115. 4 The nurse shows an understanding of the client's needs by not totally restricting the handwashing. (3) (MH; IM; PS; PR)
 1 At this time, the client is still too anxious and is incapable of dealing with the reasons for handwashing.
 2 Continued handwashing does not reveal an understanding of the problem or a sign of progress.
 3 This denies the client's feelings, is untrue, and will close off any communication.

116. 2 Toxoids are modified toxins that stimulate the body to form antibodies, lasting up to 10 years, against the specific disease. (3) (PE; AN; TC; BI)
 1 Passive immunity is temporary; even the natural type derived from the mother does not last longer than the first year of life.
 3 Only by having the disease can lifelong natural immunity become possible; toxoids confer artificial active immunity.
 4 Toxoids give artificial active immunity.

117. 4 Optic nerve inflammation is an early effect of multiple sclerosis caused by lesions in the optic nerves or their connections. (1) (ME; IM; ED; NM)
 1 At present there is no evidence of viral infection of the eyes in multiple sclerosis.
 2 Tumors of the brain, not multiple sclerosis, cause increased intracranial pressure because the skull cannot expand.
 3 This causes blindness as a result of increased intraocular pressure, not inflammation of the optic nerve.

118. 4 This lessens anxiety, promotes verbalization, reduces guilt, and helps the family feel useful. (2) (MH; IM; PS; TR)
   1 This is a generalized personal opinion; the nurse at this time does not know about family relationships.
   2 This is false reassurance.
   3 The "why" creates defensiveness; the information is incorrect, and crying helps to relieve tension.

119. 4 The cervix is 50% effaced and 6 cm dilated; these finding are typical midway through the first stage of labor. (2) (CW; AS; PA; HC)
   1 When the cervix is 6 cm dilated the individual is beyond the early stage of labor.
   2 The transitional phase of labor begins when the cervix is 8 cm dilated.
   3 In the second stage of labor the cervix is fully dilated and 100% effaced.

120. 4 Anxiety and stress tend to close communication; this in turn intensifies the reaction to illness and death. (3) (MH; PL; PS; CS)
   1 The family system could not solve all its problems at this time because of the emotional turmoil of its members.
   2 This is false; the family must begin to deal with feelings before death occurs.
   3 This is true, but the focus should be on mutual understanding by all members.

121. 2 When clients in obvious crisis appear depressed, anxious, and desperate, the nurse should question them regarding the presence of suicidal thoughts. (2) (CW; IM; PS; WH)
   1 Further assessment and exploration is needed before encouraging clients to admit themselves to a psychiatric facility.
   3 Running away from problems does not help solve them, nor will escaping bring lasting relief.

4 When the client is overwhelmed with problems, it is difficult to think positively and to focus on the good things in life.

122. 2 When a client has perforated viscera, barium could leak out of the intestinal tract and cause inflammation and/or an abscess. (2) (ME; AN; TC; GI)
   1 Although it may be irritating, this does not contraindicate barium studies.
   3 Serum potassium would be unaffected; barium is insoluble and would not affect blood content.
   4 Barium studies are not contraindicated and could be useful in diagnosing ulcerative colitis and Crohn's disease.

123. 1 To avoid symptoms, these clients often refuse to eat and become malnourished; a high-calorie, high-protein diet is advised. (1) (ME; PL; ED; GI)
   2 This is not a problem in Crohn's disease.
   3 Same as answer 2.
   4 This is a secondary problem that results from malnutrition; correcting the malnutrition will increase strength.

124. 2 This is the definition of a positive CST result. (3) (CW; AN; TC; HP)
   1 Other fetal assessment methods should be used before labor is induced.
   3 A normal fetal heart rate is 120 to 160.
   4 A positive CST result does not dictate a cesarean delivery; an expeditious vaginal delivery may be attempted.

125. 3 This rejects the behavior, not the client; it helps separate the client from the behavior. (3) (MH; IM; PS; SD)
   1 This does not help the client learn self-control; it rejects both the client and the behavior.
   2 Isolating this client limits learning more acceptable responses.
   4 Part of recovery is learning acceptable behavior; ignoring inappropriate behavior does not help.

126. 1 Hard candy may produce salivation, which helps alleviate the anticholinergic-like side effect of dry mouth that is experienced with phenothiazines. (2) (MH; PL; ED; DR)
2 Fluids should be encouraged, not discouraged; fluids may alleviate the dry mouth.
3 This is unnecessary.
4 This is unnecessary; although these drugs can cause leukopenia and agranulocytosis, they do not cause thrombocytopenia.

127. 2 Stopping the flow reduces cramping caused by distension. (1) (SU; IM; TC; GI)
1 There is no need to discontinue the enema; flow should be interrupted temporarily until discomfort subsides; an effective enema must be administered before surgery.
3 This would result in the administration of a Harris flush; the purpose of the preoperative enema is to evacuate the bowel of feces, not flatus.
4 This is unsafe; this would increase the discomfort.

128. 3 Severe edema is usually present, and change of position is necessary to prevent breakdown of tissue. (3) (PE; PL; TC; IT)
1 Fluids are not forced and may even be restricted during periods of edema.
2 Play periods would be permitted during remission but not during the edema phase to limit energy expenditure.
4 A high-protein diet minimizes negative nitrogen balance; a low-protein diet is used in renal failure with azotemia.

129. 4 The pinworm emerges when the client is asleep to lay its eggs; these can be collected from the perianal area by applying tape upon awakening. (1) (PE; PL; ED; GI)
1 Any larvae on the perianal area would have been removed by the bath.
2 The larvae would not have been deposited yet because the adult pinworm would still be in the bowel; it emerges when the client is asleep.
3 Any larvae that were present in the morning would probably have been wiped away.

130. 4 As the lower uterine segment stretches and thins, tearing and bleeding occurs at the lower implantation site. (2) (CW; AS; PA; HP)
1 This is usually associated with abortion or an ectopic pregnancy.
2 This is usually associated with abruptio placentae rather than placenta previa.
3 This is associated with abortions, but cramping and backache are usually present.

131. 4 This presents the reality of the situation and helps support the client during a threatening hallucination. (2) (MH; IM; PS; SD)
1 Clients cannot be distracted from hallucinations without competing stimuli.
2 This would have little effect on the client's behavior and would not stop the hallucinations.
3 This would encourage withdrawal and isolation and would not stop the hallucinations.

132. 3 Regression to a more immature, helpless developmental level is normal and should be supported at this point. (2) (SU; PL; PS; EH)
1 Denial is not the response described.
2 The client's behavior is inconsistent with the need for more control.
4 The client's behavior does not indicate anger.

133. 3 Fluid may shift from the intravascular space to the abdomen as fluid is removed, leading to hypovolemia and compensatory tachycardia. (3) (SU; EV; PA; GI)
1 The fluid shift can cause hypovolemia with resulting hypotension, not hypertension.
2 A paracentesis should decrease the degree of abdominal distention.
4 This sign of dehydration may occur, but it is not as vital or immediate as signs of shock.

134. 1 This is done to reduce the possibility of bladder puncture. (1) (CW; IM; TC; HP)
2 The mother may eat and drink before the test; a hungry mother may cause a restless fetus.

3 Medications are not given because of their effect on the fetus.

4 This procedure is not done via the colon, so fecal material does not have to be expelled.

135. 1 Heat causes vasodilation and an increased blood supply to the area. (2) (CW; PL; PA; HC)

2 This is not the purpose of the sitz baths.

3 Cleansing is done immediately after voiding and defecating with a perineal bottle filled with cleansing solution.

4 Relaxation of the rectal sphincter is promoted by the sitz bath; this will provide comfort but will not increase healing.

136. 2 Yogurt, which contains calcium, is easily digested because it contains the enzyme lactase, which breaks down milk sugar. (1) (SU; AN; PA; GI)

1 These are deficient in calcium.

3 Same as answer 1.

4 Same as answer 1.

137. 4 Mood changes can occur as a side effect of steroid therapy. (3) (ME; EV; TC; DR)

1 This denies the value of the client's statement and provides false reassurance.

2 The client has already stated he does not know why this is happening.

3 This is difficult to do, because the direction a situation will take cannot always be anticipated.

138. 1 This acknowledges the client's apprehension and encourages further communication. (1) (SU; IM; PS; EH)

2 This negates the client's feelings and promotes false reassurance.

3 This does not address the client's feelings and may cause more anxiety.

4 This is perhaps true, but it does not foster communication; the client may focus on the word pain.

139. 1 This points out reality and does not support the client's hallucinations. (2) (MH; IM; PS; SA)

2 This feeds into the client's hallucination and provides false reassurance.

3 Same as answer 2.

4 The client has hallucinations, not illusions.

140. 4 This is responsible for the effectiveness of alkylating agents, of which nitrogen mustard is one. (3) (ME; AN; TC; DR)

1 Some drugs are believed to act in this way, but nitrogen mustard does not.

2 This is the mechanism of action of antimetabolites.

3 Antibiotics used in cancer chemotherapy are believed to act in this way.

141. 2 Cerebellar astrocytomas, unlike those in the cerebrum, are slow growing and benign, with a cure rate of 80% to 90% after surgery. (2) (PE; IM; PA; NM)

1 Other infratentorial tumors, such as medulloblastomas, are more rapid growing and highly malignant.

3 This is not true of a cerebellar astrocytoma.

4 Same as answer 3.

142. 1 This frequently begins with what parents describe as clumsiness that becomes progressively worse; the cerebellum controls coordination. (2) (PE; AS; PA; NM)

2 Seizures usually occur with cerebral or supratentorial tumors.

3 This is a very late sign of tumor involvement.

4 At this age, sutures are completely closed and the tumor would be contained in the cranium.

143. 4 Sexual anxiety and conflict occur with schizophrenia; uncertainty is projected onto others to defend the ego. (2) (MH; IM; PS; SD)

1 This avoids the issue and is a threatening response; this could increase anxiety.

2 This validates ideas of reference and is an inappropriate response.

3 The anxious client may not be able to handle being confronted with feelings; this may precipitate a panic reaction.

144. 4 This is the correct flow rate; 500 units of insulin added to 500 ml of IV fluid results in a solution where 1 ml contains 1 unit of the drug; therefore 60 ml must be administered in 30 minutes; 120 ml per hour ÷ 2 = 60 units of insulin in 30 minutes. (2) (ME; AN; TC; DR)

1 This would deliver an inadequate amount of insulin.
2 Same as answer 1.
3 Same as answer 1.

145. 3 Absence of peptidase results in an inability to metabolize the gliadin component of grains; this results in excessive glutamine that is toxic to the mucosal cells. (1) (PE; AN; PA; GI)

1 This is unrelated; meconium is present in the first bowel movements before the introduction of food.
2 This does not occur.
4 Fluid balance is not the basic problem with celiac disease; however, dehydration can occur in celiac crisis.

146. 4 Skin-to-skin contact between mother and baby is most effective in maintaining the baby's body temperature; heat is transferred by conduction. (1) (CW; IM; PA; NN)

1 Oxygen is not administered unless the baby is experiencing respiratory and cardiac difficulties; oxygen has a cooling effect.
2 This is not very effective and leaves much of the baby exposed; a blanket and warmer would also be necessary.
3 Bathing the baby should be delayed until the body temperature is stabilized.

147. 4 An objective examiner confirms the fetal movements; this eliminates subjectivity by the client. (2) (CW; AS; PA; HC)

1 This is a softening of the lower uterine segment, a presumptive sign of pregnancy.
2 This could be caused by a variety of situations other than pregnancy; it is a probable sign of pregnancy.
3 This is only a probable sign of pregnancy because of possible false negative readings.

148. 1 This is an accurate and concise explanation of Haldol's effects; it blocks postsynaptic dopamine receptors in the brain. (1) (MH; IM; ED; DR)

2 This is not true; it is a tranquilizer, and it does not alter mood.
3 This drug lowers the seizure threshold.
4 Same as answer 2.

149. 4 Inadequate protein decreases colloidal osmotic pressure within the vascular space, allowing fluid to shift into the interstitial spaces. (2) (CW; EV; PA; HP)

1 Petechiae result from an abnormality in the clotting mechanism such as thrombocytopenia.
2 Protein does not affect heart rate.
3 Bleeding gums are due to a deficiency in vitamin C or platelets, not protein.

150. 2 SGA infants have little subcutaneous fat or glycogen stores. (2) (CW; AS; PA; HN)

1 Intestinal bleeding is not common in SGA infants.
3 This would provide no therapeutic value for this SGA infant.
4 Hydrocephalus is not characteristic of SGA infants.

151. 4 Preschoolers are active, sociable individuals who enjoy the company of peers and become bored when isolated. (3) (PE; IM; PA; GD)

1 Preschoolers have a limited ability to understand complex explanations of cause and effect; they employ concrete thinking.
2 This will increase agitation and be punitive.
3 Although this would provide some distraction, it is better to permit peer contacts.

152. 1 The client will be unable to speak because a tracheostomy tube is in place to prevent edema from blocking the airway; writing provides an alternate form of communication. (1) (SU; IM; PS; RE)

2 The client cannot speak with a tracheostomy tube in place.

3   This has no effect; the client's ability to hear or understand is not affected.

4   Same as answer 3.

153. 1   Without trust, the nurse-client relationship will achieve nothing. (1) (MH; AN; PS; TR)

2   Although this is important, trust must be developed first.

3   Same as answer 2.

4   Open communication will not occur until trust is developed.

154. 3   Eating in a semirecumbent position slows gastric emptying, thereby preventing premature gastric dumping of contents. (3) (SU; PL; ED; GI)

1   This would speed gastric emptying and should be avoided.

2   Same as answer 1.

4   Same as answer 1.

155. 2   Children, because of the demands of growth and their dietary indiscretions, have a more fragile glucose balance. (1) (PE; IM; ED; EN)

1   This is untrue; it is more often associated with non-insulin dependent diabetes mellitus.

3   The fragility of glucose balance is not due to resistance to treatment, but rather to the changing requirements associated with growth.

4   This is untrue; hypersensitivity is unrelated to either type of diabetes mellitus.

156. 3   Saccharin is a non-nutritive substitute; aspartame is made of two amino acids, phenylalanine and aspartic acid, and is metabolized as such. (2) (PE; IM; ED; EN)

1   Honey, a fructose, provides 1.3 times as many Kcal as does table sugar and must be calculated into the diet.

2   Simple sugars may be used in controlled amounts and must be calculated into the diet.

4   Foods do not have to taste sweet to contain sugar.

157. 1   Ataxia is a side effect of phenytoin, and drug continuation may cause cerebellar damage. (3) (ME; IM; ED; DR)

2   This sign of toxicity should be reported.

3   Massaging the gums should be done regularly to prevent gingival hyperplasia, which can result from phenytoin therapy.

4   The client should report the rash but keep taking the drug; withdrawal may precipitate a seizure.

158. 2   Prevention of infection continues as a priority both before and after the repair of the sac. (2) (PE; PL; TC; NM)

1   A neurologically impaired infant would not be given sedatives because it would interfere with accurate assessment.

3   This is unrealistic; newborns lose weight in the first few days of life.

4   This is not the priority at this time.

159. 3   The caloric distribution of the "Prudent Diet" proposed by the American Heart Association is 30% fat (less than 10% saturated fat), 50% carbohydrates (35% complex carbohydrates), and 20% protein. (1) (ME; IM; ED; CV)

1   Fried foods are not advocated on the "Prudent Diet"; peanut oil is a monounsaturated fatty acid; these acids should not exceed 15% of the kilocalories of the diet.

2   This is untrue; this would be discouraging and encourage noncompliance.

4   Same as answer 2.

160. 2   This drug suppresses activity in key regions of the subcortical area of the CNS; it also has antihistaminic and anticholinergic effects. (1) (MH; EV; TC; DR)

1   These symptoms are not associated with Vistaril.

3   Same as answer 1.

4   Same as answer 1.

161. 4   Hyperextension of the neck places tension on the suture line. (2) (SU; AN; TC; RE)

1   The cervical vertebrae are designed to flex and hyperextend; there should be no ill effects.

2   Hyperextension would not cause this.

3   Same as answer 2.

656   CHAPTER 7

162. 4 This reduces pressure on the cord, increasing oxygen to the fetus. (1) (CW; IM; TC; HP)
1 Although this may eventually be done, the priority is to relieve pressure on the cord.
2 This promotes placental perfusion but would not relieve pressure on the cord.
3 Same as answer 1.

163. 4 This expands collapsed alveoli and enhances surfactant activity, thereby preventing atelectasis. (3) (SU; PL; PA; RE)
1 This promotes exhalation, not inhalation.
2 This clears accumulated secretions from the pulmonary tree; it does not directly promote alveolar expansion.
3 This promotes collapse of, not expansion of, alveoli.

164. 3 The lack of a social support system can precipitate feelings of isolation. (1) (MH; AN; PS; AX)
1 The data do not support this nursing diagnosis.
2 Same as answer 1.
4 Same as answer 1.

165. 3 Intestinal antibiotics and a complete cleansing of the bowel with enemas until returns are clear are necessary to reduce the possibility of fecal contamination when the bowel is resected. (1) (SU; PL; TC; GI)
1 The bladder will be removed, so there is no need for a Foley catheter.
2 A clear liquid diet is usually prescribed for several days with npo for at least 8 hours before surgery.
4 This is not necessary; there is no evidence of urinary infection.

166. 2 This provides for release of tension with no element of competition; success in a simple project increases the sense of accomplishment and worth. (2) (MH; PL; TC; MO)
1 This allows the client to withdraw further.

3 The client has psychomotor retardation and may not be able to cope with fine details at this time.
4 This is too cheerful; this could result in excessive stimuli and increase the client's irritation.

167. 3 This is an iron-rich food appropriate for slight anemia, which has probably occurred from blood loss into the tissues at the site of the injury. (2) (PE; IM; TC; BI)
1 This is not necessary unless there is a marked decrease.
2 Same as answer 1.
4 If internal bleeding occurred there would have been earlier signs other than a reduction in hemoglobin and hematocrit.

168. 1 A gown and gloves must be worn to prevent contamination of the nurse from blood or body secretions. (1) (CW; IM; TC; HP)
2 This is not sufficient protection for the nurse.
3 Same as answer 1.
4 A mask is not needed because the virus is not airborne.

169. 2 This fat-binding agent would also bind and eliminate the fat-soluble vitamins such as vitamins A, D, E, and K. (3) (ME; EV; TC; DR)
1 This is not a fat-soluble vitamin and would be unaffected.
3 Same as answer 1.
4 Same as answer 1.

170. 4 Taking the drug in the early morning mimics normal adrenal secretions; food and/or antacid helps reduce gastric irritation. (1) (ME; EV; ED; DR)
1 Diurnal rhythms may be altered, and steroids are ulcerogenic; they should be taken with more than just a snack.
2 Steroids cause gastric irritation and should be taken with food.
3 The food helps decrease gastric irritation; however, normal diurnal rhythms could be altered.

171. 4 Lack of symmetry and palpation of a thickening are signs of a possible breast mass. (1) (CW; EV; TC; WH)
   1 Engorgement is an expected response to menstrual hormones.
   2 Premenstrual engorgement may cause the breast to feel lumpy.
   3 This is a common deviation that is within normal limits.

172. 4 Because the client is feeling a loss of control, it would be important to include the client in revision of the plan. (2) (MH; PL; TC; CS)
   1 This does not consider changes in the client or the client's feelings.
   2 This is unnecessary; planning nursing care is within the nurse's function and judgment, not the physician's.
   3 This is very authoritarian and places total control with the nurse.

173. 2 Greenish fluid is indicative of meconium, which is released by the fetus; it is considered a possible indicator of fetal distress unless the fetus is in breech position. (1) (CW; PL; TC; HP)
   1 A bloody show is normally present and may increase at the end of the first stage of labor; this is not indicative of any problem.
   3 This is normal; it is not indicative of any problem.
   4 This is a normal occurrence as labor progresses; it is not indicative of any problem.

174. 3 With abruptio placentae there is uterine bleeding that results in massive internal hemorrhage, causing hypovolemic shock. (2) (CW; AS; PA; HP)
   1 Jaundice occurs only when there is a deposition of bilirubin into subcutaneous tissues and skin; this is not associated with abruptio placentae.
   2 It is more likely that with internal bleeding, blood pressure will fall rather than increase.
   4 Convulsions are associated with pregnancy-induced hypertension; there is no information indicating the presence of this condition.

175. 4 Familiarity with situations and continuity add to the client's sense of security and foster trust in the relationship. (2) (MH; PL; PS; DD)
   1 Although this helps individualize care, continuity is the priority.
   2 Some degree of flexibility by the nurse would help to individualize care.
   3 Detailed explanations will be forgotten; instructions should be simple and to the point and given when needed.

176. 2 A continuous flushing of the bladder dilutes the bloody urine and empties the bladder, preventing clots. (1) (SU; AN; TC; RG)
   1 Only the kidneys form urine; fluid instilled into the bladder does not affect kidney function.
   3 Urinary output can be easily measured regardless of the amount of fluid instilled.
   4 The continuous drip does not exert any additional pressure within the bladder.

177. 3 Tetanus immune globulin should not cause anaphylaxis because it is derived from human serum. (2) (PE; AN; TC; BI)
   1 Tetanus immune globulin is not as effective as the antitoxin, but it is not derived from horse serum and should not cause anaphylaxis.
   2 It is necessary to perform skin tests for both types of medications to determine the presence of sensitivity.
   4 These medications always carry the risk of hypersensitivity; it cannot be assumed they can be safely given to everyone.

178. 3 This prevents the spread of infection to others; isolation is a priority that should be immediately implemented. (1) (PE; IM; TC; NM)
   1 There is no indication that the child is dehydrated; fluid maintenance is a continuing goal.
   2 There is no indication that the child needs oxygen, and it would not be given routinely.
   4 This would not be given because these children are sensitive to stimuli and movement causes increased discomfort.

179. 4 Furniture and loose rugs can interfere with crutch walking and should be removed to prevent further injury. (1) (SU; PL; ED; SK)
1 The client may shower if the cast is protected from becoming wet.
2 Calcium, rather than vitamin C, would be encouraged to enhance bone healing; vitamin C prevents capillary fragility.
3 This is a medical, not a nursing, decision.

180. 4 Nerve and vascular injury and significant blood loss may be present. (2) (SU; AS; PA; SK)
1 This is a medical decision that has not yet been made; closed fractures generally are reduced by manipulation.
2 False reassurance is never appropriate.
3 Closed fractures generally do not require operative reduction; they are usually reduced by manipulation.

181. 2 Improving ventilation provides comfort, maintains existing lung function, and prevents further lung damage. (1) (ME; AN; PA; RE)
1 Maintaining hydration thins secretions so that there is less interference in achieving the goal of improved ventilation.
3 Some decrease in hypoxia will promote comfort, but the primary problem is too much carbon dioxide rather than too little oxygen; oxygen should not exceed 2 liters per minute.
4 Correcting the bicarbonate deficit will not help ventilation but will correct the accompanying respiratory acidosis.

182. 1 The shift of fluid predisposes to hypovolemia; an increased thready pulse and hypotension are signs of shock. (3) (PE; AS; PA; RG)
2 Tubular reabsorption of sodium is increased to replenish vascular volume; therefore potassium would be excreted.
3 This is not a complication of nephrotic syndrome, although pulmonary effusion may occur.
4 This does not usually occur as an early complication of this disease; it is a major complication of glomerulonephritis.

183. 3 Pelvic rocking on the first postoperative day would be very painful and could traumatize the wound site. (1) (CW; EV; ED; HP)
1 Leg bends promote circulation in the lower extremities and help to alleviate gas pains.
2 Foot circles promote circulation in the lower extremities.
4 Shoulder circles relieve neck stiffness and tension that may be present after delivery.

184. 3 This would give the client a familiar gauge in estimating the amount of bleeding she is experiencing. (1) (CW; AS; PA; HP)
1 The presence of clots does not indicate the amount of bleeding.
2 This may indicate a problem but does not relate to the amount of bleeding.
4 Weakness is a subjective symptom and may not truly reflect blood loss.

185. 2 A sharing of views helps to support the client's trust in self and others; participation increases self-esteem. (3) (MH; EV; PS; SD)
1 Clients are sensitive to others' feelings; this may be viewed as a lack of trust.
3 Pressuring the client to explain behavioral changes increases anxiety and the need to use defenses.
4 Asking clients to defend their point of view is threatening.

186. 2 This therapy permits relative isolation of the tumor area and saturation with the drug(s) selected. (2) (SU; AN; TC; GI)
1 This is not true; this procedure requires medical and nursing supervision.
3 These effects cannot be confined completely to the treated area; some migration still occurs.
4 Combinations of drugs also can be administered via IV or oral routes.

187. 3 Laryngeal spasms can occur abruptly; patency of the airway is determined by constant assessment for symptoms of respiratory distress. (1) (PE; AS; TC; RE)
1 This is important, but maintenance of respiration has priority.

2 The fever should be treated, but it is not critical at 103°F; maintenance of respiration has priority.

4 Same as answer 1.

188. 2 Hypoglycemia stimulates the production of ACTH, glucagon, glucocorticoids, growth hormone, and catecholamines; this produces glycogenolysis and gluconeogenesis and results in hyperglycemia. (2) (ME; AN; PA; EN)

1 This would result in hyperglycemia, not hypoglycemia.

3 Same as answer 1.

4 Excessive glucose intake causes hyperglycemia, not gluconeogenesis.

189. 1 This is a prime time for symptoms of a pulmonary embolus to appear. (2) (SU; EV; TC; SK)

2 This would not require nursing intervention; a productive cough would indicate a respiratory infection.

3 This could result from the inflammatory process; the temperature-regulating mechanisms in the aged may be slightly compromised, and they may show a slight elevation in body temperature for a longer period of time after surgery.

4 Weight bearing is being done by the unoperative leg at this time, and fatigue may be expected.

190. 3 The fontanels, anterior and posterior, are both open at birth. (2) (CW; AS; PA; NN)

1 Closed sutures are abnormal and may prevent normal brain growth during the first year.

2 This would indicate dehydration.

4 This is cephalohematoma, an abnormal but common finding, indicating injury to the head during the labor process.

191. 2 The Centers for Disease Control have determined that health professionals should use gloves when coming into direct contact with body fluids and blood of HIV-infected individuals because these fluids contain the virus. (1) (PE; PL; TC; BI)

1 Approaching the bedside does not expose the health care worker to the virus.

3 Contact should not be limited; this does not allow for optimal care of the client.

4 A mask and an impervious gown are needed in addition to gloves only when there is a potential for the health worker to be splashed with body fluids or blood.

192. 3 These are the classic symptoms of neuroleptic malignant syndrome, which is caused by neuroleptic-induced blockage of dopamine receptors. (3) (MH; EV; TC; DR)

1 These are side effects of Haldol, but they are not signs of neuroleptic malignant syndrome.

2 Same as answer 1.

4 Same as answer 1.

193. 3 The increased circulating plasma volume during pregnancy requires more protein to sustain the plasma protein level essential for the normal capillary fluid shift mechanism and correction of hypovolemia. (3) (CW; PL; TC; HP)

1 Caloric intake should not be restricted during pregnancy because of the associated increased BMR and the needs of the developing fetus.

2 It is impossible to eliminate all salt; salt is usually not restricted in hypertensive disorders of pregnancy; only excessive salt intake is discouraged.

4 The person is hypervolemic, not hypovolemic; iron promotes RBC production, not an increased circulating blood volume.

194. 1 A rising reticulocyte count indicates accelerated erythropoietic activity that may reflect increased RBC destruction; increased RBC destruction raises the bilirubin level, causing jaundice. (3) (CW; AN; PA; HN)

2 In this instance the sedimentation rate or WBCs, not the reticulocytes, would be elevated.

3 Although the reticulocyte count may be elevated with chronic blood loss, there are no data to indicate the baby is bleeding.

4 This test does not reflect respiratory functioning; however, ultimately with hemorrhage the respiratory rate will be elevated.

195. 4 The client needs to feel in control to prevent ego deterioration. (3) (MH; PL; PS; CS)
 1 It is too soon after the rape to discuss this.
 2 Although the nurse should always be available and supportive, feelings of anger are usually not the initial response.
 3 Same as answer 1.

196. 1 Subcutaneous emphysema refers to the presence of air in the tissue that surrounds an opening in the normally closed respiratory tract; the tissue appears puffy, and a crackling sensation is detected under the fingertips as trapped air is compressed between the tissue. (2) (SU; AS; TC; RE)
 2 The lungs are not affected.
 3 Gas exchange, and thus blood gases, are not affected.
 4 Same as answer 2.

197. 2 The client is nervous and afraid of leaving home; the priority is provision for safety and security needs. (3) (MH; PL; PS; AX)
 1 Unless the client is provided with a sense of security, adjustment is likely to be unsatisfactory because the anxiety will most likely escalate.
 3 This cannot be done until anxiety is reduced.
 4 The client is experiencing memory loss and may not be able to remember what precipitated admission to the hospital; some memory loss may be due to high anxiety and thought blocking.

198. 2 Gastric secretions, which are electrolyte rich, are lost through the NG tube; the imbalances that result could prove life threatening. (1) (SU; EV; TC; FE)
 1 This is unnecessary and could damage the suture line.
 3 This is unsafe; this could result in suture line disruption.
 4 This is unsafe; if respiratory intubation has occurred, aspiration will result.

199. 2 School-age children are most concerned about school, if not for the academics, for the social aspects. (2) (PE; AS; ED; GD)
 1 This may be of some concern, but not as much as is school.

 3 School-age children generally look at physicians as authority figures and do not doubt their competence.
 4 School-age children are generally not this future oriented.

200. 4 Baseline vital signs are extremely important; physical assessment precedes diagnostic measures and intervention. (2) (ME; AS; PA; RE)
 1 This might be done after it is determined if a specimen for blood gases is needed; this is not usually an independent function of the nurse; oxygen is only administered independently by the nurse in an emergency situation.
 2 This would be done after the physician makes a medical diagnosis; this is not an independent function of the nurse.
 3 A sputum specimen should be obtained after vital signs and before administration of antibiotics.

201. 2 Because more people are living longer, this problem of the elderly, especially elderly women, is increasing. (3) (SU; AN; ED; GD)
 1 This is unrelated to osteoporosis; the fat that is removed in skim milk does not contain calcium.
 3 This is unrelated to osteoporosis.
 4 Early retirement does not necessarily imply inactivity or immobility.

202. 1 Buck's traction is an example of traction applied directly to the skin by traction tape or a foam boot. (2) (SU; AN; PA; SK)
 2 There is no such traction.
 3 Skeletal traction is applied directly to the bony skeleton.
 4 Balanced suspension traction keeps the affected extremity elevated off the bed.

203. 1 During detoxification this provides safety and prevents suicide, which is a real threat. (2) (MH; PL; TC; SA)
 2 Bright light is preferable to dim light, which creates shadows and increases illusions and misinterpretations.

3 This type of client does not usually lose the sense of hearing, so there is no need to shout.

4 Restraints tend to upset the client further; if at all possible, they should not be used.

204. 1 This is a plant alkaloid that is cell-cycle specific; it affects cell division during metaphase by interfering with spindle formation and causing cell death. (3) (ME; IM; ED; DR)

2 This is typical of antimetabolites such as Fluorouracil.

3 Alkylating agents such as nitrogen mustard act in this way.

4 Antibiotics such as Dactinomycin act in this way.

205. 3 This is an emergency situation that exerts sudden pressure on the third cranial nerve on the affected side from displacement of the tentorium or uncus. (3) (PE; AN; PA; NM)

1 Response to severe pain is generally equal in both eyes.

2 An autonomic response to fear would affect both pupils equally.

4 This is inaccurate; reduced pressure would not cause one pupil to dilate; more likely, increasing pressure would cause this response.

206. 2 The longest and strongest contractions occur at the end of the first stage; a backache is common. (1) (CW; AS; PA; HC)

1 In this stage contractions are well spaced, with time to relax in between.

3 This is the period between the birth of the baby and the delivery of the placenta.

4 In this stage the fetal head begins to crown and would be seen at the perineum.

207. 2 The loss of a job can bruise the ego and decrease self-esteem. (1) (MH; PL; PS; AX)

1 Feelings should be expressed, not limited; attempting to decrease crying frequently increases it.

3 The crying is not necessarily an expression of sadness; there are other feelings involved.

4 The focus should be on the client's self-acceptance.

208. 3 Intravenous analgesics will be used because after major surgery an infusion will be in place avoiding the discomfort of an injection. (3) (PE; PL; TC; NM)

1 Oral analgesics are not as effective as IV analgesics.

2 IM analgesics are not necessary because circulatory access will be available.

4 This is false reassurance; it is rarely possible to relieve all pain immediately postoperatively.

209. 1 The client may become injured in many ways during a seizure, and trauma prevention is a priority. (2) (ME; PL; ED; NM)

2 Especially early in therapy, many anticonvulsants can cause GI disturbances; they should be taken with food.

3 Others should be aware of the condition and taught how to help in case of a seizure.

4 This is untrue; symptoms and treatment of seizure disorders vary greatly.

210. 4 Gastric returns would indicate correct placement. (1) (PE; IM; TC; GI)

1 Further assessment is necessary.

2 This could cause undue trauma regardless of where the tube is.

3 This is unsafe until correct placement is verified; feeding could enter the lung if the tube is not in the stomach.

211. 4 Toxicity can result because the action of calcium ions is similar to that of digitalis. (3) (ME; AN; TC; DR)

1 Calcium gluconate cannot be added to a solution containing carbonate or phosphate because a dangerous precipitation will occur.

2 If calcium infiltrates, sloughing of tissue will result.

3 Calcium can be added to this solution.

212. 2 Decreased sodium intake can accelerate lithium retention, with subsequent toxicity. (3) (MH; IM; ED; DR)

1 This is unrelated to the administration of lithium.

3 Same as answer 1.

4 Same as answer 1.

213. 4 Because of the anatomic position of the parathyroids, they may be accidentally removed during surgery. (3) (SU; EV; TC; EN)
1 This is unlikely; the thoracic cavity is not entered.
2 This is unlikely; the thyroid is nearer to the trachea.
3 This is unlikely; this usually results from a blunt blow.

214. 4 The newborn does not have intestinal flora to synthesize vitamin K, a precursor to prothrombin that is necessary for clotting. (2) (CW; AN; PA; NN)
1 This is not affected by vitamin K.
2 Same as answer 1.
3 Same as answer 1.

215. 3 Nasogastric suction is maintained to prevent pressure on the intestinal anastomoses; no oral fluids are permitted until peristalsis resumes and nasogastric suction is stopped. (3) (SU; IM; TC; GI)
1 This drains immediately unless it is a continent conduit; this has no bearing on when oral fluids can be started.
2 This would be too long to wait; sips of water are permitted when peristalsis returns and the nasogastric tube is removed; this usually takes 2 to 3 days.
4 This has no bearing; the return of peristalsis and removal of the nasogastric tube are determinants.

216. 1 Initiating interactions demonstrates that the depressed person is attempting to change behavior patterns. (2) (MH; EV; PS; MO)
2 Avoiding people is a reinforcement of the depressed lifestyle.
3 Clients who attempt to modify behavior to please others make only superficial changes.
4 Solitary activities are nonthreatening but do not deal with the problem of impaired relationships.

217. 3 This prevents the pelvis and hips from rotating and places equal stress on the growing extremities. (2) (PE; IM; ED; SK)
1 This is a balanced suspension traction that is used for a fractured femur in adults.

2 This is a description of Russell traction.
4 This is a description of Buck's traction.

218. 4 The virus disintegrates rapidly on contact with soap. (2) (CW; EV; ED; HP)
1 The lesion is in the genital area, not on the lips; kissing will not affect the infant.
2 This is unnecessary; only meticulous hand washing is required.
3 This is not necessary, because soap effectively disintegrates the virus.

219. 4 This provides the family member with an opportunity to express feelings. (1) (MH; IM; PS; CS)
1 Although true, this statement really does not address the family member's concerns.
2 This is false reassurance and cuts off communication.
3 This shuts off communication and abdicates nursing responsibility toward the client.

220. 4 This demonstrates the client's diminished anger and is a realistic assessment and acceptance of present capabilities and limitations. (2) (MH; EV; PS; CS)
1 This shows dependency; either the client has given up or is being sarcastic.
2 Anger is still apparent at loss of decision making; there is no real evidence of sharing.
3 This shows dependency and suggests the client has given up.

221. 4 Urinary retention and distention are common problems after a cystoscopy because of urethral edema. (2) (SU; EV; TC; RG)
1 Fluids dilute the urine and reduce the chance of infection after cystoscopy.
2 Although this can occur, an inability to void deserves further investigation because infection can follow retention of urine.
3 More conservative methods such as running water or a sitz bath should be attempted; catheterization carries a risk of infection.

222. 3 The formula is drop factor (60) ÷ time in minutes (60) × desired hourly volume (800 ÷ 24) = drops per minute; the correct answer is 33 drops per minute. (2) (PE; AN; TC; FE)
1 This is too slow; a rate of 3 drops/min would deliver 72 ml in 24 hours.

2   This is too slow; a rate of 6 drops/min would deliver 144 ml in 24 hours.

4   This is too fast; a rate of 60 drops/min would deliver 1440 ml in 24 hours.

223. 2   Stable vital signs are the major indicators that transfer will not jeopardize the client's condition; apprehension and complaints of pain do not place the client in jeopardy. (2) (SU; AS; TC; CV)

1   Restlessness may be a sign of shock; the client needs further assessment.

3   The vital signs are not stabilized, and transfer at this time is contraindicated.

4   These are signs of increased intracranial pressure, and the client should not be transferred at this time.

224. 1   Low concentrations of oxygen do not reduce the stimulus to breathe and prevent carbon dioxide narcosis. (1) (ME; IM; PA; RE)

2   Sedatives would further depress respirations and increase the carbon dioxide level.

3   Chronic hypercapnia is present; additional carbon dioxide only adds to the problem and results in carbon dioxide narcosis.

4   Respiratory obstruction causes difficulty on expiration; deep breathing will aggravate this situation.

225. 1   In grand multiparas observation for failure of the uterus to contract after delivery is a priority. (3) (CW; PL; TC; HP)

2   This is not a priority goal immediately after delivery; it also is not common after abdominal delivery.

3   This is an important goal, but it is not primary or lifethreatening.

4   This can be done only after the mother is in stable condition.

226. 3   These are signs of increasing hypoxia; a tracheotomy may be necessary to maintain an open airway. (2) (PE; IM; TC; RE)

1   The symptoms are not indicative of increased secretions; suctioning can precipitate sudden laryngospasm.

2   This is ineffective for laryngeal spasms.

4   Increased O_2 therapy can induce carbon dioxide narcosis.

227. 2   The client's major concern at this time is pain caused by inappropriate handling. (2) (SU; IM; PS; SK)

1   This is not the major concern, and false reassurance should not be given.

3   The number of personnel will not necessarily ensure careful handling; this does not address the client's primary concern.

4   Diversion at this time would not be an appropriate response to the client's primary concern.

228. 3   Most injuries to abused children are not life threatening; protection takes priority over immediate treatment. (3) (MH; PL; TC; CS)

1   Treatment of medical injuries is the physician's primary responsibility.

2   An accurate diagnosis of child abuse may take time and must be fully investigated.

4   The nurse is often the first individual to see the abused child and must establish protection even before the physician arrives.

229. 2   The disease is most common in this age group; it has a slight predilection for men. (2) (ME; AN; ED; EH)

1   This is not completely accurate; sometimes it is possible.

3   The opposite is true.

4   Incidence is not limited to any age group.

230. 2   Pressure of the uterus against major blood vessels reduces circulation; decreased perfusion of the placenta can result. (1) (CW; AN; PA; HC)

1   This is false; it can lead to supine hypotension.

3   This does not interfere with the movement of the symphysis pubis.

4   This could possibly prolong labor, but this is not the most essential reason; it is known that women who stand and walk during labor have shorter labors.

231. 2 Application of cold relieves discomfort, and the binder provides support and aids in pressure atrophy of acini cells so that no more milk will be produced. (3) (CW; IM; TC; HC)
1 This is suitable for the engorged breast-feeding mother because it promotes comfort and stimulates milk production.
3 Same as answer 1.
4 Severe restriction of fluid will not prevent engorgement and might cause dehydration.

232. 2 Anemia may result because of the possible bone marrow depressant effect of this drug. (1) (ME; IM; TC; DR)
1 This would be unsafe; a physical examination and blood studies are necessary to determine the cause of the client's symptoms.
3 This is unsafe; this is not the role of the nurse.
4 An increase may result in toxic effects if the client is taking the maximum dose.

233. 2 Changes in an ECG will reflect the area of the heart that has been damaged because of hypoxia. (1) (ME; AN; ED; CV)
1 A stethoscope is used to detect heart sounds.
3 Medical interventions such as cardioversion or cardiac medications, not an ECG, can alter heart rhythm; an ECG will reflect heart rhythm, not change it.
4 This is accomplished through a stress test; this uses an ECG in conjunction with physical exercise.

234. 4 No bowel sounds are present; therefore the client must remain npo. (2) (SU; IM; PA; IT)
1 The urinary output is adequate; there is no need to increase IV fluids.
2 This is unsafe; the client must be kept npo until bowel sounds are present.
3 Same as answer 2.

235. 3 Maintaining a patent airway is the priority; inhalation burns may have occurred. (1) (SU; AN; PA; RE)
1 This is extremely important but not the first priority.

2 Same as answer 1.
4 Same as answer 1.

236. 4 It is necessary to assess behavior changes that clue the nurse to impending suicidal acting out. (2) (MH; IM; TC; MO)
1 Because there has been no overt acting out, continuous observation may threaten the client's ability to maintain self-control.
2 The depressed client cannot follow involved interesting activities because of psychomotor retardation.
3 Detailed explanations are inappropriate and overwhelming for a client with psychomotor retardation.

237. 4 A change in behavior may indicate the client has worked out a plan for suicide; the potential for acting out on suicide increases when physical energy returns. (2) (MH; IM; TC; MO)
1 The client should not be considered for discharge simply because of a change in behavior.
2 This is not indicated at this time.
3 The client needs to be supervised, not complimented, at this time.

238. 1 Grief reactions to the impending loss and security present in the one-to-one relationship need to be anticipated. (3) (MH; EV; PS; TR)
2 This phase occurs early in the one-to-one relationship, not at termination.
3 There should not be a disintegration of the personality.
4 This behavior may occur in the early phase of a working relationship.

239. 3 Talking about what actually happened helps the client sort out the truth from confused thoughts and begins to help the client accept what happened as a part of the history. (2) (MH; IM; PS; CS)
1 The victim should be told of the legal services available; legal counsel should come from a legal authority.

2   Most rapes are planned in advance and are violent acts of the perpetrators, who are responsible for their behavior; nevertheless, the victim often feels unjustified guilt related to the incident.

4   If the client does not want to discuss intimate details, this should be respected.

240. 4   This objective includes observable client behavior, which is specified by amount and time and therefore is measurable. (2) (SU; AN; TC; RE)

1   This objective is not stated in measurable terms.

2   Same as answer 1.

3   This is a statement, not an objective.

241. 4   This technique is required when a wound is infected to prevent the spread of infection to others. (2) (SU; IM; TC; IT)

1   This technique is used when changing dressings to protect the client from infection.

2   This may be used with clients who are immunosuppressed and at risk for infection.

3   Wound or peritoneal infections are transmitted through incisional drainage, not feces.

242. 3   The data presented indicate an infectious process within the lung. (1) (ME; AN; PA; RE)

1   The cardinal signs would be pain in the lower lobe at the height of inspiration and a pleural friction rub.

2   Although fever and chills can occur later in the disease, the cardinal signs are irritating cough, chest pain, and shortness of breath.

4   The cardinal signs would be barrel chest, resonance on percussion, and thick tenacious sputum.

243. 2   This is a reflective statement that conveys acceptance and encourages further communication. (2) (SU; IM; PS; EH)

1   This is false reassurance that does not lessen anxiety.

3   The reliance on a pill to help the client in this instance evades the problem and cuts off further communication.

4   This is too direct; this statement does not encourage the client to discuss feelings.

244. 3   Sleep deprivation alone can cause these disturbances. (2) (SU; IM; PA; NM)

1   Lack of contact with significant others increases anxiety and feelings of isolation and can lead to disturbances in rest.

2   Pain limits or interrupts periods of sleep and rest.

4   Constant light limits sleep.

245. 3   This diet is low in fiber, and after digestion and absorption, there is very little substance to be eliminated. (2) (SU; AN; TC; GI)

1   This diet does not affect the bacterial milieu of the intestine.

2   This diet does not promote peristalsis, the products of digestion remain in the intestine longer, and flatus is increased.

4   Although a low-residue diet is less irritating, this is not the primary reason for use before surgery.

246. 2   This is an open-ended question that should elicit the desired information. (2) (PE; AS; PS; GD)

1   This may establish that the child knows where she is but does not elicit why she knows why she is there.

3   This question can be answered with a yes or no and does not elicit what the child thinks about the situation.

4   This is not an open-ended question because it can be answered with a yes or a no response.

247. 4   Leakage of fluid could be caused by ruptured membranes, predisposing to an ascending infection and infection of the fetus. (1) (CW; EV; ED; HP)

1   This is a common discomfort of pregnancy caused by the shift in the center of gravity because of the enlarged uterus.

2   Leukorrhea is common during pregnancy because of increased vascularity of the cervix and increased production of mucus.

3   Braxton-Hicks contractions are painless contractions of the uterus occurring at irregular intervals throughout pregnancy.

248. 1 Digoxin slows the heart rate, which is reflected in a slowing of the pulse; it also increases kidney perfusion, which promotes urine formation, resulting in diuresis and decreased edema. (2) (ME; EV; TC; DR)
2 Digoxin does not decrease the pulse pressure or directly influence the blood pressure; diuresis will lower the weight and blood pressure
3 Digoxin lowers the pulse rate and produces diuresis as a result of improved cardiac output.
4 Digoxin will not affect a defective valve or reduce a heart murmur.

249. 3 This reduces energy requirements, allows for rest, and lessens the demand for oxygen. (2) (PE; IM; PA; RE)
1 Although this loosens secretions in the lungs, it should not be used when the infant is in distress.
2 This is not done unless respiratory distress is extremely severe; it increases restlessness and energy demands.
4 This positional change will not reduce energy and oxygen demands.

250. 2 The function of sucking requires more oxygen and therefore tires the infant. (2) (PE; PL; PA; RE)
1 Laryngospasm, or spasmodic closing of the glottis, which results from edema, is not related to oral feedings.
3 IVs have no effect on vagal stimulation.
4 Intravenous fluids do not provide for complete caloric needs.

251. 2 This is caused by manipulation of abdominal contents and the depressant effects of anesthesia and analgesics. (1) (SU; AN; PA; GI)
1 Edema would not totally interfere with peristalsis; edema may cause peristalsis to be less effective but some output would still result.
3 An absence of fiber has a greater impact on decreasing peristalsis than fluids do.
4 A nasogastric tube decompresses the stomach; it does not cause cessation of peristalsis.

252. 1 A cancerous mass can grow into the lumen of the intestine, altering the shape of the stool; stools may be ribbon-like or pencil thin. (1) (SU; AS; PA; GI)
2 This is not specific to intestinal cancer.
3 Same as answer 2.
4 Same as answer 2.

253. 4 Care for an infant after croup should be directed toward personal care, proper nutrition, and stimulation. (1) (PE; PL; ED; RE)
1 The infant does not require additional fluids if all feedings are consumed.
2 Young infants need environmental stimuli.
3 Croup is not directly related to antigen-antibody responses.

254. 3 Redness and pain are signs of phlebitis; the site should be changed to avoid further inflammation and possible thrombus formation. (3) (PE; IM; TC; CV)
1 Continuing administration can lead to further irritation and even permanent damage to the vein.
2 Although this is generally true, there is no indication that this is what is occurring in this situation.
4 Same as answer 1.

255. 1 This would numb the nerve endings and reduce pain; cold also produces vasoconstriction, limits edema, and prevents hemorrhage. (1) (PE; PL; ED; NM)
2 Aspirin has anticoagulant properties that could increase the risk of bleeding and should therefore be avoided.
3 Hard candies can scratch the operative site and dislodge the clot and should therefore be avoided.
4 This could dislodge a clot and cause bleeding.

256. 1 The client needs positive relationships with other adults, but clear, consistent limits must be presented to minimize attempts at manipulation. (1) (MH; PL; PS; PR)
2 This is not a therapeutic approach.
3 This is not a therapeutic approach; clear, consistent limits are necessary to prevent manipulation.
4 This is a judgmental attitude that should be avoided.

257. 1   Most child abusers have been abused themselves; they do not know how to deal with the rage they feel. (2) (MH; PL; PS; CS)
   2   Parents in abusing parent groups have already admitted and begun to seek help for their problem.
   3   This type of presentation usually alienates individuals who are struggling with their own present difficulties.
   4   Therapy should focus on and encourage the sharing of feelings, not personal parenting information.

258. 4   The muscular action during ambulation facilitates the return of venous blood to the heart. (1) (CW; IM; PA; HP)
   1   Early ambulation would not prevent this complication.
   2   Same as answer 1.
   3   This is unrelated; the baby is usually given to the mother in the delivery room to begin the bonding process.

259. 2   A frequent complication of a cerebrovascular accident (CVA) is an inability to control emotional affect; clients may be depressed or apathetic and have a lability of mood. (2) (ME; IM; ED; NM)
   1   There are no data to support this conclusion.
   3   Same as answer 1.
   4   Same as answer 1.

260. 3   The heart muscle begins to fail, and the muscle does not contract with enough strength to pump sufficient blood to meet the body's metabolic needs. (3) (ME; AN; PA; CV)
   1   Hypertension and arteriosclerosis can add stress to this situation, but they are not the reason for this client's congestive heart failure.
   2   Hypervolemia can precipitate congestive heart failure in individuals with a diseased heart, but it is not specific to rheumatic heart disease.
   4   Heart valves can become stenotic or regurgitant as a result of rheumatic fever; however, left ventricular failure will occur only when the heart can no longer pump an adequate amount of blood to maintain cardiac output.

261. 3   Steroids are used for their antiinflammatory, vasoconstrictive, and antipruritic effects. (2) (ME; EV; ED; DR)
   1   Steroids increase the incidence of infections by masking symptoms.
   2   Steroids increase fluid retention.
   4   Although steroids have an antipruritic effect, their major purpose after surgery is the antiinflammatory effect.

262. 2   Pinworms emerge nocturnally to lay eggs in the perianal area; eggs are caught on cellophane tape in the morning before toileting. (1) (PE; IM; TC; GI)
   1   A stool culture will not reveal presence of parasites.
   3   There is no such test to diagnose pinworms.
   4   The ova cannot be seen with the naked eye; the parasite is rarely observed in the stool.

263. 4   Many closures require the use of two hands, and some clothing requires movement of both sides of the body when dressing. (1) (ME; AP; PA; NM)
   1   The client can continue to use the right hand to perform this activity.
   2   Same as answer 1.
   3   Same as answer 1.

264. 1   Panting and blowing keep the glottis open so the client cannot hold the breath and bear down. (2) (CW; EV; ED; HC)
   2   While this pattern keeps the pressure of the diaphragm off the contracting uterus, it does not reduce the urge to push.
   3   Shallow chest breathing interferes with adequate oxygenation of fetus because it limits the mother's O_2 intake.
   4   Same as answer 2.

265. 4   Air drying nipples several times a day hardens the nipples and reduces soreness; changing the position of neonate while nursing will also relieve sore nipples. (1) (CW; PL; TC; HC)
   1   This would cause vasoconstriction and lead to milk suppression.
   2   This may reduce the discomfort, but it will not help the nipples to dry and harden.
   3   This would inhibit lactation; the baby must suckle and empty the breasts regularly for milk production to continue.

How to Use Worksheet 1: Errors In Processing Information

Common errors in processing information are listed in the left-hand column of this worksheet. At the top of the worksheet is a row of blank spaces for inserting the number of the question missed. Directly below each number, check any errors you made in answering that question. You may have made more than one type of error in an answer.

Worksheet 1: Errors in Processing Information

Question number																				
Did not read situation/ question carefully																				
Missed important details																				
Confused major and minor points																				
Defined problem incorrectly																				
Could not remember terms/ facts/concepts/principles																				
Defined terms incorrectly																				
Focused on incomplete/incorrect data in assessing situation																				
Interpreted data incorrectly																				
Applied wrong concepts/ principles in situations																				
Drew incorrect conclusions																				
Identified wrong goals																				
Identified priorities incorrectly																				
Carried out plan incorrectly/ incompletely																				
Was unclear about criteria for evaluating success in achieving goals																				

How to Use Worksheet 2: Knowledge Gaps

Types of common knowledge gaps are listed along the top of this worksheet. Write a brief description of topics you want to review in the spaces provided. For example, if you missed a question on administration of a particular drug, write the drug name and problem (e.g., dosage) in the appropriate space under the column labeled *Pharmacology*.

Worksheet 2: Knowledge Gaps

Basic science	Skills/ procedures	Basic human needs	Growth and develop- ment	Normal nutrition	Psycho- social factors	Clinical area/ topic	Stressors/ coping mechanisms	Patho- physiology	Pharma- cology	Therapeutic nutrition	Legal implications	Other

Instructions for Disk Start-up

System Requirements

A computer with at least 324K of RAM (Random Access Memory) available is needed for this program. This computer must be IBM PC or 100% compatible. This program operates on a high density (HD) disk only.

For these examples we assume that your A drive is your floppy drive, and your C drive is your hard drive. Please substitute the letter of your floppy drive for A if your floppy drive letter is different. Substitute the letter of your hard drive for C if your hard drive letter is different.

Start-up (floppy drive)

1. Turn your computer on
2. At the prompt, insert the disk into your A drive
3. Type A: and press <Enter>
4. Type **MOSBY** and press <Enter>
5. Follow the instructions on the screen

Start-up (hard disk)

1. Turn your computer on
2. At the prompt, insert the disk into your A drive
3. Type C: and press <Enter>
4. Type **MD\MOSBY** and press <Enter>
5. Type **CD\MOSBY** and press <Enter>
6. Type **COPY A:*.*** and press <Enter>

The software is now installed on your hard drive. Once the software is installed, start the software by following these directions:

1. Type **CD\MOSBY** and press <Enter>
2. Type **MOSBY** and press <Enter>
3. Follow the directions on the screen

**REMEMBER THE NAME THAT YOU HAVE ENTERED.
YOUR DISK WILL BE BRANDED WITH THIS INITIAL NAME.**